Manual of Anaesthesia

C. Y. Lee
Department of Anaesthesiology & Intensive Care
Faculty of Medicine
Universiti Kebangsaan Malaysia

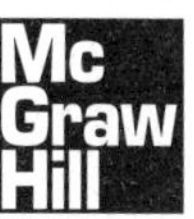

Singapore • Boston • Burr Ridge, IL • Dubuque, IA • Madison, WI
New York • San Francisco • St. Louis • Bangkok • Bogotá • Caracas
Kuala Lumpur • Lisbon • London • Madrid • Mexico City • Milan
Montreal • New Delhi • Santiago • Seoul • Sydney • Taipei • Toronto

The McGraw-Hill Companies

Notice

Medicine is an ever-changing science. As new research and clinical experience broaden our knowledge, changes in treatment and drug therapy are required. The authors and publisher of this work have checked with sources believed to be reliable in their efforts to provide information that is complete and generally in accord with the standards accepted at the time of publication. However, in view of the possibility of human errors or changes in medical sciences, neither the authors nor the publisher nor any other party who has been involved in the preparation or publication of this work warrants that the information contained herein is in every respect accurate or complete, and they disclaim all responsibility for any errors or omissions or for the results obtained from use of the information contained in this work. Readers are encouraged to confirm the information contained herein with other sources. For example, and in particular, readers are advised to check the product information sheet included in the package of each drug they plan to administer to be certain that the information contained in this work is accurate and that changes have not been made in the recommended dose or in the contraindications for administration. The recommendation is of particular importance in connection with new or infrequently used drugs.

Manual of Anaesthesia

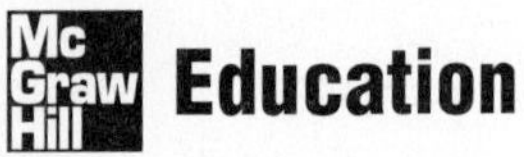

1 2 3 4 5 6 7 8 9 10 BJE 09 08 07 06

When ordering this title, use ISBN 007-124807-2

Printed in Singapore

To the loves of my life,

Teong Yong, Cheryl and Cheryn

Without you this will not be possible.

Contents

Foreword

Comprehensive coverage and practical focus are not qualities normally found in anaesthetic textbooks. Dr CY Lee has achieved a remarkable feat – meeting these challenges and providing a concise, systematic approach to the practice of anaesthesia.

The contents of this book have undergone extensive revision to incorporate advances in new drugs, techniques, equipment, guidelines and concepts to reflect modern standards and evidence based practice.

Readers will find in this book the advice and skills they use from day to day. They will identify the needs and knowledge gaps, which they have not previously acknowledged, and they will find inspiration for good practice and continuing search for new knowledge.

Trainees will also find this book useful for crystallising their thoughts and knowledge for their examinations. Indeed, both trainees and specialists will have found a true soul mate in this book.

Peter C.A. Kam
MBBS, MD, FANZCA, FRCA, FCARCSI, FHKCA (Hon)
Professor of Anaesthesia
University of New South Wales
St George Hospital
Kogarah, NSW, Australia

Preface

This manual started off as a guidebook written specifically for the anaesthesia trainees in the Department of Anaesthesiology, Hospital Kuala Lumpur.

Over the years, new developments, drugs and anaesthetic techniques have modified our present day anaesthetic practice, and it has become imperative that the book should be revised and updated. But what started off as merely "rearranging and updating facts in the book" became a major undertaking of sorts, because there is just no end to the details that can and should be included here.

From the feedback received, the appeal of the first book was largely attributable to its simplicity and practicality. It was raw and somewhat flawed, as seen through the eyes of a young specialist fresh from exams. While retaining the practical aspects, more facts are included in this book because it is felt that with more background knowledge available, it would help the reader to understand not just *what to do* and *how to do it*, but also the rationale in our anaesthetic management.

The chapters in *Manual of Anaesthesia* are arranged in 5 sections:

A. **Introduction:** highlights on various general topics.

B. **Clinical Conditions:** common medical problems encountered in patients coming for anaesthesia and surgery.

C. **Anaesthesia for Specific Surgery:** anaesthetic management for specific surgical procedures.

D. **Issues in Anaesthesia:** new developments and issues in the field of anaesthesia.

E. **Problems in Anaesthesia:** untoward events encountered during the peri-operative period.

As the name implies, this is far from being a textbook of anaesthesia. It is meant to be a source of quick reference when the reader is unsure of certain aspects of anaesthetic management and help is not immediately at hand. The emphasis of this book is on the practical guidelines for solving problems that the reader may encounter during the course of anaesthesia.

Anaesthesiology is a challenging and fascinating field. It is much more than putting patients to sleep and waking them up at the end of the surgery. This is especially true in patients with a multitude of medical problems, or in surgical procedures which result in major physiological derangement and massive blood loss. It has often been quoted that *"Anaesthesia is hours of boredom and moments of terror"*. Those who have been involved in anaesthetic misadventures can surely testify to that!

Anaesthesiology is also a field where there is tremendous scope for new development and refinement of technique. The anaesthesiologist is certainly not a technician but a perioperative physician, an integral member of the medical team that aims to provide optimal patient care. The anaesthesiologist is looking beyond the confines of the operating theatre and becoming more involved in the perioperative management of the patient. Examples of these include anaesthesia preoperative evaluation clinic, acute and chronic pain service, as well as obstetric anaesthesia and analgesia service. More and more patients (surgeons, too!) are aware of the essential services provided by the anaesthesiologist — we are more than nameless faces underneath caps and masks!

Despite the fact that anaesthesia can be stressful at times, I hope that many will be inspired to take up anaesthesiology for post-graduate studies. However, even if one does not fancy being an anaesthesiologist for the rest of one's life, this is still a useful skill worth acquiring. It is always better to know *how* to manage a difficult patient, *why* we do things the way we do, and *what* to do when something unexpected happens. This knowledge is essential in whichever specialty of medicine one decides to embark on. When one is equipped with such knowledge, one will become more prepared to handle crisis situations, less likely to panic under stress, and more rational in one's approach to overcome the crisis.

I wish to thank Dr Peter Kam, my *si-fu*, mentor and source of inspiration, for kindly consenting to write the Foreword to this book.

I would also like to acknowledge the contribution by Professor Dr Felicia Lim for co-writing the chapters on "Paediatric and Neonatal Anaesthesia" and "Cardiac Arrest". Your help and encouragement are much appreciated.

I hope that this book will be informative and beneficial to all.

Lee Choon Yee
MBBS (Mal), M. Med (Anaesth) UKM, FANZCA, AMM
Associate Professor and Consultant Anaesthesiologist
Department of Anaesthesiology & Intensive Care
Faculty of Medicine
Universiti Kebangsaan Malaysia

Abbreviations

AAA	Abdominal aortic aneurysm
ABC	Airway, breathing, circulation
ABG	Arterial blood gases
ABT	Autologous blood transfusion
ACE	Angiotensin-converting enzyme
ACLS	Advanced cardiac life support
ACT	Activated clotting time
ACTH	Adrenocorticotropic hormone
ADH	Antidiuretic hormone
AEP	Auditory evoked potential
AF	Atrial fibrillation
AHA	American Heart Association
ALS	Amyotrophic lateral sclerosis
ANH	Acute normovolaemic haemodilution
APL	Adjustable pressure limiting
APS	Acute Pain Service
APTT	Activated partial thromboplastin time
AR	Aortic regurgitation
ARDS	Acute respiratory distress syndrome
ARF	Acute renal failure

AS	Aortic stenosis
ASA	American Society of Anesthesiologists
ASD	Atrial septal defect
ASIS	Anterior superior iliac spine
AT	Antithrombin
ATLS	Advanced Trauma Life Support
ATP	Adenosine triphosphate
AV	Arteriovenous; Atrioventricular
AVF	Arteriovenous fistula
AVM	Arteriovenous malformation
BIPAP	Biphasic positive airway pressure
BIS	Bispectral index
BMI	Body mass index
BMR	Basal metabolic rate
BP	Blood pressure
BSA	Body surface area
CABG	Coronary artery bypass graft
CAD	Coronary artery disease
CCU	Coronary care unit
CEA	Carotid endarterectomy
CFM	Cerebral function monitor
CICU	Cardiothoracic intensive care unit
CMR	Closed manipulation and reduction
$CMRO_2$	Cerebral metabolic rate for oxygen
CNS	Central nervous system
COHb	Carboxyhaemoglobin
COPA	Cuffed oropharyngeal airway
COPD	Chronic obstructive pulmonary disease

COX	Cyclooxygenase
CPAP	Continuous positive airway pressure
CPB	Cardiopulmonary bypass
CPP	Cerebral perfusion pressure
CPR	Cardiopulmonary resuscitation
C&S	Culture and sensitivity
CSE	Combined spinal-epidural
CSF	Cerebrospinal fluid
CT	Computed tomography
CTEV	Congenital talipes equinovarus
CTG	Cardiotocography
CVA	Cerebrovascular accident
CVC	Central venous catheter
CVP	Central venous pressure
CVS	Cardiovascular system
CXR	Chest X-ray
DASI	Duke Activity Status Index
DBS	Double burst stimulation
DCR	Dacrocystorhinostomy
DDAVP	Desmopressin (deamino D-arginine vasopressin)
DIC	Disseminated intravascular coagulation
DLT	Double lumen tube
DVT	Deep vein thrombosis
εACA	Epsilon-aminocaproic acid
EBV	Estimated blood volume
ECG	Electrocardiography
ECMO	Extracorporeal membrane oxygenation
ECT	Electroconvulsive therapy

EDTA	Ethylene diamine tetraacetic acid
EEG	Electroencephalography
ELMS	Endoscopic laryngoscopy and microsurgery
EMD	Electromechanical dissociation
EMLA	Eutectic mixture of local anaesthetics
ENT	Ear, nose and throat
ERCP	Endoscopic retrograde cholangio-pancreatoscopy
ESWL	Extracorporeal shock wave lithotripsy
$ETCO_2$	End-tidal carbon dioxide
ETC	Oesophageal-tracheal Combitube
ETT	Endotracheal tube
EVD	External ventricular drainage
FBC	Full blood count
FDA	(US) Food and Drug Administration
FDP	Fibrinogen degradation products
FE(S)	Fat embolism (syndrome)
FESS	Functional endoscopic sinus surgery
FEV_1	Forced expiratory volume in one second
FFP	Fresh frozen plasma
FGF	Fresh gas flow
FiO_2	Fractional inspired oxygen content
FRC	Functional residual capacity
FSH	Follicle-stimulating hormone
FTCA	Fast-track cardiac anaesthesia
FVC	Forced vital capacity
GA	General anaesthesia
GCS	Glasgow Coma Scale
GFR	Glomerular filtration rate

GH Growth hormone
GIK Glucose-insulin-potassium
GIT Gastrointestinal tract
G&S Group and screen
GTN Glyceryl trinitrate or nitroglycerin
GXM Group and cross-match

Hct Haematocrit
HDU High dependency unit
HELLP Haemolysis, elevated liver enzymes, low platelets
HES Hydroxyethyl starch
HIV Human immunodeficiency virus
HITS Heparin-induced thrombocytopaenic syndrome
HME Heat and moisture exchanger

IABP Intraarterial blood pressure; intraaortic balloon pump
ICA Internal carotid artery
ICD Implantable cardioverter-defibrillator
ICP Intracranial pressure
ICU Intensive care unit
IDDM Insulin dependent diabetes mellitus
I:E ratio Inspired : expired ratio
IgG Immunoglobulin G
IHD Ischaemic heart disease
ILMA Intubating laryngeal mask airway
IM Intramuscular
INR International normalized ratio
IOP Intraocular pressure
IPPV Intermittent positive pressure ventilation
IRDS Idiopathic respiratory distress syndrome

IV	Intravenous
IVC	Inferior vena cava
IVRA	Intravenous regional anaesthesia
JVP	Jugular venous pressure
LA	Local anaesthetic; left atrium
LAP	Left atrial pressure
LH	Luteinizing hormone
LMA	Laryngeal mask airway
LMWH	Low molecular weight heparin
LOR	Loss of resistance
LOS	Lower oesophageal sphincter
LSCS	Lower segment caesarean section
LTH	Luteotropic hormone
LV	Left ventricle
LVEDP	Left ventricular end-diastolic pressure
LVH	Left ventricular hypertrophy
LVRS	Lung volume reduction surgery
MAC	Minimal alveolar concentration; Monitored anaesthesia care
MAOI	Monoamine oxidase inhibitor
MAP	Mean arterial pressure
MEN	Multiple endocrine neoplasia
MEP	Motor evoked potential
MH	Malignant hyperthermia
MI	Myocardial infarction
MIDCAB	Minimally invasive direct-access coronary artery bypass
MLAER	Middle latency auditory evoked response
MLT	Microlaryngeal tube
MR	Mitral regurgitation

MRI	Magnetic resonance imaging
MS	Mitral stenosis
MSBOS	Maximum surgical blood order schedule
MVP	Mitral valve prolapse
NEC	Necrotizing enterocolitis
NIBP	Non-invasive blood pressure
NIDDM	Non-insulin dependent diabetes mellitus
NMS	Neurolept malignant syndrome
NSAID	Non-steroidal antiinflammatory drug
NYHA	New York Heart Association
OCP	Oral contraceptive pills
OCR	Oculocardiac reflex
OHS	Obesity hypoventilation syndrome
OLV	One-lung ventilation
OMF	Oral and maxillofacial
O&G	Obstetrics and Gynaecology
OPCAB	Off-pump coronary artery bypass
OSA	Obstructive sleep apnoea
OT	Operating theatre
PA	Pulmonary artery
PACU	Post-anaesthesia care unit
$PaCO_2$	Arterial partial pressure of carbon dioxide
PaO_2	Arterial partial pressure of oxygen
PAP	Pulmonary artery pressure
PARS	Post-anaesthetic Recovery Score
PCA	Patient-controlled analgesia
PCEA	Patient-controlled epidural analgesia
PCNL	Percutaneous nephrolithotripsy

PCS	Patient-controlled sedation
PCWP	Pulmonary capillary wedge pressure
PDA	Patent ductus arteriosus
PE	Pulmonary embolism; Preeclampsia
PEA	Pulseless electrical activity
PEEP	Positive end-expiratory pressure
PEFR	Peaked expiratory flow rate
PFC	Perfluorocarbon
PIH	Pregnancy-induced hypertension
PONV	Postoperative nausea and vomiting
PSIS	Posterior superior iliac spine
PT	Prothrombin time
PTC	Post-tetanic count
PTCA	Percutaneous transluminal coronary angioplasty
PTE	Pulmonary thromboembolism
PTH	Parathyroid hormone
PTT	Partial thromboplastin time
PVC	Polyvinyl chloride
PVR	Pulmonary vascular resistance
QA	Quality assurance
RA	Regional anaesthesia; Right atrium
RAP	Right atrial pressure
RBC	Red blood cell
REM	Rapid eye movement
RTI	Respiratory tract infection
RV	Right ventricle
SAH	Subarachnoid haemorrhage
SaO_2	Arterial oxygen saturation

SBE	Subacute bacterial endocarditis
SC	Subcutaneous
SH	Standard heparin
SIADH	Syndrome of inappropriate antidiuretic hormone secretion
SLE	Systemic lupus erythematosus
SNP	Sodium nitroprusside
SpO_2	Oxygen saturation (based on pulse oximeter reading)
SSEP	Somatosensory evoked potential
SVC	Superior vena cava
SVR	Systemic vascular resistance
SVT	Supraventricular tachycardia
TAA	Thoracic aortic aneurysm
TAAA	Thoracoabdominal aortic aneurysm
TCI	Target-controlled infusion
TEE / TOE	Transoesophageal echocardiography
TENS	Transcutaneous electrical nerve stimulation
TIA	Transient ischaemic attack
TIVA	Total intravenous anaesthesia
TMJ	Temporomandibular joint
TNS	Transient neurologic syndrome
TOF	Train of four; Tetralogy of Fallot; Tracheo-oesophageal fistula
TPN	Total parenteral nutrition
TRALI	Transfusion-related acute lung injury
TSH	Thyroid-stimulating hormone
TURBT	Transurethral resection of bladder tumour
TURP	Transurethral resection of prostate
U	Unit
UPPP	Uvulopalatopharyngoplasty

VA	Ventriculo-atrial
VAE	Venous air embolism
VAS	Visual analogue scale
VATS	Video-assisted thoracoscopic surgery
VEP	Visual evoked potential
VF	Ventricular fibrillation
VIMA	Volatile induction and maintenance of anaesthesia
VP	Ventriculo-peritoneal
V/Q	Ventilation / perfusion
VSD	Ventricular septal defect
VT	Ventricular tachycardia
WPW	Wolff-Parkinson-White

A

Introduction

Chapter 1

Practical Considerations

- **Getting Started**
- **Universal Precaution and Management of Needlestick Injury**
- **Induction of Anaesthesia**
- **Maintenance of Anaesthesia**
- **Emergence and Recovery**
- **Postanaesthesia Follow-Up**
- **Further Reading**

GETTING STARTED

— The anaesthesiologist should arrive at the operating theatre (OT) early to prepare for the day's work in an unhurried manner. This includes a thorough check of the anaesthetic equipment including monitors, and preparation of anaesthetic and resuscitation drugs. If a regional anaesthetic technique is planned for the first case, the procedure should be performed early to ensure that the surgery commences at the scheduled time.

— All syringes should be clearly labelled stating both the name and dilution of the drug. Drug ampoules should be retained for drug checks in the event of an anaesthetic mishap. To avoid undue drug wastage, only the amount required for a particular patient should be drawn into the syringe from a multi-dose vial. It is recommended that the contents of a single-dose ampoule be used for one patient only. *Syringes must not be shared among patients.*

— Before performing a regional anaesthetic technique, the anaesthesiologist should prepare a resuscitation tray with the following drugs diluted and drawn into syringes.
  - Thiopentone for induction of general anaesthesia or as an anticonvulsant.
  - Vasopressor (ephedrine or phenylephrine) for treatment of hypotension.
  - Atropine for treatment of bradycardia.
  - Suxamethonium to facilitate rapid tracheal intubation.

— Introduce yourself to the patient you are about to anaesthetize. Verify the patient's identity, nature and site of the planned surgical procedure. Ensure that the consent form for surgery and anaesthesia has been duly signed by the patient and/or the next-of-kin and witnessed. Do a quick reassessment of the patient and review the most recent investigation results. Enquire about duration of fasting. Spend time to answer the patient's queries as this would help to further allay his/her anxiety towards the impending surgery and anaesthetic.

— Establish monitoring on the patient before induction of anaesthesia. The extent of monitoring depends on the patient's condition and the nature of surgery. Certain painful procedures, such as cannulation for invasive haemodynamic monitoring, can be performed under general anaesthesia in some patients. If it is deemed necessary to perform such procedures in a conscious patient, these should be supplemented with local anaesthetic infiltration and/or intravenous sedation.

— Intravenous cannulae larger than 20G should be inserted under local anaesthesia unless venous access appears difficult, as local anaesthetic infiltration may sometimes render the vein more difficult to identify. Older children may be coaxed into accepting an intravenous anaesthetic induction if the pain associated with intravenous cannulation can be reduced by local anaesthetic, specifically by using a eutectic mixture of local anaesthetic (EMLA) cream. Identify the vein for cannulation during the premedication round, and instruct the ward staff to apply EMLA cream on the area and cover with an occlusive dressing. Time this approximately 45 minutes to 1 hour before the procedure.

UNIVERSAL PRECAUTION AND MANAGEMENT OF NEEDLESTICK INJURY

— It is important that one should practise *universal precaution* in order to reduce the risk of disease transmission through blood and body fluids. Examples of universal precaution, in which every patient is regarded as potentially infected with a blood-borne virus, are listed here.
  - Frequent hand washing before handling a new patient or equipment to be used on a new patient, after leaving a patient, whenever the hands become contaminated and before any invasive procedure.
  - Cover existing cuts and skin abrasions with waterproof dressing.
  - Wear gloves when contact with blood, saliva or any other body fluid is anticipated, such as intravenous cannulation or venepuncture for blood sampling, airway instrumentation, and transfusion of blood and blood products.
  - Change gloves after a procedure to minimize contamination of the workplace.
  - Change gloves in between patients to minimize cross-infection from one patient to another.

— Take precaution to prevent needlestick injury.
  - Use blunt drawing-up cannulae instead of hypodermic needles to draw up drugs.
  - Use plastic rather than glass ampoules if both types are available in the OT.
  - Wear gloves for intravenous cannulation. The total amount of inoculum is decreased by gloves should a needlestick injury occur.
  - Use protected stylet cannulae if available; otherwise immediately dispose of the used stylet into a sharps disposal container.
  - Do not recap the needle if a standard syringe and needle is used.
  - Use intravenous infusion sets with needleless injection ports, or attach a 3-way tap to the IV set so that needles are not required for drug administration.
  - Dispose of needles, glass ampoules and other sharp objects in appropriate puncture-proof sharps disposal containers.

— Policy for accidental needlestick injury should be drawn up and adapted to the setting of individual institutions. In the event of an accidental exposure:
  - Immediately wash the wound with soap and water.
  - Try to express blood from the puncture wound.
  - Report the exposure to Occupational Health Department.
  - Commence treatment according to specific regimes for postexposure prophylaxis in the institution. This is necessary in view of a seroconversion rate of 0.2–0.4% for human immunodeficiency virus (HIV).

   - Hepatitis B: depending on history of prior immunization, either hepatitis B vaccine booster or a full course plus hepatitis B immunoglobulin.
   - HIV: zidovudine 200 mg tds, lamivudine 150 mg bd, and indinavir 800 mg tds for a duration of 4 weeks. These drugs are associated with a high rate of unpleasant gastrointestinal and other side-effects.
   - Hepatitis C: no prophylaxis is currently available.
- Consider obtaining consent from the patient for blood test to check the hepatitis B/hepatitis C/HIV status. This can be taken only with patient's consent.
- Check for seroconversion 6 months later.

INDUCTION OF ANAESTHESIA

— Anaesthesia may be induced by means of intravenous or inhalational induction. The technique of rapid sequence induction is utilized in patients with increased risks of gastric regurgitation and aspiration. In selected cases, intubation may be achieved by means of fibreoptic laryngoscopy with the patient either awake or anaesthetized and breathing spontaneously.

— Intravenous induction of anaesthesia is by far the commonest induction technique in the adult patient. Advantages of this technique are ease of administration, rapid loss of consciousness (within one arm-brain circulation time) and clear end-point. Intravenous induction agent is injected slowly in titrated doses until the patient loses consciousness as manifested by a loss of eyelash reflex. In contrast, a precalculated dose of intravenous induction agent is administered in rapid sequence induction. Cricoid pressure is applied by the anaesthetic assistant and a rapid-onset neuromuscular blocker, usually suxamethonium, is administered to facilitate tracheal intubation.

— Inhalational induction of anaesthesia tends to take a longer time and may be complicated by breath-holding, laryngospasm and hypoventilation. Common indications for inhalational induction include:

- Babies, young children or needle-phobic adults.
- Upper airway obstruction, such as acute epiglottitis and laryngeal tumour.
- Superior vena cava obstruction.
- Patients with difficult venous access.

— For a paediatric patient, the parent or guardian is often permitted to accompany the child to the OT and be present during induction of anaesthesia. This helps to allay the child's anxiety and enhance cooperation with the anaesthesiologist.

However, there are some parents who are extremely anxious or distressed; it is probably better for such individuals not to be present in the OT.

MAINTENANCE OF ANAESTHESIA

— *Be vigilant at all times.* It is particularly difficult to maintain full alertness in "routine" anaesthesia for healthy patients, if surgery is a long drawn-out procedure or takes place after working hours. There may also be distraction from clinical monitoring of the patient by having too much gadgetry around, or when the anaesthesiologist is deep in conversation with the surgeon or OT staff. These factors impair the anaesthesiologist's response in the event of an anaesthetic mishap.

— The anaesthesiologist should not leave an anaesthetized patient unattended at any time especially when the patient is ill and unstable, or if airway maintenance is of particular concern. If there is an unavoidable need to leave the patient for a brief period of time, the anaesthesiologist should request for another colleague (if available) to take over temporary management, or delegate observation of the patient to an appropriately qualified person deemed competent for the task.

— If it is necessary for a permanent handover of responsibility for the case, this should be done in a detailed and systematic manner. Essential information includes any relevant medical, surgical and anaesthetic history, health status of the patient, anaesthetic technique and drugs administered, monitoring and venous access, any intraoperative problem encountered or anticipated, current state of the surgical procedure, any special requirement for the procedure, and plans for further intraoperative and postoperative management.

— The anaesthesia record is a medico-legal document. It should be treated with respect. Relevant details should be written legibly, and all perioperative complications should be clearly documented in the record. This would be useful for future anaesthetic management if the patient should undergo another surgery and anaesthetic.

EMERGENCE AND RECOVERY

— At the end of the surgery, ensure that the patient demonstrates partial recovery of neuromuscular function before reversal of neuromuscular blockade. Suction the pharynx and oral cavity to clear secretions, and administer 100% oxygen while allowing the patient to awaken.

— If the patient is at risk of regurgitation and aspiration, it would be prudent to remove the endotracheal tube when the patient is awake and with full return of protective airway reflexes. This is also true for the patient whose intubation has been difficult, as awake extubation would minimize the need for reintubation due to depressed level of consciousness or inadequate ventilation.

— It is advisable in certain situations to extubate the patient "deep" – for example, the patient with reactive airways, cardiovascular disease or intracranial pathology – in order to reduce the risks of bronchospasm, hypertension, tachycardia or increased intracranial pressure. Care must be taken not to remove the endotracheal tube early before airway reflexes return.

— The anaesthesiologist should accompany the patient during transport from OT to the Post-Anaesthesia Care Unit (PACU) or Intensive Care Unit (ICU). Information for the PACU nurse on handing over includes the surgical procedure, anaesthetic technique, any intraoperative complications and any anticipated problems in the immediate postoperative period. The anaesthesiologist should ensure that patient's condition is stable before leaving the patient to the nurse's care. Do not commence the next anaesthetic until you are satisfied that the patient in PACU is stable.

— The patient should be promptly reviewed if any complications should arise in PACU. Problems in PACU include excessive pain, hypoventilation, airway obstruction, hyper- or hypotension and hypoxia. Appropriate treatment should be instituted accordingly when the underlying cause is diagnosed. A second anaesthesiologist should be available if the anaesthesiologist concerned is unable to attend to the patient immediately.

— The patient should be reviewed before discharge to the ward. He/she should be awake, comfortable, breathing adequately and having stable haemodynamic parameters on discharge. Specific instructions (for example, oxygen therapy, observation following regional anaesthesia, management by Acute Pain Service) should be clearly documented in the patient's case notes and conveyed to the ward staff.

POSTANAESTHESIA FOLLOW-UP

— In the ideal situation, all patients should be followed up in the wards because post-anaesthesia rounds are just as relevant as premedication rounds. Notable features include the adequacy of pain relief, postoperative fluid management, haemodynamic and respiratory status, and any complications arising from general or regional anaesthesia. Other than having the welfare of the patient in mind, this is an opportunity to heighten the public profile of the role of the anaesthesiologist as a perioperative physician.

— Unfortunately this is often not feasible in view of the heavy workload faced by the anaesthesiologist. Postanaesthesia follow-up is often confined to patients being managed by the APS team, and those who develop intra- and postoperative problems.

— Parturients who received epidural analgesia during labour are often followed up in the postpartum period before discharge from the hospital. In this way the anaesthesiologist can obtain feedback from the parturients on epidural analgesia, and elicit any immediate complications arising from the central neuraxial blockade.

FURTHER READING

1. Avidan MS, Jones N, Pozniak AL. The implications of HIV for the anaesthetist and the intensivist. Anaesthesia 2000;55:344–54.
2. Parker MRJ. The use of protective gloves, the incidence of ampoule injury and the prevalence of hand laceration amongst anaesthetic personnel. Anaesthesia 1995;50:726–8.

Chapter 2

Anaesthesia Preoperative Evaluation Clinic

INTRODUCTION

The Anaesthesia Preoperative Evaluation Clinic (APEC or "Anaesthetic Clinic") is an anaesthesia-based outpatient clinic to assess surgical patients before elective surgery. The scope of coverage of the APEC varies from hospital to hospital; it ranges from surgeons' referral of selected patients with significant medical or anaesthetic problems for in-depth assessment and preoperative counselling, to preoperative screening of *every* patient scheduled for surgery.

As the trend of surgical patient management increasingly shifts towards day-care or same-day admission surgery, many patients are no longer admitted to the hospital before surgery. It is therefore important for the anaesthesiologist to be involved in the preoperative assessment of the patient at an earlier stage, ideally as the patient is scheduled for the planned surgical procedure. The ultimate goal of preoperative assessment is to provide thorough, timely, and cost-effective evaluation of surgical patients. The inability to meet these criteria can result in costly operating room delays, surgical case cancellations and decreased patient satisfaction.

OBJECTIVES

Initially created to reduce postponement rate of elective surgical cases resulting from inadequate preoperative assessment and preparation, APEC has evolved to include other objectives and benefits.

— Shorter period of hospitalization by continuing the medical treatment and optimization on an outpatient rather than inpatient basis.
— Identification of potential problems which may arise during perioperative anaesthetic management.
— Education and explanation about the anaesthetic procedure, risks and benefits, anaesthetic options, and consequent reduction of patient anxiety towards anaesthesia and surgery.
— Increase patient awareness of the role and responsibilities of the anaesthesiologist in perioperative patient care.

ASSESSMENT

The timing for referral to APEC depends on the length of waiting list for the scheduled surgery, but should neither be too early when the patient's medical condition may have altered by the time he/she presents for surgery, nor too late when there may not be sufficient time for further assessment and optimization of treatment. An interval of 4–6 weeks would be a good compromise between the two extremes.

Written protocols and clinical pathway guidelines on criteria for referral (if APEC is meant for specific patients only), mechanisms for ordering further investigations or referring for subspecialty consultations, and further communication and feedback to the surgeon should be available. The objective is to keep the preoperative process as streamlined as possible to minimize the patient's waiting time or unnecessary visits to subspecialty clinics.

Appropriate staffing of APEC is important for it to function efficiently. This is especially so if APEC is used for preoperative screening of every patient scheduled for surgery. There should be adequate medical (anaesthesiology trainees and consultants) and nursing staff to handle the workload. The nurses can be trained to help with preoperative screening using structured questionnaires and refer more complex patients to the anaesthesiologist.

Assessment of the patient includes:

— Type of surgery scheduled.

— History pertaining to the cardiovascular, respiratory, endocrine and any other relevant systems.
— Detailed history of the patient's medication – current and past – and compliance to treatment.
— Thorough physical examination including airway assessment.
— Review of results of any investigations that were carried out.

Based on the above assessment, further investigative procedures and referral for subspecialty consultation may be necessary. Patients do not "pass" or "fail" their preoperative assessment. This is just a means to identify patients who are fit to proceed for surgery, and those who need more time for adjustment of current treatment or referral for further assessment.

Education is possible at APEC when the patient is receptive. Information on the scheduled procedure and its expected outcome, anaesthetic and pain relief options, and postoperative management (which may include ICU or HDU care) can be given in the knowledge that the patient has time to assimilate it. Questions from the patient are encouraged so that preoperative anxiety may be allayed with suitable explanation and reassurance.

The anaesthesiologist assessing a particular patient in APEC should ideally be involved in the anaesthetic management of the same patient at the time of surgery. This is, however, not always feasible. Therefore a summary of the patient's problems should be clearly documented in the patient's case notes. When the patient presents for surgery, the anaesthesiologist in charge of the OT list can then refer to the record and be forewarned about the potential anaesthetic problems.

FURTHER READING

1. Pollard JB. Economic aspects of an anesthesia preoperative evaluation clinic. Curr Opin Anaesthesiol 2002;15:257–61.
2. Kopp VJ. Preoperative preparation: value, perspective, and practice in patient care. Anesthesiol Clin North Am 2000;18:551–74.
3. Parker BM, Tetzlaff JE, Litaker DL, Maurer WG. Redefining the preoperative evaluation process and the role of anesthesiologist. J Clin Anesth 2000;12:350–6.
4. Klafta JM, Roizen MF. Current understanding of the patient's attitudes toward and preparation for anesthesia: A review. Anesth Analg 1996;83:1314–21.

Chapter 3

Premedication Round

GENERAL CONSIDERATIONS

Preanaesthetic evaluation is the process of clinical assessment that precedes the delivery of anaesthesia care for surgery and non-surgical procedures. It is the responsibility of the anaesthesiologist and is an integral part of safe anaesthetic practice.

A properly conducted preanaesthetic evaluation is accomplished through:

— Thorough assessment of the patient's medical condition by means of detailed history, physical examination and relevant investigations.

— Optimization of the patient's medical condition for anaesthesia and surgery.

— Identification of anaesthetic risk factors and, if significant, conveyance of such risks to the patient.
— Planning of anaesthetic technique and perioperative management.
— Establishment of rapport between the patient and the anaesthesiologist in order to allay anxiety and facilitate conduct of anaesthesia.
— Information and education of the patient on anaesthesia, perioperative care and pain management.

The premedication visit is an important aspect of anaesthetic management and should not be glossed over or hurried through. As far as possible, preanaesthetic assessment should be performed by the same anaesthesiologist scheduled to conduct the anaesthesia. This should be carried out at an appropriate time before surgery to allow adequate preparation of the patient.
— Inpatients scheduled for elective surgery are usually reviewed the day before the planned procedure.
— Same-day admission and day-care surgery patients are assessed on the day of surgery itself.
— As far as possible, all ill patients presenting for emergency surgery should be assessed in the ward prior to surgery. If surgery cannot be delayed in spite of increased anaesthetic risks, this should be documented clearly in the patient's anaesthesia record.

THE PREMEDICATION VISIT

These are carried out during the premedication visit.
— Confirmation of patient identification, review of diagnosis, proposed surgical procedure and consent for surgery and anaesthesia.
— Assessment through history-taking, physical examination and review of relevant investigation results, with emphasis on previous anaesthetic history, drug allergies, past and current medications, potential anaesthetic problems such as difficult airway, obesity, significant cardiopulmonary disease.
— Classification of physical status according to American Society of Anesthesiologists (ASA); see Table 3–1.
— Relevant preoperative preparation, such as optimization of medical treatment,

preoperative chest physiotherapy and breathing exercises, group and cross-match (GXM) blood and/or blood products.

— Informing the patient of the planned anaesthetic technique and perioperative management, including risk assessment and explanation.
— Giving clear instruction on medications: whether to continue or omit the dose, and when to take the medication on the day of surgery.
— Prescription of premedicant drugs.

Table 3–1. American Society of Anesthesiologists physical status classification and overall mortality rate

Category	Description of Patient	Mortality (%)
I	Healthy patient	0.06–0.08
II	Mild systemic disease with no functional limitation	0.3–0.4
III	Severe systemic disease with definite functional limitation	1.8–4.3
IV	Severe systemic disease that is a constant threat to life	7.8–23.4
V	Moribund patient unlikely to survive 24 hours with or without operation	9.4–50.7
"E"	Denotes emergency surgery	

Instructions for the ward staff on the preparation of the patient for OT must be written clearly. These are some examples.

— Repeat investigations if necessary.
— GXM blood and/or blood products: type of blood product and quantity.
— Time to commence fasting especially for children.
— Medications to be continued or omitted on the day of surgery.
— Preoperative nebulization of bronchodilator for patient with asthma or chronic obstructive pulmonary disease (COPD).

— Commencement of dextrose infusion or glucose-insulin-potassium (GIK) regime for diabetic patients.
— Premedicant drugs: dose, route and time of administration.

The surgeon should be informed if surgery has to be deferred. Specific reasons should be stated, and recommendations – such as referral to physician for further assessment and optimization, correction of abnormal biochemical results – should be documented clearly in the patient's case notes and anaesthesia record. Discuss with the surgeon if any changes to the sequence in the OT list are preferred to facilitate anaesthetic management, such as early scheduling of babies, diabetic patients or those with significant medical or anaesthetic problems. Inform the OT if the surgeon agrees to the change.

RECOMMENDED PREANAESTHETIC INVESTIGATIONS

The nature and extent of preanaesthetic investigations depend on the patient's age, presence of any co-morbid condition, as well as the nature and extent of the planned surgical procedure.

Routine investigations, listed in Table 3–2, are solely based on age and nature of surgery for asymptomatic patients without abnormal clinical findings. Major surgery is empirically defined as one in which the cranium, thorax or abdomen is opened or when the anticipated blood loss is significant and exceeds 15% of total blood volume.

Table 3–2. Routine investigations for patients undergoing anaesthesia

Routine Investigation	Indication
Urinalysis	All patients (check blood glucose concentration if urine sugar is positive)
FBC	All females; males > 40 years; all major surgery
Urea, creatinine, electrolytes	Major surgery
ECG	Age > 50 years
CXR	Age > 60 years
Liver function test	Major surgery in patients > 50 years

If a medical condition is present, relevant investigations irrespective of age and type of operation should be ordered. For example, ECG and CXR are indicated for a 20-year-old patient with mitral stenosis and atrial fibrillation presenting for a hernia operation.

Some preanaesthetic investigations and their indications are listed here.

1. **Full blood count (FBC)**
   - Anaemia and other haematological disease.
   - Renal disease.
   - Patient on chemotherapy.

2. **Urea, creatinine and electrolyte concentration**
   - Renal and liver diseases.
   - Metabolic disease, e.g., diabetes mellitus.
   - Abnormal nutritional states.
   - History of diarrhoea, vomiting.
   - Preoperative bowel preparation.
   - Drugs that may alter electrolyte balance or exhibit enhanced toxic effects in the presence of electrolyte abnormality, e.g., digitalis, diuretics, antihypertensives, corticosteroids, hypoglycaemic agents.

3. **Blood glucose concentration**
   - Diabetes mellitus.
   - Severe liver disease.

4. **Electrocardiogram (ECG)**
   - Heart disease, hypertension or chronic pulmonary disease.
   - Diabetes mellitus.

5. **Chest X-ray (CXR)**
   - Significant respiratory disease.
   - Cardiovascular disease.

6. **Arterial blood gases (ABG)**
   - Debilitated or septic patients.
   - Moderate to severe pulmonary disease.
   - Patients in respiratory difficulty.
   - Morbidly obese patient.
   - Patient scheduled for thoracotomy.

7. **Lung function test**
   - Patient scheduled for thoracotomy.
   - Moderate to severe pulmonary disease, such as COPD, bronchiectasis, restrictive lung disease.

8. **Coagulation screen**
   - Haematological disease.
   - Severe liver disease.
   - Coagulopathy due to any cause.
   - Anticoagulant therapy, e.g., oral anticoagulant (warfarin) or heparin.

9. **Liver function test**
   - Hepatobiliary disease.
   - History of alcohol abuse.
   - Tumour with possible metastases to the liver.

10. **Thyroid function tests**
    - Thyroid surgery.
    - History of thyroid disease.
    - Suspected endocrine abnormalities, e.g., pituitary tumour.

11. **Tests to assess cardiac function**
    - These are elaborated in Chapter 12.

Normal investigation results are valid for varying periods of time, ranging from 1 week (FBC, urea, creatinine, electrolyte concentration, blood glucose concentration), 1 month (ECG) to 6 months (CXR). Investigations should be repeated under the following circumstances:

- Appearance of fresh symptoms, such as chest pains, diarrhoea, vomiting.
- Assessment for effectiveness of therapy, such as potassium supplement for hypokalaemia, insulin therapy for hyperglycaemia, dialysis for patients with renal failure, blood products for correction of coagulopathy.

CONSENT

Both legal and ethical considerations mandate a competent adult patient to provide consent prior to any planned anaesthetic and surgical procedure. It is highly desirable that a separate, written consent for anaesthesia should be obtained by the anaesthesiologist after due explanation and risk information.This avoids the problem of misinformation or miscommunication when the surgeon is saddled with the task of obtaining a common surgical and anaesthetic consent.

Consent should be obtained from the parent or guardian for an underaged patient, while explanation and discussion should involve the patient's next-of-kin if the patient is in no condition to provide consent for treatment. In an emergency, it is often not practical to delay life-saving procedures on account of the issue of consent. Similarly, unconscious patients may be given essential emergency treatment without consent.

Sufficient information should be provided during the preoperative visit to allow the patient to make a considered decision. These should be discussed with the patient:

— The planned anaesthetic procedure.

— Alternative anaesthetic options, if applicable.

— Possible risks and complications pertaining to anaesthesia.

— Benefits versus risks.

Anaesthetic risk disclosure is a rather contentious issue because it is not possible to have firm practice guidelines for the anaesthesiologist to adhere to. Furthermore, the actual risks of anaesthesia are not readily listed anywhere, and anaesthesiologists differ widely in their approach to conveying risk information. It is not always easy to strike a balance between inadequate information which hinders informed decision-making, and excessive information which creates unwarranted doubt and anxiety. These points are generally agreed upon as necessary for discussion with the patient.

— Complications with reported incidence greater than 1:100 constitute material risks and should be discussed with the patient.

— For better understanding and to place the risks in proper perspective, these should be compared with the relative risks of everyday events (Table 3–3).

— The severity of a particular complication (e.g., one which results in permanent disability or death) should be considered in the discussion even though it may be unlikely to occur.

— Patients with significant co-morbid conditions and high anaesthetic risks should be counselled about such risks, and alternative surgical and anaesthetic options should be discussed with the patient and/or next-of-kin.
— It is important for the discussion to be documented, and the written consent to be signed, witnessed and dated.

Table 3–3. Examples of everyday and clinical risks

Everyday Risks	Risk Level	Clinical Risks
	1:1 **Very High**	Postoperative nausea and vomiting (1:4) Dizziness (1:5)
	1:10 **High**	Oral trauma following intubation (1:20) Difficult intubation (1:50)
Deaths per year (1:100)	1:100 **Moderate**	Perioperative death (1:200) Failed intubation (1:500)
Traffic deaths per year (1:8,000)	1:1,000 **Low**	Aspiration (1:3,000) Failure to intubate and ventilate (1:5,000)
Death by accident at home per year (1:11,000)	1:10,000 **Very Low**	Anaphylaxis (1:10,000) Spontaneous epidural abscess (1:10,000)
Rail accidents per year (1:140,000)	1:100,000 **Minimal**	Epidural haematoma (1:150,000–200,000) Death due solely to anaesthesia (1:180,000)
	1:1,000,000 **Negligible**	Spontaneous epidural haematoma (1:1,000,000)
Death by lightning strike per year (1:10,000,000)	1:10,000,000 **Minute** 1:100,000,000	

FASTING GUIDELINES

Patients scheduled for surgery are fasted to avoid the risks of regurgitation and aspiration of gastric contents under anaesthesia. Such fasting guidelines should be observed even when the patient is scheduled for local or regional anaesthesia, in case general anaesthesia becomes necessary for various reasons during surgery. Recent evidence has demonstrated the adverse effects of prolonged fasting especially in the obstetric, paediatric and geriatric populations. Provision of clear fluids up to two hours before surgery does not increase aspiration risks and is now an accepted practice.

Guidelines for preoperative fasting before surgery, applicable for patients with no known risk factors for aspiration, are given in Table 3–4.

Table 3–4. Guidelines for preoperative fasting

Age of Patient	Nature of Oral Intake	Length of Fasting (hr)	Amount of Fluid Allowed
< 6 months	Clear fluid* Breast milk Formula milk	2 3 4	20 ml/kg
6 months – 5 years	Clear fluid* Formula milk Solids	2 4 6	10 ml/kg
> 5 years	Clear fluid* Solids	2 6	10 ml/kg
Adult, morning list	Clear fluid* Solids	2 Fast from 12 midnight	
Adult, afternoon list	Clear fluid* Solids	2 Fast from 8 am after light breakfast**	

* Water, clear fruit juice, glucose water; *not* carbonated drinks, soup, milk, coffee or tea.

** A maximum of 2 slices of bread or 4 pieces of biscuits with milk, tea or coffee for adults; or a slice of bread and a cup of milk for children.

PREMEDICATION

Any premedication ordered must be clearly written, stating:

— Name and dose of the premedicant drug (in actual dose in milligrams rather than "tab" or "ml").

— Route of administration.

— Time of administration.

The name and signature of the anaesthesiologist should be legible so that he or she can be consulted should any queries arise.

Some premedication guidelines are listed below:

1. **No sedative premedication**
   - Ill, septic, elderly patients.
   - Patients with potential airway problems (consider antisialogogue to facilitate fibreoptic intubation).
   - Day-care surgery patients.
   - Most neurosurgical patients.
   - Neonates and infants less than 6 months.

2. **Oral benzodiazepine** (e.g., midazolam, diazepam, temazepam)
   - Night sedation where indicated.
   - Most elective surgical patients.
   - Patients for whom a regional anaesthetic technique is planned.

   The oral premedication should be timed such that it can be served 2 hours before the scheduled operation.

3. **Opioids**

   IM pethidine 1 mg/kg with IM promethazine 12.5–25 mg.

   IM papaveratum 0.2–0.3 mg/kg with IM scopolamine 0.008 mg/kg.
   - Healthy patients undergoing major cases.
   - Preexisting painful conditions, e.g., fracture of femur.
   - Patients in whom absorption of orally administered drugs is unreliable, e.g., oesophageal stricture.

No intramuscular injections should be given for patients with coagulation problems (e.g., haemophiliacs) or patients on anticoagulants.

The premedication should be timed such that it can be given 1 hour before surgery.

Note that oral premedication is preferred to intramuscular injection unless the parenteral route is specifically indicated.

4. **Paediatric patients**

   Avoid intramuscular injections as far as possible.

   — *Omit premedication* in any ill babies, neonates and infants less than 6 months especially those with history of prematurity.

   — **Small children < 15 kg**
   - Syrup trimeprazine 3–4 mg/kg.
   - Syrup diazepam 0.2 mg/kg.

   — **Bigger children > 5 years or > 15 kg**
   - Oral diazepam 0.2 mg/kg.
   - Oral midazolam 0.5–0.7 mg/kg.
   - EMLA cream on dorsum of hand 1 hour before surgery; cover with a clear transparent dressing.

5. **Obstetric patients**

   — Oral ranitidine 150 mg nocte and on morning of operation.

   — 0.3M sodium citrate 30 ml.

   — For emergency caesarean section or postpartum procedures, administer IV ranitidine 50 mg as soon as decision for the procedure is made.

6. **Patients at risk of regurgitation and aspiration**

   — These include morbidly obese patients, all obstetric patients and those with known history of hiatus hernia or reflux oesophagitis.

   — Drugs prescribed as prophylaxis against acid aspiration include H_2 receptor antagonists (e.g., ranitidine, cimetidine), proton-pump inhibitors (e.g., omeprazole), non-particulate antacids (e.g., 0.3M sodium citrate) and gastrokinetic agents (e.g., metoclopramide), given in combination.

MEDICATIONS

— Most medications should be continued as usual, and oral medications should be taken with sips of water on the morning of surgery. For patients in whom oral administration may not be suitable (e.g., oesophageal disease, gastric outlet obstruction), alternative drug or alternative routes of drug delivery should be considered.

— The anaesthesiologist should have a working knowledge of the pharmacology of the patient's medication. Potential adverse interactions of these drugs with anaesthetic agents should be recognized and the anaesthetic technique modified if necessary.

— The perioperative use of herbal medicines may be associated with adverse effects and drug interactions, such as enhanced potential for bleeding, hypertension or untoward cardiovascular effects, potentiation of anaesthetic agents, electrolyte disturbances, hepatotoxicity, and hormonal effects. Their use should be specifically asked for during preoperative assessment. No guidelines have been formalized as yet, but it seems prudent to discontinue these products at least 2 weeks before elective surgery.

— Most cardiovascular drugs should be continued. A few pertinent points:
  - Diuretics are usually withheld unless they are used in the treatment of chronic renal failure.
  - Angiotensin-converting enzyme (ACE) inhibitors are associated with higher incidence and greater magnitude of hypotension on induction but usually respond well to intravenous fluids and/or vasopressor.
  - Antiarrhythmic agents should be continued; but ensure that plasma concentrations of the drugs are within therapeutic range and correct any electrolyte abnormalities which may potentiate drug toxicity.

— When it is deemed necessary to withhold medication preoperatively, sufficient time (3–5 half-lives) should be allowed for metabolic clearance. Drugs which should be withheld include insulin and oral hypoglycaemic agents, drugs that affect haemostasis (e.g., anticoagulants, fibrinolytics), and certain psychotropic drugs (e.g. monoamine oxidase inhibitors).

FURTHER READING

1. Practice advisory for preanesthesia evaluation: A report by the American Society of Anesthesiologists Task Force on Preanesthesia Evaluation. Anesthesiology 2002;96:485–96.

2. Jenkins K, Baker AB. Consent and anaesthetic risk. Anaesthesia 2003;58:962–84.
3. White SM, Baldwin TJ. Consent for anaesthesia. Anaesthesia 2003;58:760–74.
4. Adams AM, Smith AF. Risk perception and communication: Recent developments and implications for anaesthesia. Anaesthesia 2001;56:745–55.
5. Hodges PJ, Kam PCA. The peri-operative implications of herbal medicines. Anaesthesia 2002;57:889–99.
6. Ang-Lee MK, Moss J, Yuan CS. Herbal medicines and perioperative care. JAMA 2001;286:208–16.
7. Practice guidelines for preoperative fasting and the use of pharmacologic agents to reduce the risk of pulmonary aspiration: Application to healthy patients undergoing elective procedures: A report by the American Society of Anesthesiologists Task Force on Preoperative Fasting. Anesthesiology 1999;90:896–905.
8. Splinter WM, Schreiner MS. Preoperative fasting in children. Anesth Analg 1999;89:80–9.

Chapter 4

Perioperative Fluid Therapy

INTRODUCTION

Fluid therapy is an important aspect of perioperative management and should be tailored to the individual patient. Optimal fluid therapy begins with clinical assessment of the patient to determine the amount, the nature as well as the speed at which the fluid should be administered. This is aided by laboratory investigations as well as invasive haemodynamic monitoring in selected cases.

Intraoperative fluid therapy should take into account the preexisting deficit, maintenance requirement and on-going losses. Choices of fluid include various types of crystalloid and colloid solutions. In the presence of significant blood loss, blood and blood products are required to restore intravascular volume.

Postoperative fluid therapy should be individualized as well. Consideration should be given to the length and complexity of surgery, the organ system involved in the surgery, the patient's general status, and expected time to recommencement of oral intake.

These patient groups require careful monitoring of fluid status.

— Extremes of age groups.
— Patients with abnormal losses of blood or plasma (e.g., trauma, burns), body fluids (e.g., vomiting, diuresis, excessive sweating) or fluids from the third space (e.g., intestinal obstruction).
— Patients with reduced fluid intake due to various causes, such as malignancy or gastrointestinal diseases, reduced level of consciousness, excessive vomiting.
— Patients in whom fluid overload is undesirable, such as those with poor cardiac function, renal failure or neurosurgical conditions.
— Patients undergoing major surgical procedures that are prolonged or complicated with significant fluid shifts and haemodynamic changes.

EVALUATION OF INTRAVASCULAR VOLUME

The intravascular volume is best assessed clinically. Laboratory tests and haemodynamic measurements confirm the clinical impression and serial readings are useful to evaluate the adequacy of fluid therapy.

1. **Clinical evaluation**

   The history enables one to identify the patients at risk, and to assess the nature of fluid loss, the extent and severity of dehydration.

   These signs are noted in physical examination.

   — Mental status.
   — Skin turgor, tension of anterior fontanelle in babies < 18 months, hydration of mucous membrane.
   — Character of peripheral pulse, resting heart rate and blood pressure, effect of postural changes.
   — Urine output.
   — Evidence of overt or occult blood or fluid loss.

   As shown in Table 4–1, the degree of dehydration is empirically divided into mild (fluid loss of approximately 5% of body weight), moderate (10%) and severe (15% or more). This serves as an approximate guide to indicate the urgency and aggressiveness of fluid therapy.

Table 4–1. Signs of fluid loss

Sign	Mild (5%)	Moderate (10%)	Severe (> 15%)
Mucous membrane	Dry	Very dry	Parched
Sensorium	Normal	Lethargic	Obtunded
Postural changes in heart rate or BP	Absent or mild	Present	Marked
Urine output	Mildly decreased	Decreased	Markedly decreased
Pulse rate	Normal or increased	Increased	Markedly increased
Blood pressure	Normal	Mildly decreased	Decreased

2. **Laboratory investigations**

   Laboratory tests are neither sensitive nor specific indicators of the intravascular volume status. Furthermore, not all the test results can be immediately available, and we must rely on our clinical acumen to assess the patient's intravascular volume status.

   — Full blood count
   - Low haemoglobin in blood loss.
   - High haematocrit in losses of body fluids other than blood.

   — Blood urea and electrolyte concentrations
   - High blood urea in dehydration.
   - Abnormalities in sodium or potassium concentration depending on clinical scenario.

   — Arterial blood gases
   - Metabolic acidosis in shock states with poor organ perfusion and anaerobic metabolism.
   - Increased serum lactate concentration.

   — Urine examination
   - Specific gravity may be high (> 1.010).
   - Urine sodium may be low (< 20 mEq/ml) in an attempt to conserve sodium and water.

3. **Haemodynamic measurements**
   - Central venous pressure (CVP)
     This measures the right heart pressure as opposed to pulmonary artery pressure that indicates the left heart pressure. Serial readings are more useful than a single reading for assessing adequacy of fluid therapy.
   - Pulmonary artery pressure (PAP)
     Pulmonary artery catheterization is mainly done in the intensive care setting. It is rarely, if ever, employed in the initial resuscitation stage. It is indicated in patients with significant cardiac disease since the right heart pressure may not correlate with the left heart pressure. Again serial readings are more useful than a single reading.

SOME FACTS ON INTRAVENOUS FLUIDS

- Crystalloid solutions (Table 4–2) are aqueous solutions of low molecular weight ions (salts) with or without glucose. They rapidly equilibrate with, and distribute throughout, the extravascular space. Replacement of intravascular volume deficit with crystalloid solutions generally requires approximately 3 times the volume of estimated deficit.
- Colloid solutions (Table 4–3) are solutions containing high molecular weight substances such as proteins or large glucose polymers. They maintain plasma oncotic pressure and remain intravascularly for longer periods. Colloid solutions can replace blood loss in a ratio of 1:1–1.5; hence severe intravascular fluid deficits can be more rapidly and efficiently corrected using colloid solutions.
- The colloid-crystalloid controversy in resuscitation and intensive care has been in existence for more than 30 years. Reservations regarding colloid solutions exist in situations associated with increased capillary permeability, such as burns, anaphylaxis and multiple trauma. Colloid particles may diffuse into the interstitial space across the leaky capillaries, worsening interstitial oedema and hindering fluid resorption from the interstitium.
- A definitive answer on the best solution for resuscitation and maintenance does not exist, neither is there an "ideal" intravascular fluid volume replacement strategy. One suspects that the "middle ground" approach is probably the safest: a mixture of crystalloid and colloid solutions, the proportion of each depends very much on the severity of fluid deficit, nature of fluid loss, cost considerations, availability and personal preference.

Table 4–2. Composition of crystalloid solutions

Solution	Osmolality (mosm/kg)	Sodium (meq/L)	Chloride (meq/L)	Potassium (meq/L)	Calcium (meq/L)	Lactate (meq/L)	Glucose (g/L)
Dextrose 5%	253						50
Normal saline	308	154	154				
Ringer's lactate	273	130	109	4	3	28	
Dextrose saline	561	154	154				50

Table 4–3. Composition of colloid solutions

Solution	Molecular Weight	Osmolality (msom/kg)	Albumin (g/L)	Polysaccharide (g/L)	Sodium (meq/L)	Potassium (meq/L)	Calcium (meq/L)	Chloride (meq/L)
25% albumin	50,000		250					
Haemacel®	35,000	300–306	35		145	5.1	12.5	145
Dextran 40*	40,000	346–368		100	150			150
Dextran 70**	70,000	335–337		60				
Hydroxyethyl starch (HES)	70,000–550,000#	310		60–100	154			154

* 10% dextran 40 in 0.9% saline.
** 6% dextran 70 in 5% dextrose.
# Different molecular weights in different generations of HES (Voluven® 130,000; Hemohes® 200,000; Hetastarch® 450,000; Hextend® 550,000).

Crystalloid Solutions

Crystalloid solutions can be classified into:

— *Hypotonic solutions* (maintenance-type solutions) for correction of deficits primarily due to water loss.

— *Isotonic solutions* (replacement-type or balanced salt solutions) for replacement of deficits due to both water and electrolyte losses.

— *Hypertonic solutions* (e.g., dextrose 30%, dextrose 50%, hypertonic saline 3%) for total parenteral nutrition (dextrose solutions); treatment of severe hyponatraemia, e.g., in TURP syndrome (hypertonic saline). The role of hypertonic saline in fluid resuscitation is still controversial and being investigated.

Glucose solutions are given to prevent hypoglycaemia and ketosis during fasting. They are not recommended for use in resuscitation during cardiac arrest and cerebral ischaemia, as hyperglycaemia is found to be associated with adverse cardiovascular and neurological outcomes. Specific indications for glucose solutions include:

— Documented hypoglycaemia due to any cause.

— Patients at risk for hypoglycaemia, such as:

- Diabetic patients on long-acting hypoglycaemic agents.
- Newborns, particularly preterm neonates and babies of diabetic mothers.
- Patients with severe liver disease in whom glycogen store may be depleted.

Colloid Solutions

Colloid solutions are either synthetic or derived from blood. Examples of each are:

— Synthetic colloid solutions: dextrose starches (e.g., hydroxyethyl starch, dextran solutions), gelatin solutions (e.g., Haemaccel®, Gelafundin®, Gelafusine®).

— Blood-derived colloid solutions: human albumin 5% or 25%, plasma protein fraction (e.g., Plasmanate®, Plasmatein®).

Colloid solutions are indicated in these clinical situations:

— Severe intravascular fluid deficits, such as haemorrhagic shock before blood is available for transfusion.

— Severe hypoalbuminaemia and large protein losses, seen in severe liver disease and burns respectively.

— Improvement of microcirculation in vascular surgery or reimplantation of limb or digits with dextran solutions, especially Dextran 40 for its "anti-sludging" properties.

Problems of colloid solutions include:

— Cost, in particular the newer HES solutions.
— Allergic reactions, estimated to be in the range of 0.033–0.22%.
— Interference with blood-typing (dextran > 20 ml/kg/24 hr).
— Association with acute renal failure.
— Coagulopathy as a result of interference of platelet function and dilutional effect.

INTRAOPERATIVE FLUID THERAPY

Three aspects of fluid therapy should be considered.

1. **Maintenance requirement**
   — This is required to replace losses from urine, gastrointestinal tract secretions, perspiration and insensible loss via the respiratory tract.
   — Maintenance requirement may be higher in certain situations, e.g., fever, hypermetabolic states, tachypnoea.
   — A rough estimation of the maintenance requirement can be obtained by applying the formula:
   - first 10 kg: 4 ml/kg/hr
   - 11–20 kg: 40 ml/hr + 2 ml/hr for every kg above 10 kg
   - 21 kg and above: 60 ml/hr + 1 ml/hr for every kg above 20 kg

2. **Preexisting deficit**
   — This depends on the length of fasting before surgery and is derived from normal maintenance per hour multiplied by number of hours of fasting.
   — The fluid deficit is increased when there are abnormal fluid losses, such as bleeding, vomiting, diuresis, diarrhoea, fluid sequestration, and increased insensible losses.

3. **On-going losses**

— Other than intraoperative blood loss, fluid losses include:
  - Drainage of ascitic fluid or cystic fluid.
  - Fluid sequestrated in the gastrointestinal tract.
  - Evaporation from exposed surgical field.
  - Tissue oedema when it is traumatized, inflamed or infected.

— One should keep abreast with intraoperative fluid losses, and the type of intravenous fluids administered should reflect the nature of fluids lost. For example, colloid solution should be used to replace ascitic or cystic fluid with high protein content.

— Evaporative losses from the surgical field are estimated according to the degree of surgical exposure. This is empirically classified as superficial, moderate and severe, and estimated to be 1–2 mg/kg/hr, 3–4 mg/kg/hr and 6–8 mg/kg/hr respectively.

— However, too much importance should not be placed on formulae and figures. Ultimately it depends on close monitoring and assessment of the patient's intravascular volume status by clinical means. Intraarterial BP and CVP monitoring should be employed in major surgery where significant fluid and blood losses are anticipated. Hourly urine output should be measured by means of continuous bladder drainage.

— There is no hard and fast rule as to when the patient should receive blood transfusion. While every attempt is made to avoid allogeneic blood transfusion in order to reduce the risks of disease transmission and transfusion reactions, this should not be withheld from patients who suffer massive blood loss. Autologous blood transfusion, if applicable, may be used as part of the blood conservation strategies.

POSTOPERATIVE FLUID THERAPY

The amount and nature of fluids administered again depend on the patient's status, anaesthetic and surgical factors. These guidelines should be noted.

— Surgery done under regional anaesthesia and/or sedation, not involving the gastrointestinal tract
  - No postoperative fasting is required.
  - Allow clear fluids and later solids as tolerated.

— Minor surgery done under general anaesthesia, not involving the gastrointestinal tract
  - Allow oral fluids when the patient is fully conscious and not nauseous.
  - Start with clear fluids, then soft diet and finally solids as tolerated.
  - Discontinue intravenous fluid administration when the patient can tolerate oral intake.

— Major surgery, or surgery involving the gastrointestinal tract
  - Maintain intravenous hydration of 2.5 L/24 hr in a 60-kg adult with crystalloid solutions in the form of dextrose saline, normal saline or Ringer's lactate.
  - Close haemodynamic monitoring is required.
  - Send blood samples for full blood count, glucose, urea and electrolyte concentrations.
  - Attempt early feeding if postoperative recovery is uneventful.
  - Consider total parenteral nutrition if oral intake may be delayed.

FURTHER READING

1. Rosenthal MH. Intraoperative fluid management: What and how much? Chest 1999;115:106S–112S.
2. Choi PTL, Yip G, Quinonez LG, Cook DJ. Crystalloids vs. colloids in fluid resuscitation: A systematic review. Crit Care Med 1999;27:200–10.
3. Boldt J. New light on intravascular volume replacement regimens: What did we learn from the past three years? Anesth Analg 2003;97:1595–604.
4. Boldt J. Volume replacement in the surgical patient: Does the type of solution make a difference? Br J Anaesth 2000;84:782–93.

5 Chapter

Perioperative Blood Transfusion

- Introduction
- Anaemia
- Some Facts on Blood and Blood Products
- Blood Conservation Techniques
- Massive Blood Transfusion
- Some Practical Pointers
- Appendix: Maximum Surgical Blood Order Schedule (MSBOS) for Elective Surgery
- Further Reading

INTRODUCTION

Blood and blood products are valuable resources with the potential to save lives and improve clinical outcome. As blood transfusion is not without risks, there should be definite indications for transfusion so that blood is not empirically given just to achieve a predetermined haemoglobin value. A patient scheduled for elective surgery and found to be anaemic should be investigated for the cause of anaemia. If blood transfusion is deemed necessary, it should ideally be given 36–48 hours prior to surgery in order to maximize the oxygen-carrying capacity of the transfused blood.

ANAEMIA

Anaemia, or deficiency in red blood cells, can be caused by acute or chronic blood loss, nutritional deficiency (iron, Vitamin B_{12} or folate), bone marrow failure or infiltration with tumour cells, increased haemolysis, or in association with systemic illness such as chronic renal failure, blood dyscrasia, or haemoglobinopathy. In cases where diagnosis is in doubt and investigations are necessary, it is best to withhold blood transfusion until the diagnosis is confirmed. This consideration obviously does not apply if blood transfusion is urgently warranted as a life-saving measure.

Oxygen flux is dependent on haemoglobin, oxygen saturation and cardiac output. In a normal healthy patient, haemoglobin of 7.0 g/dl is sufficient for adequate tissue oxygenation. The transfusion threshold has traditionally been recommended at a haemoglobin value 10.0 g/dl, which corresponds to a haematocrit of 30%. This has now been refuted, and one should not condone the practice of indiscriminate preoperative blood transfusion to boost the haemoglobin to 10.0 g/dl. Each patient should be assessed individually, weighing risks of blood transfusion against risks of developing complications of inadequate oxygen carriage.

Some factors that determine the need for blood transfusion are:

— *Physiological status:* lower transfusion threshold for patients at extremes of age.

— *Concomitant medical conditions:* lower transfusion threshold for patients with significant cardiopulmonary and cerebrovascular diseases.

— *Haemodynamic status:* heart rate, blood pressure, urine output, CVP; presence of cardiac failure or angina in patients with decompensated states.

— *Anticipated and actual surgical blood loss:* nature, amount and speed of blood loss; likelihood of further losses intra- and postoperatively.

Note that estimations of intraoperative blood loss are often inaccurate. Crystalloid and colloid solutions should be used for volume replacement initially. Blood transfusion is generally indicated when blood loss is greater than 10–15% of the blood volume. This threshold is lower in patients who are ill, septic, and those with borderline organ functions.

In general, red cell transfusion is not indicated in mild and asymptomatic anaemia (Hb > 8.0 g/dl) responsive to haematinic therapy. Anaemia associated chronic disease such as chronic renal failure is usually well tolerated and does not require transfusion. On the other hand, red cell transfusion should be given when there is active uncontrolled bleeding, when anaemia is symptomatic or associated with respiratory or cardiac decompensation, and when there is little time for correction of anaemia before urgent major surgery.

SOME FACTS ON BLOOD AND BLOOD PRODUCTS

1. **Whole blood**
   - It is indicated in situations of acute blood loss such as haemorrhagic shock.
   - Whole blood can be separated into various components thus allowing administration of appropriate products specific to the patient's needs.

2. **Packed red blood cells**
   - Red cells are transfused in patients with anaemia to increase the oxygen content of the blood, improve oxygen delivery and thereby prevent tissue hypoxia.
   - In a 70-kg adult with no on-going blood loss, a 250-ml packed RBC or one unit of whole blood increases the haematocrit by 3% or haemoglobin by 1 g/dl.

3. **Fresh frozen plasma (FFP)**
   - Indications for FFP transfusion.
     - Urgent reversal of anticoagulation or in known coagulation factor deficiencies.
     - Specific conditions such as pseudocholinesterase deficiency.
     - Microvascular bleeding in the presence of elevated (>1.5 times normal) prothrombin time (PT) or partial thromboplastin time (PTT), or after replacement of more than one blood volume when PT or APTT results are not available.
   - FFP is *not* meant for volume expansion or protein replacement.
   - One unit of FFP is approximately 200–250 ml; 4–8 units of FFP are required in order to produce a clinically significant increase in serum levels of clotting factors.
   - FFP is stored at –30°C. It should be thawed to body temperature and given in a dedicated transfusion set with a standard 170-μm filter.

4. **Platelet concentrate**
   - Platelet transfusion is used to arrest or prevent bleeding in patients with qualitative or quantitative platelet defects.
   - Qualitative platelet defects can exist in a patient with an apparently normal platelet count. Examples include sepsis, renal failure, use of aspirin and other antiplatelet agents.

- Platelet transfusion is recommended in these clinical situations.
    - Prior to major surgery in patients with preoperative platelet count < 50,000/µl.
    - Intra- and postoperative microvascular bleeding with platelet count < 50,000/µl.
    - Following cardiopulmonary bypass or other situations associated with platelet dysfunction with platelet count of 50,000–100,000/µl.
    - Surgery where minimal bleeding may cause major damage (e.g., neurosurgery, ophthalmic surgery) in a patient with platelet count of 50,000–100,000/µl.
- In situations where there is clinical evidence of disseminated intravascular coagulation (DIC), massive transfusion and/or platelet dysfunction, platelet transfusion may be given without laboratory confirmation. This decision should, however, be undertaken on a case-by-case basis.
- The therapeutic dose is 1 unit of platelet concentrate per 10 kg body weight. Each unit should raise the platelet count by 5,000–10,000/µl in the adult patient.
- Packs of platelet concentrates are stored at room temperature. Since platelet viability decreases with time, these should be transfused as soon as the units are received from the Blood Bank. Platelets should be given in a fresh transfusion set or a special platelet-giving set.

5. **Cryoprecipitate**

- Cryoprecipitate is rich in fibrinogen and contains factors VIII, XIII, von Willebrand (vW) factor and fibronectin.
- Its indications include:
    - Prophylaxis against bleeding for von Willebrand's disease, congenital deficiencies of factors I, VIII and vW factor in the perioperative period.
    - Massive transfusion and DIC with low fibrinogen levels.
- The volume of one bag is approximately 30 ml. The dose is 1 unit of cryoprecipitate per 10 kg body weight. In DIC, at least 6 units are required in adult patients.

6. **Cryosupernatant ("Liver plasma")**

- Cryosupernatant contains factors II, VII, IX, X (Vitamin K-dependent factors), albumin and immunoglobulins.

— It is indicated for correction of prolonged PT or APTT in a patient who is bleeding as a result of liver disease or DIC, and for urgent reversal of warfarin therapy or overdose.
— One unit of cryosupernatant is approximately 170–220 ml.

7. **Other blood products**
   — Clotting factor concentrate.
   — White cell concentrate.

BLOOD CONSERVATION TECHNIQUES

The potential for adverse effects, high costs and intermittent blood shortages mandate a wise use of allogeneic blood transfusions. Blood conservation techniques that have been developed are summarized here.

1. **Preoperative preparation**
   — Haematinics (iron, Vitamin B_{12}, folate) for specific anaemia.
   — Recombinant human erythropoietin therapy to increase red cell synthesis in chronic renal failure.
   — Prophylactic angiographic embolization to reduce tumour vascularity and intraoperative bleeding.
   — Limit blood sampling for investigations unless absolutely necessary.
   — Withhold drugs which affect haemostasis (e.g., aspirin, warfarin, heparin) in the immediate preoperative period.

2. **Surgical techniques**
   — Minimally invasive surgery with endoscopic procedures rather than open surgery.
   — Good surgical technique with gentle handling of tissue, expeditious and meticulous haemostasis.
   — Minimize duration of surgery, or plan for staged surgery for complex procedures.
   — Consider temporary packing and wound closure for non-surgical bleeding.
   — Use of haemostatic surgical instruments: electrocautery, laser, ultrasonic scalpel, argon beam coagulator, radiofrequency thermal ablation, water-jet dissector, microwave devices.
   — Use of arterial tourniquets, vascular clips, clamps during surgery.
   — Topical/local vasoconstrictors: adrenaline, cocaine, phenylephrine.

— Topical/local haemostatic agents: tissue adhesives, fibrin glue, gelatin foam (Gelfoam®), oxidized cellulose haemostat (Surgicel®).

3. **Positioning**
   — Measures to promote venous drainage and thereby reduce venous congestion and bleeding from the surgical site.
   - Head and neck surgery: slight reverse Trendelenburg position (15–20°), avoid kinking of blood vessels at the neck.
   - Spine surgery in prone position: supports at chest and pelvis to avoid abdominal compression.

4. **Anaesthetic technique**
   — Regional anaesthesia in appropriate cases.
   — Smooth induction and maintenance of adequate level of anaesthesia using volatile anaesthetics and opioids.
   — Controlled hypotensive anaesthesia using vasodilators and/or β-adrenergic blocking agents.
   — Thermal management
   - Maintain perioperative normothermia (hypothermia may predispose to platelet dysfunction and impairment of coagulation).
   - Consider controlled therapeutic hypothermia in certain clinical situation (e.g., cardiac surgery, neurosurgery) to decrease tissue oxygen consumption and protect against myocardial or cerebral ischaemia.

5. **Pharmacological agents**
   — Antifibrinolytic agents such as tranexamic acid, aprotinin, and epsilon-aminocaproic acid (ε-ACA) inhibit the fibrinolytic pathway and enhance the clotting process.
   — Desmopressin (DDAVP), a synthetic analogue of vasopressin, exerts haemostatic effect by enhancing platelet aggregation and increasing serum levels of factor VIII and vW factor.
   — Preoperative prophylactic administration of Vitamin K increases levels of Vitamin K-dependent clotting factors.
   — Clotting factor replacement therapy: factors VIIa, VIII, IX are available as recombinant products; activated recombinant factor VII is emerging as novel therapy for treatment of acquired coagulopathies presenting with intractable life-threatening haemorrhage.

6. **Autologous blood transfusion** (see Chapter 55)
   — Autotransfusion in various forms depending on availability of resources and suitability of patient and surgical conditions – preoperative autologous blood donation, acute normovolaemic haemodilution, intra- or postoperative cell salvage.

7. **Red cell substitutes**
   — Perfluorocarbon emulsions and haemoglobin-based oxygen carriers.
   — These products do not have the same ability to bind to oxygen as haemoglobin and have reported side-effects such as anaphylaxis (in PFC) and hypertension (in haemoglobin solutions).

MASSIVE BLOOD TRANSFUSION

Many definitions for massive blood transfusion have been proposed. It is often referred to as allogeneic transfusion in any of these situations.

— Replacement of more than 1 blood volume in 24 hours.
— Transfusion of more than 6 units of blood in 24 hours.
— Transfusion of more than 50% of blood volume in 1 hour.

Massive blood transfusion is associated with a myriad of complications.

1. **Hypothermia**

   This occurs frequently in massive transfusion when there is inadequate time for warming the blood and blood products. If severe, it can result in cardiac arrhythmias, impaired coagulation and prolonged action of anaesthetic drugs.

2. **Fluid overload**

   This occurs in overzealous resuscitation or when blood loss estimation is difficult, particularly in paediatric patients, the elderly and those with poor left ventricular compliance.

3. **Coagulopathy**

   There is significant loss and dilution of platelets and clotting factors, particularly factors V and VIII. DIC usually develops when 1.5–2 times the blood volume have been replaced. It is characterized by widespread activation of coagulation that results in microcirculatory thrombosis, and consumption of coagulation factors and platelets that results in bleeding. Clinically it presents as oozing from multiple areas including wounds and venepuncture sites. Replacement with cryoprecipitate, platelets and FFP is indicated (see Chapter 23).

4. **Hypocalcaemia**

   Citrate toxicity occurs with massive transfusion and presents with features of hypocalcaemia as citrate binds to calcium. Besides being an essential co-factor in the coagulation pathway, calcium is also required to maintain myocardial contractility and conduction of electrical impulses. There is little evidence on the optimal time and dose of calcium; most sources suggest 10 ml of 10% calcium chloride after transfusion of a single blood volume.

5. **Potassium**

   Hyperkalaemia occurs transiently following transfusion of stored blood rich in potassium. Hypokalaemia ensues when potassium re-enters red cells after being warmed to body temperature.

6. **Acid-base imbalance**

   Metabolic acidosis may occur as a result of the clinical condition that warrants resuscitation (hypovolaemic shock, poor perfusion states) rather than the blood *per se*. Routine administration of sodium bicarbonate is not recommended since excessive bicarbonate therapy may worsen the situation by causing fluid overload, alkalosis and intracellular acidosis. Sodium bicarbonate may be given if profound metabolic acidosis is suspected or documented on ABG analysis.

7. **Blood incompatibility**

   Signs of major incompatibility reactions are often masked in the anaesthetized patient. Increased blood oozing from surgical and venepuncture sites may offer a clue. If left undetected, profound shock and even cardiac arrest may result.

8. **Transfusion-related acute lung injury (TRALI)**

   TRALI is defined as a non-cardiogenic pulmonary oedema temporally related to transfusion therapy. The pathophysiology of TRALI remains uncertain; antibodies to neutrophils and biologically active lipids may cause the lung injury. It is characterized by chills, fever, cough, dyspnoea and hypotension. The chest X-ray is characterized by widespread pulmonary infiltrates. Treatment is mainly supportive. Differential diagnoses include trauma, aspiration, sepsis, volume overload and cardiogenic pulmonary oedema.

9. **Transmission of infectious diseases**

   The risk of disease transmission is increased several-fold due to the increased quantity of blood products transfused. These include human immunodeficiency virus (HIV), hepatitis C virus, hepatitis B virus, parasites and bacteria.

SOME PRACTICAL POINTERS

— Be prepared for volume resuscitation by securing venous access with large bore cannulae. These are easier to locate when the patient is haemodynamically stable rather than in the shocked, vasoconstricted state. Even though central venous access by means of triple lumen catheter is useful for CVP monitoring, the catheter lumens are not large enough for rapid transfusion.

— Rapid transfusion devices with counter-current heating mechanism, allowing transfusion of up to 600 ml/min at body temperature, should be utilized when massive blood loss and transfusion are anticipated. The blood-giving set containing a standard 170-μm filter should be primed with normal saline before blood transfusion. Microfilters slow down the flow rate and are not suitable for rapid transfusion.

— For every ml of blood loss, 3 ml of crystalloid or 1–1.5 ml of colloid solution should be infused. By virtue of their longer intravascular half-lives, colloid solutions are more efficient volume expanders but are more costly and have a small risk of allergic reactions. Remember that volume replacement is just as important as red cell replacement, and the central circulating blood volume should be maintained to ensure optimal filling of the heart.

— The use of autologous blood transfusion should be advocated whenever possible.

— Group-specific blood can be matched in 5–10 min at the Blood Bank and is preferred over Rhesus-negative Group O unmatched blood even in emergency situations. The logistics of transport should be arranged and every effort should be made to shorten transit time.

— All blood products to be administered should be checked against the patient's name, identity and hospital registration number. The blood product number, blood group and expiry date should also be checked and confirmed. This verification should be documented.

— Whenever possible, blood should be warmed to body temperature prior to transfusion. This may not always be feasible especially in emergency situations of massive blood loss. Avoid overheating the blood, which can result in haemolysis.

— If the situation permits, blood should be transfused one unit at a time, followed by an assessment of benefit and need for further transfusion. Again this may not be feasible during massive blood transfusion. When a range of blood products must be given in quick succession, transfuse cryoprecipitate first, followed by platelets and then FFP.

— The on-going surgical blood loss and the patient's haemodynamic status should be closely monitored to gauge the adequacy of blood transfusion and volume resuscitation. Haematocrit, electrolytes, ABG and coagulation screen should be checked from time to time and abnormalities corrected if present.

— A high index of suspicion for transfusion reaction is needed since the clinical features are masked in anaesthetized patients. Suggestive signs include hypotension, tachycardia, urticaria, bronchospasm, oozing at the surgical and venepuncture sites, haemolysis, or haemoglobinuria. If this is suspected, stop the transfusion and alert the Blood Bank. Send the patient's blood sample and all the blood packs for analysis, and give supportive treatment as indicated.

APPENDIX

MAXIMUM SURGICAL BLOOD ORDER SCHEDULE (MSBOS) FOR ELECTIVE SURGERY

The MSBOS is a guideline for surgical procedures to eliminate unnecessary cross-matching and to increase the efficiency of blood usage. For many surgical procedures a transfusion is unlikely and group and antibody screen (G&S) is adequate. If unexpected bleeding occurs and the antibody screen is negative, cross-matched blood will be available from the Blood Bank in 10 minutes compared to 45 minutes if G&S has not been performed.

This list indicates the type of surgery and the units of blood or G&S recommended.

1. **General surgery**

abdomino-perineal resection	4
cholecystectomy	G&S
gastrectomy	2
hemicolectomy	G&S
small bowel resection	G&S
mastectomy	G&S
oesophagectomy	4
pancreatectomy	4
portocaval shunt	4
splenectomy	2
hepatectomy	5
thyroidectomy	G&S
parathyroidectomy	G&S
varicose veins	G&S
vagotomy	G&S
Whipple's procedure	4
hiatus hernia repair	
— abdominal	G&S
— transthoracic	2
inguinal hernia repair	G&S
laparotomy	G&S
— perforated viscus	2

2. **Cardiothoracic**

aortic valve replacement	3
coronary artery bypass graft	3
mitral valve replacement	3
cardiac surgery & weight < 50 kg	5
cardiac transplantation	5
re-do cardiac surgery	5
bronchoscopy & mediastinotomy	G&S
thoracotomy	2
open lung biopsy	G&S

3. **Vascular**

elective aortic surgery	2
bypass grafts	
— aorto-femoral	G&S
— femoro-popliteal	G&S
endarterectomy	
— carotid, femoral	G&S
sympathectomy	
— lumbar	3
— cervical	G&S
amputation	Individualized

4. **Plastic**

burns, grafts, debridement	Individualized

5. **Gynaecology**

hysterectomy	
— abdominal, vaginal	G&S
— Wertheim	2
myomectomy	2
ovarian cystectomy	G&S
termination, D&C	G&S
vaginal repair	G&S
vulvetomy	2

6. **Neurosurgery**

Craniotomy, cerebral aneurysam	2	laminectomy, spincal fusion	2

7. **Urology**

cystectomy	4	— complicated or large calculus	2
nephrectomy	G&S	renal transplant	G&S
percutaneous nephrolithotomy	G&S	retropubic prostatectomy	2
pyelolithotomy		TURP	G&S
— simple	G&S	ureterolithotomy	G&S

8. **ENT**

cancer of jaw or neck	6	tonsillectomy and adenoidectomy	G&S
laryngectomy	2		
mandibulectomy	4		

9. **Orthopaedic**

femoral osteotomy	2	Putti-Platt shoulder repair	G&S
fractured humerus	G&S	total hip replacement	3
fractured neck of femur	G&S	total knee replacement	2
laminectomy, spinal fusion	2	total shoulder replacement	G&S
Harrington rods	4		

10. **Miscellaneous**

cardiac catheterization	G&S	liver, renal biopsy	G&S
coronary angiogram	G&S	pacemaker insertion	G&S

FURTHER READING

1. Spahn DR. Strategies for transfusion therapy. Best Prac Res Clin Anaesthesiol 2004;18:661–73.
2. Chen AY, Carson JL. Perioperative management of anaemia. Br J Anaesth 1998;81:20–4.
3. Goldhill D, Boralessa H, Boralessa H. Anaemia and red cell transfusion in the critically ill (Editorial). Anaesthesia 2002;57:527–9.

4. Waschke KF, Frietsch T. Modified hemoglobins and perfluorocarbons. Curr Opin Anaesthesiol 1999;12:195–202.
5. Spahn DR, Casutt M. Eliminating blood transfusions: New aspects and perspectives. Anesthesiology 2000;93:242–55.
6. Porte RJ, Leebeck FW. Pharmacological strategies to decrease transfusion requirements in patients undergoing surgery. Drugs 2002;62:2193–211.
7. Looney MR, Gropper MA, Matthay MA. Transfusion-related lung injury: A review. Chest 2004;126:249–58.
8. Hardy JF, de Moerloose P, Samama M. Massive transfusion and coagulopathy: Pathophysiology and implications for clinical management. Can J Anesth 2004;51:293–310.

Chapter

Perioperative Temperature Control

- **Introduction**
- **Consequences of Inadvertent Perioperative Hypothermia**
- **Temperature Monitoring**
- **Thermal Management**
- **Therapeutic Hypothermia**
- **Further Reading**

INTRODUCTION

In an awake individual, the thermoregulatory centre usually maintains the core body temperature to within 0.2–0.4°C of normal (about 37°C). However, central thermoregulatory control is impaired during anaesthesia, redistribution of body heat occurs, and hypothermia commonly ensues. This is particularly so in long surgical procedures involving extensive areas exposed to cold ambient OT temperature. On the other hand, the patient's body temperature may rise precipitously in conditions such as malignant hyperthermia and thyrotoxic crisis.

Selected patients with specific clinical conditions may benefit from induced or therapeutic hypothermia. Moderate hypothermia between 32–34°C may be associated with improved outcome postcardiac arrest and may confer protection against cerebral ischaemia and myocardial infarct. Patients undergoing cardiac surgery frequently require cardiopulmonary bypass or full circulatory arrest under hypothermia.

Temperature monitoring is therefore an essential part of monitoring for at-risk patients presenting for anaesthesia and surgery. Attempts must be made to maintain body temperature within the normal range, or, in the case of induced hypothermia, ensure that the patient's temperature returns to normal during rewarming.

CONSEQUENCES OF INADVERTENT PERIOPERATIVE HYPOTHERMIA

The problems of inadvertent perioperative hypothermia are summarized here.

— Cardiac morbidity
  - Cold-induced sympatho-adrenal activation causes haemodynamic stresses, which result in increased cardiac workload; this may predispose to myocardial ischaemia in compromised individuals.
  - There is an increased incidence of cardiac arrhythmias, with initial sinus tachycardia followed by bradycardia, and ventricular arrhythmias.
  - Systemic vascular resistance is increased as a result of peripheral vasoconstriction.

— Coagulopathy
  - Increased surgical bleeding may occur secondary to impaired platelet and clotting factor function.
  - Fibrinolysis remains normal during mild hypothermia.

— Wound complications
  - Immune function may be impaired by suppression of inflammatory response.
  - Tissue hypoperfusion may occur secondary to hypothermia-induced vasoconstriction.
  - These changes predispose to delayed wound healing and wound infection; they may contribute to wound dehiscence or anastomotic breakdown.

— Pharmacokinetics and pharmacodynamics
  - Hypothermia results in delayed drug metabolism and clearance, with prolonged effect and slow recovery from anaesthetic agents and neuromuscular blocking drugs.
  - Enhanced drug effects are shown by reduced minimal alveolar concentration (MAC) of volatile anaesthetics.

- Postoperative shivering
  - This results in patient discomfort, increased oxygen consumption and metabolic demand, disruption of skin grafts or surgical wounds.
  - Hypothermia is the commonest, but not the only, cause for postoperative shivering. It may also be associated with the use of volatile anaesthetic (especially halothane), epidural anaesthesia, sepsis, drug allergy and transfusion reactions.
- Venous stasis
  - It is plausible thsat vasoconstriction may promote deep vein thrombosis (DVT) by producing venous stasis; however this hypothesis awaits confirmation by clinical trials.

TEMPERATURE MONITORING

Core temperature usually decreases by 1°C in the first 30 minutes following induction of anaesthesia as a result of anaesthetic-induced vasodilatation. Devices for intraoperative temperature monitoring should be made available to all patients but are of particular importance in these situations.

- Patient groups
  - Extremes of age group.
  - Preoperative fever or hypothermia.
  - Patients with burns.
  - Risk of malignant hyperthermia or thyrotoxic crisis.
- Surgery
  - Long surgical procedure with major fluid shifts and large exposed body areas.
  - Procedures requiring cardiopulmonary bypass.
  - Surgical procedures carried out under induced hypothermia.

Temperature Monitoring Sites

The body is arbitrarily divided into a core thermal compartment and a peripheral thermal compartment. The core thermal compartment is composed of highly perfused tissues in which the temperature is uniform and high compared to the rest of the body. Core temperature can be measured in the pulmonary artery, nasopharynx, tympanic membrane and the distal oesophagus. Sites outside the core thermal compartment include the skin, axilla, bladder and rectum.

— Nasopharynx
  - The probe is positioned behind the soft palate and depth of insertion is approximately the distance between tragus of ear and angle of mouth.
  - This is less accurate than oesophageal temperature.

— Tympanic membrane
  - This is an almost ideal temperature monitoring site because it is likely to accurately reflect brain temperature as a result of its close proximity.
  - Temperature is monitored by means of an infrared thermometer or a disposable aural probe with thermocouple at its tip.

— Oesophagus
  - Temperature at the distal quarter of the oesophagus approximates blood and cerebral temperature provided that the chest is not open.

— Pulmonary artery
  - This provides accurate measurement of core temperature via thermistor incorporated at the tip of the pulmonary artery catheter.
  - It is of limited practical application because of its invasiveness and cost.

— Rectum
  - This is reasonably accurate under steady-state conditions, but is unsuitable for rapidly changing temperatures (e.g., rewarming after cardiopulmonary bypass) because of its slow response.

— Bladder
  - This is reasonably accurate provided urine flow is high; lags behind actual core temperature when urine flow is low.

— Skin and axilla
  - This is most unreliable and gives no information other than the temperature of the area of skin the probe is in contact with.
  - The arm must be kept adducted for temperature monitoring at the axilla.

THERMAL MANAGEMENT

Thermoregulatory defence mechanisms are impaired during anaesthesia. Heat loss occurs by means of radiation, conduction, convection and evaporation from exposed tissue at surgical sites. Efforts should be made to maintain core temperature above 36°C unless hypothermia is specifically indicated. The OT temperature is often increased to 24°C for neonates and small infants and 22°C for older children. This is effective in reducing heat loss but is limited by discomfort to OT personnel when ambient temperature exceeds 23°C.

Various methods for maintaining perioperative normothermia are described here.

1. **Cutaneous warming**
   - This may be achieved by active warming or passive insulation.
     - Active warming by means of forced-air warming (the most effective, commonly available and non-invasive warming method) or circulating-water mattress.
     - Passive insulation by means of blankets, wrapping extremities with cotton wool and covering the head with a cap (for babies and small children).
   - Additional measures for neonates and small children include:
     - Use of incubator during transport and at PACU.
     - Use of overhead radiant heater during anaesthetic induction and emergence.

2. **Fluid warming**
   - Heat loss becomes significant when large amounts of intravenous fluids or blood are administered; these should be warmed to body temperature before transfusion.
   - Special rapid infusion systems incorporated with heaters should be used in major surgery where massive fluid and blood losses are anticipated.
   - Warm abdominal packs and irrigation fluids should be used during surgery.

3. **Heating and humidification of airway gases**
   - This has minimal impact in maintaining normothermia since less than 10% of metabolic heat production is lost via the respiratory tract.
   - This method is more effective in paediatric patients than in adults.
   - Methods include use of heat and moisture exchangers, and paediatric humidifier circuit to warm and humidify the anaesthetic gases.
   - Low-flow anaesthesia with circle breathing system contributes to preservation of heat and humidity especially in long surgical procedures.

— Heating and humidification also prevent drying of respiratory tract mucosa, maintain normal ciliary function and reduce likelihood of bronchospasm.

4. **Prewarming and postoperative warming**
   — Actively warming patients before induction of anaesthesia helps to reduce likelihood of hypothermia under anaesthesia.
   — Aim to prevent hypothermia or restore normothermia before emergence from anaesthesia.
   — Prevent and treat shivering if it occurs.

THERAPEUTIC HYPOTHERMIA

Controlled therapeutic hypothermia may be useful in certain surgical procedures to decrease tissue oxygen requirement and protect against myocardial or cerebral ischaemia. These are mainly in the realm of cardiac surgery and neurosurgery, for example, clipping of cerebral aneurysm, carotid endarterectomy and cardiac procedures under cardiopulmonary bypass. Other non-surgical clinical situations that may benefit from therapeutic hypothermia include cardiopulmonary resuscitation, myocardial infarction, traumatic brain injury and stroke.

Hypothermia is induced by surface cooling and/or infusion of cold intravenous fluids to a target temperature of 32–34°C. In patients with raised intracranial pressure, it is advocated that return to normothermia should be attempted only when ICP has been below 20 mmHg for at least 24 hours.

FURTHER READING

1. Lenhardt R. Monitoring and thermal management. Best Prac Res Clin Anaesthesiol 2003;17:569–81.
2. Leslie K, Sessler DI. Perioperative hypothermia in the high-risk surgical patient. Best Prac Res Clin Anaesthesiol 2003;17:485–98.
3. De Witte J, Sessler DI. Perioperative shivering: Physiology and pharmacology. Anesthesiology 2002;96:467–84.
4. Sessler DI. Complications and treatment of mild hypothermia. Anesthesiology 2001;95:531–43.

5. Sessler DI. Perioperative heat balance. Anesthesiology 2000;92:578–96.
6. Kabon B, Bacher A, Spiss CK. Therapeutic hypothermia. Best Prac Res Clin Anaesthesiol 2003;17:551–68.
7. Hachimi-Idrissi S, Huyghens L. Resuscitative mild hypothermia as a protective tool in brain damage: Is there evidence? Eu J Emerg Med 2004;11:335–42.

Chapter

Checking the Anaesthetic Equipment

INTRODUCTION

Since failure of anaesthetic equipment is one of the known and preventable causes of anaesthetic mishap, it is imperative that the anaesthesiologist checks anaesthetic equipment as a matter of routine before commencement of each case, be it under general or regional anaesthesia. This is akin to the routine check performed by a pilot before take-off. In addition, the anaesthetic machine must be serviced by a skilled technician at regular and specified intervals, and the service record should be prominently displayed at each anaesthetic machine.

Modern-day anaesthetic machines are often incorporated with self-check and self-calibration; the anaesthesiologist merely follows instructions on the display screen to complete the checklist. However, this should not detract the anaesthesiologist from learning how to perform checks on an anaesthetic machine which is not equipped with such features.

The anaesthesiologist should be familiar with the checking sequence so that the procedure can be carried out smoothly and systematically. Equipment in the checklist should include the anaesthetic machine, breathing system, scavenging system, all apparatus required in airway management, suction device, monitoring devices and other adjuncts.

There are three different levels of checks on the anaesthetic machine. Level one check is a detailed check performed by the service personnel and is required on a new anaesthetic machine before it is commissioned for use. Level two check is a thorough check performed at the start of each anaesthesia session while level three check refers to a quick abbreviated check immediately before commencement of each anaesthetic. Always remember to check the anaesthetic equipment (among other things) if something untoward happens during the course of anaesthesia.

CHECKS BEFORE COMMENCEMENT OF ANAESTHESIA SESSION

1. Anaesthetic Machine

A. Gas supply

— Wall supply

- Check that the piped gas supplies are at the specified pressures and that the bulk gas warning lights are not activated.
- The oxygen, air and nitrous oxide hoses are labelled, colour coded and fitted with specific connectors at the wall outlets. Check that the hoses from the wall outlets are correctly connected to the respective inlets on the machine. Use a multi-gas analyzer to check gas composition at the common gas outlet, inspiratory limb or the Y-piece.

— Cylinders

- Open and close each cylinder valve in turn, observe the respective cylinder pressure gauge. Replace oxygen cylinders which are less than quarter full.
- A falling pressure on the pressure gauge indicates a high pressure leak which needs to be rectified.
- Reopen each cylinder valve in turn and then, with the piped gas supply hose disconnected, turn on the appropriate flowmeter to check that gas is able to pass from the cylinder through the flowmeter.
- Make sure the cylinders are turned off after checking.

— Oxygen failure warning device
  - With nitrous oxide and oxygen flowing at 2 L/min, disconnect oxygen supply and depress the oxygen bypass button to release oxygen from the machine.
  - The audible alarm should be activated. For an anaesthetic machine fitted with a device to cut off the flow of nitrous oxide, this should do so within 10 seconds.
  - The alarm should stop when oxygen supply is restored.

— One gas test
  - This is carried out to eliminate the possibility of crossed pressure hoses.
  - Check that the oxygen analyzer is correctly calibrated and that the low oxygen alarm is working.
  - With the oxygen supply "on", disconnect all other gas sources.
  - After other gases have been bled from the machine, open all flowmeter controls and check that only oxygen flows as detected by the oxygen analyzer.
  - Connect the high pressure gas hose for nitrous oxide from the anaesthetic machine to the correct wall outlet. Restore nitrous oxide flow to the machine and check that nitrous oxide flows in the correct flowmeter.
  - If the machine is fitted with air flowmeter, check oxygen analyzer. With air flowing at 6 L/min, it should show 21%.

B. Flowmeters

— Ensure that each flowmeter bobbin rotates freely within the column and does not stick to the sides of the column.

— Turn off each flowmeter control and see that the bobbin is at zero position when no gas flows (there may be a minimum oxygen flow of approximately 0.25 L/min in some machines).

— In a machine fitted with antihypoxic device, check that as the nitrous oxide flow is increased the oxygen flow is automatically increased to maintain the ratio of nitrous oxide to oxygen at 3:1.

— Turn off all flowmeter controls after checking.

C. Vaporizer

— Check that the vaporizer is seated correctly and locked securely in place.

- Ensure that sufficient volatile anaesthetic is present and that the filling and emptying ports are closed.
- Check that the vaporizer can be turned on and off easily. Make sure that it is turned off.
- Ensure that power is available for electrically operated vaporizers.

D. Precircuit leaks

- Turn on the oxygen flowmeter to 2 L/min and occlude the common gas outlet for 10 seconds. The oxygen bobbin should dip when back pressure is built up. If the rotameter bobbin does not fall, take steps to detect sites of leakage.
- Test with each vaporizer turned on and off in turn.
- More precise testing for leaks should be performed if gas flows of less than 1 L/min are to be used in low-flow anaesthesia (see Chapter 56).

2. Breathing System

- Check that the gas supply is connected to the selected breathing system.
- Check that the size of the tube used to make this connection is adequate to cope with anticipated gas flows, and that the length of the tubing is adequate for the particular surgical procedure. This is important when the head end of the patient is away from the anaesthetic machine, e.g., in head and neck surgery.

A. Circle system

- Check by visual inspection that the system is correctly assembled and firmly connected. Observe the colour of the carbon dioxide absorbent and replace if necessary.
- Check valve function and leaks in the breathing system.
  - Close the adjustable pressure limiting (APL) valve and attach a reservoir bag on the patient limb of the Y-piece.
  - Depress the oxygen bypass button to fill the reservoir bags.
  - Alternately squeeze the two bags to ensure that oxygen passes freely from one bag to another, checking visually that each unidirectional valve functions correctly.

- Squeeze both bags and maintain pressure at 30 cmH_2O for 5 seconds. The bags should remain distended and no audible hiss should be noted.
- Open the APL valve and check that gas spills easily to atmosphere when both the reservoir bags are squeezed.

— If a spare reservoir bag is not available, check for leaks by closing the expiratory valve, occluding the patient end and depressing the oxygen bypass button to pressurize the circuit. Maintain the pressure at 30 cmH_2O for 5 seconds. The reservoir bag should remain distended and no audible hiss should be heard.

— A more thorough test for leaks should be carried out if low-flow anaesthesia is employed (see Chapter 56).

B. Bain circuit

— Visual inspection for cracks, kinks, discontinuity or absence of the inner tube.

— Close the expiratory valve and turn on oxygen flow at 2 L/min. The bobbin should dip when the inner tube is occluded.

— Pethick test

- Turn off oxygen flow and keep the expiratory valve closed. Occlude the patient end and pressurize the circuit by depressing the oxygen bypass button. The reservoir bag should remain distended.
- Continue depressing the oxygen bypass button while releasing the patient end. As oxygen flows out through the inner tube, a low pressure area is created in its vicinity, based on the Venturi effect. Oxygen is drawn out from the reservoir bag via the outer tube to this low pressure area and the reservoir bag is seen to collapse.

3. Scavenging System

— Ensure that the scavenging system is correctly assembled and connected to the selected breathing system and ventilator outlet.

— Check that all components of the system are unencumbered to allow free gas flow.

— If negative pressure is used to aid scavenging, check that this does not empty the breathing system.

4. Other Apparatus

- "MALES": Masks, Airways, Laryngoscopes, Endotracheal tubes, Suction devices.
- Ventilator and alarms (especially the disconnection and high pressure alarms) should be checked according to manufacturer's recommendations.
- Emergency ventilation system (e.g., self-inflating bag) as an alternative means of providing oxygen and controlled ventilation.
- Monitoring equipment.
- Miscellaneous equipment: warming devices, breathing system humidifiers and filters, infusion devices.

CHECKS IN BETWEEN CASES

A quick check should be made on the following:

- *Gas Supply:* Check the pressure gauges for the main supply; or pressure gauges for the cylinders if these have been in use. Replace the cylinders if necessary.
- *Flowmeter:* Make sure that the bobbins move freely within the flowmeter columns. Turn the flowmeter off after checking.
- *Vaporizer:* Check the level of liquid agent in the vaporizer and refill if necessary.
- *Breathing System:* Check for disconnection, misconnection, leaks in the system and colour of carbon dioxide absorbent for exhaustion.
- *Other Apparatus:* Prepare the appropriate-sized mask, airway, laryngoscope and endotracheal tube for the next patient. Check that the suction device is functioning and that the suction catheter/rigid sucker have been changed.

FURTHER READING

1. Protocol for checking the anaesthetic machine. ANZCA Professional Document PS31 (2003).
2. Crosby WM. Checking the anaesthetic machine, drugs and monitoring devices. Anaesth Intens Care 1988;16:32–5.

Chapter

Monitoring in Anaesthesia

- Introduction
- Patient Monitors
- Machine Monitors
- Summary
- Further Reading

INTRODUCTION

Monitors used during anaesthesia are established with patient safety in mind. The monitoring devices are able to do so by yielding useful information about the patient's condition and providing early warning of any physiological derangement. However, they should be used in conjunction with careful clinical observation of the patient. Anaesthetic mishaps have occurred when the clinical signs of deterioration in the patient go undetected while the anaesthesiologist becomes engrossed in rectifying a faulty monitoring equipment or gets distracted by a piece of novel monitoring gadget.

The common monitoring devices are briefly described in this chapter. The reader should be aware of their indications, uses, limitations and pitfalls. It must be remembered, however, that regardless of how complex and sophisticated the monitoring equipment may be, there can be no substitute for the "ultimate" monitor – a well-trained, vigilant anaesthesiologist.

PATIENT MONITORS

A. Electrocardiography (ECG)

The ECG should be continuously displayed throughout the anaesthetic. It is widely accepted because the ECG monitor is relatively cheap; the electrodes are non-invasive and easy to apply on the patient.

Uses

- Lead II is the most commonly used ECG lead, ideal for detection of cardiac arrhythmias and inferior ischaemia. The configurations are:
  - Negative electrode: right arm or right infraclavicular region.
  - Positive electrode: V_5 position (fifth left intercostal space at anterior axillary line).
  - Indifferent electrode: left arm or left infraclavicular region.
- Modified bipolar limb leads are used to detect antero-lateral ischaemia. The configurations for the various leads, monitored on Lead I, are as follows:
  - Positive electrode: V_5 position.
  - Indifferent electrode: anywhere, usually at left infraclavicular region.
  - Negative electrode: CM_5 lead on right sternal border at second intercostal space; CB_5 lead on right scapula posteriorly; CS_5 lead on right infraclavicular region at midclavicular line.

  The CM_5 lead is most commonly used since it detects ST-segment changes more frequently than other three-lead configurations.

Limitations

- A normal ECG pattern does not exclude awareness, hypoxia, hypercarbia or hypotension. It provides information about the electrical activity of the heart but does not indicate adequacy of oxygenation or peripheral circulation.
- Inaccuracies in the interpretation of myocardial ischaemia are further compounded by errors such as:
  - Poor contact between the skin and electrode.
  - Improper placement of electrodes.
  - Improper selection of leads.
  - Selection of monitor mode (narrower bandwidth of 0.5–30 Hz) instead of diagnostic mode (bandwidth of 0.05–100 Hz).
  - Interference from electrocautery.

- Lack of paper print-out to quantify the ST-segment changes.

Newer computerized systems with ST-segment trend analysis are able to monitor changes indicative of myocardial ischaemia, even though ECG changes are neither sensitive nor specific for this purpose.

B. Blood Pressure

Non-invasive blood pressure (NIBP) monitoring

Blood pressure monitoring is mandatory in patients undergoing anaesthesia. Most commonly an automated blood pressure monitoring device (e.g., Dinamap™) is used. A manual sphygmomanometer should also be available in the OT in case the automated blood pressure reading needs to be counterchecked.

Limitations

— It is inaccurate if an inappropriate cuff size is selected for the patient. Underreading occurs if the cuff is too large while the opposite occurs if the cuff is too small. The correct-sized cuff should have a width of about 40% of the arm circumference.

— It is inaccurate in extremes of blood pressures. Errors may range from –30% to +40%. Low mean arterial pressures are usually overestimated and high mean pressures underestimated.

— It is inaccurate in the presence of cardiac dysrhythmias such as atrial fibrillation, frequent atrial and ventricular ectopics.

— It does not provide continuous, beat-to-beat monitoring of BP.

— Nerve palsies may be produced with frequent BP measurements for prolonged periods.

Invasive or intraarterial blood pressure (IABP) monitoring

Arterial cannulation allows continuous BP monitoring. The arterial cannula is connected to a pressure transducer system and the pressure waveforms are displayed on the monitor.

Uses and indications for IABP

— Patient-related: critically ill patients or those with significant cardiac disease or hypertension.

- Surgery-related: major surgery with large volume shifts and sudden haemodynamic disturbances; long, protracted surgery.
- Anaesthetic-related: controlled hypotensive anaesthesia, use of potent vasodilator or inotrope.
- The presence of an arterial cannula facilitates blood sampling for ABG, haematocrit, biochemical studies, blood for further group and cross-matching.

Sites of arterial cannulation

1. **Radial artery**
   - The radial artery is most commonly used as it is often accessible to the anaesthesiologist during surgery.
   - As far as possible, artery on the non-dominant hand should be used for cannulation.
   - The adequacy of collateral circulation from the ulnar artery is checked by a simple bedside test called the modified Allen's test.
     - Exsanguinate the hand by asking the patient to make a fist.
     - Occlude the radial and ulnar arteries simultaneously by applying digital pressure on the arteries.
     - Ask the patient to relax the blanched hand.
     - Release pressure on the ulnar artery and check the time taken for the colour to return.

       Normal: < 5 seconds
       Equivocal: 5–10 seconds
       Insufficient collaterals: > 10 seconds
     - The modified Allen's test is easily carried out but may not be completely reliable.

2. **Dorsalis pedis artery**
   - Systolic pressure measured in the dorsalis pedis artery is 10–20% higher and diastolic pressure is 15–20% lower than those recorded in the radial artery. The mean arterial pressure is similar in both arteries.
   - Cannulation is not advisable in patients with diabetes mellitus and peripheral vascular disease.

3. **Brachial artery**
   - This is the major source of blood supply to the lower arm, and may result in limb ischaemia if it is occluded or thrombosed.

— Avoid brachial artery cannulation in anticoagulated patients who have increased risk of uncontrolled bleeding into the fascial planes around the cubital fossa. This may compress on the median nerve and result in Volkmann's ischaemic contracture.

4. **Femoral artery**
   — This artery is located at the midpoint between the pubic tubercle and anterior superior iliac spine (ASIS) between the femoral nerve laterally and femoral vein medially.
   — It is frequently palpable even in shocked, hypotensive patients.
   — The artery should be punctured below the inguinal ligament to lessen the risk of retroperitoneal haemorrhage.
   — There is an increased risk of contamination and sepsis, as such alternative sites for cannulation should be sought once the blood pressure improves.

5. **Less common cannulation sites**
   — These include the axillary, popliteal and posterior tibial arteries.

Complications in IABP monitoring

— Thrombosis, with a reported incidence of 15–20% but is usually not clinically significant.
— Distal embolization of thrombus, air or catheter tip.
— Bruising, haematoma, arteriovenous fistula or aneurysm formation at the site of puncture.
— Local or systemic sepsis.
— Accidental intraarterial injection of drugs.
— Accidental disconnection leading to exsanguination.
— Fluid overload in susceptible patients, as a result of frequent flushing of the catheter-transducer system.

C. Pulse Oximetry

Pulse oximetry utilizes the differences in light absorption spectra of oxyhaemoglobin (HbO_2) and deoxyhaemoglobin (HHb) to determine their relative proportions and hence the oxygen saturation (SpO_2). In addition to SpO_2 measurement, pulse rate can be computed from the number of plethysmographic pulsations detected per unit time in the vascular bed.

It is non-invasive, simple to use and provides continuous information about the degree of oxygen saturation and adequacy of peripheral circulation. Its use is now mandatory for all patients under anaesthesia.

Uses and indications

- Routine perioperative use
- Cases where oxygen delivery may be unreliable
  - Shared airway with the surgeon, such as ENT surgery, dental surgery.
  - Major thoracic surgery with one lung ventilation.
  - Head and neck surgery.
- Cases where clinical assessment for detection of cyanosis may not be possible
  - Dark room anaesthesia, such as anaesthesia in the radiology department, or during eye surgery.
  - Poor accessibility of the patient.
  - Patient with deeply pigmented skin.
- Patients with increased risks of hypoxia
  - Pregnancy.
  - Obesity.
  - Poor cardiorespiratory status.
  - Risk of gas, air or fat embolism.
- Miscellaneous uses
  - Checking for adequacy of circulation in reimplanted limb or digit.
  - Checking for efficacy of cardiopulmonary resuscitation.
  - Adjunct to Allen's test for checking adequacy of collateral circulation to the hand.

Limitations

- Adequate pulse volume is needed for the signal to be produced. Hence problems arise with:
  - Hypotension (systolic BP < 50 mmHg).
  - Hypothermic, vasoconstricted patients.
  - Venous congestion at the digits.
  - Peripheral vascular disease.
- Problems with dyshaemoglobinaemia and intravascular dyes.
  - Methaemoglobin (metHb): corresponds to saturation of 85%, thus underreading may occur.

- Carboxyhaemoglobin (COHb): overestimates the actual oxygen saturation.
- Methylene blue, indocyanine green: underestimates the actual oxygen saturation.
- Gross anaemia itself (Hb < 5 g/dl) may generate inadequate signal.

— Artefacts may occur with patient movement and shivering, electrocautery, ambient light.

— Both hyperoxia and histotoxic hypoxia are not detected.

— Changes in the shape and position of the oxygen dissociation curve may necessitate a change in interpretation of SpO_2 readings in relation to arterial oxygen tensions (PaO_2).

D. Capnography

Rapid analysis of carbon dioxide in the OT is achieved by infrared spectrophotometry. Two types of analyzers are available in the market: "main-stream" and "side-stream" analyzers. There are advantages as well as problems associated with both types of analyzers.

Capnography provides much more information than a quantitative measurement of end-tidal carbon dioxide ($ETCO_2$). Changes in the shape of the waveform, the inspired and $ETCO_2$ values, and the trend of $ETCO_2$ over a period of time are all important indicators. Its routine use during anaesthesia is strongly recommended.

Uses and indications

— **As a respiratory monitor**

- Hypoventilation gives rise to high $ETCO_2$ level, but may result in low $ETCO_2$ level if impaired CO_2 excretion occurs secondary to poor respiratory efforts.
- Hyperventilation gives rise to low $ETCO_2$ level.
- Presence of $ETCO_2$ tracing is the most accurate confirmation of endotracheal intubation.
- Other endotracheal tube problems may be detected, such as oesophageal or endobronchial intubation, kinking or obstruction of endotracheal tube, accidental disconnection or extubation.
- "Curare cleft" indicates wearing off of neuromuscular blockade.

— **As a cardiovascular monitor**

- Presence of $ETCO_2$ tracing indicates adequate pulmonary perfusion required for CO_2 excretion.

- Exponential decrease in $ETCO_2$ is seen in cardiac arrest and significant pulmonary embolism (air, thrombus, gas, particulate or amniotic fluid).
- Adequacy of cardiopulmonary resuscitation can be assessed by checking the capnograph tracing.

— **As a metabolic monitor**

- Rapid increase in $ETCO_2$ is one of the earliest signs of malignant hyperthermia (MH).
- Transient increase may be observed after administration of intravenous sodium bicarbonate, or after release of vascular clamps or limb tourniquets.
- Reduction in $ETCO_2$ level occurs during hypothermia or low metabolic states.

— **As an equipment monitor**

- Increase in inspired CO_2 level occurs in rebreathing, which may be secondary to problems with unidirectional valves in circle system, exhaustion of carbon dioxide absorbent or inadequate fresh gas flows.
- Sudden drop in $ETCO_2$ can be seen in breathing circuit disconnection.

Problems

These are mainly related to the different types of analyzers.

— Side-stream analyzers

- Lag-time between true airway CO_2 concentration and detection by the system.
- Blockage of sampling tube by water or secretions.
- Scavenging is needed for exhaust gases.
- High sampling flow rate may not be suitable for neonates and small children.
- Exhaust gases need to be returned to the breathing system in low-flow anaesthesia.

— Main-stream analyzers

- Bulky, heavy sensors located at the patient's end increase risk of accidental extubation.
- Sensors are prone to be damaged by trauma or abuse.
- The presence of dead space in sensors may be significant in small children.

E. Neuromuscular Blockade

Muscle paralysis by means of neuromuscular blockade is widely practised as part of the balanced anaesthetic technique. Compared to older drugs, the newer neuromuscular blocking drugs are less cumulative and easier to reverse, so most patients recover from neuromuscular blockade without problems. However there remains a group of patients who require special attention when neuromuscular blockade is instituted.

Uses and indications

Monitoring of neuromuscular blockade should ideally be carried out whenever a neuromuscular blocking drug is administered during anaesthesia. While this may be impractical and indeed unnecessary in a healthy patient undergoing short- or medium-length procedures, this form of monitoring is particularly useful in these situations.

— Assurance that adequate muscle relaxation is achieved prior to airway instrumentation, particularly important in patients with reactive airway disease, cardiovascular disease, intracranial or intraocular pathology.

— Surgery in which maintenance of adequate neuromuscular blockade is paramount: ophthalmic surgery, neurosurgery, laser surgery or any surgery under the microscope.

— Prolonged surgical procedure with neuromuscular blockade, to prevent overdosage arising from cumulative effects of neuromuscular blocking drugs.

— Patients whose response to neuromuscular blockade may be unpredictable or prolonged, such as those with neuromuscular disease, severe hepatic or renal disease.

— Patients in whom residual paralysis is highly undesirable: morbid obesity, severe cardiac or respiratory disease, the very young and the very old.

— Assessment of recovery of neuromuscular function to facilitate reversal at the end of surgery.

— Differential diagnosis of postoperative apnoea or hypoventilation, to exclude possibility of residual curarization.

— Differentiation between depolarizing block and non-depolarizing block; diagnosis of dual block.

Many peripheral nerve stimulators (e.g., TOF-Guard™) come with programmable stimulation patterns. Many of them are also equipped with low current outputs (less than 3 milliamperes) meant for precise localization of the nerve(s) during nerve or plexus blocks in regional anaesthesia.

Types of stimulation pattern

1. **Single twitch**
   - This consists of single stimuli at 1-second intervals, i.e., 1 cycle/second or 1 hertz (Hz).
   - It can be tolerated by conscious patients and is used to determine stimulation threshold and supramaximal stimulus.
   - It is the least sensitive method in demonstrating a partial neuromuscular blockade.

2. **Tetany**
   - This is a sustained stimulus at 50 or 100 Hz for 5 seconds.
   - It is painful and should not be used on conscious patients.
   - It is used in combination with single twitch in an anaesthetized patient to elicit posttetanic count.

3. **Train of four (TOF)**
   - This consists of four successive supramaximal stimuli at 0.5-second intervals.
   - A progressive decrease in twitch height ("fade") is seen with non-depolarizing block; this is absent in depolarizing block.
   - *TOF ratio* (T_4/T_1) is the ratio between heights of the fourth response to the first response. Subjective tactile evaluation of the TOF ratio is inaccurate as it is difficult to detect the presence of fade once the TOF ratio exceeds 0.4. Many newer generations of nerve stimulators (e.g., TOF-Guard™) provide objective measurement of the TOF ratio using acceleromyography together with a piezoelectric transducer.
   - *TOF count* is the number of responses to the four stimuli, in which
     - 3 TOF counts = 75% block
     - 2 TOF counts = 80% block
     - 1 TOF count = 90% block
     - no TOF count = > 95% block

- Clinical relaxation usually requires 75–95% neuromuscular blockade.
- TOF count should return to 4 before reversal of neuromuscular blockade is attempted.

4. **Posttetanic count (PTC)**
   - PTC makes use of the phenomenon of posttetanic facilitation in non-depolarizing block and is used to assess the degree of neuromuscular blockade at a deeper plane during maintenance of anaesthesia.
   - Stimulus pattern consists of 50-Hz tetanic stimulation for 5 seconds, pause for 3 seconds, followed by single twitch at 1 Hz.
   - The number of PTCs desired depends on the type of surgery and the degree of neuromuscular blockade required.
     - Peripheral surgery: 8–10
     - Abdominal surgery: 4–6
     - Profound relaxation: 2–4
   - Time to return of TOF is inversely related to the PTC: the more the PTCs, the shorter time it takes for TOF to return.

5. **Double burst stimulation (DBS)**
   - DBS is more sensitive than TOF in the clinical evaluation of fade by visual and tactile means.
   - Two main stimulus patterns are designed.
     - $DBS_{3,3}$: three high-frequency, short-lasting bursts at 50 Hz; pause for 750 milliseconds then three more stimuli at 50 Hz.
     - $DBS_{3,2}$: similar to $DBS_{3,3}$ except that the second set of stimuli consists of two bursts instead of three.

Practical guidelines

- The ulnar nerve is most commonly used. Stimulation of the ulnar nerve causes contraction of adductor pollicis seen as adduction of the thumb. Movement of the fingers should be disregarded as this may be due to direct muscle stimulation. Alternative sites of stimulation include the posterior tibial nerve applied behind the medial malleolus (flexor hallucis brevis giving rise to plantarflexion of the foot) and the ocular branch of facial nerve (orbicularis oculi giving rise to twitching of the eyelid).

- Attach electrodes to the ulnar aspect of the wrist in the conscious patient. There must be good contact between the skin and electrodes. Check the proximal and distal connections of the cables to make sure that the polarity is correct.
- Explain to the patient that he/she will experience a mild tingling sensation in the hand. Put on *single twitch*. Increase the current strength until adduction of the thumb is just perceived. This is the *initial threshold for stimulation (ITS). Supramaximal stimulus* is 2.75 times the stimulation threshold. In some monitors the default current strength is set at 40 milliamperes (mA).
- Induction of anaesthesia is carried out in the usual manner. Check *TOF count* at supramaximal current strength when the patient loses consciousness. Programme the TOF to repeat at 12-second intervals. When TOF disappears, neuromuscular blockade is sufficiently profound for tracheal intubation to be carried out.
- Maintain neuromuscular blockade by means of continuous infusion or intermittent bolus doses of neuromuscular blocking drug. Check TOF count. If TOF is not elicited, check *PTC*.
- At the end of the surgery, check TOF count. The TOF count should return to 4 before reversal of neuromuscular blockade is attempted. The presence of fade is better appreciated by using *DBS*.
- If adequacy of reversal is in doubt in the PACU, recheck the *TOF count* and *DBS*. All four TOF counts should be present and there should be no visible fade on DBS. Administer half an initial dose of reversal agent if necessary and reassess.

Limitations

- Useful information is derived only if the above guidelines are followed. The stimulation threshold is often not elicited before induction of anaesthesia; hence the supramaximal stimulus used may not be appropriate.
- There should be good contact between the skin and electrodes. This may not be the case if the patient is hirsute or obese.
- Nerve conduction is affected by temperature; hence the readings may not be accurate if the patient is hypothermic.
- Different muscle groups have different onset, sensitivity and recovery characteristics. For example, the onset of paralysis at adductor pollicis is slower than at the larynx or the diaphragm, but is more sensitive to neuromuscular blockade than laryngeal adductors or diaphragm. This makes it a poor choice to indicate onset of laryngeal muscle paralysis but is suitable for detection of postoperative residual block.

F. Central Venous Pressure

The central venous pressure (CVP) or right atrial pressure (RAP) estimates the right ventricular (RV) filling pressure and allows assessment of RV function. In the absence of significant cardiorespiratory disease, there is a reasonable correlation between the right and left filling pressures, and therefore the state of left ventricular function can also be inferred from CVP measurements.

Central venous cannulation can be achieved via the internal jugular, external jugular, subclavian, basilic and femoral veins. In both anaesthesia and intensive care practice, the most common route of central venous access is the internal jugular vein.

Insertion of central venous catheter (CVC) is not without complications especially if the practitioner is inexperienced and unsupervised, and in patients who are likely to be "difficult": those with short and broad necks, goitre or other tumours, the obese, those with a history of neck surgery or previous difficulty in CVC insertion. Under such circumstances, it is extremely useful to perform the CVC insertion under ultrasound guidance to accurately locate the vein. However, this technique requires some training and experience, and the ultrasound device may not be freely available in all hospitals.

Uses and indications of CVC

CVP measurement is a major indication for CVC in order to assess cardiac performance and guide fluid therapy in selected patients, particularly those with cardiovascular instability, and those undergoing major surgery with large fluid shifts and haemodynamic changes.

Other uses for CVC include:

— Rapid administration of blood and fluid (if large bore cannulae are used).
— Infusion of vasoactive drugs or irritant drugs.
— Aspiration of air in venous air embolism.
— Access for total parenteral nutrition.
— Conduit for placement of transvenous pacemaker and pulmonary artery catheter.
— Venous access in patients with poor peripheral veins.

Complications

Complications can occur during the procedure itself and become immediately evident, or they may not be apparent until a few hours later. It is therefore important that the patient should be closely monitored after the procedure. A check CXR should be reviewed to assess the correct positioning of the CVC and to rule out pneumo-, haemo- or hydrothorax. There are also late complications mainly pertaining to sepsis and thrombosis.

— Trauma during CVC insertion may result in:
  - Pneumo- or haemothorax.
  - Hydrothorax if intravenous fluid is infused.
  - Bleeding with haematoma formation, especially when an adjacent artery is inadvertently punctured.
  - Cardiac perforation with tamponade.
  - Laceration of thoracic duct with chylothorax.
  - Injury to surrounding structures, e.g., nerves.

— Air or catheter embolism.

— Improper positioning of catheter tip giving inaccurate readings.

— Sepsis.

— Venous thrombosis, thrombophlebitis.

G. Pulmonary Artery Pressures

In patients with compromised cardiac function, the RAP may not accurately reflect left atrial pressure (LAP). At times, in fact, changes of RAP and LAP are in opposite directions to each other. Therefore, it would be disastrous to base management decision on CVP reading alone.

The most widely used pulmonary artery (PA) catheter is the Swan-Ganz catheter. It consists of 4 lumens.

— Proximal port (CVP): 31 cm from the tip.

— Distal port (PAP): at the tip of the catheter.

— Inflation port for balloon, with a lock for volume-limited syringe of 1.5 ml; the balloon is immediately proximal to the tip.

— Thermistor: 3.5 cm proximal to the tip, for measurement of cardiac output by thermodilution technique.

Even though PA catheterization is best achieved via the internal jugular vein (the most direct route), the right subclavian vein may also be used. The procedure should be done under strict asepsis. The patient's ECG, blood pressure (direct intraarterial BP), oxygen saturation and pressure waveform changes during insertion of PA catheter should be closely monitored.

Uses

Information derived from PA catheterization includes:

— Pulmonary artery pressure: indicates pulmonary artery hypertension if the value is high.
— Pulmonary capillary wedge pressure: may be used to deduce left ventricular end-diastolic pressure (LVEDP) and hence left ventricular function.
— Cardiac output measurement: most commonly by means of thermodilution technique.
— Derived haemodynamic parameters from cardiac output studies: systemic and pulmonary vascular resistances, LV stroke volume and stroke index, right and left ventricular stroke work indices.
— Means to obtain mixed venous oxygen saturation: determine intrapulmonary shunt, oxygen consumption.
— Central venous pressure.

Indications

PA catheterization is useful in these clinical situations.

— To aid in differential diagnosis of low cardiac output states, where the underlying causes may be hypovolaemia or fluid overload, heart failure, pulmonary embolism or cardiac tamponade.
— To evaluate effectiveness of therapeutic intervention in terms of fluid resuscitation, vasoactive drug therapy and mechanical ventilation.
— As a form of haemodynamic monitoring for poor cardiac risk patients undergoing major vascular or cardiac surgery.

Contraindications

— Unfamiliarity with the procedure or lack of supervision.
— Inadequate monitors or equipment.
— Coagulopathy (relative contraindication).
— Abnormal cardiac anatomy (relative contraindication), such as atrial or ventricular septal defect, tricuspid or pulmonary valve disease.

Complications

Complications associated with CVC insertion may be seen with PA catheterization. These can occur during the procedure or manifest some time later.

- Complications during insertion
  - Cardiac arrhythmias.
  - Knotting or kinking of PA catheter.
  - Trauma to heart valve or chamber.
  - Thromboembolism.
- Delayed complications
  - Thrombosis.
  - Catheter embolization.
  - Pulmonary artery rupture.
  - Pulmonary infarction.
  - Sepsis at insertion site, endocarditis, septicaemia.

PA catheterization is an invasive procedure which should not be undertaken lightly. The benefits and information derived from PA catheterization should be weighed against the risks of complications mentioned above. One should be aware of these problems and complications, and the catheter should not be left in the patient for longer than is necessary.

I. Other Patient Monitors

- Temperature monitoring (see Chapter 6).
- Urine output measurement.
- Oesophageal or precordial stethoscope.
- Neurological monitoring
  - Electroencephalography (EEG).
  - Evoked potentials: somatosensory (SSEP), motor (MEP), auditory (AEP), visual (VEP).
  - Internal carotid artery stump pressure in carotid endarterectomy.
- Monitoring of "depth of anaesthesia" (see Chapter 53).
- Transoesophageal echocardiography (TEE/TOE).

MACHINE MONITORS

A. Oxygen Analyzer

This device provides continuous monitoring of the oxygen concentration in the patient's inspired gas, and gives an audible alarm if a hypoxic mixture is delivered.

It is a monitor for the gas delivered by the anaesthetic machine and breathing system.

Pulse oximeter, by measuring the patient's oxygen saturation, monitors the oxygen delivery at the tissue level. If a hypoxic mixture is delivered, pulse oximetry can only give a late warning when the patient starts to desaturate. These two monitors are, therefore, not mutually exclusive and both are essential for the safe conduct of anaesthesia.

The use of the oxygen analyzer is recommended during normal conduct of anaesthesia, and is mandatory during low-flow anaesthesia. Inspired oxygen can either be measured independently or incorporated into the multi-gas analyzer as one of the gases measured, in which case both the inspired and end-tidal oxygen concentrations can be measured and displayed simultaneously.

Besides safeguarding against delivery of hypoxic gas mixture to the patient, an unexpected increase in FiO_2 may also be detected provided that the high level alarm limit has been set. This protects against awareness during anaesthesia as well as the hazards of oxygen toxicity in susceptible individuals. The free-standing oxygen analyzer may also act as a disconnect alarm even though it is not designed specifically to detect disconnection, and is neither sensitive nor reliable for this purpose.

A free-standing oxygen analyzer should be placed in the inspiratory limb upstream to the humidifier (if in use) so that it is at an area of lowest humidity in the breathing system. It should be placed upright or tilted slightly to prevent water from accumulating in the sensor probe.

Most oxygen analyzers are incorporated on modern anaesthetic machines and are self-calibrating. If manual calibration is done, the oxygen analyzer should be calibrated on room air as well as in 100% oxygen each morning before use. Alarm limits should be set and the audible alarm should be checked to see that it is functioning.

B. Anaesthetic Concentration Monitor

An anaesthetic concentration monitor is desirable whenever inhalational anaesthetic agents are used. Its use is mandatory in low-flow anaesthesia since it is important to monitor both the inspired as well as the end-tidal anaesthetic concentrations to avoid under- or overdosage.

There are different types of anaesthetic concentration monitors in the market; many of them utilize the principle of infrared absorption similar to that for a capnometer. Automatic anaesthetic agent identification is available on newer monitors. The sensor probe is located at the patient end, and there is minimal interference from water vapour. For low-flow anaesthesia, the gases extracted through the anaesthetic concentration monitor should be returned to the breathing system.

C. Breathing System Disconnection Alarm

A disconnection alarm is a low pressure alarm which is activated when the pressure within the gas delivery and breathing systems falls below a predetermined value. It can either be incorporated into an anaesthesia ventilator or be a free-standing alarm (e.g., HAMA™ alarm) connected in the breathing system. In many studies of critical incident reporting, the disconnection alarm has been found to be sensitive and useful in detecting breathing system disconnection. It is often the first monitor to alert the anaesthesiologist that the breathing system integrity is breached. Since the disconnection alarm is an integral part of a ventilator, it should be automatically activated and should not be disarmed either temporarily or permanently.

D. Airway Pressure Monitor

The airway pressure monitor is either incorporated into the ventilator or attached to the breathing system. No audible alarm is present in the latter, hence the anaesthesiologist must be vigilant and check the pressure reading from time to time.

High airway pressure reading may be caused by these.

- — The patient coughing or gagging on the endotracheal tube.
- — Inadequate muscle relaxation and/or depth of anaesthesia.
- — Increase in airway resistance, e.g., due to bronchospasm.
- — Decreased lung or chest wall compliance.
- — Kinking or obstruction of the breathing system or endotracheal tube.

Low airway pressure may be caused by these.

- — Disconnection or significant leak in the breathing system.
- — Ventilator failure.

SUMMARY

Various types of patient and machine monitors have been highlighted in this chapter. The value of monitors in detecting untoward anaesthetic events has been well substantiated in several critical incident reports. However, before one becomes caught up with gadgets and technological advances, one must remember that such monitors are, at best, pieces of equipment that may be prone to inaccuracy and failure. Too many monitors may in fact be disadvantageous if they distract the anaesthesiologist from monitoring the clinical signs of the patient under his or her care. These monitors cannot, and should not, replace a knowledgeable and vigilant anaesthesiologist.

FURTHER READING

1. Viby-Morgensen J. Neuromuscular monitoring. Curr Opin Anaesthesiol 2001;14:655–9.
2. Torda TA. Monitoring neuromuscular transmission. Anaesth Intens Care 2002;30:123.
3. Poelaert JIL. Haemodynamic monitoring. Curr Opin Anaesthesiol 2001;14:27–32.
4. Hall AP, Russell WC. Toward safer central venous access: Ultrasound guidance and sound advice (Editorial). Anaesthesia 2004;60:1–4.
5. Sakka S, Reinhart K, Wegschneider K, Meier-Hellman A. Is the placement of a pulmonary artery catheter still justified solely for the measurement of cardiac output? J Cardiothorac Vasc Anesth 2000;14:119–24.
6. Banoub M, Tetzlaff JE, Schubert A. Pharmacologic and physiologic influences affecting sensory evoked potentials: Implications for perioperative monitoring. Anesthesiology 2003;99:716–37.

Chapter

Common Drugs in Anaesthesia

- Introduction
- Premedication
- Intravenous Induction Agents
- Inhalational Anaesthetic Agents
- Neuromuscular Blocking Drugs
- Reversal Agents
- Local Anaesthetics
- Analgesic Agents
- Inotropic and Sympathomimetic Agents
- Hypotensive Agents
- Other Cardiovascular Drugs
- Miscellaneous Drugs
- Further Reading

INTRODUCTION

Drugs commonly used in anaesthesia and resuscitation are included in this chapter. Drug dosages listed here are meant to be rough guides because the actual dose depends on the specific indication as well as clinical condition of the patient. It is always advisable to titrate the drug against response in order to avoid inadvertent overdosage. This is particularly so when we anaesthetize shocked, debilitated individuals, patients with significant medical problems (e.g., cardiovascular, neuromuscular, liver or renal disease), obese patients and those in extremes of age group.

PREMEDICATION

Drugs which are often used for premedication are benzodiazepines, phenothiazines, opioids, anticholinergics and drugs used for acid aspiration prophylaxis.

Benzodiazepines are drugs with sedative, hypnotic, anxiolytic, anticonvulsant and amnesic properties. They produce light sedation and are the mainstay of premedicant drugs since the oral route of administration is generally preferred to intramuscular injection.

— Diazepam: 0.1–0.2 mg/kg oral
— Midazolam: 0.2 mg/kg oral; adult dose 3.75–15 mg
— Temazepam: 0.5 mg/kg oral; adult dose 10–30 mg

Opioids are used for their analgesic effect and are given in combination with phenothiazines or anticholinergics which have antiemetic properties. They are particularly useful in healthy individuals with preexisting painful conditions, for example, fracture of femur.

— Pethidine: 1.0–1.5 mg/kg IM
— Morphine: 0.15–0.2 mg/kg IM
— Papaveratum: 0.2–0.3 mg/kg IM

Phenothiazines are antihistamines with sedative and antiemetic properties. They may be administered orally or intramuscularly in combination with an opioid, usually pethidine.

— Promethazine: 0.25–0.5 mg/kg IM; adult dose 12.5–25 mg
— Trimeprazine: 3–4 mg/kg oral (in syrup form)

Anticholinergics are agents prescribed predominantly for their antisialogogue effects. Three drugs – hyoscine, atropine and glycopyrrolate – are commonly used, each with its distinct pharmacological effects. Hyoscine produces sedation, amnesia and antiemesis but should be avoided in elderly patients because of its central nervous system (CNS) excitatory effects. Atropine produces tachycardia and crosses the blood-brain barrier to produce central effects. Large doses of atropine can cause central anticholinergic syndrome, characterized by ataxia, excitement, tremors, hallucinations and drowsiness. Glycopyrrolate, on the other hand, has no CNS side-effects and produces less tachycardia compared to atropine.

- Atropine: 0.02 mg/kg IM
- Hyoscine/scopolamine: 0.008 mg/kg IM
- Glycopyrrolate: 0.004–0.008 mg/kg IM

Acid aspiration prophylaxis is indicated in patients who are prone to regurgitation under anaesthesia. The H_2 receptor antagonist (e.g., ranitidine, cimetidine) or proton-pump inhibitor (e.g., omeprazole) is used in combination with an antacid to reduce gastric volume and acidity. The addition of a gastrokinetic agent (e.g., metoclopramide) shortens gastric emptying time and decreases gastric volume during anaesthetic induction and emergence.

- Ranitidine: 150 mg oral; 50 mg IV
- Cimetidine: 200 mg 6-hourly, 400 mg nocte oral; 200 mg IV
- Omeprazole: 40 nocte oral and day of surgery
- 0.3M sodium citrate: 30 ml
- Metoclopramide: 10 mg

INTRAVENOUS INDUCTION AGENTS

Intravenous anaesthetic agents can be used for induction of anaesthesia and for maintenance in total intravenous anaesthesia (TIVA). Most anaesthetic agents produce unconsciousness within one arm-brain circulation time even though the speed of onset may be delayed in elderly and debilitated individuals. As many of these drugs cause myocardial depression, peripheral vasodilatation and depression of airway reflexes, the patient's cardiovascular system should be closely monitored and the ventilation assisted following drug administration.

Thiopentone is an ultra short-acting barbiturate most frequently used for induction of anaesthesia. Induction is smooth and rapid but is often associated with hypotension, reflex tachycardia and apnoea. The drug is irritant: extravasation may cause tissue necrosis, and accidental intraarterial injection results in vasospasm, pain and ischaemia to the affected limb.

— Thiopentone: 4–5 mg/kg

— Methohexitone: 1–1.5 mg/kg

Propofol is 2,6-diisopropyl phenol with properties suitable for day-care anaesthesia and TIVA, notably smooth emergence, minimal hangover effect and antiemesis. Airway reflexes are depressed to a greater extent compared with thiopentone, allowing for excellent condition for insertion of laryngeal mask airway. Lignocaine is frequently added to reduce pain during injection. Propofol-®Lipuro, a new propofol formulation in a fat emulsion consisting of medium- and long-chain triglycerides, is said to produce less injection pain.

— Propofol: 2–2.5 mg/kg; 2.5–4 mg/kg in children < 8 years

Ketamine is a phencyclidine derivative used to produce a clinical state of "dissociative anaesthesia". Its sympathetic effects are useful in hypotensive patients, but may be deleterious in patients with hypertension and coronary artery disease. As it also causes increases in intracranial and intraocular pressures, ketamine is contraindicated in patients with raised ICP or IOP. Its profound analgesic properties are useful for painful procedures such as change of burns dressing. Ketamine also causes bronchodilation and is the induction agent of choice in patients with acute exacerbation of asthma. Its effects of increased bronchial secretions and postoperative hallucinations can be counteracted by atropine and midazolam respectively.

— Ketamine: 2 mg/kg IV, 5 mg/kg IM

Fentanyl is often used together with other intravenous anaesthetic agents during induction. When used alone or in combination with midazolam, there is much inter-individual variation in induction dose and onset of action. As fentanyl results in more cardiovascular stability compared to thiopentone or propofol, relatively large doses – up to 50 μg/kg – can be used for induction of anaesthesia in cardiac patients ("opioid-based anaesthesia"). Other opioid analgesics, for example, alfentanil, sufentanil, remifentanil, can also be used for intravenous induction. Similarly, midazolam may be used in combination with another induction agent in a technique termed co-induction in order to reduce the dose of the principal induction agent.

— Fentanyl: 1–5 μg/kg
— Alfentanil: 5 μg/kg
— Midazolam: 0.2 mg/kg

Etomidate is a carboxylated imidazole derivative characterized by cardiovascular stability, minimal histamine release and minimal respiratory effects. Incidence of myoclonus can be reduced by benzodiazepine premedication and use of an opioid during induction. There is a transient suppression of cortisol synthesis following a single induction dose, but cortisol levels are restored after 2–6 hours. There is little risk of adrenal suppression on single-dose administration.

— Etomidate: 0.25–0.3 mg/kg

INHALATIONAL ANAESTHETIC AGENTS

Nitrous oxide is frequently administered together with oxygen in a 2:1 ratio. It is a weak anaesthetic with fair analgesic properties. Due to its higher solubility compared to nitrogen, it should be avoided in patients with pneumothorax or bowel distension, certain middle-ear and retinal surgery, and procedures with increased risk of venous air embolism.

Volatile anaesthetic agents include halothane, enflurane, isoflurane, sevoflurane and desflurane. They cause myocardial depression, peripheral vasodilatation, respiratory depression and bronchodilation in varying degrees. Undesirable side-effects include cardiac arrhythmias and autoimmune hepatitis with halothane, and epileptiform electroencephalography (EEG) discharges with enflurane. These older volatile anaesthetics have been superseded by isoflurane, sevoflurane and desflurane.

Despite earlier findings of "coronary steal" phenomenon attributed to isoflurane, it is now recognized that volatile anaesthetics have myo-protective properties by limiting infarct size and improving functional recovery from myocardial ischaemia. Sevoflurane has replaced halothane as inhalational induction agent of choice because of its non-irritant properties and rapid onset and offset of action. Desflurane, despite its excellent pharmacologic profile, is less popular because it requires a special electrically heated vaporizer for delivery.

NEUROMUSCULAR BLOCKING DRUGS

Suxamethonium, a depolarizing muscle relaxant, is the agent of choice in emergency anaesthesia and suspected airway difficulties. It has rapid onset (within 45 seconds), short duration of action (5–7 minutes) and produces profound muscle relaxation for an excellent intubating condition. Adverse effects include myalgia, bradycardia, hyperkalaemia, and increased intracavity pressures (intracranial, intraocular, intragastric). It is a triggering agent for malignant hyperthermia in genetically susceptible individuals. Prolonged apnoea can occur as a result of dual block (mixed depolarizing and non-depolarizing block), or deficiency in pseudocholinesterase, the enzyme required for hydrolysis of suxamethonium.

— Suxamethonium (succinylcholine): 1.0–1.5 mg/kg

The older non-depolarizing neuromuscular blocking drugs (e.g., curare, alcuronium, pancuronium, gallamine) have been replaced by agents with fewer side-effects and better pharmacologic profile. Monitoring of the degree of neuromuscular blockade is highly recommended in long procedures and susceptible individuals.

— Atracurium: 0.3–0.6 mg/kg
— Vecuronium: 0.1–0.15 mg/kg
— Rocuronium: 0.6–0.9 mg/kg
— Mivacurium: 0.15–0.2 mg/kg
— Cisatracurium: 0.1–0.15 mg/kg

REVERSAL AGENTS

Neuromuscular blockade produced by a non-depolarizing neuromuscular blocker is reversed by a mixture of two drugs, an anticholinesterase (usually neostigmine) and an antimuscarinic agent (atropine or glycopyrrolate). Suxamethonium does not require reversal of block; the reversal agents may in fact create a dual block if inadvertently administered.

— Neostigmine: 0.05 mg/kg
— Atropine: 0.02 mg/kg
— Glycopyrrolate: 0.004 mg/kg

LOCAL ANAESTHETICS

Local anaesthetics are used in many forms of locoregional anaesthesia. They may be used as sole agents or in combination with opioids (commonly fentanyl or sufentanil) in central neuraxial blockade. Adverse effects include cardiotoxicity, CNS excitation with seizures, and respiratory depression when these agents are inadvertently injected into the systemic circulation. Bupivacaine has been the most commonly used local anaesthetic agent, newer agents include ropivacaine and levobupivacaine (a chiral derivative of bupivacaine). Ropivacaine, though less potent than bupivacaine, is less cardiotoxic and produces less lower limb motor block when used in the epidural route.

The often quoted maximum safe doses are:

- bupivacaine: up to 2 mg/kg of plain solution in any 4-hour period, or 3 mg/kg with adrenaline
- lignocaine: plain solution 3 mg/kg; with adrenaline 7 mg/kg
- prilocaine: plain solution 5–6 mg/kg; with adrenaline 8 mg/kg
- ropivacaine: 3–4 mg/kg

ANALGESIC AGENTS

Narcotic analgesics are commonly used at induction, during maintenance and for postoperative analgesia following major surgery. They can be administered parenterally (usually IV, occasionally IM), epidurally or intrathecally. These include:

- Fentanyl: 1–5 μg/kg IV; 10–50 μg/kg IV as sole induction agent for cardiac anaesthesia; 15–25 μg (in combination with local anaesthetic) intrathecally; 50–100 μg epidural bolus or 2 μg/ml (in combination with local anaesthetic) for postoperative analgesia.
- Pethidine: 1 mg/kg IM as premedication or postoperative analgesia; 25–50 mg IV bolus; 25–50 mg epidural bolus for postoperative analgesia.
- Morphine: 0.1–0.2 mg/kg IV; 2.5–10 mg SC; 0.1–0.2 mg intrathecally; 3–5 mg epidural bolus for postoperative analgesia.
- Alfentanil: 5 μg/kg IV.
- Remifentanil: 0.5 μg/kg/min, range 0.05–0.5 μg/kg/min by intravenous infusion.
- Nalbuphine: 0.2 mg/kg; usual dose 10 mg in adult.

Non-narcotic analgesics consist of a miscellaneous group of drugs which are efficacious in treating mild to moderate postoperative pain. They are useful as adjuncts to opioid analgesics and have some opioid-sparing effect, thereby reducing the incidence and severity of some opioid-related side-effects. Non-steroidal inflammatory drugs (NSAIDs) which are selective cyclooxygenase-2 (COX-2) inhibitors cause fewer gastrointestinal and haematological side-effects compared to non-selective COX-1 and

COX-2 inhibitors, even though renal side-effects remain a problem. Here are examples of these drugs.

— Ketorolac: 10–30 mg IM or IV.
— Diclofenac: 0.5–1 mg/kg rectally.
— Celecoxib: 100–200 mg bd oral.
— Parecoxib: 40 mg IM or IV; maximum dose 80 mg/day.
— Etoricoxib: 120 mg daily oral.
— Meloxicam: 7.5 mg bd oral.
— Paracetamol: 15–20 mg/kg oral; 20–30 mg/kg rectally.

The initial enthusiasm for COX-2 inhibitors has been somewhat dampened by adverse effects shown by rofecoxib. In 2004, rofecoxib was withdrawn from the market worldwide following reports of increased relative risk for confirmed cardiovascular events such as myocardial infarction, sudden cardiac death and stroke. The safety of other COX-2 inhibitors awaits further study.

Dosages of drugs which are commonly used in anaesthesia and resuscitation are given in the next section. The reader is strongly advised to be familiar with the drugs, not only the appropriate dosages but their pharmacological actions, side-effects and contraindications.

INOTROPIC AND SYMPATHOMIMETIC AGENTS

— Adrenaline
  - Intravenous bolus
    — For severe anaphylactic reaction: 1 mg diluted to 10 ml (1:10,000 solution), 0.5–1 ml (50–100 μg) at a time, titrate against BP and heart rate.
    — For cardiac arrest (adult): 1 mg repeat every 3–5 minutes, doses up to 0.1 mg/kg every 3–5 minutes have been used.
    — For cardiac arrest (paediatric): 10 μg/kg (0.1 ml/kg of 1:10,000 solution).
  - Intravenous infusion
    — Dilution [0.3 × body weight (kg)] mg in 50 ml (1 ml/hr = 0.1 μg/kg/min).
    — Dose range: 0.1–1 μg/kg/min.
  - Subcutaneous infiltration
    — 1:100,000 solution: not more than 10 ml in 10 minutes.

    - 1:200,000 solution: not more than 20 ml in 20 minutes.

- Dopamine and dobutamine
  - Dilution [3 × body weight (kg)] mg in 50 ml (1 ml/hr = 1 μg/kg/min).
  - Dose range: 2.5–20 μg/kg/min.
- Ephedrine: 5–10 mg repeated doses.
- Phenylephrine: 50–100 μg repeated doses.
- Isoprenaline: 0.5–5 μg/min IV infusion (3 mg in 50 ml at 0.5–5 ml/hr).
- Noradrenaline
  - Only by intravenous infusion via a central vein, *no* intravenous bolus should be given.
  - Essential to have continuous haemodynamic monitoring.
  - Dose range: 0.01–0.2 μg/kg/min.
- Salbutamol
  - Nebulizer: 2.5–5 mg (0.5–1 ml of 0.5% solution), dilute to 2.0–2.5 ml with normal saline.
  - Subcutaneous: 8 μg/kg (500 μg in adult) 4-hourly.
  - Intravenous injection: 4 μg/kg (250 μg in adult) slowly.
  - Infusion 0.05–0.5 μg/kg/min.
- Terbutaline
  - Inhaler: 0.25 mg per puff.
  - Subcutaneous: 0.5–0.75 μg/kg 6-hourly.

HYPOTENSIVE AGENTS

- Esmolol: 0.5–1 mg/kg each dose, 50–300 μg/kg/min infusion for controlled hypotensive anaesthesia.
- Diazoxide: 1–3 mg/kg fast IV bolus, maximum single injection 150 mg.
- Hydralazine: 5 mg each dose titrating to BP.
- Labetalol: 5–10 mg repeated doses.
- Metoprolol: 2 mg doses IV titrating to BP, do not exceed 10 mg.
- Nifedipine: 10 mg sublingual.
- Nitroglycerin: Dose range 0.1–1 μg/kg/min, starting dose 0.1 μg/kg/min.
- Sodium nitroprusside
  - Starting dose: 0.5 μg/kg/min, titrate according to BP.

- Average dose: 3 μg/kg/min (dose range 0.5–8 μg/kg/min).
- Do not exceed 3 mg/kg.

OTHER CARDIOVASCULAR DRUGS

— Adenosine
- 6 mg fast bolus, repeat 12 mg after 1–2 minutes.
- Third dose of 12 mg may be given in 1–2 minutes.

— Amiodarone
- For treatment of atrial fibrillation: 10–20 mg/kg/day, infusion 0.5–0.7 mg/kg/hr.
- For shock-resistant ventricular fibrillation: 5 mg/kg.

— Amrinone: 0.75 mg/kg bolus over 5–10 minutes, infusion 5–15 μg/kg/min.

— Digoxin
- 2.5–5 μg/kg daily.
- Reduce dose in the elderly and patients with renal failure.
- Correct hypokalaemia which enhances digoxin toxicity.

— Diltiazem: 0.2 mg/kg bolus over 1 minute, infusion 5–15 μg/kg/min.

— Milrinone
- Loading dose: 50 μg/kg administer slowly over 10 minutes.
- Maintenance dose: 0.5 μg/kg/min (range 0.375–0.75 μg/kg/min).

— Vasopressin
- For persistent or recurrent ventricular tachycardia or fibrillation: 40 IU, single, one-time dose.

— Verapamil: 0.05–0.1 mg/kg bolus over 2–3 minutes.

MISCELLANEOUS DRUGS

— Aminophylline: 5 mg/kg bolus over 20 minutes, 0.5–0.7 mg/kg/hr infusion.

— Calcium chloride: 5–10 ml of 10% solution slow IV.

— Dantrolene: 2.5 mg/kg initial dose, maximum dose 20 mg/kg.

— Dexamethasone: 0.15–0.2 mg/kg.

— Dexmedetomidine: 1 μg/kg loading dose over 10–20 minutes, 0.2–0.7 μg/kg/hr maintenance.

— Droperidol: 0.625–1.25 mg IV.

— Ergometrine: 0.25–0.5 mg.
— Flumazenil: 0.2 mg initial dose, 0.1 mg per dose at 1-minute intervals titrating to response, maximum dose 1.0 mg.
— Frusemide: 0.5–1.0 mg/kg.
— Heparin: 3 mg/kg for cardio-pulmonary bypass;
  1 mg/kg for vascular surgery (1 mg = 100 U).
— Hydrocortisone: 25–150 mg for steroid replacement therapy.
— Lignocaine: 1.0–1.5 mg/kg.
— Magnesium sulphate: 2–4 g slow IV over 10 minutes, followed by IV infusion 1 g/hr.
— Mannitol: 0.5–1.0 gm/kg.
— Naloxone: 0.01 mg/kg (neonate), 0.1 mg per dose; maximum 0.4 mg (adult).
— Nimodipine: 0.1–1 μg/kg/min IV infusion.
— Ondansetron: 4–8 mg IV, 8 mg oral.
— Protamine: 1–3 mg/kg, equi-dose with heparin.
— Sodium bicarbonate: 1 mEq/kg of 8.4% solution, dilute to 4.2% solution in neonates.
— Syntocinon: 5 U stat dose, 40–80 U in 500 ml infusion if indicated.

FURTHER READING

1. Splinter W. Halothane: The end of an era? (Editorial) Anesth Analg 2002;95:1471.
2. Wong SF, Chung F. Succinylcholine-associated postoperative myalgia. Anaesthesia 2000;55:144–52.
3. Moore EW, Hunter JM. The new neuromuscular blocking agents: Do they offer any advantages? Br J Anaesth 2001;87:912–25.
4. Lee C. Structure, conformation, and action of neuromuscular blocking drugs. Br J Anaesth 2001;87:755–69.
5. Whiteside JB, Wildsmith JAW. Developments in local anaesthetic drugs. Br J Anaesth 2001;87:27–35.
6. Tarkkila P, Rosenberg PH. Perioperative analgesia with non-steroidal analgesics. Curr Opin Anaesthesiol 1998;11:407–10.
7. Gajraj NM. Cyclooxygenase-2 inhibitors. Anesth Analg 2003;96:1720–38.
8. Fitzgerald GA, Patrono C. The coxibs, selective inhibitors of cyclooxygenase-2. N Engl J Med 2001;345:433–42.

Chapter 10

Post-Anaesthesia Care Unit

- Introduction
- Requirements
- Management in PACU
- Problems Encountered in PACU
- Discharge from PACU
- Appendix: Postanaesthetic Recovery Score (PARS)
- Further Reading

INTRODUCTION

Post-Anaesthesia Care Unit (PACU), or the Recovery Ward, is an area located adjacent to or within the OT complex and is designated for management of patients recovering from the effects of anaesthesia.

This area is no less important than the operating room itself, as many of the anaesthetic mishaps are found to occur in the immediate postoperative period. The incidence of PACU morbidity in adults ranges from 18% to 30% in various studies.

In the day-care surgery setting, the recovery phase consists of two stages: immediate recovery from the effects of anaesthesia, and further recovery until the patient has regained "street fitness". The first stage is no different from recovery for inpatients while the second stage is usually managed in the Day Care Unit.

REQUIREMENTS

1. **Location and design features**

   The PACU should be located within the OT complex, ideally in the centre of the complex with accessibility to all the operating rooms, ICU and CCU. Easy access for medical staff from inside and outside the OT complex is essential to maintain supervision and care. Facilities such as laboratory, radiology and Blood Bank should also be readily available and accessible at all hours.

   The number of bed spaces in the PACU depends on the number of operating rooms in the OT complex. It should be sufficient to deal with peak loads and there should be at least 1.5 spaces per operating room. The layout of bed spaces should allow the staff to have an uninterrupted view of several patients at once.

   The space allocated per bed should be at least 9 m^2. There must be easy access to the patient's head in case emergency airway management is necessary.

2. **Equipment**

   The equipment listed here should be available. The ones marked with an asterisk should be available in every bed while the others may be shared among patients.

   — Trolley*: should be equipped with firm base and mattress, brakes, hand rails; should be easy to manoeuvre, tiltable for at least 15° both head up and head down, and have provision for sitting the patient up.

   — Oxygen source*: oxygen flowmeter and oxygen delivery systems, masks of different types and sizes, tracheostomy masks, tubings and connectors.

   — Suction device*: vacuum source, suction catheters, rigid suction, e.g., Yaunkeur sucker.

   — Monitors: blood pressure monitor and pulse oximeter should be available at every bed; ECG monitor at least one per three beds. Monitors that should be easily available include pressure transducer sets for invasive BP or CVP monitoring, capnograph and peripheral nerve stimulator.

   — Warming devices: radiant heater, blankets, forced air warming devices, blood warmer, incubator or Infant Resuscitaire for babies.

   — Airway equipment: oro- and nasopharyngeal airways, face masks of different types and sizes, self-inflating bags, laryngoscopes with different sizes of blades, different sizes of endotracheal tubes with stylets, laryngeal mask airways, emergency cricothyroromy sets. Tracheostomy sets should be easily available.

- Equipment for intravenous therapy: drugs and intravenous fluids, needles, syringes, infusion sets, syringe pumps, pressure bags for rapid transfusion.
- Resuscitation equipment: resuscitation drugs, defibrillator (connected to the mains supply and ready for use), cardiac boards.
- Light source* to allow accurate assessment of patient's colour.
- Power outlets*: 2–4 sockets per bed.
- Means to perform simple bedside investigations: glucometer, blood gas analyzer, ECG and X-ray facilities.

3. **Personnel**

It would be ideal to have an anaesthesiologist in PACU at all times; failing which the anaesthesiologist should be easily contactable and immediately available should any problem arise.

The quality and level of expertise of the PACU staff will directly affect the quality of care and safety of patients recovering from anaesthesia. Ideally the nurses should be dedicated PACU staff and not from the common pool of OT nurses. The practice of delegating the most junior nurses (those "unable to scrub") to work in PACU should not be condoned. Trainee nurses and those inexperienced in taking care of patients recovering from anaesthesia must be supervised. The nurse to patient ratio should be flexible – one to one during the initial period when the patient is drowsy or unconscious; and one to two or three patients thereafter.

The nursing staff should be adequately trained in observation, monitoring and general care of the unconscious patient, as well as in emergency procedures and resuscitation. They should be vigilant enough to identify problems, institute immediate remedial measures and quickly alert the anaesthesiologist. The anaesthesiologist should review the patients promptly if any complications should arise. Resuscitative measures should be started while the underlying cause is being worked out.

MANAGEMENT IN PACU

The anaesthesiologist should accompany the patient from the operating room to the PACU. Relevant information regarding the patient, the surgery and any problems encountered intraoperatively or expected postoperatively should be passed over clearly to the nursing staff.

The patient should receive oxygen by mask, his/her blood pressure, heart rate and oxygen saturation checked on arrival at PACU. The anaesthesiologist should only leave the patient to the care of the nursing staff when the patient's condition is stable.

The patient should be observed and the BP, heart rate, SpO_2 recorded every 5 minutes. Other parameters to be noted include the state of consciousness, colour and respiratory function. The staff should stay with a patient who is drowsy or unconscious to provide airway support if necessary.

The nurses may also perform care and assessment of pressure areas, limbs, wounds, dressings and drains. However, the nurses' main areas of responsibility are observation and life support of the patient; these take precedence over the other tasks described above.

PROBLEMS ENCOUNTERED IN PACU

Problems that may be encountered in PACU are listed here. Some of these problems are elaborated further in Chapter 61.

— Central nervous system: failure to awaken, confusion, restlessness.

— Cardiovascular system: hyper- or hypotension, cardiac dysrhythmias, acute myocardial infarction, heart failure, shock of any pathology.

— Respiratory system: hypoventilation, aspiration, upper airway obstruction, laryngo- or bronchospasm, hypoxaemia, acute pulmonary oedema.

— Others: pain, nausea and vomiting, bladder distension, shivering, hypothermia, bleeding from surgical site.

DISCHARGE FROM PACU

The patient should be observed for at least 30 minutes in PACU. This period can be shortened if the surgery has been done under regional anaesthesia and the intraoperative course has been uneventful.

Alternatively, the patient should be observed for a longer period if the intraoperative course has been stormy or the surgery has been protracted or complicated. If the patient is to remain in the PACU for a prolonged period, it is important that the surgeon should be informed and be involved in the on-going management of the patient.

Responsibility for discharging the patient from PACU lies with the anaesthesiologist. Checklists such as Post-Anaesthetic Recovery Score (PARS) can be used to document the patient's condition on discharge (see Appendix). At the time of discharge, the patient should be conscious, have adequate respiratory effort, be haemodynamically stable, and be reasonably comfortable and pain-free.

Postoperative instructions to the ward staff should be documented in the case notes and verbally passed over to the staff receiving the patient from the OT. Such instructions include oxygen therapy in the ward, postoperative pain management if the patient is under Acute Pain Service (APS), instructions following spinal anaesthesia, special investigations, for example, chest X-ray, 12-lead ECG in the ward.

APPENDIX

POSTANAESTHETIC RECOVERY SCORE (PARS)

Criteria	Score
1. ACTIVITY	
— able to move 4 extremities voluntarily or on command	2
— able to move 2 extremities voluntarily or on command	1
— unable to move extremities voluntarily or on command	0
2. RESPIRATION	
— able to breathe deeply and cough easily	2
— dyspnoeic or with limited breathing	1
— apnoeic	0
3. CIRCULATION	
A. Blood Pressure	
— blood pressure ± 20% preanaesthetic level	2
— blood pressure ± 20% to 50% preanaesthetic level	1
— blood pressure ± 50% preanaesthetic level	0
B. Pulse	
— regular	2
— irregular	1
C. Heart Rate	
— heart rate ± 20% preanaesthetic level	2
— heart rate ± 20% to 50% preanaesthetic level	1
— heart rate ± 50% preanaesthetic level	0

4. CONSCIOUSNESS	
— fully awake	2
— arousable on calling	1
— not responding	0
5. COLOUR	
— pink	2
— pale, dusky, blotchy, jaundiced	1
— cyanotic	0
Total	

FURTHER READING

1. Rose DK, Cohen MM, De Boer DP. Cardiovascular events in the postanesthesia care unit. Anesthesiology 1996;84:772–81.
2. Van Der Walt JH, Webb RK, Osborne GA, Morgan C, MacKay P. Recovery room incidents in the first 2000 incident reports. Anaesth Intens Care 1993;21:650–2.

B

Clinical Conditions

Chapter 11

Anaesthesia and Hypertension

- **Introduction**
- **Classification of Hypertension**
- **Drug Therapy for Hypertension**
- **Preoperative Assessment**
- **Anaesthetic Management**
- **Further Reading**

INTRODUCTION

Hypertension is a disorder in which the basal level of arterial pressure is higher than that expected for the age and gender of the person. It is one of the commonest forms of co-morbidity encountered by the anaesthesiologist among the patients presenting for surgery and anaesthesia.

As a rule of thumb, normal systolic BP in mmHg is approximately [Age (years) + 100]. The diagnosis of hypertension should be based on two or more readings taken at separate occasions, since a single reading may be erroneously high for some reason. The so-called "white-coat" hypertension, in which BP is persistently elevated in the hospital setting despite a normal ambulatory BP, may further complicate matters. The patient's normal BP reading should ideally be sought from the general practitioner. Unfortunately this information is not always available, and the anaesthesiologist often has to make a perioperative management decision on the basis of two or three readings taken over a period of hours in the hospital.

The significance of hypertension for the anaesthesiologist is 2-fold.

- Hypertensive patients are likely to have co-morbidities which add to the anaesthetic risk, such as accelerated atherosclerosis leading to coronary artery disease or cerebrovascular disease, renal and endocrine disorders.
- Untreated or poorly treated hypertensive patients show exaggerated cardiovascular responses and BP lability during anaesthesia, which may precipitate adverse myocardial or cerebrovascular events intraoperatively.

Despite the high prevalence of hypertension among the population, there have not been clear guidelines on perioperative management of hypertension, specifically whether a patient with uncontrolled hypertension should be anaesthetized or should have the surgery deferred. It has been the traditional teaching that such patients should have anaesthesia and surgery deferred until BP is controlled, but there is no clear evidence that in doing so the perioperative risks are significantly reduced. It is also unclear for how long treatment should be given before the patient can be rescheduled for surgery.

CLASSIFICATION OF HYPERTENSION

Hypertension can be categorized according to the underlying aetiology or in terms of severity.

1. **Aetiology**
   - *Primary or essential hypertension* is by far the commonest, occurring in > 90% cases.
   - *Secondary hypertension* is associated with these medical conditions.
     - Cardiovascular: coarctation of aorta, renal artery stenosis.
     - Renal: chronic pyelonephritis, chronic glomerulonephritis, polycystic disease, renin-producing tumours.
     - Endocrine: phaeochromocytoma, Conn's syndrome (primary hyperaldosteronism), Cushing's syndrome, acromegaly, congenital adrenal hyperplasia, hyperparathyroidism.
     - Neurogenic: acute intracranial hypertension, autonomic hyperreflexia (e.g., tetanus).

A relatively young patient presenting with hypertension, particularly if it is paroxysmal in nature, warrants thorough investigations to rule out secondary causes of hypertension.

— A third subclass of **systolic hypertension** can be seen in high cardiac output states (e.g., thyrotoxicosis, arteriovenous fistula) and when the aorta is atherosclerotic and rigid.

2. **Severity**

— Various classifications from the Seventh Joint National Committee on the Detection, Evaluation and Treatment of High Blood Pressure (JNC 7) and the World Hypertension Society/International Society of Hypertension (WHO/ISH) are available. Classification under JNC 7, for adults aged 18 years or older, is based solely on arterial pressure readings (Table 11–1). Patients with prehypertension are at increased risk for progression to hypertension; those in the 130/80 to 139/89 mmHg BP range are at twice the risk to develop hypertension as those with lower values.

Table 11–1. JNC 7 classification of hypertension according to severity

Category	Systolic BP (mmHg)	Diastolic BP (mmHg)
Normal	< 120	< 80
Prehypertension	120–139	80–89
Stage 1 hypertension	140–159	90–99
Stage 2 hypertension	160	100

DRUG THERAPY FOR HYPERTENSION

Oral antihypertensive drugs can be classified according to their modes of action.

— Diuretics: thiazide diuretics (chlorothiazide, hydrochlorothiazide), loop diuretics (bumetanide, frusemide), potassium-sparing diuretics (amiloride).

— Adrenergic receptor blockers:

- α_1-blocker: prazosin, phenoxybenzamine.

- α- and β-blocker: labetalol.
- β-blocker: metoprolol, atenolol, propranolol, acebutolol.

— Angiotensin-converting enzyme (ACE) inhibitors: captopril, enalapril, lsinopril.
— Angiotensin II receptor antagonists: losartan, valsartan.
— Direct vasodilators: hydralazine, minoxidil.
— Calcium channel blockers: amlodipine, felodipine, nifedipine, diltiazem, verapamil.
— Central α_2-agonists and other centrally-acting drugs: clonidine, methyldopa, reserpine.

Many hypertensive patients require two or more antihypertensive medications to achieve BP control, either as separate prescriptions or in fixed-dose combinations. Drugs from different classes with different modes of action generally have additive effects on blood pressure when they are prescribed together.

New antihypertensive agents are constantly being developed and introduced into clinical practice. Examples include angiotensin II receptor antagonists and centrally-acting agents (e.g., urapidil, ketanserin, moxonidine, mivazerol). The anaesthesiologist should be familiar with the pharmacology of these drugs including their side-effects and potential interaction with anaesthetic agents.

Patients who are on antihypertensive therapy should be instructed to continue taking their medications up to and including the day of surgery, and treatment should be restarted as soon as possible in the postoperative period. There is evidence that the cardiovascular risks can be reduced by perioperative β-blockade. However, ACE inhibitors and in particular angiotensin II receptor antagonists have the potential to interact with anaesthetic agents to produce hypotension, and cases of severe hypotension following central neuraxial blockade have been reported. This has prompted some anaesthesiologists to suggest withholding these classes of antihypertensive agents on the morning of surgery, especially so if the preoperative BP is not markedly elevated, if postural hypotension is present, and if central neuraxial blockade is the planned anaesthetic technique.

PREOPERATIVE ASSESSMENT

These aspects require in-depth evaluation.

— Assessment of blood pressure control
- History of hypertension: age of onset, presenting symptoms, investigations for secondary causes of hypertension (if applicable).

- Medication history: nature of antihypertensive medication, past and present treatment, compliance in taking medication, other medications.
- Erect and supine BP, presence of postural hypotension, 4-hourly BP observation in the ward.

— Assessment of target organ damage and associated medical conditions
- Cardiovascular system: hypertensive heart disease (left ventricular hypertrophy, diastolic dysfunction), heart failure, coronary artery disease with symptomatic or silent myocardial ischaemia. Mandatory tests are 12-lead ECG and CXR, and further tests are indicated in selected cases.
- Renal system: note that even mild hypertensives may have a degree of renal impairment. Check serum urea, creatinine and electrolyte concentrations.
- Central nervous system: cerebrovascular disease (transient ischaemic attacks, ischaemic stroke, focal cerebral haemorrhage). Perform fundoscopic examination for hypertensive changes.
- Other concomitant diseases such as diabetes mellitus, hypercholesterolaemia, obesity, peripheral vascular disease.

— Acceptability for surgery
- The presence of significant target organ damage is more of a concern to the anaesthesiologist than a diagnosis of hypertension *per se.*
- Elective surgery should be deferred if BP is persistently elevated, with diastolic BP > 110 mmHg or systolic BP > 180 mmHg. The presence of target organ damage adds weight to the decision to defer, and medical treatment should be started or escalated to optimize antihypertensive therapy.
- The risks of delaying emergency surgery may outweigh those of proceeding in the face of uncontrolled hypertension. Intravenous antihypertensive agents such as esmolol, labetalol or hydralazine may be required to achieve rapid BP control. However, dramatic acute reductions in BP may also be fraught with risk and should be avoided.

ANAESTHETIC MANAGEMENT

Premedication

— It is necessary to provide adequate sedation and anxiolysis to prevent anxiety-induced tachycardia and hypertension.

— Antihypertensives should be continued on the morning of surgery. ACE inhibitors and angiotensin II receptor antagonists may be omitted as explained earlier.

Monitoring

- Mandatory monitors include ECG (CM_5 the preferred lead to monitor for myocardial ischaemia), BP (non-invasive or intraarterial depending on nature of surgery), pulse oximetry, capnography.
- Include central venous cannulation for CVP monitoring and/or pulmonary artery catheterization in patients with poor left ventricular function undergoing major surgery.
- Others include peripheral nerve stimulator, urine output, temperature where indicated.

No particular anaesthetic agent or technique has been found to be superior; the choice depends on surgical requirements and the skill, experience and preference of the anaesthesiologist.

Regional Anaesthesia

- Regional anaesthesia, in the form of central neuraxial blockade and peripheral nerve blocks, obviates the problems of wide haemodynamic fluctuations common during general anaesthesia. Furthermore, catheter techniques are able to provide effective analgesia to minimize haemodynamic stresses arising from postoperative pain.
- Hypotension secondary to spinal anaesthesia may be deleterious for hypertensive patients with significant target organ disease. This can often be minimized by judicious fluid preloading, frequent BP measurements and early use of vasopressor.
- Hypotension following central neuraxial blockade should be treated with intravenous fluids and/or vasopressor such as ephedrine or phenylephrine. Such patients may be resistant to conventional vasopressors, and in extreme cases may require vasopressin to reverse refractory hypotension.
- It is important to ascertain that regional blockade is effective before the surgeon is allowed to proceed: pain resulting from inadequate block is a potent stimulus for hypertension and tachycardia.
- Be prepared to convert to general anaesthesia if the regional block is not adequate. Do not supplement inadequate block with heavy sedation.
- Extremely anxious patients may need verbal reassurance and/or sedation in the form of midazolam or propofol infusion or bolus doses.

General Anaesthesia

Induction of anaesthesia

— The surgeon should be ready to begin surgery soon after induction of anaesthesia. This minimizes the time interval between induction and surgical incision when the BP is likely to sag.

— Use a combination of opioid (e.g., fentanyl) with thiopentone or propofol for induction; avoid ketamine as it causes hypertension and tachycardia. Opioid-based anaesthesia confers more cardiovascular stability than thiopentone or propofol, but may give rise to postoperative respiratory depression in short- and medium-length procedures. Etomidate may be advantageous in this aspect.

— An intravenous antihypertensive (e.g., esmolol, hydralazine) may be required if BP remains high despite adequate premedication and antihypertensive medication.

— Ensure adequate depth of anaesthesia by achieving an end-tidal concentration of inhalational anaesthetic greater than 1 MAC before laryngoscopy and intubation.

— Allow adequate time for neuromuscular blockade before attempting laryngoscopy and intubation; monitor the degree of muscle relaxation by using the peripheral nerve stimulator.

— Drugs that can obtund the sympathetic responses during airway instrumentation include IV lignocaine 1–1.5 mg/kg and IV esmolol 0.5–1 mg/kg. These should be given approximately 90 seconds before laryngoscopy and intubation.

Maintenance

— Maintain normocarbia and adequate oxygenation.

— Maintain adequate depth of anaesthesia using opioid and volatile anaesthetic; isoflurane and sevoflurane are preferred to halothane as they are less myocardial depressant.

— Neuromuscular blocking agents which are cardiovascularly stable (e.g., vecuronium, rocuronium) are preferred.

— The lower limit for autoregulation of cerebral blood flow is higher than that in normal patients. This should be taken into account if controlled hypotensive anaesthesia is required during surgery.

Emergence and recovery

— This phase is often neglected even though it is just as important as induction and maintenance.

- An additional dose of IV lignocaine or esmolol helps to obtund the sympathetic responses during emergence and extubation.
- The patient should be extubated early – as soon as protective airway reflexes return – in order to avoid coughing and gagging on the endotracheal tube.
- Blood pressure and heart rate should be closely monitored in PACU, and treatment for hypertension should be instituted if necessary.
- Monitoring should continue into the postoperative period until it is clear that the patient is cardiovascularly stable. It may be appropriate to manage the patient in HDU in the immediate postoperative period.
- Recommence antihypertensive therapy as soon as possible; patients who require prolonged fasting should be given alternative antihypertensive medications in parenteral form.

FURTHER READING

1. Howell SJ, Sear JW, Foex P. Hypertension, hypertensive heart disease and perioperative cardiac risk. Br J Anaesth 2004;92:570–83.
2. Chobanian AV, et al. The seventh report of the Joint National Committee on Prevention, Detection, Evaluation, and Treatment of High Blood Pressure. JAMA 2003;289:2560–71.
3. Fleisher LA. Preoperative evaluation of the patient with hypertension. JAMA 2002;287:2043–6.
4. Howell SJ. Anaesthesia and hypertension. Curr Anaesth Crit Care 2003;14:100–7.
5. Makris R, Coriat P. Interactions between cardiovascular treatments and anaesthesia. Curr Opin Anaesthesiol 2001;14:33–9.
6. Bertrand M, Godet G, Meersschaert K, et al. Should the angiotension II antagonists be discontinued before surgery? Anesth Analg 2001;92:26–30.

Chapter 12

Coronary Artery Disease and Anaesthesia for Non-Cardiac Surgery

INTRODUCTION

Coronary artery disease (CAD), also known as ischaemic heart disease (IHD), is one of the commonest medical problems in surgical patients above the age of 40. The patient may present in any of these ways:

— "Chest pains" which are non-specific or atypical, and may or may not be associated with ECG changes of myocardial ischaemia. This presents a problem of diagnosis; further tests may be necessary to determine whether the patient indeed has CAD.

— Typical symptoms of angina which may be stable or unstable.

- Previous history of myocardial infarction, currently with or without angina.
- Cardiac failure or dysrhythmias associated with CAD.
- Asymptomatic as a result of autonomic neuropathy, typically seen in diabetes mellitus.

The risk of perioperative mortality is high for patients with unstable angina and those with acute or recent myocardial infarction (MI). Elective surgery should be deferred in these high-risk patients. Emergency surgery entails consideration of the benefits of surgery against the anaesthetic risks, and conveying these risks to the patient and close relatives. In view of the patient's unstable cardiac status, the surgeon should consider modifying the surgical procedure to one which is shorter, less extensive or invasive.

Traditionally, risk assessment for non-cardiac surgery following MI has been based on the time interval between MI and surgery. However, this may no longer be valid in the current era of thrombolytics and angioplasty, where more emphasis is placed on functional status during convalescence rather than the age of MI *per se*. Risk of reinfarction is low if the patient has made an uneventful recovery with no evidence of residual myocardium at risk on stress test. Essential non-cardiac surgery may be allowed to proceed at 6 weeks following MI in such patients.

PREOPERATIVE ASSESSMENT

History

- Previous MI, if any
  - Details include the use of thrombolytic agent (e.g., streptokinase) in acute management, any complications during the acute period, length of Coronary Care Unit (CCU) and hospital stay. Examine old hospital records if available.
  - Inquire about further symptoms such as chest pains, arrhythmias or decreased effort tolerance following MI.
- Cardiac symptoms
  - Angina: quantify the frequency, severity, site, character, aggravating and relieving factors, bearing in mind that on-going myocardial ischaemia may be silent in patients with autonomic neuropathy.
  - Heart failure: elicit presence or history of pedal oedema, orthopnoea, paroxysmal nocturnal dyspnoea.
  - Symptomatic arrhythmias: elicit history of palpitations or syncope.

— Functional status
  - Effort tolerance specifies the amount of physical activity tolerated before symptoms of angina or cardiac insufficiency sets in but may not be accurate in the presence of significant pulmonary, orthopaedic or peripheral vascular disease.
  - The patient's functional status is commonly quantified according to the classifications proposed by the New York Heart Association (Table 12–1) or the Canadian Cardiovascular Society (Table 12–2).
  - Functional capacity can also be expressed in metabolic equivalent (MET) levels. One MET represents the oxygen consumption of a resting adult (3.5 ml/kg/min). Both perioperative cardiac and long-term risks are increased in patients who are unable to meet a 4-MET demand during most normal daily activities. (Table 12–3). These criteria are based largely on the Duke Activity Status Index (DASI), which comprises a simple 12-item yes/no questionnaire. Scoring the DASI involves multiplying a weighted score for each item then summing the results for the 12 items (see Appendix I).

Table 12–1. New York Heart Association (NYHA) functional classification

Class	Functional Status	One Year Mortality
Class I	No limitations of physical activity. No symptoms with ordinary exertion.	5–10%
Class II	Slight limitation of physical activity but comfortable at rest. Ordinary activity results in fatigue, palpitation, dyspnoea or angina.	10–15%
Class III	Marked limitation of physical activity. Less than ordinary activity leads to symptoms. Asymptomatic at rest.	15–20%
Class IV	Inability to carry on any physical activity without discomfort. Symptoms of cardiac insufficiency are present at rest. With any activity, increased discomfort is experienced.	20–50%

Table 12–2. Canadian Cardiovasular Society classification

Class	Functional Status
I	Ordinary physical activity, such as walking and climbing stairs, does not cause angina. Angina occurs with strenuous or rapid or prolonged exertion at work or recreation.
II	Slight limitation of ordinary activity. Angina occurs with walking or climbing stairs rapidly, walking uphill, walking or stair climbing after meals, or in cold, or in wind, or under emotional stress, or only during the few hours after awakening. Angina occurs when walking more than two blocks on the level or climbing more than one flight of ordinary stairs at a normal pace and in normal conditions.
III	Marked limitation of ordinary physical activity. Angina occurs with walking one or two blocks on the level and climbing one flight of stairs in normal conditions and at a normal pace.
IV	Inability to carry on any physical activity without discomfort. Angina may be present at rest.

Table 12–3. Estimated energy requirement for various activities from the Duke Activity Status Index

1–4 MET*	Take care of oneself (eat, dress or use the toilet) Do light work around the house (dusting or washing dishes) Walk indoors around the house Walk a block or two on level ground at 3–5 km/hr
5–9 MET*	Climb a flight of stairs or walk up a hill Walk on level ground at > 6 km/hr Run a short distance Do heavy work around the house (scrubbing floors or lifting heavy furniture) Participate in moderate recreational activities (golf, bowling, dancing, doubles tennis, throwing a baseball or football)
≥ 10 MET*	Participate in strenuous sports (e.g., swimming, singles tennis, football, basketball, skiing)

* Metabolic equivalent.

— Past and present treatment
  - Identify nature of medication; assess compliance and response to treatment.
  - Patient may also receive treatment for concomitant medical conditions such as hypertension, diabetes mellitus, hypercholesterolaemia and/or hyperuricaemia.
  - Patient may have implanted pacemaker or automatic implantable cardioverter-defibrillator (ICD).
  - Previous coronary revascularization in the form of coronary artery bypass graft (CABG) presents with an attenuated risk of cardiac events during subsequent non-cardiac surgery if the patient is asymptomatic and functionally active, and if the surgery is performed within 6 years post-CABG.
  - Percutaneous transluminal coronary angioplasty (PTCA) with intraluminal stenting is associated with an increased risk of stent thrombosis and infarction if surgery is performed within 6 weeks post-PTCA. Surgery should be deferred until 3 months later.

— Risk factor identification, with increased risks of perioperative morbidity/mortality associated with:
  - Demographics such as gender (male or post-menopausal female), age > 70 years.
  - Obesity.
  - Smoking.
  - Co-morbid conditions such as diabetes mellitus, hypertension, hypercholesterolaemia, peripheral vascular disease, renal dysfunction, chronic pulmonary disease, cerebrovascular disease.
  - Family history of CAD or cardiac death.

Physical Examination

— A thorough examination of the cardiovascular system is necessary even though no abnormal physical signs can be elicited in many patients.

— Features of significance include uncontrolled hypertension or cardiac arrhythmia, signs of heart failure (raised jugular venous pressure, oedema, hepatomegaly, cardiomegaly, pulmonary oedema), presence of sternotomy scar.

Investigations

— Routine investigations include full blood count, serum creatinine, urea and electrolyte concentrations, blood glucose concentration, 12-lead ECG and chest X-ray.

— Further investigations are indicated in these cases:
  - Patients with atypical symptoms which pose a problem to diagnosis.
  - Patients with symptoms of heart failure or frequent chest pains.
  - History of recent myocardial infarction (< 6 months).
  - Candidates for CABG or major surgery with significant haemodynamic disturbances.

— Echocardiography
  - This enables assessment of the chamber size, valve function, wall motion abnormalities and to estimate ejection fraction in a semi-quantitative manner.
  - Echocardiography can be done at rest, during exercise or under dobutamine stress.

— Exercise ECG
  - This test, an inexpensive and widely available method of screening for CAD, depends on the patient's exercising capability.
  - A positive stress test enables the physician to diagnose the presence of ischaemia and determine the workload at which ischaemia is present.
  - It may not be feasible if the patient has co-existing peripheral vascular disease (e.g., intermittent claudication) or orthopaedic problems, in which case pharmacologic stress test using dobutamine may be carried out.
  - Interpretation is also difficult in patients on β-blockers since the heart rate response is attenuated.

— Dipyridamole-thallium scintigraphy
  - This is a form of radionuclide scan in which thallium is taken up by viable myocardial cells as myocardial perfusion is increased with dipyridamole, a coronary vasodilator.
  - Infarcted areas remain as fixed defects whereas ischaemic myocardium appears as defects which are reversible on reperfusion later.

— Preoperative ambulatory ECG
  - The patient is put on a 24-hour Holter monitoring to detect the frequency and type of arrhythmias and/or periods of myocardial ischaemia.
  - High-risk patients may have baseline ECG abnormalities that preclude interpretation.

— Coronary angiography
  - This is the "gold standard" to quantify the cardiac status, delineate involvement of the coronary arteries and identify patients suitable for coronary revascularization.

- Due to its invasive nature which carries its own morbidity and mortality (0.03–0.25% and 0.01–0.05% respectively), this procedure is indicated only in unstable coronary syndromes, of uncertain stress tests in high-risk patients for major surgery, and in potential candidates for coronary revascularization.
- The optimal role of coronary revascularization prior to non-cardiac surgery is debatable, but patients with strong indications for CABG (e.g., left main stem, three-vessel, significant left anterior descending artery stenosis) should be recommended to do so before elective non-cardiac surgery.

Risk Stratification

Several risk indices have been developed on the basis of multivariate analyses, one of the earliest and most widely quoted index being the Goldman Multi-factorial Cardiac Risk Index (see Appendix II). However, formal scoring according to the risk indices is very rarely documented or used in clinical practice.

According to the American College of Cardiologists/American Heart Association (ACC/AHA) practice guidelines, these are clinical predictors of increased perioperative cardiovascular risk in terms of myocardial infarction, congestive heart failure or death.

1. **Major predictors**
   - Unstable coronary syndromes
     - Acute (within 7 days) or recent (7–30 days) myocardial infarction, presence of clinical symptoms or positive non-invasive study.
     - Unstable or severe angina (Canadian Class III or IV); or "stable" angina in patients who are unusually sedentary.
   - Decompensated heart failure.
   - Significant arrhythmias
     - High-grade atrioventricular block.
     - Symptomatic ventricular arrhythmias in the presence of underlying heart disease.
     - Supraventricular arrhythmias with uncontrolled ventricular rate.
   - Severe valvular disease.

2. **Intermediate predictors**
   - Mild angina (Canadian Class I or II).
   - Prior myocardial infarction by history or pathological Q waves on ECG.

- — Compensated or prior heart failure.
- — Diabetes mellitus (particularly insulin dependent).
- — Renal insufficiency.

3. **Minor predictors**
   - — Advanced age.
   - — Abnormal ECG (left ventricular hypertrophy, left bundle branch block, ST-T abnormalities).
   - — Rhythm other than sinus (e.g., atrial fibrillation).
   - — Low functional capacity (e.g., inability to climb a flight of stairs with a bag of groceries).
   - — History of stroke.
   - — Uncontrolled systemic hypertension.

The type of surgical procedure the patient is scheduled to undergo should be considered as it may also influence cardiac risk. They are stratified as:

1. **High-risk procedures** (cardiac complication rate > 5%): Emergent major surgery, particularly in the elderly; aortic and other major vascular surgery; peripheral vascular surgery; anticipated prolonged surgical procedures associated with large fluid shifts and/or blood loss.

2. **Intermediate risk procedures** (cardiac complication rate 1–5%): Carotid endarterectomy; head and neck surgery; intraperitoneal and intrathoracic surgery; orthopaedic surgery; prostatectomy.

3. **Low-risk procedures** (cardiac complication rate < 1%): Endoscopic procedures; superficial procedures; cataract surgery; breast surgery.

Based on preoperative cardiac evaluation and risk stratification, these options may be pertinent:

- — Defer surgery for further treatment including coronary revascularization if appropriate.
- — Forego elective surgery because of prohibitive risks.
- — Proceed with surgery, with modifications to surgery (shorter, less extensive or invasive surgical procedure), anaesthetic management (anaesthetic technique,

intraoperative monitoring and postoperative care) and location of care (inpatient rather than outpatient).

The risks of undergoing anaesthesia and surgery should be conveyed to the patient and family.

— **Mild CAD:** reassure and allay anxiety.
— **Moderate to severe CAD**
  - Explain anaesthetic risks to the patient and immediate family members.
  - Obtain high-risk consent.
  - Optimize medical treatment.
  - Discuss with the surgeon whether it is possible to limit the duration and extent of surgery.
  - Institute close perioperative monitoring in ICU, CCU or HDU.
  - Ensure early detection and aggressive treatment of haemodynamic disturbances.

Premedication

— Evidence for the prophylactic use of β-adrenergic antagonists to reduce myocardial ischaemia is compelling, and should be considered in all high-risk patients undergoing non-cardiac surgery. They should be started 2 weeks before surgery and continued in the postoperative period.
— The use of α_2-adrenoreceptor agonists, such as clonidine and dexmedetomidine, has also been advocated as they are shown to reduce perioperative mortality and myocardial ischaemia following cardiac and non-cardiac surgery.
— At this juncture, the recommendation is that perioperative β-blockade is indicated in all high-risk patients; α_2-agonists should be considered an alternative in those who cannot tolerate β-blockers.
— The patient's usual medication should be served on the morning of surgery. All cardiovascular drugs, except aspirin and perhaps diuretics, should be continued.
— The patient may bring along glyceryl trinitrate (GTN) tablets to the OT.
— It is desirable that the patient should be adequately sedated to avoid anxiety-induced hypertension and tachycardia. This should, however, be weighed against the risk of oversedation and respiratory depression.
— Premedication should be omitted in poor risk patients. Others should receive adequate premedication with night sedation and oral benzodiazepine prior to surgery.

INTRAOPERATIVE MANAGEMENT

Optimal anaesthetic management aims to achieve these.

— Maintain or improve myocardial oxygen supply versus demand ratio.
— Avoid extremes of blood pressure. Hypertension increases oxygen demand while hypotension reduces coronary perfusion pressure.
— Avoid tachycardia which decreases oxygen supply (by shortening diastole) and increases oxygen demand (by increasing myocardial work).
— Avoid a high preload which increases left ventricular end-diastolic pressure.
— Maintain adequate oxygen flux by optimizing cardiac output, haemoglobin and oxygen saturation.
— Avoid factors which may cause coronary vasospasm.

Monitoring

— Mandatory monitoring include ECG (CM_5 lead for detection of anterolateral myocardial ischaemia, and lead II for arrhythmia recognition and detection of inferior myocardial ischaemia), non-invasive BP, pulse oximetry, capnograph.
— When indicated, institute invasive haemodynamic monitoring (intraarterial BP, CVP, pulmonary artery pressure); also consider monitoring of urine output, temperature, neuromuscular blockade by means of peripheral nerve stimulator.

Anaesthetic Options

Considerable debate still remains over the advantages and disadvantages of regional compared to general anaesthesia for this category of patients. It appears that no clear-cut answer is forthcoming as no definitive study has proven that one approach is superior to the other. The “best technique” in any anaesthesiologist’s hand is very much dependent on his/her experience and expertise. Perhaps there is actually no “technique of choice” as long as the patient’s haemodynamic parameters are aggressively maintained. Perhaps the judicious combination of regional anaesthesia with light general anaesthesia is the key to the answer, even though large-scale studies have not demonstrated that combined regional and general anaesthesia offers any significant benefits either.

Regional anaesthesia

Advocates of regional anaesthesia contend that this technique causes a greater reduction in intraoperative stress responses. Thoracic epidural anaesthesia is postulated to convey additional benefits by blocking cardiac afferent and efferent fibres, thus preventing the unwanted effects of sympathetic stimulation (tachycardia, hypertension, increased myocardial oxygen consumption). It is also shown to cause coronary vasodilatation and improve global ventricular function, effects which are particularly relevant in patients with CAD.

The choice of any particular regional anaesthetic technique depends on the site, extent and duration of surgery. Certain techniques which allow catheter insertion have the additional advantage of providing effective postoperative analgesia. However, the anaesthesiologist should minimize sudden haemodynamic changes such as hypotension following sympathetic blockade, which may reduce coronary perfusion to a critical level.

These criteria must be met.

— The procedure must be explained to the patient who should be willing and co-operative; otherwise anxiety-induced tachycardia may obviate the advantages of the regional anaesthetic technique.
— Surgical anaesthesia provided by the regional block must be effective, otherwise alternative techniques of anaesthesia should be utilized. Do not allow surgery to carry on despite inadequate regional block and supplement with heavy sedation.
— The anaesthesiologist must be experienced with the technique – no learning to do blocks on such patients!
— The patient should be closely monitored at all times. Any haemodynamic disturbances should be treated early and aggressively.

General anaesthesia

The cardiovascular responses to noxious stimuli are exaggerated in such patients. The stress of tracheal intubation and emergence from anaesthesia in particular can result in unacceptably high levels of sympathetic stimulation, resulting in increases in heart rate, BP, myocardial contractility and left ventricular afterload. Our aim in anaesthesia is to obtund such responses and provide stable haemodynamic conditions during this period.

Many of the anaesthetic considerations are similar to the perioperative management of hypertensive patients. The reader is referred to Chapter 11 for further details. Only issues pertaining to anaesthesia and the ischaemic myocardium will be presented here.

— Choice of anaesthetic agents
- Anaesthetic agents which are cardiovascularly stable are preferred for obvious reasons.
- These include fentanyl, midazolam, etomidate, rocuronium, vecuronium.
- Thiopentone and propofol can be used in small titrating doses and are usually used in combination with opioid and/or midazolam.

— Volatile anaesthetic agents and myocardial ischaemia
- A series of reports published in the mid-1980s suggested that isoflurane may be capable of producing an abnormal redistribution of coronary blood flow away from ischaemic towards normal myocardium, the so-called "coronary steal" phenomenon. This was attributed to its coronary vasodilating properties which occur primarily in arterioles of less than 100 μm in diameter.
- This hypothesis was subsequently dispelled by several investigations conducted in animal models and humans with coronary artery disease.
- Since then many studies have convincingly shown that volatile anaesthetics *protect* the heart against ischaemia and reperfusion injury, limiting infarct size and improving functional recovery from myocardial ischaemia.
- Other advantages include coronary vasodilatation and afterload reduction by systemic vasodilatation.
- Isoflurane is now regarded as the anaesthetic agent of choice for patients with CAD.

Detection of Intraoperative Ischaemia

These monitoring devices are discussed in order of decreasing sensitivity.

— Transoesophageal echocardiography (TEE)
- TEE is the most sensitive monitor for detection of myocardial ischaemia.
- It is expensive, requires extensive training to ensure accurate interpretation, and is not freely available in locations other than the cardiac OT. The TEE probe is inserted in anaesthetized patients, hence is not available for monitoring during the crucial period at induction, and is not available for high-risk patients under regional anaesthesia.

  - Myocardial ischaemia is shown as diastolic dysfunction and/or regional wall motion abnormality. Mitral valve incompetence as a result of papillary muscle dysfunction may also be seen.
  - Development of myocardial ischaemia can result in "myocardial stunning" (continued decrease in contractile function despite resolution of ischaemia). This is manifested as persistent wall motion abnormalities on TEE even after ischaemia has resolved.

— Pulmonary capillary wedge pressure (PCWP)

  - Pulmonary artery (PA) catheterization is an invasive procedure and should be used only if the benefits derived justify the risk of complications.
  - It is not widely available and is only indicated for selected patients.
  - Myocardial ischaemia is manifested as an increase in PCWP even though this increase is not specific to ischaemia alone.
  - The sensitivity of PCWP changes for ischaemia detection is poor; but additional information derived from PA catheterization may guide fluid and vasopressor management.

— Electrocardiography

  - This method is simple, non-invasive and freely available. Computerized ST-segment trend analysis has become standard in modern monitors.
  - Diagnosis of myocardial ischaemia is focused mainly on ST-segment changes. Arrhythmias such as ventricular ectopics and ventricular tachycardia may also be of significance.
  - ECG changes have small sensitivity and specificity, with demonstrable changes occurring relatively late in the event of myocardial ischaemia.

— Other haemodynamic monitors (CVP, BP, heart rate) are neither sensitive nor specific in detecting myocardial ischaemia.

Management of Intraoperative Ischaemia

— Management of intraoperative ischaemia depends on the clinical scenario and possible underlying causes. A rational approach is shown in Figure 12–1.

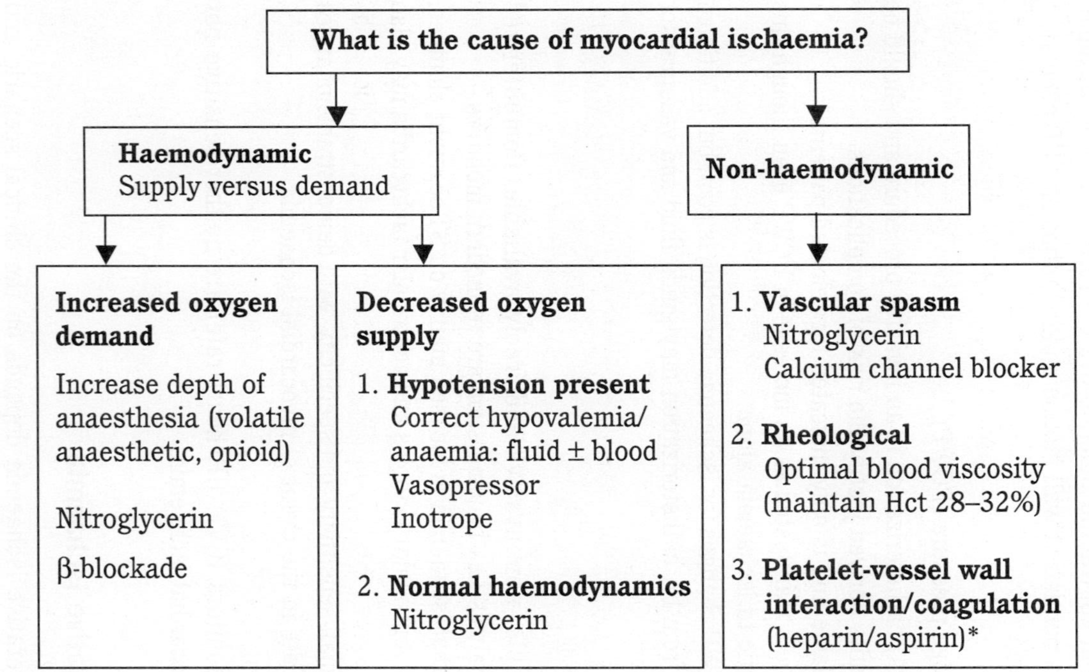

Figure 12–1. Management of intraoperative myocardial ischaemia

POSTOPERATIVE MANAGEMENT

— It must be realized that the occurrence of ischaemic events does not conclude with surgery or anaesthesia but persists with even greater frequency during the postoperative period.

— The highest risk for myocardial ischaemia was previously thought to occur on the third postoperative day. Recent studies have shown that this actually occurs on the day of surgery and the first postoperative day. Most cases of myocardial ischaemia are silent and only a small percentage of patients develop typical symptoms of angina, hence the importance of close monitoring and early aggressive treatment.

— Whether the patient is managed in ICU, CCU, HDU or general ward depends on these factors.

- Preoperative assessment of the patient's general condition and severity of cardiac disease.
- Nature, duration and complexity of surgery.
- Occurrence of significant intraoperative events.

— High-risk patients with unstable haemodynamic status require continued cardiovascular and ventilatory support in ICU.

— Continue close haemodynamic monitoring. Correct anaemia, hypoxia, hypovolaemia, acid-base and electrolyte imbalance as appropriate. Repeat 12-lead ECG and observe for fresh changes in ECG.

— Diagnosis of acute MI is based on history, ECG changes, a rise in the plasma creatinine kinase-MB fraction (CK-MB) or cardiac Troponin I concentration. The latter is by far the most specific marker of postoperative MI and its value is not influenced by muscle damage. The Troponin I concentration rises within 3 hours of myocardial necrosis and remains high 5–7 days thereafter.

— Optimal postoperative pain management is paramount to prevent the deleterious effects of sympathetic activation secondary to inadequate pain relief.

APPENDIX I

DUKE ACTIVITY STATUS INDEX

Each patient is asked if he/she can do the following. Answers are expressed as a YES (1 point) or NO (0 point) response. The points are then multiplied by the weight value for each question and a composite score obtained.

Activity	Weight
1. Can you take care of yourself, that is, eating, bathing or using the toilet?	2.75
2. Can you walk indoors, such as around your house?	1.75
3. Can you walk a block or two on level ground?	2.75
4. Can you climb a flight of stairs or walk up a hill?	5.50
5. Can you run a short distance?	8.00
6. Can you do light work around the house like dusting or washing dishes?	2.70
7. Can you do moderate work around the house like vacuuming, sweeping floors or carrying in groceries?	3.50
8. Can you do heavy work around the house like scrubbing floors or moving heavy furniture?	8.00
9. Can you do yardwork like raking leaves, weeding or pushing a power mower?	4.50
10. Can you have sexual relations?	5.25
11. Can you participate in moderate recreational activities like golf, bowling, dancing, doubles tennis or throwing a baseball or football?	6.00
12. Can you participate in strenuous sports like swimming, singles tennis, football, basketball or skiing?	7.50

APPENDIX II

GOLDMAN'S MULTI-FACTORIAL CARDIAC RISK INDEX

Variable	Point
1. History	
— Myocardial infarction within 6 months	10
— Age > 70 years old	
2. Physical examination	
— S_3 gallop rhythm or raised jugular venous pressure	11
— Severe aortic stenosis	
3. ECG	
— Rhythm other than sinus or premature atrial contractions	7
— Premature ventricular contractions, > 5/min at any time	7
4. General medical status	
— PaO_2 < 60 mmHg	
— $PaCO_2$ > 50 mmHg	
— Urea > 6.5 mmol/L	
— Potassium < 3.0 mmol/L	
— Bicarbonate < 20 mmol/L	
— Creatinine > 3.0 mg/dL	
— Abnormal serum aspartate aminotransferase	
— Chronic liver disease or patient bedridden	3
5. Surgery	
— Emergency	4
— Peritoneal or intrathoracic	3
Total possible points	**53**

Scoring

Class	Points	Morbidity	Mortality	Recommendations
I	0–5	0.7%	0.2%	Normal
II	6–12	5%	2%	Critical
III	13–25	11%	2%	Needs specific consult for cardiac problems
IV	> 26	22%	56%	Surgery not justified

FURTHER READING

1. Eagle KA, Berger PB, Calkins H, Chaitman BR, et al. ACC/AHA guideline update for perioperative cardiovascular evaluation for non-cardiac surgery: Executive summary. A report of the American Heart Association/American College of Cardiology Task Force on Practice Guidelines. Circulation 2002;105:1257–67.
2. Fleisher LA. Evaluation of the patient with cardiac disease undergoing noncardiac surgery: An update on the original AHA/ACC guidelines. Int Anesthesiol Clin 2002;40:109–120.
3. Chassot PG, Delabays A, Spahn DR. Preoperative evaluation of patients with, or at risk of, coronary artery disease undergoing non-cardiac surgery. Br J Anaesth 2002;89:747–59.
4. Davies SJ, Wilson RJT. Preoperative optimization of the high-risk surgical patient. Br J Anaesth 2004;93:121–8.
5. Mangano DT. Assessment of the patient with cardiac disease: An anesthesiologist's paradigm. Anesthesiology 1999;91:1521.
6. Warltier DC, Pagel PS, Kersten JR. Approaches in the prevention of perioperative myocardial ischemia. Anesthesiology 2000;92:253–9.
7. Auerbach AD, Goldman L. β-blockers and reduction of cardiac events in noncardiac surgery: JAMA 2002;287:1435–44.
8. Wijeysundera DN, Naik JS, Beattie WS. Alpha-2 adrenergic agonists to prevent perioperative cardiovascular complications: A meta-analysis. Am Med J 2003;114:742–52.

9. Katsuya T, Ludwig L, Kersten JR, Pagel PS, Warltier DC. Mechanisms of cardioprotection by volatile anesthetics. Anesthesiology 2004;100:707–21.
10. Agnew NM, Pennefather SH, Russell GN. Isoflurane and coronary heart disease. Anaesthesia 2002;57:338–47.
11. Toller WG, Kersten JR, Pagel PS, Waltier DC. Ischemic preconditioning, myocardial stunning and anesthesia. Curr Opin Anesthesiol 2000;13:35–40.
12. Mollhoff T, Theilmeier G, Van Aken H. Regional anaesthesia in patients at coronary risk for noncardiac and cardiac surgery. Curr Opin Anaesthesiol 2001;14:17–25.
13. Meissner A, Norbert R, Van Aken H. Thoracic epidural anesthesia and the patient with heart disease: Benefits, risks, and controversies. Anesth Analg 1997;85:517–28.
14. Fleisher LA. Real-time intraoperative monitoring of myocardial ischemia in noncardiac surgery. Anesthesiology 2000;92:1183–8.

Chapter 13

Anaesthesia in Valvular and Congenital Heart Diseases

INTRODUCTION

Patients with valvular or congenital heart diseases may present for any form of surgery, be it cardiac or non-cardiac. Their ages range from infancy to adulthood and the cardiac lesions may be uncorrected, palliated or totally corrected. These patients represent a spectrum from completely well patients with normal physiology to those with severely deranged physiology.

The lesion in valvular disease can be stenotic, or regurgitant, or mixed, and any of the four heart valves – mitral, aortic, tricuspid or pulmonary – may be involved. Even though many of the lesions are rheumatic in origin, a clear-cut history of acute rheumatic fever is not often obtainable.

Congenital heart lesion can be cyanotic or acyanotic, the common ones are listed here.

Acyanotic lesions
- Ventricular septal defect (VSD)*
- Atrial septal defect (ASD)*
- Patent ductus arteriosus (PDA)*
- Pulmonary stenosis
- Coarctation of aorta*
- Aortic stenosis
- Atrioventricular septal defect

Cyanotic lesions
- Tetralogy of Fallot (TOF)*
- Complete transposition of the great arteries
- Total anomalous pulmonary venous connection (TAPVD)
- Eisenmenger's syndrome*

Detailed descriptions of each valvular and congenital heart disease are beyond the scope of this book, and only the more common ones (*marked with asterisks*) will be highlighted. Optimal anaesthetic management entails an understanding of the pathophysiological changes associated with the cardiac defect, assessment of the patient's functional status and anticipation of the likely perioperative stresses.

ANAESTHETIC MANAGEMENT: GENERAL GUIDELINES

Preoperative Management

The information below should be elicited during preoperative assessment of the patient.

1. **History**
   - Age of onset of cardiac disease.
   - Past history suggestive of rheumatic fever.
   - Past history of surgical correction of cardiac defect and its details, including complications and immediate and/or long-term sequelae.
   - History of cyanosis or hypercyanotic spells, aggravating and relieving factors.
   - Effort tolerance and degree of physical impairment.
   - Symptoms of heart failure, angina, syncope.
   - Consequence of thromboembolic phenomenon, e.g., neurological deficit.

— Past and present treatment, compliance to medication.

2. **Physical examination**
   — General status: body size, pallor, polycythaemia, cyanosis, oedema, respiratory pattern.
   — BP: supine, sitting or standing.
   — Peripheral pulses: volume, rhythm, regularity, characteristics, delayed or absent pulses.
   — Heart size, characteristics of apex beat, heart sounds and murmurs.
   — Signs of heart failure: jugular venous pressure, fourth heart sound, peripheral oedema, hepatomegaly, acute pulmonary oedema.
   — Lung examination for reduced breath sounds, crepitations, rhonchi, signs of pleural effusion.
   — Evidence of previous cardiac surgery: sternotomy or thoracotomy scar.

3. **Investigations**
   — Full blood count.
   — Urea, creatinine, electrolyte concentrations.
   — 12-lead ECG.
   — Chest X-ray.
   — Coagulation screen if the patient is on anticoagulant therapy.
   — Further cardiac evaluations such as echocardiogram, coronary angiography as indicated.

4. **Preoperative preparation**
   — Consultation with the physician or cardiologist is essential and treatment should be optimized before surgery.
   — High-risk consent should be obtained if significant anaesthetic risks are involved. The anaesthetic options and postoperative management should be explained to the patient and/or immediate family.
   — Arrange for the patient to be managed in the intensive care unit (ICU), coronary care unit (CCU) or high dependency unit (HDU) as appropriate during the postoperative period.
   — Begin antibiotic prophylaxis for infective endocarditis in those patients at risk (*vide infra*).
   — Usual fasting guidelines apply. Commence intravenous maintenance fluids in patients with polycythaemia secondary to cyanotic heart disease to avoid the

risks of dehydration, hyperviscosity and thrombosis. Consider scheduling these patients early in the OT list to minimize the duration of fasting.

— Give clear instruction regarding the patient's medication – whether it should be served or omitted on the morning of surgery – and document this in the anaesthesia record.
— Premedication may be prescribed as appropriate based on the general condition of the patient and the nature of surgery.

5. **Endocarditis prophylaxis** (see Appendix)
   — Endocarditis is a serious illness associated with significant mortality.
   — It may develop in individuals with preexisting cardiac disorders who undergo procedures expected to produce bacteraemia with organisms likely to cause endocarditis.
   — Blood-borne bacteria may lodge on damaged or abnormal heart valves, endocardium or endothelium near anatomic defects.
   — These factors should be considered in endocarditis prophylaxis.
   - Type of underlying cardiac lesion.
     — High risk: prosthetic heart valves, past history of endocarditis, complex cyanotic congenital heart disease, surgically constructed systemic-pulmonary shunts.
     — Moderate risk: most other congenital cardiac malformation, acquired valvular dysfunction, hypertrophic cardiomyopathy, mitral valve prolapse with mitral regurgitation and/or thickened valve leaflets.
   - Type of procedure with apparent risk of bacteraemia.
   - Potential adverse reaction to the prophylactic antimicrobial agent to be used.
   - Cost-benefit aspects of recommended prophylaxis regimen.

Intraoperative Management

As in coronary artery disease, the preferred anaesthetic technique has long been a subject of debate. In general, the sicker the patient, the safer it is to choose general anaesthesia over regional anaesthesia, since the haemodynamic parameters as well as PaO_2, $PaCO_2$ can be more easily controlled under GA.

Our anaesthetic management should be geared towards achieving stable haemodynamics and avoiding changes that are known to be deleterious to the heart condition. Mandatory monitors include ECG, non-invasive BP, pulse oximetry and capnography.

Depending on the nature of the surgery and the condition of the patient, other monitors include intraarterial BP, CVP, pulmonary artery pressure, urine output, temperature and peripheral nerve stimulator. The monitors should preferably be established while the patient is awake in order to closely monitor the haemodynamic parameters during induction of anaesthesia. This may not always be feasible particularly in young fretful children.

Postoperative Management

Usual criteria for reversal of neuromuscular blockade and extubation apply. If the cardiac lesion is severe, the patient should be managed in ICU, CCU or HDU where the patient's cardiovascular system can be closely monitored. The patient should be reviewed and followed up by the physician or cardiologist during the perioperative period.

These are important aspects of management.

- Supplemental oxygen should be administered and the patient's oxygenation monitored by means of pulse oximetry and/or ABG samplings.
- Effective postoperative analgesia is essential to prevent pain-induced sympathetic activation. It also enables early chest physiotherapy to prevent lung atelectasis and retention of secretion, as well as early mobilization to reduce the risk of thromboembolism.
- Relevant investigations should be repeated and any abnormalities corrected. The fluid and electrolyte balance should be closely monitored. Blood transfusion is warranted if haematocrit is lower than 30%.

VALVULAR HEART DISEASE

Aortic Stenosis (AS)

Aortic stenosis may be congenital, resulting in calcification of the bicuspid or tricuspid aortic valve, or rheumatic in origin. The natural history of AS in the adult consists of a prolonged latent period of several decades with minimal morbidity and mortality. When symptoms of angina, syncope or heart failure develop, the outlook changes dramatically. Appearance of symptoms signifies critically severe narrowing of the aortic valve, and correlates well with mortality. The 50% mortality rates are reported at five years from the onset of angina, three years from the onset of syncope and two years from the onset of heart failure.

As a result of narrowing of the aortic valve, there is systolic pressure overload on the left ventricle (LV). This results in concentric LV hypertrophy with high LV systolic pressure which increases myocardial oxygen demand, and decreased LV compliance which results in poor LV filling during diastole. A decrease in LV compliance also results in significant elevation of LV end-diastolic pressure. This may reduce coronary perfusion pressure and myocardial oxygen supply giving rise to myocardial ischaemia.

Anaesthetic considerations

Anaesthesia for patients with AS carries a high risk of morbidity and mortality as indicated by the prominence it receives in Goldman's Multi-factorial Cardiac Risk Index. This is attributed to its fixed cardiac output state and its poor tolerance to significant haemodynamic changes during anaesthesia and surgery.

These are haemodynamic goals for optimal management.

1. **Heart rate and rhythm**
   - Maintain sinus rhythm: LA systole may contribute up to 40% to LV diastolic volume (instead of 15–20% in normal individuals).
   - Avoid tachycardia: this decreases myocardial oxygen supply, increases myocardial oxygen demand and worsens ischaemia.
   - Avoid bradycardia: cardiac output may be heart rate dependent since stroke volume is relatively fixed.

2. **Preload**
   - "Better full than empty" assuming good LV function, with adequate vascular access and sufficient volume loading.
   - Avoid central neuraxial blockade which results in sympathetic blockade causing vasodilatation and reduced preload.
   - Arteriolar vasodilators should be used judiciously, if at all, as they cause vasodilatation and reflex tachycardia.

3. **Afterload**
   - It is important to maintain afterload to ensure adequate coronary perfusion; hypotension is poorly tolerated since coronary blood flow decreases when diastolic pressure is reduced.
   - Early and aggressive treatment of hypotension with an alpha-agonist is imperative; phenylephrine may be used.

- Avoid vasodilators and central neuraxial blockade because of their deleterious effects on afterload.

4. **Contractility**
   - Maintain myocardial contractility.
   - Avoid myocardial depressant drugs.

General anaesthesia is preferred over regional anaesthesia since GA offers a better control of the intravascular volume status than RA. An opioid-based GA confers more haemodynamic stability than conventional GA using intravenous induction agents, nitrous oxide and volatile anaesthetic agents.

Mitral Stenosis (MS)

Mitral stenosis is almost always rheumatic in origin although a positive history of acute rheumatic fever is seldom obtained. This lesion may occur in conjunction with other cardiac valve involvement (e.g., aortic valve), or the mitral valve itself may be incompetent at the same time. Only 25% of patients present with pure MS.

The normal mitral valve area is 4–5 cm^2. Symptoms usually do not develop until the valve area becomes < 2.5 cm^2, while symptoms at rest occur when the mitral valve area decreases to < 1.5 cm^2. The first symptoms of dyspnoea are usually precipitated by exercise, emotional stress, pregnancy, intercurrent infection or atrial fibrillation with rapid ventricular response. Dyspnoea arises mainly from elevated LA pressures and volumes with pulmonary venous congestion rather than from reduced cardiac output itself.

Atrial fibrillation may develop secondary to atrial dilatation. Formation of LA thrombus with systemic thromboembolism may occur and may result in neurological deficits. The patient may be placed on long-term oral anticoagulant therapy.

As a result of narrowing of the mitral valve, there is diastolic pressure overload of LA while LV becomes pressure and volume underloaded. These changes can be observed.

- Volume overload of LA and pulmonary vasculature, with resultant LA enlargement and pulmonary congestion.
- Pulmonary hypertension.
- Right ventricular (RV) enlargement progressing to RV failure.
- Tricuspid incompetence.
- Atrial fibrillation.

Anaesthetic considerations

Other than the cardiac pathology *per se*, patients who are on oral anticoagulant therapy should be assessed and managed accordingly (see Chapter 23).

These are the haemodynamic goals.

1. Heart rate and rhythm
   — Maintain sinus rhythm, or control ventricular rate in atrial fibrillation.
   — Avoid tachycardia which shortens the time for blood flow across the stenotic mitral valve.

2. Preload should be "appropriately full", in order to prevent tachycardia secondary to hypovolaemia.

3. Afterload should be maintained, and increases in pulmonary vascular resistance should be avoided.

4. LV contractility should be maintained at normal or near normal, and RV failure should be treated if it occurs.

Aortic Regurgitation (AR)

The onset of aortic regurgitation may be acute or chronic. These exhibit different time course and symptomatology.

Acute AR, secondary to bacterial endocarditis, aortic dissection, connective tissue disorders or trauma, causes acute LV volume overload. There is insufficient time for compensatory mechanisms to develop, resulting in LV failure, pulmonary oedema, systemic hypoperfusion and heart failure. Mortality is high even with intensive medical management, and early surgical intervention is recommended.

Chronic AR, seen in rheumatic heart disease, hypertension and syphilis, has a long latent period where the patient is asymptomatic. As the disease progresses, recruitment of preload reserve and compensatory hypertrophy enable a normal LV ejection performance to be maintained. Onset of symptoms signifies exhaustion of the compensatory mechanisms of the LV. As a result of incompetent aortic valve, the LV is volume-overloaded during diastole. This gives rise to LV dilatation and eccentric hypertrophy, with large end-diastolic volume but normal end-diastolic pressure.

Anaesthetic considerations

1. Heart rate and rhythm
   - Avoid bradycardia since a slow heart rate increases regurgitant flow.
   - A modest degree of tachycardia may be beneficial because it decreases LV size, decreases regurgitant flow and augments forward flow.

2. Preload should be "appropriately full" except in acute AR where volume overload is prominent.

3. Afterload reduction may be beneficial. Avoid increases in afterload which increase regurgitant flow.

4. Contractility should be maintained and supported if there is evidence of LV dysfunction.

Mitral Regurgitation (MR)

As in the case of AR, mitral regurgitation may be acute or chronic. The causes of MR include:

- Rheumatic fever.
- Dilatation of mitral annulus secondary to LV dilatation.
- Mitral valve prolapse.
- Papillary muscle dysfunction secondary to ischaemia (acute MR).
- Rupture of chordae tendinae following myocardial infarction or trauma (acute MR).

Symptoms are associated with LV failure, resulting in weakness and easy fatigue. In acute MR, there is insufficient time for LA enlargement to develop. This causes acute increases in LA pressure, pulmonary venous pressure, acute pulmonary oedema and congestive heart failure.

Anaesthetic considerations

1. Heart rate and rhythm
   - Maintain sinus rhythm.
   - Maintain appropriate ventricular response rates when atrial fibrillation is present.

— Avoid bradycardia which increases regurgitant flow.

2. Preload should again be "appropriately full".

3. Afterload increases cause LV distension, ischaemia and failure. Hence slight reduction (without causing excessive hypotension) is beneficial.

4. Contractility should be maintained and inotropes should be started early in LV failure.

Mitral Valve Prolapse (MVP)

In this condition, the redundant mitral valve leaflet prolapses into the left atrium during closure of the mitral valve. The posterior valve leaflet is most commonly involved.

This condition may arise from an anatomical variation of a normal mitral valve, or may be associated with certain connective tissue disorders (e.g., Marfan's syndrome, Ehlers-Danlos' syndrome). In the older age group, it may arise from pathological changes in the chordae tendinae or mitral valve leaflets.

The patient is frequently asymptomatic or may complain of non-specific symptoms such as atypical chest pain, palpitations or dizziness. There is an increased risk of infective endocarditis with a small risk of systemic embolism.

Clinical examination may reveal a mid-systolic click with late systolic murmur. If gross mitral regurgitation occurs, then left atrial dilatation and left ventricular hypertrophy may be present. Atrial and ventricular arrhythmias may occur.

Anaesthetic considerations

1. Infective endocarditis prophylaxis is recommended for most patients with MVP, especially those with evidence of MR. This also includes patients with echocardiographic evidence of a higher-risk profile for endocarditis, such as thickening and/or redundancy of the valve leaflets, LA enlargement or LV dilatation.

2. The degree of prolapse is increased by factors that reduce ventricular volume thus accentuating redundancy of mitral valve leaflet, for example,
   — Increased myocardial contractility.
   — Decreased preload due to hypovolaemia or sympathetic blockade.
   — Tachycardia, which reduces time for ventricular filling.
   — High airway pressure produced by straining and coughing.

3. There may be unexpected atrial and ventricular arrhythmias. Occasionally ventricular fibrillation or profound bradycardia may occur. These should be treated accordingly.

Summary

— Sinus rhythm should be maintained if possible, or ventricular rates controlled in atrial fibrillation.
— Tachycardia may be beneficial in regurgitant lesions but not in stenotic lesions.
— Bradycardia is especially deleterious in AS.
— Preload and myocardial contractility should be maintained in all cases.
— Afterload reduction is beneficial in regurgitant lesions, but deleterious in AS.
— The haemodynamic parameters should be kept on the "straight and narrow" in AS where the safety margin is extremely small.

CONGENITAL HEART DISEASE

Ventricular Septal Defect (VSD)

This is one of the most common congenital cardiac lesions. Abnormalities in ventricular function can be expected in the uncorrected VSDs, and may be present even in corrected VSDs if the corrective surgery was performed later than the fifth year of life.

Blood flows from LV to RV across the defect and then to the pulmonary circulation. The direction of flow is from left to right. Chronic volume overload is associated with increased pulmonary blood flow and varying degrees of pulmonary arterial hypertension. Reversal of shunt occurs in severe cases, blood flows from right to left and results in development of Eisenmenger's syndrome.

Atrial Septal Defect (ASD)

Simple ostium secundum ASDs permit survival into late adulthood. The defect often goes undetected in early life because the patients are asymptomatic and clinical signs are subtle.

Atrial tachyarrhythmias, particularly atrial fibrillation, are more common in adulthood and are often the precipitating causes of heart failure. As in VSD, increased pulmonary blood flow may result in pulmonary artery hypertension and reversal of shunt in severe cases, giving rise to Eisenmenger's syndrome.

Patent Ductus Arteriosus (PDA)

In this condition, there is failure of closure of the duct connecting the pulmonary artery and the aorta. If the PDA is not surgically ligated, part of the blood from the aorta continues to be shunted to the pulmonary artery, increasing blood flow to the pulmonary circulation and eventually giving rise to pulmonary hypertension. If PDA ligation is done early in life, there are no surgical sequelae and such patients can be treated as normal individuals.

Coarctation of Aorta

Severe coarctation may present with heart failure in the first weeks of life, but most patients who live beyond infancy survive until adulthood. Mortality in such patients usually results from left ventricular failure, ruptured cerebral aneurysm or dissection of aorta from a postcoarctation aneurysm.

This condition is associated with increased incidence of hypertension and premature coronary artery disease. There may be a co-existing bicuspid aortic valve which may be normal, stenotic or incompetent but always susceptible to infective endocarditis. Mitral valve abnormalities may also be seen, of which about 20% are functionally significant.

Tetralogy of Fallot (TOF)

This is a cyanotic heart lesion consisting of right ventricular outlet obstruction (in the pulmonary valve or infundibular level), ventricular septal defect, overriding aorta and right ventricular hypertrophy.

Cyanosis develops as a result of reduced pulmonary blood flow secondary to RV outflow obstruction and right-to-left shunting across VSD. Cyanosis or desaturation is exaggerated ("hypercyanotic spells") in these situations.

- Increased pulmonary vascular resistance: airway obstruction, acidosis, crying.
- Reduced systemic vascular resistance: peripheral vasodilatation, hypovolaemia.
- Increased oxygen requirements: infection, sepsis.

Patients may present for surgery as uncorrected or fully corrected TOF. They may also present with a history of palliative surgery, in which an aorto-pulmonary shunt (e.g., Blalock-Taussig shunt) has been placed to increase pulmonary blood flow, but no complete reparative surgery has been done.

The perioperative course is relatively uncomplicated if the patient has had an adequate repair. For others, there may be significant haemodynamic or electrophysiologic sequelae such as right ventricular dysfunction or cardiac dysrhythmias. This contributes to problems in the anaesthetic management and increases the risks of perioperative morbidity.

Eisenmenger's Syndrome

This syndrome was originally designated for patients with non-restrictive VSDs, pulmonary vascular disease and reversed shunt. It has subsequently been extended to include any condition in which there is a communication between pulmonary and systemic circulation (at arterial, atrial or ventricular level) that produces pulmonary vascular disease of such severity that right-to-left shunting occurs.

There is decreased cross-sectional area of the pulmonary arteriolar bed with irreversible pulmonary hypertension. This is in contrast with Tetralogy of Fallot in which the pulmonary vascular bed is relatively oligaemic and "protected" by reduced pulmonary perfusion.

The degree of right-to-left shunting depends on the magnitude of pulmonary vascular resistance (PVR) and systemic vascular resistance (SVR). Factors which decrease SVR relative to PVR cause an increase in right-to-left shunting and a worsening of arterial hypoxaemia. Our anaesthetic management aims to reduce PVR while maintaining SVR in order to minimize right-to-left shunt.

ANAESTHETIC CONSIDERATIONS FOR CYANOTIC HEART DISEASE

In addition to the general guidelines, these should be considered.

1. **Hyperviscosity**
   - The patient is often polycythaemic as a result of chronic hypoxaemia; but this increase in oxygen carrying capacity achieved by an increase in haematocrit may be offset by its deleterious effects on blood flow and cardiac load.
   - Phlebotomy has been shown to reduce the thrombosis and bleeding complications but should be carried out with appropriate replacement of blood volume using crystalloid or colloid solutions.

— The hyperviscosity state may be worsened by preoperative fasting and fluid restriction; hence the patients should not be fasted for long periods. An intravenous infusion of maintenance fluid should be commenced in the ward if prolonged fasting is unavoidable.

2. **Infective endocarditis prophylaxis**
   — Appropriate antibiotics should be administered during the perioperative period for prophylaxis against infective endocarditis.
   — Orotracheal intubation is preferred to nasotracheal intubation to reduce the risks of bacteraemia and bleeding associated with the latter approach.

3. **Premedication**
   — Heavy premedication is usually well tolerated.
   — Adequate premedication reduces the incidence of crying and possibility of hypercyanotic spells in a child. It also enables the dose of induction agent to be kept to a minimum.

4. **Paradoxical air embolism**
   — Since blood flows from right to left across the shunt, any venous air embolus can pass across the shunt to the systemic circulation, resulting in paradoxical air embolism.
   — Meticulous care should be taken to avoid such hazard, by the anaesthesiologist while administering intravenous drugs and fluids, and by the surgeon when opening large veins or venous sinuses to minimize the risk of vascular air entrainment.

5. **Choice of anaesthetic technique**
   — General anaesthesia is preferable for such patients. Opioid-based anaesthesia may be more suitable than anaesthesia using inhalational agents.
   — Central neuraxial blockade, associated with sympathetic blockade and peripheral vasodilatation, would seem to be potentially hazardous. However, there have been case reports in the literature where epidural anaesthesia was employed without adverse effects or complications. Low-dose sequential combined spinal-epidural (CSE) is another regional anaesthetic technique which seems promising.

6. **Monitoring**
   — All patients should be monitored by means of ECG, non-invasive BP, pulse oximetry and capnography. The patient's initial oxygen saturation should be noted so that increasing desaturation can be detected and treated.
   — Arterial cannulation may be used for continuous measurement of blood pressure and for blood sampling.
   — Pulmonary artery (PA) catheterization is rarely indicated because the benefits derived do not justify the risks of catheter-related complications such as PA rupture, embolism or haemorrhage. Furthermore, the abnormal cardiac anatomy and flow dynamics can pose technical difficulties during flotation of the PA catheter.

7. **Induction of anaesthesia**
   — Intravenous induction occurs rapidly since the arm-brain circulation is shortened by the right-to-left shunt.
   — Barbiturates should be used with caution (if at all) because they cause a fall in blood pressure by depressing cardiac output and decreasing SVR. Ketamine is preferred because it maintains SVR.
   — Systemic hypotension, should it occur during induction, should be treated early with intravenous fluids and/or vasopressor.
   — Inhalational induction takes longer than in normal patients. Volatile anaesthetics should be used cautiously since they cause varying amounts of myocardial depression and reduction in SVR.

8. **Maintenance**
   — Nitrous oxide should be avoided because of these deleterious effects.
   - Decreasing the amount of oxygen delivered.
   - Myocardial depression.
   - Increasing pulmonary vascular resistance.
   - Worsening effects of air embolism.

   — If the occurrence of increasing cyanosis is attributable to infundibular spasm, this can be treated by using a β-blocker.

9. **Reversal of neuromuscular blockade and postoperative management**
   — These are according to the usual guidelines mentioned above.
   — Such patients should be managed in the ICU, CCU or HDU, with intensive

monitoring because significant morbidity and mortality may occur during the postoperative period.

HEART DISEASE IN PREGNANCY

— This deserves a special mention because heart disease continues to be an important cause of maternal death in many parts of the world.

— The anaesthesiologist is likely to encounter such pregnant cardiac patients at various stages of pregnancy, labour, delivery and postdelivery. Examples include anaesthesia for incidental surgery or termination of pregnancy, provision of labour epidural analgesia, anaesthesia for caesarean delivery or postpartum procedures, and resuscitation of such patients *in extremis*.

— Extensive physiological changes occur in the cardiovascular system during pregnancy. While these are well tolerated in healthy women, those with heart disease can decompensate, resulting in significant morbidity and mortality.

— Cardiac evaluation during pregnancy is notoriously difficult because many clinical features of normal pregnancy can mimic heart disease. Examples are dyspnoea, orthopnoea, peripheral oedema, tachycardia, distended jugular veins, displaced apex beat and ejection systolic murmur due to a hyperdynamic circulation.

— A wide range of cardiac conditions may be encountered during pregnancy. Prognosis depends on the specific cardiac condition, the patient's functional class and the degree of cardiac dysfunction during pregnancy. Peripartum cardiomyopathy is a condition of unknown aetiology that occurs in relation to pregnancy in women with no prior history of heart disease. Conditions that carry a grave prognosis include Eisenmenger's syndrome, primary and secondary pulmonary hypertension, complex cyanotic congenital heart disease, Marfan's syndrome with aortic root dissection, and severe LV dysfunction.

— A multi-disciplinary team approach consisting of cardiologist, obstetrician, anaesthesiologist and neonatologist, combined with early anaesthetic assessment and a carefully managed delivery are essential for optimal maternal and fetal outcome.

— Epidural analgesia during delivery is particularly useful in providing effective pain relief to minimize sympathetic stimulation during painful contractions. This option should be offered to all parturients provided contraindications to central neuraxial blockade have been excluded.

— The principles of anaesthetic management for surgical procedures are as outlined earlier. It seems prudent to opt for general anaesthesia for patients with fixed cardiac output states or elevated pulmonary arterial pressures, even though cases successfully managed under epidural anaesthesia or low-dose sequential CSE have been reported in the literature.

APPENDIX

SUGGESTED REGIME FOR ENDOCARDITIS PROPHYLAXIS

A. **For dental, oral, respiratory tract or oesophageal procedures**

- *Standard general prophylaxis:* oral amoxicillin 2 gm (adults); 50 mg/kg (children) 1 hour before the procedure.
- *Unable to take oral medications:* IV or IM ampicillin 2 gm (adults); 50 mg/kg (children) 30 minutes before the procedure.
- *On long-term penicillin or are allergic to penicillin:* clindamycin 600 mg (adults); 20 mg/kg (children) orally 1 hour before the procedure, or intravenously 30 minutes before the procedure.

B. **For genitourinary and non-oesophageal gastrointestinal procedures**

- *High-risk patients:* ampicillin plus gentamicin
  - IV or IM ampicillin 1 gm (adults); 50 mg/kg (children) *and* IV gentamicin 1.5 mg/kg (maximum 120 mg) 30 minutes before the procedure *plus*
  - IV or IM ampicillin 1 gm or oral amoxicillin 1 gm (adults); IV or IM ampicillin 25 mg/kg or oral amoxicillin 25 mg/kg (children) 6 hours later.
- *High-risk patients allergic to penicillin:* vancomycin plus gentamicin
  - IV vancomycin 1 gm (adults); 20 mg/kg (children) over 1–2 hours *and* IV gentamicin 1.5 mg/kg (maximum 120 mg), complete infusion 30 minutes before the procedure.
- *Moderate risk patients:* amoxicillin or ampicillin
  - oral amoxicillin 2 gm (adults); 50 mg/kg (children) 1 hour before the procedure *or*
  - IV or IM ampicillin 2 gm (adults); 50 mg/kg (children) 30 minutes before the procedure.
- *Moderate risk patients allergic to penicillin:* vancomycin
  - IV vancomycin 1 gm (adults); 20 mg/kg (children) over 1–2 hours complete infusion 30 minutes before the procedure.

FURTHER READING

1. Bonow RO, et al. ACC/AHA guidelines for the management of patients with valvular heart disease: Executive summary. A report of the American College of Cardiology/ American Heart Association Task Force on Practice Guidelines Circulation 1998;98:1949–84.
2. Lovell AT. Anaesthetic implications of grown-up congenital heart disease. Br J Anaesth 2004;93:129–39.
3. Vongpatanasin W, Brickner ME, Hills LD, Lange RA. The Eisenmenger's syndrome in adults. Ann Intern Med 1998;128:74–55.
4. Raines DE, Liberthson RR, Murray JR. Anesthetic management and outcome following noncardiac surgery in nonparturients with Eisenmenger's physiology. J Clin Anesth 1996;8:341–7.
5. Dajani AS, et al. Prevention of bacterial endocarditis: Recommendations by the American Heart Association. JAMA 1997;277:1794–801.
6. Weiss BM, Hess OM. Pulmonary vascular disease and pregnancy: Current controversies, management strategies, and perspectives. Eur Heart J 2000;21:104–115.
7. Tan JYL. Cardiovascular disease in pregnancy. Curr Obstet Gynaecol 2004;14: 155–65.

Chapter 14

Cardiac Pacemaker and Anaesthesia

INTRODUCTION

Cardiac pacemakers are usually implanted to treat symptomatic bradycardia, complete heart block and sick sinus syndrome. Current pacemakers are smaller, more dependable, longer lasting and have more adaptive features. Other devices such as implantable cardioverter-defibrillator (ICD) and ventricular assist device (VAD) have advanced pacing capabilities and can be life-saving.

The anaesthesiologist may have to anaesthetize a patient with a permanent pacemaker. It is thus important to have a basic understanding of the pacemaker in order to appreciate the likely problems and solutions during the perioperative period.

SOME INFORMATION ON PACEMAKERS

A pacemaker consists of three parts:

— Pulse generator: the energy source (battery) for both sensing and pacing functions.

— Lead: the insulated wire connecting the electrode and the generator.

— Electrode: the exposed metal at the tip of the lead that is in contact with the myocardium.

Pacing can be unipolar or bipolar. In unipolar pacing, the negative (stimulating) electrode is in the atrium or ventricle, and the positive (ground) electrode is distant from the heart, typically the metallic portion of the implanted generator. In bipolar pacing, both the electrodes are located at the heart chamber that is being paced. Bipolar pacing generally applies to temporary ventricular pacing.

The site of pacing can be either endocardial or epicardial. In the former, the lead/electrode system is passed through a vein to the right atrium or right ventricle. The pulse generator is usually located at the infraclavicular region. In epicardial pacing, the electrode is inserted through the epicardium into the myocardium. The pulse generator is usually located at the hypochondrium.

There are various systems of classifications for pacemakers. The North American Society of Pacing and Electrophysiology (NASPE) and the British Pacing and Electrophysiology Group (BPEG) initiated a generic code for describing pacemaker functions (Table 14–1). This is a five-letter system in which the first three letters describe the basic antibradycardia functions and the last two letters describe programmability and antitachycardia functions. Clinically, the first three letters are often used alone if the pacemaker has no designated additional features.

The commonest pacemaker mode is VVI, whereby the pacing and sensing activities occur in the ventricle, and the pulse generator is inhibited each time the patient's own impulse is detected by the generator. Physiological pacemakers are rate-adaptive or dual-chamber devices. The former have motion sensors that can result in increased basal heart rate, while the latter have programmable atrioventricular (AV) delays. Claimed advantages of dual-chamber pacemakers include preservation of AV synchrony and maintenance of normal ventricular activation in patients with intact AV conduction, improved cardiac output and decrease in pacemaker syndrome.

Table 14–1. NASPE/BPEG Generic (NBG) pacemaker code

Position	**I**	**II**	**III**	**IV**	**V**
Category	**Chamber(s) Paced**	**Chamber(s) Sensed**	**Response to Sensing**	**Programmability or Rate Modulation**	**Antitachycardia Functions**
	0 = None	0 = None	0 = None	0 = None	0 = None
	A = Atrium	A = Atrium	T = Triggered	P = Simple programmable	P = Pacing
	V = Ventricle	V = Ventricle	I = Inhibited	M = Multi-programmable	S = Shock
	D = Dual (A + V)	D = Dual (A + V)	D = Dual (T + I)	C = Communicating R = Rate modulation	D = Dual (P + S)
	D = Dual (A + V)	D = Dual (A + V)	D = Dual (T + I)		D = Dual (P + S)

ANAESTHETIC CONSIDERATIONS

These factors are of particular concern to the anaesthesiologist.

— The nature and severity of the underlying cardiac condition which necessitated pacemaker insertion should be thoroughly assessed and given due consideration during anaesthetic management.

— The pacemaker function should be evaluated preoperatively to ensure that it is functioning properly.

— Interference with the proper working of the pacemaker may originate from extrinsic (electromagnetic interference) or intrinsic (electrolytes, drugs, myopotentials from exercise, shivering, fasciculation following suxamethonium) sources. This may affect the stimulation threshold, alter the programming in the pacemaker, or change the mode of the pacemaker from demand (synchronous) to fixed rate (asynchronous).

ANAESTHETIC MANAGEMENT

Preoperative Evaluation

Besides the routine assessment, one needs to evaluate both the pacemaker function and the cardiac condition that necessitated pacemaker insertion. The patient should also be reviewed by the cardiologist.

1. **History:** The following information should be elicited.
   — Indication, type and time of pacemaker insertion: lifespan for lithium-powered pulse generator is at least 5 years.
   — Rate at pacemaker insertion: a pacemaker rate of 10% below the preset rate is indication for generator replacement.
   — Return of prepacemaker symptoms of syncope, palpitations, chest pain, congestive heart failure
   - Consider pacemaker malfunction unless proven otherwise.
   - May be due to myopotentials inhibiting the pacemaker impulse if symptoms occur during exercise.

2. **Physical examination**
   — Palpate for the rate and regularity of peripheral pulse: present rate should not be more than 10% below the preset pacemaker rate.

- While palpating the pulse, check the ECG for
  - Frequency of paced beats: whether there is any intrinsic cardiac rhythm or if the patient is pacemaker dependent.
  - One-to-one capture: each paced beat should correspond to a pulse.
- It may be necessary to slow down the patient's intrinsic rate to check for pacemaker function. Valsalva manoeuvre is preferred to carotid massage as the latter has the potential to dislodge atheromatous plaque from the carotid artery into the cerebral circulation.

3. **Investigations:** These should be reviewed in addition to routine investigations.
   - Chest X-ray for position of the pulse generator, integrity of the leads, electrode tip position, heart size and pulmonary vasculature.
   - Serum electrolyte concentration, especially potassium.

Intraoperative Management

The theatre environment is potentially hazardous for patients with pacemakers. Any of these factors can cause the pacemaker to malfunction.

- Drugs.
- Physiological changes during anaesthesia and surgery.
- Electrical equipment: electrocautery, monitors, defibrillators.

Electrocautery, in particular, poses additional problems to the patient. Besides its potential to interfere with pacemaker function, it may also interfere with monitoring devices making it difficult to observe the patient's cardiovascular status just when it is most needed.

The application of a magnet above the pulse generator converts most pacemakers from demand mode to fixed or asynchronous mode. This renders the pacemaker less susceptible to electrical interference, but makes some pacemakers more vulnerable to reprogramming by external stimuli. Various responses may be elicited in different pacemakers depending on manufacturer and model; hence it is advisable to confirm magnet behaviour from the manufacturer before its use.

Generally, basic antibradycardia modes must be preserved in the perioperative period, but rate-adaptive modes, antiarrhythmia therapies and other complex features should be disabled. These modes can be reactivated and reprogrammed postoperatively.

Discuss with the surgeon the problems of electrocautery interfering with the pacemaker function and whether its use can be avoided altogether. If this were not feasible, a bipolar would be preferable to a unipolar diathermy.

Take these precautions if a unipolar diathermy is to be used.

- Place the ground plate as far away from the pacemaker generator as possible in a position that will ensure current flow does not traverse the chest.
- Use the lowest effective energy output.
- Minimize diathermy to short bursts of 1–2 seconds duration.
- Monitor pacemaker output at all times by observing the ECG, blood pressure, and keeping a finger on the patient's pulse.
- Keep isoprenaline available to start an infusion if pacemaker output fails.
- Keep an emergency transvenous pacing kit available if this becomes a necessity.

Practical Recommendations

- Antibiotics for infective endocarditis prophylaxis are indicated.
- Apply the pads for transcutaneous pacing on the patient. Note that its efficacy is highly dependent on electrode position and the chest wall thickness. If this is in doubt it is advisable to have a temporary transvenous pacing wire inserted before the procedure.
- Prepare atropine and isoprenaline infusion. Isoprenaline should be used with caution. It has potent inotropic and chronotropic properties, increases myocardial oxygen consumption and may precipitate myocardial ischaemia. In the event of pacemaker failure, isoprenaline should be used as a temporizing measure before transcutaneous pacing is activated.
- Establish monitoring before induction of anaesthesia. If pulmonary artery catheterization is strongly indicated, PA catheter should be inserted with caution in the presence of a pacemaker with endocardial electrode especially if this has been inserted less than 4–8 weeks ago.
- Essentially all standard anaesthetic techniques can be used for induction and maintenance of anaesthesia. One should be aware that induction of anaesthesia might depress cardiac conduction and result in the triggering of a previously inhibited pacemaker.
- Avoid the use of suxamethonium if possible since suxamethonium-induced fasciculations may inhibit pacemaker output.

— Avoid hypercarbia and hypoxaemia as these predispose to ventricular ectopics or tachyarrhythmias, which may result in competition between the intrinsic rhythm and the pacemaker.

— Avoid shivering by maintaining normothermia.

— Isoflurane is preferred over halothane since the latter can raise the stimulation threshold and lead to loss of capture.

— If pacemaker malfunction occurs
  - Ensure normal oxygenation and ventilation.
  - Begin cardiopulmonary resuscitation if the intrinsic heart rate is too slow to maintain cardiac output and if the pacemaker is unable to pace the heart within 10 seconds.
  - Infuse isoprenaline at 1–3 μg/min to increase the ventricular rate and decrease the pacemaker threshold.
  - Activate transcutaneous pacing.
  - Consider the possibility of an acute myocardial infarction, with the electrode in the infarcted area resulting in loss of capture.

— If the patient needs to be defibrillated
  - Place the paddles at least 12 cm away from the pacemaker generator.
  - The pacemaker is likely to be destroyed if the energy exceeds 400 J.
  - Immediately establish emergency temporary pacing if the pacemaker no longer functions after the shock.

Postoperative Management

The patient should be closely monitored in HDU and reviewed by the cardiologist. The pacemaker function – settings and thresholds – should be checked especially if electrical devices have been used.

OTHER DEVICES

1. Implantable cardioverter-defibrillators (ICDs)
   — These are devices which sense and abort arrhythmias (VTs/VFs) that may cause sudden death and are useful in patients with coronary artery disease, low ejection fraction and a history of ventricular arrhythmia.
   — As in the case of pacemakers, the major intraoperative concern for ICD is the risk of electromagnetic interference from electrocautery.

- The ICD should be reprogrammed to suspend arrhythmia detection before the use of diathermy but only after the patient is in the OT and is fully monitored; it should be reactivated before leaving the OT.
- Facilities for external defibrillation should be available immediately after the device is disabled.

2. Left ventricular assist devices (LVADs)
   - These are *not* pacemakers but devices which take over the functions of the damaged ventricle to restore normal haemodynamics and end-organ blood flow.
   - They function as mechanical pumps that collect blood returning to the heart and eject it downstream of the failing ventricle.
   - They are used either as an interim measure to recovery (short- or intermediate-term LVADs), or while awaiting heart transplantation (long-term LVADs).
   - The patient may be on long-term anticoagulant therapy with warfarin, which should be converted to intravenous heparin therapy before elective surgery. Heparin should be discontinued during the immediate preoperative period and resumed when the risk of postoperative bleeding has diminished. Newer devices are generally maintained with chronic aspirin therapy alone, and excess perioperative bleeding may require platelet transfusion to obtain adequate haemostasis.
   - Once the patient has arrived in the OT it is prudent to convert the battery-powered LVAD to an alternating current power source in order to secure a reliable power supply to assure its continuous operation.
   - The potential for electromagnetic interference with LVAD function by external defibrillation or electrocautery should be recognized and steps taken to minimize the risk.
   - The pump function of LVAD depends on both filling volume and outflow resistance; hence it is critically important to maintain adequate preload and avoid increase in afterload.

FURTHER READING

1. Salukhe TV, Dob D, Sutton R. Pacemakers and defibrillators: Anaesthetic implications. Br J Anaesth 2004;93:95–104.
2. Bourke ME. Healey JS. Pacemakers, recent directions and developments. Curr Opin Anaesthesiol 2002;15:681–6.

3. Bourke ME. The patient with a pacemaker or related device. Can J Anaesth 1996;43:R24–32.
4. Deroy R, Graham TR. Pacemakers and anaesthesia. Curr Anaesth Crit Care 1995;6:171–9.
5. Kam PCA. Anaesthetic management of a patient with an automatic implantable cardioverter defibrillator *in situ.* Br J Anaesth 1997;78:102–6.
6. Stone ME, Soong W, Krol M, Reich DL. The anesthetic considerations in patients with ventricular assist devices presenting for noncardiac surgery: A review of eight cases. Anesth Analg 2002;95:42–9.
7. Nicolosi AC, Pagel PS. Perioperative considerations in the patient with a left ventricular assist device. Anesthesiology 2003;98:565–70.

Chapter 15

Respiratory Disease and Anaesthesia

INTRODUCTION

Anaesthesia causes profound changes in respiratory function. Such changes are magnified in patients with preexisting pulmonary diseases who are at increased risk of developing intra- and postoperative respiratory complications. Postoperative pulmonary complications occur as frequently as cardiac complications; these include atelectasis, pneumonia, bronchospasm, acute exacerbation of underlying chronic lung disease and respiratory failure with the need for mechanical ventilation.

Our objectives in the preoperative assessment of these patients are 3-fold.

— Recognition of the underlying chronic pulmonary disease.
— Assessment of the patient's functional reserve.
— Treatment of any reversible acute problems.

Intraoperative anaesthetic management includes these aspects.

— Selection of the anaesthetic technique least likely to interfere with pulmonary function.
— Close monitoring of the patient's ventilation and oxygenation, ensuring normocarbia and adequate oxygenation.
— Prompt recognition and treatment of any intraoperative adverse events, such as bronchospasm, hypoxaemia, inability to ventilate.

Postoperative management is no less important. These aspects are essential.

— Supplemental oxygen and/or ventilatory support.
— Adequate postoperative analgesia.
— Regular chest physiotherapy and breathing exercises.
— Early diagnosis and aggressive treatment of pulmonary complications.

PULMONARY RISK FACTORS

These risk factors are associated with increased postoperative respiratory morbidity.

— Preexisting pulmonary disease
  - Risk increases with poor lung function tests of < 50% predicted value, low PaO_2 (< 50 mmHg), high $PaCO_2$ (> 60 mmHg).

— Age > 70 years
  - Pulmonary complications are more strongly related to the increase in prevalence of pulmonary disease than to chronological age *per se.*
  - Increase in closing capacity which may be greater than functional residual capacity predisposes to airway closure and atelectasis even in normal individuals.

— Smoking
  - Smoking increases risk even among those without chronic pulmonary disease.
  - Increased airway irritability predisposes to bronchospasm.
  - Decreased mucociliary action reduces ability to clear secretions.

    - Increased bronchial secretions predispose to sputum retention and atelectasis.
    - Smoking is also associated with an increased prevalence of chronic obstructive pulmonary disease (COPD).
- Surgical factors
    - The surgical site is the most important predictor of pulmonary risk.
    - Thoracic and upper abdominal surgery results in diaphragmatic dysfunction and restrictive ventilatory defect.
    - Vertical incisions are worse than horizontal ones.
    - Other factors include prolonged general anaesthesia (> 3 hours) and emergency surgery particularly in a patient with sepsis.
- Obesity
    - This is associated with decreased chest wall compliance, decreased functional residual capacity and increased work of breathing, more so in morbid obesity with Pickwickian syndrome.
    - Despite a common assumption that obesity increases the risk of pulmonary complications, most studies have found no such association.
- Other contributing factors
    - Other contributing factors include ineffective postoperative pain relief, residual effects of anaesthetics and incomplete reversal of neuromuscular blockade.

TYPES OF RESPIRATORY DISEASE

Chronic respiratory diseases are broadly classified into two main groups: obstructive and restrictive. Acute exacerbations of the chronic lung disorder may be brought about by respiratory infection, air pollutant, industrial exposure or allergens (in asthma). These acute insults may tip the patient into acute respiratory failure.

1. **Obstructive respiratory disease:** characterized by narrowing of the conducting airways, as in
    - Asthma, in which reversible bronchospasm occurs.
    - Chronic bronchitis and emphysema, generally termed COPD.

    The pathology in COPD varies from partially reversible obstruction with excessive mucus secretion, to irreversible airway collapse during expiration.

    Typical pulmonary function test results show
    - decreased FEV_1 (forced expiratory volume in 1 second)
    - decreased FVC (forced vital capacity)
    - decreased FEV_1/FVC ratio

2. **Restrictive respiratory disease:** characterized by reduction in lung volumes, as in:
   - Abnormalities of the alveolar-capillary membrane, e.g., pulmonary fibrosis, pulmonary oedema.
   - Abnormalities of respiratory muscle function, e.g., myasthenia gravis, poliomyelitis, muscular dystrophy.
   - Extrinsic compression on the lung parenchyma, e.g., obesity, kyphoscoliosis, pleural effusion, intrathoracic masses.

   Typical pulmonary function test results show
   - decreased FEV_1
   - decreased FVC
   - normal or slightly increased FEV_1/FVC ratio

3. **Acute respiratory dysfunction:** actually a mixed bag of conditions which may cause respiratory embarrassment during the perioperative period. Examples include respiratory tract infection, chest injuries with lung contusion, airway obstruction, pulmonary oedema, acute respiratory distress syndrome (ARDS).

ASTHMA

Asthma is a reactive airway disorder characterized by increased airway responsiveness to chemical, pharmacological and physical stimuli, resulting in reversible bronchoconstriction and airway obstruction.

Preoperative Assessment

1. **History**
   - Elicit details of the disease, such as age of onset, frequency, severity, triggering and relieving factors, past history of hospital admission or need for respiratory support, past and current medications, and compliance to treatment.
   - Enquire about history of atopy and known allergies to food or drug.
   - Determine whether there are cough, sputum or symptoms of intercurrent infection.

2. **Physical examination**
   - Assess the general condition of the patient: colour, posture, respiratory rate and

pattern, ability to speak in complete sentences, audible wheeze, tachycardia, sweating, chest movement, use of accessory muscles of respiration.
- Auscultate the chest for breath sounds, prolonged expiratory phase, rhonchi or crepitations.
- In severe cases, look for presence of cyanosis, pulsus paradoxus, silent chest, pneumothorax.
- Check the patient's peak expiratory flow rate (PEFR) at the bedside.

3. **Investigations**
   - Arterial blood gas (ABG) analysis is rarely indicated as a routine evaluation in asthmatics in remission; but may be useful as baseline reading for patients with severe respiratory dysfunction.
   - Lung function test is done in selected patients to assess the severity of airway constriction and its reversibility in response to bronchodilator therapy.
   - The value of chest X-ray is questionable in young asthmatics in remission. It may be indicated in the presence of infection and if pneumothorax is clinically suspected.

4. **Premedication**
   - The patient's usual medication should be served on the morning of surgery.
   - Nebulized bronchodilator (terbutaline or salbutamol) may be given 1 hour before surgery.
   - Frequent users of metered-dose inhalers should bring these to the OT.
   - Prescribe oral benzodiazepine for night sedation and premedication.
   - Use pethidine rather than morphine if an opioid premedication is indicated.

The asthmatic patient can be broadly classified as:
- **Mild asthma:** very infrequent attacks, not on regular medication. No problem with anaesthesia as long as precautions are taken not to induce bronchospasm.
- **Asthma in remission:** on regular medication but currently asymptomatic.
  - Continue usual medication on morning of surgery.
  - Watch out for acute exacerbation intra- and postoperatively.
- **Asthma in acute exacerbation:** postpone elective surgery. For emergency surgery
  - Initiate bronchodilator therapy preoperatively.
  - Select anaesthetic drugs with bronchodilator properties, such as ketamine, volatile anaesthetics.

- Continue bronchodilator therapy in OT and postoperatively.
- Consider postoperative ICU management for severe cases.

Intraoperative Management

Anaesthetic techniques

— Regional anaesthesia in the form of central neuraxial blockade or peripheral nerve block is the anaesthetic technique of choice wherever feasible.

— If general anaesthesia is indicated, use of face mask or airway adjunct (e.g., laryngeal mask airway) is preferable to endotracheal intubation.

— If general anaesthesia with endotracheal intubation and IPPV is necessary, steps must be taken not to provoke bronchospasm during airway manipulation.

Choice of anaesthetic agent

A proper anaesthetic technique is more important in preventing bronchospasm than choice of anaesthetic agent *per se*.

1. **Intravenous induction agents**

   — Thiopentone is not contraindicated in an asthmatic in remission as it does not precipitate bronchospasm. However, because it only provides a light plane of anaesthesia, laryngo- or bronchospasm may be triggered during airway instrumentation under thiopentone anaesthesia alone.

   — Ketamine has bronchodilator properties and is useful in patients with acute exacerbation of asthma undergoing emergency surgery.

   — Propofol depresses airway reflexes to a greater extent than thiopentone and hence may be advantageous in asthma.

   — IV lignocaine 1–2 mg/kg may be used to attenuate reflex bronchoconstriction during airway manipulation. The intravenous route is preferred over lignocaine spray onto the upper airway structures, which in itself may trigger airway reaction.

2. **Volatile anaesthetics**

   — All currently available volatile anaesthetics demonstrate smooth muscle relaxation *in vitro*; but desflurane may cause airway irritation *in vivo* which renders it less suitable for use in reactive airway disease. Halothane, enflurane,

isoflurane and sevoflurane are equally effective in preventing and attenuating reflex bronchoconstriction in equi-MAC doses.
— Halothane has the drawback of arrhythmogenicity especially in the presence of hypercarbia and toxic plasma aminophylline concentrations. Its use has been superceded by other volatile anaesthetics which are non-arrhythmogenic.

3. **Neuromuscular blocking drugs**
   — Older agents such as curare and alcuronium are known to release histamine; drugs with minimal histamine release include vecuronium and rocuronium.
   — Atracurium is known to release histamine even though most manifestations are cutaneous rather than respiratory. This effect has not been seen with cisatracurium.
   — Reversal of neuromuscular blockade with anticholinesterases may give rise to increases in secretion, bronchial tone and reactivity. This should be borne in mind although these effects are partially antagonized by co-administration of atropine or glycopyrrolate.

Management of Intraoperative Bronchospasm (See Chapter 65)

It is important to realize that not all wheezes point to asthma. Other causes of bronchospasm (e.g., mechanical problems involving the endotracheal tube or breathing system, aspiration, anaphylaxis, pneumothorax) should be excluded before the bronchospasm is attributed to an acute exacerbation of asthma.

1. **Mild cases**
   — Ensure adequate oxygenation and ventilation.
   — Manual ventilation to assess compliance.
   — Increase depth of anaesthesia with volatile anaesthetic and/or propofol.

2. **If *not* resolved**
   — Increase FiO_2 if oxygenation is compromised.
   — Administer bronchodilator, e.g., salbutamol via endotracheal tube or intravenously.
   — Consider use of inhaled corticosteroid or ipratropium bromide.
   — IV adrenaline 0.1 mg (1 ml of 1:10,000 solution) or ketamine may be used in refractory cases.

- Reassess patient and recheck for other causes of bronchospasm.
- Continue bronchodilator treatment until bronchospasm resolves.

Recovery and Postoperative Management

- The timing of reversal of neuromuscular blockade and extubation is often tricky. As far as possible, one should strive for early extubation to prevent the patient from coughing and gagging on the endotracheal tube, a potent stimulus for bronchospasm. This should be balanced against the risk of aspiration if extubation is done before airway reflexes have completely returned. In a patient with full stomach or increased risk of aspiration, it is more prudent to remove the endotracheal tube when the patient is fully awake.
- An additional dose of IV lignocaine 1–2 mg/kg may be administered prior to extubation in an effort to prevent reflex bronchoconstriction.
- The patient should be given supplemental oxygen and closely monitored in PACU during the immediate postoperative period.
- Patients who are comfortable with no evidence of respiratory difficulty can be managed in the ward. Severe cases may require ICU or HDU admission.
- Bronchodilator therapy, chest physiotherapy and breathing exercises should be carried out and any postoperative bronchospasm should be treated accordingly.

CHRONIC OBSTRUCTIVE PULMONARY DISEASE

The prevalence of chronic obstructive pulmonary disease (COPD) increases with age and is strongly associated with cigarette smoking. Many of the patients are asymptomatic or mildly symptomatic, the course of the disease being punctuated by acute exacerbations precipitated by lung infections, changes in ambient temperature or air pollutants.

Traditionally, cases of COPD have been categorized into either chronic bronchitis or emphysema. Many patients, however, present with features of both diseases. Hence chronic bronchitis and emphysema can be regarded as two ends of the disease spectrum, while features of both diseases can be found anywhere in between.

1. **Chronic bronchitis:** A *clinical* diagnosis defined by the presence of a productive cough on most days of 3 consecutive months for at least 2 consecutive years.
2. **Emphysema:** A *pathologic* diagnosis based on irreversible enlargement of the airway distal to the terminal bronchioles. The alveolar septae are destroyed.

The features of both diseases are summarized in Table 15–1.

Table 15–1. Features of chronic obstructive pulmonary disease

Feature	Chronic Bronchitis	Emphysema
	(*"Blue bloaters"*)	(*"Pink puffers"*)
Cough	Frequent	With exertion
Sputum	Copious	Scanty
Elastic recoil	Normal	Decreased
Airway resistance	Increased	Normal or slightly increased
Cor pulmonale	Early feature	Late feature
Haematocrit	Increased	Normal
PaO_2 (mmHg)	Usually < 60	Usually > 60
$PaCO_2$ (mmHg)	Often elevated > 40	Usually < 40
Chest X-ray	Increased lung markings	Hyperinflation

Anaesthetic Management

As with asthmatics, these patients should be optimally prepared before elective surgery. Preoperative preparation includes these actions.

- Cessation of smoking.
- Treatment of underlying chest infection, in which the choice of antibiotics is based on sputum culture and sensitivity.
- Treatment of reversible component of bronchoconstriction using bronchodilators.
- Chest physiotherapy and breathing exercises: postural drainage, incentive spirometry.
- Treatment of associated cor pulmonale and right heart failure.
- Oxygen therapy if indicated.
- Relevant tests in addition to routine investigations: FBC, CXR, lung function test, ABG.

Unlike asthmatics, only limited improvement in respiratory function may be seen in patients with COPD after such preparation since most of the components of the disease conditions are irreversible. However, postoperative respiratory complications have been shown to be significantly reduced with preoperative optimization of such patients.

High-risk cases are those with these features.

— Dyspnoea at rest.
— Cyanosis.
— Cor pulmonale.
— Preoperative pulmonary function test < 50% of predicted value.
— Hypoxaemia with CO_2 retention.

The high anaesthetic risks should be conveyed to the patient and relatives, and postoperative ventilation in ICU planned beforehand.

The selection of anaesthetic technique, the anaesthetic agents employed and intraoperative management of the patient with COPD are similar to those concerning the asthmatic patient. These points should be noted.

— Preoxygenation is essential prior to induction of general anaesthesia as this prevents rapid desaturation during airway instrumentation.
— There may be enhanced respiratory depression from anaesthetic agents especially in moderate to severe cases of COPD. Nitrous oxide should be used with caution and should be avoided in patients with large bullae and significant pulmonary hypertension.
— Anaesthetic gases should be humidified in prolonged surgery. This prevents bronchial secretion from being inspissated and difficult to remove.
— Intraoperative bronchospasm may only be partially reversed by bronchodilators since only the reversible component of airflow obstruction responds to bronchodilator therapy.
— Pressure-controlled ventilation is the preferred mode of ventilation, with a slow respiratory rate and a long inspiratory to expiratory ratio (I:E ratio) to avoid air trapping and provide sufficient time for expiration to occur. This may result in hypercapnia which is usually well tolerated (permissive hypercapnia).
— The gradient between end-tidal and arterial PCO_2 is increased by an unpredictable amount; hence serial ABGs are required to measure $PaCO_2$. Ventilatory parameters and FiO_2 should be adjusted accordingly.
— In emphysematous patients, the substantial dead space, ventilation-perfusion inequality and air trapping may prolong the effects of residual anaesthetic gases and delay emergence.

— Patients with poor respiratory function should be electively ventilated post-operatively, while those with borderline respiratory function should be observed in the ICU or HDU. Only those patients with mild form of COPD should be managed in the general ward. As a guide,
- preoperative normal PaO_2 and $PaCO_2$: provide general supportive therapy
- preoperative decreased PaO_2 with normal $PaCO_2$: provide oxygen therapy
- preoperative decreased PaO_2 with increased $PaCO_2$: provide ventilatory support

RESTRICTIVE RESPIRATORY DISEASE

Restrictive respiratory diseases are characterized by reduction in lung volume and vital capacity while the expiratory flow rates are relatively normal. As a result, the work of breathing is increased and the patient typically breathes in a rapid and shallow fashion.

Anaesthetic Management

Preoperative assessment and preparation of the patient follow similar procedures described above. Patients with acute pulmonary oedema and acute respiratory distress syndrome may be acutely ill and require intensive therapy before the planned surgery. Given the side-effects of general anaesthesia with endotracheal intubation, regional anaesthesia would appear to be the technique of choice in appropriate cases.

These factors are pertinent.

— Close haemodynamic monitoring is essential for acutely ill patients.

— High inspired oxygen concentration and positive end-expiratory pressure (PEEP) may be required to achieve adequate oxygenation.

— High peak inspiratory airway pressures with risks of barotrauma may complicate ventilation as a result of decreased lung compliance. This can be minimized by using small tidal volumes (6 ml/kg) and high respiratory rates (16 breaths/min or more).

RESPIRATORY TRACT INFECTION

When a patient presents with symptoms of respiratory tract infection, the anaesthesiologist is often faced with the dilemma of whether to "pass" the patient, often a child, for surgery or to defer surgery until later.

The term "upper respiratory tract infection" or URTI should be discarded in favour of "respiratory tract infection" or RTI, since the pathology involves the *whole* respiratory tract, from the nose down to the alveoli. Changes include reductions in FEV_1, FVC and VC, increase in bronchial reactivity and sensitized airway receptors. These effects last for up to 6 weeks following the acute infection.

The anaesthesiologist may be faced with these problems.

— Increased inflammation, secretions and oedema of the nasal mucosa, pharynx and larynx causing nasal obstruction and an irritable airway.

— Systemic effects of pyrexia, myalgia, malaise, toxaemia.

— Possibility of a viral toxaemia causing a pancarditis.

— Increased incidence of perioperative respiratory complications such as stridor, laryngo- or bronchospasm, breath-holding, coughing, retention of secretions with atelectasis.

Recommendations

1. ***Each patient should be** assessed individually. **No "blanket ruling" is possible or advisable.***
2. **Elective surgery**
   — It is reasonable to proceed with minor surgery if the RTI is mild and not associated with systemic effects or evidence of lung involvement.

   — These cases should be postponed.
   - Moderate to severe RTI.
   - Presence of systemic symptoms, such as fever, chills, rigors, malaise, myalgia.
   - Preexisting pulmonary disease such as asthma, COPD.
   - Patients at the extremes of age.
   - Major surgery, or surgery involving the airway.
   - Procedures requiring tracheal intubation.

   — Ideally such cases should be deferred for 4–6 weeks after the respiratory symptoms have subsided. This may not be possible in every case as some patients may have frequent RTIs. Each patient should be considered individually.
3. **Emergency or urgent surgery**
   — If the procedure does not require tracheal intubation, the patient can be

maintained on spontaneous ventilation via a face mask. However, this technique is often not feasible in emergency situations in the presence of full stomach.
- Although the role of laryngeal mask airway in RTIs has not been properly defined, the use of a supraglottic airway device is expected to be associated with a lower incidence of airway complications compared with tracheal intubation.
- If tracheal intubation is indicated, steps must be taken to avoid airway complications, and to promptly treat them if they arise.
- Should bronchospasm and/or desaturation occur, administer a higher inspired oxygen concentration, commence bronchodilator therapy and suction through the endotracheal tube to clear the bronchial secretions.
- The patient should be extubated awake and given supplemental oxygen postoperatively. Postoperative analgesia and chest physiotherapy are important aspects of management.

SMOKING AND ANAESTHESIA

These are some adverse effects of smoking.

- Increased blood concentration of carboxyhaemoglobin, which reduces oxygen binding to haemoglobin and compromises oxygen availability at the tissue level.
- Increases in heart rate and blood pressure; peripheral vasoconstriction caused by nicotine.
- Hypersecretion of mucus, impairment of tracheobronchial clearance and small airway narrowing, with greater tendency to develop bronchospasm, atelectasis and hypoxaemia.
- Impaired immune response, affecting both humoral and cell-mediated immunity.
- Increased perioperative analgesic requirements.

Tobacco smoking is an identifiable risk factor for perioperative pulmonary complications. Patients who smoke should be encouraged to stop smoking at least 6–8 weeks before scheduled surgery. However, a smoke-free interval of 6 weeks or less is insufficient to reduce pulmonary morbidity and may paradoxically increase postoperative pulmonary complications. At the very least, smoking should not be permitted 12–24 hours before surgery. This short-term abstinence helps to reduce nicotine and carboxyhaemoglobin concentrations, improve oxygen content and availability, and reverse the adverse cardiovascular effects of smoking.

FURTHER READING

1. Warner DO. Preventing postoperative pulmonary complications: The role of the anesthesiologist. Anesthesiology 2000;92:1467–72.
2. Zollinger A, Hofer CK, Pasch T. Preoperative pulmonary evaluation: Facts and myths. Curr Opin Anaesthesiol 2001;14:59–63.
3. Smetana GW. Current concepts: Preoperative pulmonary evaluation. New Engl J Med 1999;340:937–44.
4. Groeben H. Strategies in the patient with compromised respiratory function. Best Prac Res Clin Anaesthesiol 2004;18:579–94.
5. Wong DO, Warner MA, Barnes RD, Offord KP, et al. Perioperative respiratory complications in patients with asthma. Anesthesiology 1996;85:460–7.
6. Grichnik KP, Hill SE. The perioperative management of patients with severe emphysema. J Cardiothorac Vasc Anesth 2003;17:364–87.
7. Seigne PW, Hartigan PM, Body SC. Anesthetic considerations for patients with severe emphysematous lung disease. Int Anesthesiol Clin 2000;38:1–23.
8. Akrawi W, Benumof JL. A pathophysiological basis for informed preoperative smoking cessation counseling. J Cardiothorac Vasc Anesth 1997;11:629–40.
9. Zwissler B. Should smokers stop smoking preoperatively – and if so, when? Curr Opin Anaesthesiol 2002;15:53–5.

Chapter 16

Anaesthesia and Renal Disease

INTRODUCTION

Chronic renal disease exists in various grades of severity: decreased renal reserve, renal insufficiency and renal failure. Current laboratory tests of renal function are neither sensitive nor specific enough to detect changes in the early stage of the disease process, while some may be impractical to perform on a routine clinical basis. A patient with decreased renal reserve seems normal except for a decrease in glomerular filtration rate (GFR) even though only 40% of the total nephrons are functioning. Renal failure with overt signs of uraemia sets in when over 90% of the total nephrons are destroyed. This is a progressive, irreversible deterioration of renal function resulting from a variety of disease and may be acute, chronic or acute-on-chronic.

Patients with preexisting renal disease have an increased likelihood of developing renal failure in the postoperative period, particularly after cardiac or aortic surgery. Anaesthesia affects the renal system in these aspects.

— The majority of anaesthetic agents cause a decrease in renal blood flow and hence GFR. This is well tolerated in healthy patients but may be critical in patients with renal insufficiency or established renal failure.
— The pharmacokinetics of renally excreted drugs and anaesthetic agents are altered in the presence of renal disease. Overdosage and/or drug toxicity may result if the dose is not adjusted accordingly.
— Multiple organ systems are involved in the disease process in renal failure. This poses additional problems and increases the anaesthetic risk during the perioperative period.
— Any perioperative factor that predisposes to renal ischaemia exposes the kidney to postoperative renal dysfunction. Perioperative acute renal failure (ARF) contributes significantly to postoperative mortality and should be diagnosed early and treated aggressively.

PREOPERATIVE ASSESSMENT

Preoperative evaluation is aimed at determining the extent of the disease in terms of renal function and the involvement of other organs and their functions, and at evaluating the risk of developing postoperative ARF.

These are manifestations of renal failure.

— Cardiovascular system: hypertension, coronary artery disease, congestive cardiac failure, pericarditis, pericardial effusion, cerebrovascular disease.
— Respiratory system: pneumonitis, pleural effusion.
— Acid-base and electrolytes: metabolic acidosis, electrolyte imbalance (hyperkalaemia, hypocalcaemia, hypermagnesaemia, hyponatraemia).
— Haematological system: normocytic normochromic anaemia, white blood cell/platelet dysfunction, uraemic coagulopathy, hypoalbuminaemia.
— Gastrointestinal system: nausea, vomiting, delayed gastric emptying, gastric hyperacidity.
— Neurological system: uraemic encephalopathy, peripheral or autonomic neuropathy.
— Musculoskeletal system: secondary and tertiary hyperparathyroidism, osteodystrophy, pathological fractures.

Baseline investigations include FBC, blood glucose, urea, electrolytes and creatinine concentrations, ECG, CXR and coagulation screen. Additional investigations should be ordered if necessary.

Blood

- The patient may be on recombinant human erythropoietin therapy to increase red cell synthesis.
- A lower haemoglobin concentration (down to 6 g/dl) may be accepted, and blood transfusion is only indicated if
  - The patient is symptomatic.
  - The haemoglobin level is precariously low or associated with clinical features of heart failure.
  - The patient is scheduled to undergo a major surgery with anticipation of massive blood loss.
  - The patient has concomitant illness such as severe cardiac or pulmonary disease.
- Transfuse blood during dialysis to avoid fluid overload.
- Use washed red blood cells if the patient is a potential renal transplant recipient.

Dialysis

- The patient may be on regular haemodialysis or peritoneal dialysis.
- Haemodialysis is usually done during the 24 hours preceding elective surgery. Send blood for laboratory tests (FBC, blood glucose, urea, electrolytes and creatinine concentrations) after dialysis and review the results when available.
- Peritoneal dialysis can be continued until just before surgery. The dialysate should be drained prior to surgery for optimal respiratory function.

Premedication

- The patient's medication, including antihypertensive drugs, should be continued.
- Premedication should be individualized according to the patient's general status. Opioid or benzodiazepine may be prescribed in reduced doses.
- Consider acid aspiration prophylaxis using antacid and H_2 receptor antagonist such as ranitidine.

INTRAOPERATIVE MANAGEMENT

Monitoring

— This includes ECG, non-invasive blood pressure, pulse oximetry, capnography, peripheral nerve stimulator, urine output via an indwelling urinary catheter.

— Central venous cannulation and CVP monitoring may be required to guide fluid management.

— Arterial cannulation should be avoided unless absolutely indicated, in which case the dorsalis pedis or femoral artery should be cannulated. Arteries in the upper extremity may be required for placement of arteriovenous fistula (AVF) in future.

— Take special precaution not to place the blood pressure cuff or perform intravenous cannulation on the arm with AVF. This should be carefully protected to ensure its continued patency during the perioperative period.

Anaesthetic Technique

— General anaesthesia with endotracheal intubation and IPPV are often employed.

— Brachial plexus block is a useful anaesthetic technique for placement of AVF.

— Regional anaesthesia, central neuraxial blockade in particular, should not be undertaken in the presence of coagulopathy.

— Note that metabolic acidosis may lower seizure threshold for local anaesthetics.

Induction of Anaesthesia

— Any of the commonly used intravenous induction agents may be used but should be administered in small titrated doses.

— Suxamethonium should be avoided if serum potassium concentration is in the high normal range, because drug-induced potassium release may result in dangerous hyperkalaemia. There is no contraindication to its use if the baseline serum potassium concentration is normal.

— Sympathetic responses during laryngoscopy and intubation should be attenuated by means of IV lignocaine or esmolol.

Maintenance of Anaesthesia

- Anaesthesia is often maintained with nitrous oxide combined with volatile anaesthetic agent and supplemented with opioid and neuromuscular blocking drug.
- Atracurium is the preferred neuromuscular blocking drug since it does not depend on the kidney for metabolism and excretion. This is also true for cisatracurium. Regardless of the drug selected, it is prudent to monitor the degree of neuromuscular blockade by means of a peripheral nerve stimulator.
- Isoflurane is the volatile anaesthetic of choice. The position of sevoflurane in renal disease is less clear. Compound A, formed from degradation of sevoflurane, has been shown to cause dose-related tubular necrosis in rats. However, no evidence of nephrotoxicity has been demonstrated in clinical studies.
- Analgesia is provided by regional blockade if applicable, or by means of parenteral opioids such as fentanyl and morphine. Opioids have prolonged action in renal failure.
- It is important to maintain stable haemodynamic parameters to ensure adequate renal perfusion.
- Careful monitoring of intravascular volume status is necessary to prevent fluid under- or overloading.
- Ringer's lactate solution should not be used in anuric patients because of its potassium content.

"Renal Protection" (See Chapter 73)

- This is indicated for high-risk patients undergoing major surgery such as aortic, cardiac surgery.
- Nephrotoxic drugs such as aminoglycosides, non-steroidal antiinflammatory drugs (NSAIDs) should be avoided.
- Drugs which may confer "renal protection" include mannitol and frusemide. There is no evidence to support the efficacy of "renal dose" dopamine in preventing ARF in high-risk patients or to ameliorate the clinical course in established ARF.

Reversal of Neuromuscular Blockade

— The duration of action of neostigmine is prolonged in renal failure. This is useful especially when the older neuromuscular blocking drugs (e.g., curare) are used, as it lessens the problem associated with recurarization.

— Usual criteria for reversal of neuromuscular blockade and tracheal extubation apply.

POSTOPERATIVE MANAGEMENT

— The cardiovascular system, fluid, electrolyte and acid-base status as well as urine output should be closely monitored.

— Postoperative analgesia may be provided by opioids in titrated doses or in the form of intravenous patient-controlled analgesia. Analgesia using local anaesthetic and/or opioid may be continued in patients who underwent regional anaesthetic block with indwelling catheter. NSAIDs should be avoided in such patients.

— Haemodialysis may be necessary if renal function worsens or if pulmonary oedema or hyperkalaemia becomes a problem. The patient should be jointly managed by a nephrologist.

FURTHER READING

1. Cronin DF, Shorten GD. Anesthesia and renal disease. Curr Opin Anaesthesiol 2002;15:359–63.
2. Sandovnikoff N. Perioperative acute renal failure. Int Anesthesiol Clin 2001;39:95–109.
3. Sladen RN. Anesthetic considerations for the patient with renal failure. Anesthesiol Clin N Am 2000;18:863–82.
4. Byers J, Sladen RN. Renal function and dysfunction. Curr Opin Anaesthesiol 2001;14:699–706.
5. DeBellis RJ, Smith BS, Cawley PA, Burniske GM. Drug dosing in critically ill patients with renal failure: A pharmacokinetic approach. J Intens Care Med 2000;15:273–313.

Chapter 17

Anaesthesia for Patients with Liver Disease

INTRODUCTION

Diseases of the liver and biliary tract can be categorized into parenchymal liver disease (e.g., acute and chronic hepatitis, liver cirrhosis) and cholestasis with or without obstruction to the extrahepatic biliary tree. Patients with liver disease may present for surgery unrelated to the underlying disorder. They may also undergo surgical procedures related to the liver disease, such as control of bleeding oesophageal varices by means of variceal banding, ligation, or sclerotherapy, porto-systemic shunting, as well as liver transplantation and liver resection.

Patients with significant liver disease, especially acute parenchymal liver disease, carry a substantial risk for surgery and anaesthesia. Liver and renal failure, postoperative bleeding and sepsis are common causes of poor operative outcome. These patients should not be considered for any elective surgery until their condition can be brought under control. However, they may present with upper GIT bleed or acute abdomen for emergency surgery. The surgical and anaesthetic risks should be weighed carefully against the potential benefits, and such risks should be conveyed to the patient and immediate family.

CLINICAL MANIFESTATIONS

Cirrhosis of the liver occurs as a result of a variety of chronic progressive liver diseases, which are most commonly due to excessive alcohol ingestion or chronic viral hepatitis. The patient with liver cirrhosis exemplifies the multi-system nature of chronic liver disease even though the clinical features differ from those with chronic hepatitis. The clinical manifestations of liver cirrhosis are listed here.

— Central nervous system
  - Hepatic encephalopathy of various grades, ranging from mild somnolence to coma with decorticate or decerebrate posturing.
  - Mental obtundation, asterixis, fetor hepaticus.
  - Cerebral oedema, raised ICP.

— Cardiovascular system
  - Systemic arteriovenous shunts with reduced peripheral resistance.
  - Hyperdynamic circulation with high cardiac output state leading to heart failure (late stage).
  - Cardiomyopathy presenting as congestive heart failure, typically seen in alcoholic cirrhosis.
  - Portopulmonary syndrome: right ventricular failure secondary to severe portal and pulmonary hypertension.

— Respiratory system
  - Hepatopulmonary syndrome: decreased PaO_2 due to intrapulmonary shunting, in 0.5–4% patients.
  - Decreased functional residual capacity, ventilation-perfusion (V/Q) mismatch, pleural effusion.
  - Frequent lung infection in the form of bacterial pneumonia, lung abscess, aspiration pneumonitis.

— Renal system
  - Decreased renal perfusion and GFR.
  - Toxic or ischaemic tubular necrosis.
  - Hepatorenal syndrome, a functional renal failure which carries a grave prognosis.

— Gastrointestinal system
  - Portal hypertension, giving rise to ascites, gastro-oesophageal varices, gastrointestinal bleeding, haemorrhoids.
  - Spontaneous bacterial peritonitis.
  - Associated duodenal ulcer disease, gallstones, cholangitis.
  - Increased tendency for regurgitation.

— Haematological system
  - Anaemia from gastrointestinal bleeding and/or malnutrition.
  - Coagulopathy due to decreased synthesis of clotting factors.
  - Hypersplenism with thrombocytopaenia, leukopaenia.

— Metabolism and immunity
  - Hypoglycaemia secondary to glycogen depletion and impaired gluconeogenesis.
  - Electrolyte imbalance with dilutional hyponatraemia and hypokalaemia aggravated by vomiting, diarrhoea and diuretics.
  - Metabolic acidosis from lactate accumulation.
  - Accumulation of ammonia giving rise to hepatic encephalopathy.
  - Hypoalbuminaemia from reduced synthesis.
  - Decreased pseudocholinesterase production.
  - Altered drug pharmacokinetics.
  - Impaired host-defence mechanisms.

SURGICAL RISK ACCORDING TO SEVERITY OF LIVER DISEASE

In 1964, Child and Turcotte proposed a system of classification to assess the risk of porto-systemic shunting operations in cirrhotic patients. They empirically selected five parameters (serum albumin, serum bilirubin, ascites, encephalopathy, and nutritional status) to which they attributed one of three risk levels, and assigned the composite to one of three classes. In 1972, Pugh modified the Child-Turcotte classification by substituting prothrombin time in place of nutritional status, thereby obviating the most subjective element in the classification (Table 17–1). Although not formally evaluated for its statistical accuracy, the classification has been used to assess the outcome of any form of interventional therapy, including stratifying patients on the waiting list for liver transplantation.

Poor outcomes are likely when cirrhotic patients require major surgical interventions, emergency surgery, care after trauma and treatment in which renal failure is a complicating factor.

Table 17–1. Child-Turcotte-Pugh classification of liver disease

Variables	1	2	3
Encephalopathy	None	Drowsy	Stuporous, comatose
Ascites	Absent	Moderate	Marked
Total bilirubin (µmol/L)	< 25	25–40	> 40
Albumin (g/L)	> 35	30–35	< 30
Prothrombin time (seconds prolonged)	1–4	4–6	> 6

Total score	**Surgical risk**	**Mortality (%)**
5–6	low	5
7–9	moderate risk	10
10–15	high	> 50

ANAESTHETIC MANAGEMENT

The patient should be thoroughly assessed in view of the multi-system nature of liver disease. Treatment should be optimized as much as possible before subjecting the patient for surgery. Elective surgery should be deferred in patients with acute liver disease, such as acute hepatitis, until the patient has recovered from the episode.

1. *Initial assessment* is important. In addition to clinical assessment, preoperative laboratory investigations are necessary.
   - FBC: anaemia and thrombocytopaenia may require preoperative correction if severe.
   - Coagulation screen: prothrombin time is a good marker for liver function (it is one of the Child-Turcotte-Pugh criteria). Consider administering Vitamin K and/or fresh frozen plasma if coagulation is deranged.
   - Blood glucose concentration: hypoglycaemia is a possibility and may require infusion of glucose-containing solution perioperatively.
   - Creatinine and electrolyte concentrations, urinalysis to assess renal function: urea may be falsely low because of decreased production.
   - ABG to assess the severity of arterial hypoxaemia and serve as a baseline reading.

- Liver function test: note that the tests are often normal until the liver is considerably diseased, as a result of large functional reserve in the liver.
  - Albumin, bilirubin are markers of overall liver function.
  - Liver transaminases are sensitive to even mild liver disease but are non-specific.
  - Alkaline phosphatase is increased with biliary obstruction.
- Other tests: hepatitis screening, α-fetoprotein (marker for hepatoma), ultrasound or endoscopic retrograde cholangio-pancreatoscopy (ERCP) for obstructive jaundice.

2. *Initial resuscitation* while preparing the patient for emergency surgery is important. Assess the patient for the associated systemic disorders outlined above and treat accordingly.
   - Insert wide-bore intravenous cannulae for fluid resuscitation.
   - Group and cross-match blood and blood products in preparation for surgery.
   - Establish monitoring consisting of invasive blood pressure and central venous pressure, urine output via indwelling urinary catheter to guide fluid resuscitation.
   - Obtain high-risk consent from the patient and family.
   - Admit to ICU for perioperative management.
   - Administer acid aspiration prophylaxis as the risk of regurgitation is high.

3. *Anaesthetic technique* depends on the general status of the patient and the site and extent of surgery.
   - Central neural blockade is contraindicated in the presence of coagulopathy.
   - General anaesthesia with rapid sequence induction and intubation is often indicated in emergency situations.
   - Reduce the dose of anaesthetic agents in the presence of hepatic encephalopathy or cardiovascular compromise.
   - Significant ascites results in increased intraabdominal pressure, decreased functional residual capacity, increased work of breathing and possible risks of regurgitation, aspiration and hypoxaemia. The appropriate anaesthetic technique in this case is general anaesthesia with rapid sequence induction and intubation followed by muscle paralysis and controlled ventilation.

4. Drug dosing is influenced by *altered drug pharmacokinetics*, for example:
   - Increase in volume of distribution results in the need for larger initial doses

of non-depolarizing neuromuscular blocking drugs to produce neuromuscular blockade, but the duration of action may be prolonged if these drugs depend on hepatic clearance.
- Reduced protein binding results in a larger proportion of pharmacologically active free drug, with potential for relative overdosage if the usual dose is administered.
- Reduced synthesis of certain enzymes such as pseudocholinesterase entails caution in the use of suxamethonium and mivacurium as the action may be prolonged.
- Reduced metabolism and excretion of drugs result in accumulation and increased duration of action.

5. *Drug choices* in liver disease
   - Avoid drugs that rely on the liver for metabolism and/or excretion.
   - Intravenous induction agent: thiopentone or propofol may be used in reduced dose. Ketamine is suitable in hypotensive patients.
   - Neuromuscular blocking drugs: atracurium and cisatracurium are preferred because of their non-hepatic metabolism. Suxamethonium and mivacurium are not contraindicated provided allowance is made for prolonged duration of action.
   - Volatile anaesthetic agent: isoflurane, sevoflurane or desflurane may be used. Halothane should be avoided in view of its marked effect on hepatic blood flow reduction and its potential for hepatotoxicity ("halothane hepatitis").
   - Opioid analgesic: remifentanil is safe in liver disease; fentanyl, pethidine and morphine should be used with caution.

6. The extent of *intraoperative monitoring* again depends on the severity of the liver disease, the general status of the patient and the nature of the surgery.
   - ECG, non-invasive blood pressure, pulse oximetry, capnography are mandatory.
   - Invasive pressures: intraarterial BP, CVP.
   - Urine output via indwelling urinary catheter.
   - Others: peripheral nerve stimulator, temperature, blood sampling for ABG, haematocrit, electrolytes and glucose measurement.

7. Anaesthetic concerns during *intraoperative management*
   - Universal precaution is especially important since patients with liver disease are potentially infective for hepatitis.

- A constant feature of liver cirrhosis is an increased flow resistance through the portal vein. As a result hepatic blood flow and hepatocyte oxygenation are dependent on hepatic artery blood flow. Optimal anaesthetic management entails careful selection of anaesthetic drug and technique to minimize reduction in systemic blood pressure, which compromises hepatic perfusion.
- Maintain adequate oxygenation ($PaO_2 > 100$ mmHg) and normocarbia ($PaCO_2$ 35–40 mmHg). A higher than usual FiO_2 may be needed due to the presence of intrapulmonary shunting.
- Replace ascitic fluid drainage with fluids (crystalloid and/or colloid solutions). As the ascitic fluid is in dynamic equilibrium with plasma, its rapid removal may precipitate a marked fall in blood pressure if fluid replacement is inadequate.
- Maintain adequate renal perfusion and urine output to avoid hepatorenal syndrome. Volume expansion and judicious use of diuretics such as IV mannitol 0.5–1 g/kg is recommended. Drugs known to be nephrotoxic (e.g., aminoglycosides, NSAIDs) should be avoided.
- The glycogen store of such patients may be depleted. The glucose level should be monitored regularly and hypoglycaemia, if present, corrected with bolus doses of dextrose and dextrose-containing intravenous solutions.
- Early replacement of blood, preferably fresh whole blood, may be necessary. Citrate toxicity may result from massive blood transfusion because the liver may be unable to metabolize citrate, and treatment with calcium chloride is indicated.

8. *Postoperative management* includes these.
   - Appropriate ICU or HDU management.
   - Continue supplemental oxygen therapy for 24 hours postoperatively.
   - Close haemodynamic monitoring: cardiovascular support may be necessary.
   - Adequate analgesia, best achieved using patient-controlled analgesia or epidural analgesia (if regional anaesthesia is not contraindicated).
   - Early chest physiotherapy, breathing exercises and ambulation.
   - Antibiotics are indicated in view of the increased risk of infection.
   - Accurate fluid balance and urine output monitoring. Watch out for development of hepatorenal syndrome.
   - Check FBC and coagulation profile, transfuse blood and/or blood products if necessary.

— Assess liver function clinically and biochemically. Watch out for further deterioration in the postoperative period.

ANAESTHESIA FOR LIVER TRANSPLANTATION

Liver transplantation is often carried out as a semi-emergency surgery for patients with end-stage liver disease or acute hepatic failure. Extrahepatic biliary atresia is the commonest indication for liver transplantation in children. Anaesthetic management involves the perioperative care of a patient who has multi-systemic morbidities associated with liver failure for a complex, protracted surgery with major haemodynamic, fluid, haematological and metabolic stresses.

Surgical Considerations

1. **Donor organ retrieval**

   The liver is often obtained from a brainstem dead, heart-beating donor, removed as part of multi-organ retrieval. It can also be obtained from living-related or non-related donor, from whom one segment of the liver is removed.

2. **Types of liver transplantation**

   Orthotopic liver transplantation entails replacement using a whole size graft. Split liver transplantation provides two grafts from a single donor: the left lateral segment for a child and the larger right lobe for an adult.

3. **Stages of liver transplantation**

   — **Stage one: Dissection phase**
   - The stage begins with skin incision and ends with occlusion of the hepatic artery and portal vein.
   - It involves dissection to expose the liver in preparation for transplantation.

   — **Stage two: Anhepatic phase**
   - This begins with devascularization of the liver with division of the hepatic artery and veins, portal vein and bile duct.
   - The liver is removed and the donor liver implanted. Anastomoses are made between donor and recipient inferior vena cava (IVC), and recipient and donor portal vein.
   - The stage is completed when IVC and portal vein clamps are removed.

— **Stage three: Postreperfusion phase**
  - This is the stage of re-establishment of blood flow from portal vein to IVC, and ends with completion of surgery.
  - There is usually a massive reperfusion syndrome with release of cytokines, complement activation, hypotension, arrhythmias, metabolic acidosis and transient hyperkalaemia.
  - Changes should resolve with a functioning liver graft.

Preoperative Preparation

— The patient should be assessed and optimized as far as possible prior to the surgery. This may not be feasible due to the urgent nature of surgery for cadaveric liver transplantation.

— Blood and blood products should be available.
  - Adults and children > 30 kg: 10 units packed red cells and 10 units FFP in OT; 10 units platelets in Blood Bank.
  - Children < 30 kg: 2–5 units packed red cells and 2–5 units FFP in OT; 2–5 units platelets in Blood Bank.

— Light oral premedication may be prescribed for fully conscious patients.

Monitoring

— Monitoring includes ECG, pulse oximetry, capnography, temperature, peripheral nerve stimulator, urine output and invasive haemodynamic monitors in the form of intraarterial BP, CVP and pulmonary artery catheterization.

— Transoesophageal echocardiography (TEE) is useful to monitor the ventricular filling and contractile function during surgery to guide administration of fluids and/or inotropes. It may detect intracardiac air or microthrombi during dissection or postreperfusion phases. Paradoxical air embolism may be seen to occur across a septal defect or patent foramen ovale.

— Laboratory testing for blood glucose, electrolyte, haemoglobin/haematocrit, ABG, coagulation status should be within the OT complex or readily available elsewhere. These are checked at hourly interval, and more often if indicated (every 30 minutes during anhepatic phase). Thromboelastography may be used to assess intraoperative coagulation function.

Induction and Maintenance of Anaesthesia

— It is necessary to establish adequate venous access with at least 2 large bore intravenous cannulae. Rapid infusion device with heating mechanism is extremely useful in view of anticipated massive fluid and blood transfusion. Measures should be taken to prevent hypothermia that tends to develop with surgical exposure and large volume resuscitation.

— Ensure that drugs that may be necessary during the course of the anaesthetic are available. These include adrenaline, dopamine, atropine, calcium, sodium bicarbonate, dextrose, insulin and lignocaine.

— Anaesthesia is induced using propofol, thiopentone or etomidate with fentanyl, followed by atracurium to facilitate intubation. An oral ETT should be used to avoid problems of nasotracheal intubation – such as nasal bleeding and sinusitis – in the presence of coagulopathy and immunosuppression.

— Maintenance of anaesthesia is by means of a volatile anaesthetic (isoflurane or sevoflurane) in oxygen-air mixture. Nitrous oxide is omitted to minimize bowel distension and in view of possible venous air embolism during surgery. Alternatively the total intravenous anaesthesia (TIVA) technique may be employed. Analgesia is provided by intravenous infusion of remifentanil or bolus doses of fentanyl or alfentanil.

— Veno-venous bypass is employed in some centres to facilitate venous return and lessen the severity of haemodynamic instability during the anhepatic phase. It is usually established from the femoral vein to the internal jugular or brachiocephalic vein.

Intraoperative Problems

Haemodynamic status

Hypotension may be secondary to decreased venous return, hypovolaemia, myocardial depression or peripheral vasodilatation.

Circulatory disturbances are common immediately following reperfusion of the transplanted liver as a result of the effluent from the liver, which is high in potassium and low in pH and temperature. These are manifest as hypotension, bradycardia, ventricular arrhythmias, and even cardiac arrest.

Management includes intravenous fluids, blood transfusion, use of vasopressor or inotrope according to the CVP, pulmonary capillary wedge pressure (PCWP), pulmonary artery pressure, cardiac output measurement and TEE findings.

Respiratory status

Ventilation may be compromised by decreased functional residual capacity as a result of upper abdominal retraction during surgery or placement of a large liver graft in children. Hypoxaemia may be due to intrapulmonary shunting and requires high FiO_2 to achieve adequate oxygenation.

Glycaemic status

A dextrose-containing solution is infused to maintain blood glucose concentration above 5.5 mmol/L. Hyperglycaemia may occur following reperfusion and requires changeover to infusion of dextrose-free solutions.

Haematological status

Massive blood loss is anticipated. Blood, FFP and platelets should be cross-matched in reserve. Intraoperative cell salvage is useful to reduce the use of banked blood. Haematocrit is maintained between 25–30% by blood transfusion. Antifibrinolytic agents (e.g., tranexamic acid) may be used.

Coagulopathy with thrombocytopaenia often occurs at postreperfusion and should be corrected with FFP and platelets. However, intraoperative platelet transfusion may predispose to hepatic artery thrombosis; thus transfusion should be reserved for platelet count < 50,000/μl in the presence of excessive surgical bleeding.

Fluid status

This is guided by haemodynamic measurements, estimated blood loss and urine output.

Fluid administration should be just sufficient to preserve cardiac output for adequate tissue perfusion. One should guard against overzealous administration of fluids, as this may produce intravascular hypervolaemia with oedema and congestion of the liver graft during reperfusion.

Metabolic status

Severe metabolic acidosis and hyperkalaemia are common during the postreperfusion phase but these often correct themselves when the liver graft starts to function. Treatment with sodium bicarbonate, calcium and glucose/insulin may be required if serum potassium concentration persists above 5.0 mmol/L.

Hypocalcaemia is common as calcium is chelated with unmetabolized citrate contained in the transfused banked blood during the anhepatic phase. Calcium, in the form of calcium chloride or calcium gluconate, should be administered to achieve an ionized calcium concentration of 1.1–1.2 mmol/L. This also serves to counter the cardiac effects of hyperkalaemia at the start of postreperfusion phase.

Postoperative ICU Management

— Mechanical ventilation is continued until the patient has stable circulatory and lung function, is normothermic, awake and showing adequate muscle strength. Early extubation is desirable if the intraoperative course has been uneventful and the patient's haemodynamic status is satisfactory.

— Intravenous patient-controlled analgesia is commonly employed because central neuraxial blockade is often unsuitable in view of coagulopathy. NSAIDs should not be used.

— Measures to ensure graft survival include stable haemodynamics, good oxygenation and respiratory function, optimal haematocrit (maintain at 25–30%), use of dextran to improve microcirculation, infection control, and use of immunosuppressants to prevent graft rejection.

— Postoperative complications include cardiovascular instability, coagulopathy, pulmonary oedema, pleural effusion, renal dysfunction, sepsis, poor graft function and acute graft rejection.

Even though acute complications are relatively common, long-term results are encouraging provided graft function is satisfactory. Survival with good quality of life is possible for the majority of these patients, paediatric postliver transplant patients in particular. This is made possible by improvements in organ preservation, surgical technique, perioperative care, and immunosuppression in the form of cyclosporin and low-dose steroids.

FURTHER READING

1. Ziser A, Plevak DJ. Morbidity and mortality in cirrhotic patients undergoing anesthesia and surgery. Curr Opin Anaethesiol 2001;14:707–11.
2. Lentschener C, Ozier Y. What anaesthetists need to know about viral hepatitis. Acta Anaesthesiol Scand 2003;47:794–803.
3. Patel T. Surgery in the patient with liver disease. Mayo Clin Proc 1999;74:593–9.
4. Dagher I, Moore K. The hepatorenal syndrome. Gut 2001;49:729–37.

5. Hammer GB, Krane EJ. Anaesthesia for liver transplantation in children. Paed Anaesth 2001;11:3–18.
6. Merritt WT. Issues affecting liver transplantation. Best Prac Res Clin Anaesthesiol 2005;19:17–34.

Chapter 18

Anaesthesia in Neuromuscular Disease

INTRODUCTION

Neuromuscular diseases form a heterogeneous group of illnesses. Many of them are progressive, often life-threatening, and with a limited or incomplete response to available therapies. They may be classified according to the site of abnormality.

— *Intracranial pathology:* cerebrovascular disease, Parkinson's disease, cerebral palsy.

— *Spinal cord pathology:* spinal cord injury, paraplegia and quadriplegia.

— *Motor neuron disorder:* amyotrophic lateral sclerosis, primary lateral sclerosis.

- *Peripheral neuropathy:* Guillain-Barre syndrome, diabetic neuropathy.
- *Neuromuscular junction lesion:* myasthenia gravis, myasthenic syndrome (Eaton-Lambert syndrome).
- *Muscle disorder (myopathy):* dystonia (dystrophia myotonica, myotonia congenita, paramyotonia), muscular dystrophy (Duchenne, Becker).

Anaesthesia for these patients may be especially hazardous because of these factors.

- Exaggerated hyperkalaemic response to suxamethonium, leading to ventricular arrhythmias or cardiac arrest.
- Altered response to neuromuscular blocking drugs: marked sensitivity to non-depolarizing neuromuscular blocking drugs; resistance to depolarization and delayed onset of action of suxamethonium, with increased risk of developing dual block.
- Autonomic disturbances leading to labile blood pressure changes, arrhythmias, left ventricular failure, cardiac arrest.
- Respiratory impairment as a result of respiratory muscle weakness.
- Increased susceptibility to anaesthetic agents which cause or potentiate muscle relaxation,
- Increased risk of gastric regurgitation and pulmonary aspiration if the bulbar muscles are affected by the disease process.

Many of these are rare disorders and comparatively little is known about the perioperative management of such patients. Recommendations for anaesthetic management are based largely on anecdotal reports. Some of the conditions will be elaborated further.

INTRACRANIAL PATHOLOGY: CEREBROVASCULAR DISEASE

This can be either global cerebral dysfunction or focal neurologic dysfunction ranging from transient ischaemic attack (TIA) to major stroke. The pathology can be thrombotic, embolic or haemorrhagic in nature, and cerebrovascular disease may be part of a generalized atherosclerotic process involving the coronary and peripheral vasculature. The patient may have concomitant diseases such as hypertension, coronary artery disease, peripheral vascular disease, diabetes mellitus and renal disease. These should be identified and optimized before any scheduled surgery.

Anaesthetic management of such patients is directed towards management of the concomitant medical disorders as well as measures to prevent further deterioration of neurological status. Preoperative neurologic deficit should be clearly documented as a basis for comparison with postoperative status. These anaesthetic concerns should be noted.

- The risk of postoperative stroke is increased by as much as 20-fold in patients with a stroke within 6 weeks, hence only urgent surgery should be performed within this period.
- Patients with hemiplegia of less than 6 months' duration often demonstrate an exaggerated hyperkalaemic response to suxamethonium.
- Blood pressure may be labile during surgery; thus invasive haemodynamic monitoring may be necessary.
- Hypocarbia resulting from hyperventilation should be avoided because the resultant cerebral vasoconstriction further jeopardizes cerebral perfusion. Ventilatory parameters should be adjusted to produce normocarbia and adequate oxygenation.
- Prompt emergence from anaesthesia with little residual psychomotor effect is desirable to enable early neurological assessment. New neurological signs warrant urgent referral to the neurologist so that appropriate investigation and treatment can be instituted without much delay.

SPINAL CORD INJURY

The degree of neurological deficit, respiratory muscle dysfunction and cardiovascular derangement depends on the level and extent of spinal cord injury. Table 18–1 shows the clinical features associated with the level of injury.

Clinical Manifestations

1. **Initial phase** (lasts 1–3 weeks)
    - Spinal shock, common after spinal cord lesion above T7
        - Transient period of intense neuronal discharge leading to systemic and pulmonary hypertension, cardiac arrhythmias, left ventricular failure, myocardial infarction, pulmonary oedema.

Table 18–1. Clinical features according to the level of spinal cord injury

Level of Injury	Clinical Features
Cervical Level	
Above C2–C4	Incompatible with life because of phrenic nerve paralysis
Below C5–C6	External intercostal muscles paralyzed Diaphragmatic function preserved Decreased chest wall expansion Paradoxical respiration
Thoracic Level	
Above T7	Internal intercostal and abdominal muscles paralyzed Weak cough, decreased ability to clear secretions
Below T7	Chest wall expands fully and adequately Adequate ventilatory capacity Adequate cough, able to clear secretions

  - Subsequent loss of sympathetic tone and myocardial dysfunction with venous pooling, hypotension, bradycardia worsened by unopposed vagal tone; flaccid paralysis with areflexia and sensory loss below the level of injury; loss of temperature regulation.

- — Major causes of morbidity or mortality during this period
  - Respiratory failure secondary to atelectasis, sputum retention, reduced cough effort, impaired alveolar ventilation, aspiration pneumonia resulting from depressed airway reflexes.
  - Pulmonary embolism.
  - Associated injuries in other systems.

2. **Chronic phase**
   - — Gradual return of spinal cord reflexes: may manifest as involuntary muscle spasm and spasticity.
   - — Autonomic dysreflexia in response to stimulation below the level of the cord lesion.

- Problems with immobility: chronic pulmonary infection, risk of thromboembolism, decubitus ulcers, osteoporosis, increased risk of fractures.
- Urinary stasis with urinary tract infection, renal calculi, renal failure.
- Anaemia, malnutrition.
- Mental depression.

Initial Resuscitation and Airway Management

Initial management follows the ABC of resuscitation with special attention towards preservation of spinal cord integrity and function. The spinal cord is susceptible to secondary insult in the same way as the brain. Attempts should be made to preserve adequate perfusion to the injured cord; and to avoid further mechanical disruption to the spinal cord by compression or distraction.

Airway obstruction is rapidly fatal and must be corrected at once. The initial manoeuvres for ensuring airway patency should displace the cervical spine as little as possible, by using jaw thrust rather than head tilt and chin lift, using an appropriate sized oropharyngeal airway, and keeping the cervical collar in place.

Immediate intubation is indicated in the patients with:

- Inadequate respiratory effort.
- Actual or impending airway obstruction.
- Significant maxillofacial trauma.
- Reduced level of consciousness with inability to protect the airway.
- High risk of aspiration.

The actual intubation technique depends on the urgency of the procedure, facilities available and experience of the anaesthesiologist. Direct laryngoscopy and intubation is the preferred approach if intubation is urgently indicated. Movement of the cervical spine is minimized by the use of manual in-line stabilization. In this manoeuvre, the assistant kneels at the head end of the trolley and puts one hand on each side of the skull to hold the head and neck in a neutral position during laryngoscopy and tracheal intubation. Traction on the neck is NOT indicated as this may actually distract and exacerbate certain types of spinal injury.

Ideally four persons are required for safe and efficient emergency intubation

- One applies the cricoid pressure.
- One applies manual in-line stabilization.

— One administers sedative drugs and muscle relaxant.
— One performs laryngoscopy and tracheal intubation.

The nature and dose of the hypnotic agent (fentanyl, midazolam, thiopentone, ketamine or propofol) should be titrated to the patient's age, body weight and haemodynamic status. The use of suxamethonium in the acute setting is not contraindicated because the hyperkalaemic response is not expected to be established until much later.

Fluid management may be problematic in the face of persistent hypotension, and the possibility of hypovolaemia should be excluded. If hypotension is secondary to peripheral vasodilatation in spinal shock, excessive fluids may lead to pulmonary oedema as a result of alveolar disruption that occurs with pulmonary hypertension. Central venous pressure monitoring may be unreliable as CVP may be persistently low even in the face of fluid overload. Vasopressor may be indicated and inotropic support should be commenced early to ensure adequate perfusion to vital organs.

Anaesthetic Management

Anaesthesia and surgery may be required at any stage, for example:

— Acute stage: emergency laparotomy, craniotomy or orthopaedic surgery.
— Subacute stage: stabilization of cervical spine.
— Intermediate stage: elective orthopaedic procedure, desloughing of decubitus ulcers, split skin graft.
— Chronic stage: split skin graft, rotation flaps, cystoscopy, vesicolithotomy.

The patient may also present for some other incidental surgery during the intermediate or chronic stages.

Anaesthetic management should take into account these factors.

— Level of spinal cord injury.
— Associated injury in the acute phase.
— The proposed surgical procedure.
— Time interval between spinal cord injury and surgery.

Table 18–2 summarizes the anaesthetic problems during the various stages in spinal cord injury.

Table 18–2. Anticipated anaesthetic problems in spinal cord injury

STAGE	ACUTE	SUBACUTE	INTERMEDIATE	CHRONIC
Time Interval	**0–48 hours**	**48 hours–1 week**	**1–12 weeks**	**> 3 months**
Possible Problems	Airway management: stability of cervival spine, associated neurological or maxillofacial injury	Spinal shock	Severe hyperkalaemia with suxamethonium	Hyperkalaemia with suxamethonium
	Spinal shock: hypotension, bradycardia	Increased risk of hyperkalaemia with suxamethonium	Autonomic dysreflexia	Autonomic dysreflexia
	Hypovolaemia due to acute blood loss	Increased risk of hypercalcaemia	Orthostatic pneumonia	Orthostatic pneumonia
	Full stomach, risk of regurgitation and aspiration		Sepsis	Muscle contractures
	Extent of spinal cord and associated injury not completely known			Osteoporosis

Anaesthetic Technique

Note that some form of anaesthesia is required even though the patient may have sensory deficit below the level of the lesion.

The anaesthesiologist may be requested to provide monitored anaesthesia care during procedures done under local anaesthesia or nerve block. The site of surgery, and the level and completeness of spinal cord lesion should be considered. The likelihood of autonomic dysreflexia and muscle spasm requiring anaesthesia for control during surgery should also be taken into account.

General anaesthesia: Acute phase

— Surgery during this phase is usually confined to management of life-threatening emergencies and co-existing injury. On-going resuscitation may be necessary.

— Monitoring is carried out according to the patient's condition and extent of surgery. Frequent blood pressure measurements should be made and the ECG should be closely monitored for arrhythmias. Invasive haemodynamic measurements are often indicated.

— Atropine should be available during induction of anaesthesia, as severe bradycardia or even asystole may complicate intubation.

— Reduce the dose of anaesthetic agents in view of unstable haemodynamic status and possibility of myocardial depression.

— Techniques of intubation, with attempts to minimize movement at cervical spine, are as outlined above. Suxamethonium appears to be safe within the first 72 hours of injury.

— Take steps to prevent hypothermia during surgery.

— Arrange for postoperative ICU/HDU admission for further management.

General anaesthesia: Chronic phase

— Determine whether general anaesthesia is necessary, or whether the surgery can be performed under loco-regional anaesthesia with monitored anaesthesia care.

— Sedative premedication should be avoided if respiratory function is impaired or if there is a positive history of sleep apnoea.

- Hypotension during induction of anaesthesia is common because of an absence of reflex sympathetic activity to compensate for myocardial depressant effects of intravenous induction agents. Fluid preloading with 500–1,000 ml of crystalloid prior to induction reduces the likelihood and severity of hypotension.
- Recommendations vary over the period of potential risk in using suxamethonium, though it seems prudent to avoid its use until 9 months after injury.
- Non-depolarizing neuromuscular blockers are commonly used to facilitate tracheal intubation. Subsequent doses are rarely needed if surgery is performed below the level of the lesion unless troublesome muscle spasm interferes with surgery.
- The laryngeal mask airway may be used in patients with low aspiration risks. LMA ProSeal™ may be a useful alternative.
- Care should be taken while positioning the patient in view of the problems of osteoporosis and decubitus ulcers. Pressure points should be well padded.
- All fluid losses should be diligently replaced as the patient is unable to compensate for blood loss.
- Prevention of hypothermia is just as important as in the acute phase.
- Watch out for autonomic dysreflexia and treat as outlined below if this occurs. Most episodes appear to be self-limiting and require no further treatment than temporary cessation of surgical stimulus.

Regional anaesthesia

- Spinal anaesthesia has been recommended especially for urological surgery. It is simple, safe, effective and does not affect the long-term neurological outcome. It is unlikely to result in cardiovascular instability since sympathetic tone is already low prior to the blockade. Standard doses of local anaesthetic should be used. However, it is contraindicated in the presence of local or systemic sepsis, and it is difficult to determine the success or level of blockade.
- Epidural anaesthesia is not as effective as spinal anaesthesia because of increased likelihood of missed segments (due to distortion of the epidural space from previous spinal surgery) and less satisfactory blockade of sacral segments.
- Brachial plexus block is a useful means to avoid general anaesthesia for upper limb surgery. The axillary or infraclavicular approach is preferable over the supraclavicular approach to avoid the complication of pneumothorax in a patient with borderline lung function.

Autonomic Dysreflexia

This occurs following resolution of flaccid paralysis of acute spinal cord injury, in which physical stimulus below the level of spinal cord injury triggers massive unopposed sympathetic discharge. The incidence of autonomic dysreflexia depends on the level of spinal cord lesion; its occurrence is unlikely when transection occurs below T10. The greatest responses are produced by stimuli from the most caudal root levels, hence pelvic visceral stimulation (e.g., bladder or bowel distension, anal fissure, urinary tract infection) is most commonly implicated.

Autonomic dysreflexia is manifested by:

— Hypertension: most common feature but not always present, may lead to intracranial and retinal haemorrhage, seizures, coma, myocardial ischaemia, pulmonary oedema and death.
— Reflex bradycardia.
— Vasoconstriction below and vasodilatation above level of lesion.
— Headache, sweating, nasal congestion, dyspnoea, nausea, blurred vision, anxiety.

Management includes these.

— Eliminate the precipitating cause.
— Increase depth of anaesthesia or induce general anaesthesia.
— Consider antihypertensive agents: sublingual nifedipine, sublingual or transdermal glyceryl trinitrate.

MOTOR NEURON DISORDERS

These degenerative disorders affect the neurons that lie between the motor cortex and striated muscle groups. Symptoms relate to loss of upper motor neurons (primary lateral sclerosis), lower motor neurons (progressive spinal muscular atrophy) or both upper and lower motor neurons (amyotrophic lateral sclerosis or ALS).

Recommendations on anaesthetic management of ALS are based on data which are largely anecdotal:

— Suxamethonium should be avoided because it has been reported to induce severe hyperkalaemia and cardiac arrest.
— Non-depolarizing neuromuscular blockers have prolonged effects in ALS.
— Autonomic dysfunction often leads to severe hypotension during induction of

anaesthesia and following changes in position. Intravenous fluids and vasopressor (e.g., ephedrine) are often necessary.

— Risks of pulmonary aspiration and ventilatory failure are increased in the perioperative period as a result of bulbar weakness and respiratory insufficiency.
— Regional anaesthetic techniques have been safely employed.

PERIPHERAL NEUROPATHY: GUILLAIN-BARRE SYNDROME

This is an immune-mediated polyneuropathy presenting as rapidly progressing areflexic paralysis, leading to respiratory failure requiring ventilatory support in 20–30% of the patients. Autonomic dysfunction is common, leading to labile blood pressure, tachy- and bradyarrhythmias. In some cases the onset of polyneuropathy is preceded by a bacterial or viral illness.

Anaesthesia, either regional or general, has not been reported to worsen the disease condition. Patients with lower bulbar and respiratory muscle weaknesses frequently require longer postoperative intubation and mechanical ventilation. Significant autonomic dysfunction warrants invasive haemodynamic monitoring and measures to obtund the effects of intubation and surgery. Exaggerated hyperkalaemic response to suxamethonium and increased sensitivity to non-depolarizing neuromuscular blockers have both been described. The risk of hyperkalaemia may persist for several months after clinical recovery.

NEUROMUSCULAR JUNCTION DISORDER

Myasthenia Gravis

This is an autoimmune disease in which antibodies are produced against the acetylcholine receptors in the postsynaptic membrane of the neuromuscular junction. The prevalence is estimated between 1:10,000 and 1:20,000, with young women (peak onset 20–30 years of age) most commonly affected.

The most common muscles affected are those at the orbit and mouth, pharynx, shoulder girdle and the muscles of respiration. Patients frequently complain of ptosis, diplopia and dysphagia, while severe bulbar weakness may render them at risk from pulmonary aspiration. The disease is characterized by weakness and exhaustion of voluntary skeletal muscles with repetitive use followed by partial recovery with rest.

Myasthenia gravis may be classified on the basis of the skeletal muscles involved and the severity of the symptoms, shown in Table 18–3.

Table 18–3. Classification of myasthenia gravis

Type	Clinical Manifestation
I	Extraocular muscle involvement with ocular signs and symptoms only
IIA	Slowly progressive, generalized mild muscle weakness; muscles of respiration spared; responds well to therapy
IIB	Rapidly progressive, generalized moderate muscle weakness; muscles of respiration may be involved; responds less well to therapy
III	Acute fulminating presentation and/or respiratory dysfunction, rapid deterioration (within 6 months)
IV	Late stage, severe and generalized muscle weakness, myasthenic crisis requiring artificial ventilation

Medical and surgical management

Standard treatment of myasthenia gravis includes anticholinesterase, immunosuppressive therapy and thymectomy. In addition, short-term improvement of symptoms may be obtained by means of plasmapheresis and immunoglobulins.

— Anticholinesterase
  - This is the mainstay of treatment as the anticholinesterase slows the breakdown of acetylcholine at the motor end-plate and potentiates the action of acetylcholine at receptor sites.
  - Pyridostigmine bromide (15–60 mg every 4–6 hours) and neostigmine bromide (7.5–15 mg every 4–6 hours) are most commonly used.
  - Anticholinergics may be required to control the muscarinic side effects such as bradycardia, salivation, abdominal cramps and diarrhoea.

— Immunosuppressive therapy
  - Corticosteroids may be indicated in patients whose response to anticholinesterase is suboptimal. Watch for and treat steroid-induced hypokalaemia which may aggravate muscle weakness.

  - Azathioprine has been used in conjunction with prednisolone and in refractory cases unresponsive to other measures.
  - Other drugs include cyclophosphamide and cyclosporin.
- Plasmapheresis
  - This is a temporary measure used during acute exacerbations especially in severe respiratory failure refractory to conventional treatment.
  - It produces short-term clinical improvements in patients with myasthenic crises or in selected patients being prepared for thymectomy.
- Immunoglobulins
  - Indications for intravenous immunoglobulin are similar to those for plasmapheresis.
  - Improvement occurs within days and may be sustained for months.
- Thymectomy
  - This achieves the best results especially in the presence of thymoma, in which approximately 75% cases have remission of symptoms after surgery.
  - There are various surgical techniques for thymectomy.
    - Transsternal approach via median sternotomy provides good surgical exposure and optimizes removal of all thymic tissue.
    - Transcervical approach via cervical incision and mediastinoscopy is associated with a smaller surgical incision and less postoperative pain.
    - Video-assisted thoracoscopic extended thymectomy (VATET) has also been described.

Anaesthetic management

Patients with myasthenia gravis may present for thymectomy or any other elective or emergency surgical procedures.

1. **Preoperative assessment**
   - Consultation with neurologist or physician is essential.
   - Establish the severity of the disease; take note of the muscle groups involved, duration of disease, time course, progression of symptoms and aggravating factors.
   - Inquire about symptoms of bulbar involvement such as dysphagia, drooling of saliva. Any degree of bulbar palsy indicates the need for intraoperative airway protection.
   - Look for clinical features of other co-existing autoimmune disease, such as

thyroiditis, pernicious anaemia, rheumatoid disease, scleroderma, systemic lupus erythematosis, polymyositis or dermatomyositis.

— Careful airway assessment is necessary as neck movement may be limited in the presence of associated rheumatoid disease, while a large thymoma may cause tracheal deviation or compression.
— Take a detailed drug history and assess compliance to treatment. Determine the effect that a missed dose may have on the patient, to see whether it is advisable to omit the anticholinesterase medication on the morning of surgery.
— Preoperative lung function test may be useful to identify patients likely to require postoperative ventilatory support (see Table 18–4).
— Arrange for postoperative management in ICU or HDU.
— Sedative premedication is best omitted as it may depress respiratory function.
— Controversy exists as to whether anticholinesterase should be served prior to surgery as it may interfere with the intraoperative use of neuromuscular blocking drugs. This must be weighed against the risk of muscle weakness and respiratory embarrassment if the medication is omitted. The safest approach would be to omit or reduce dose of anticholinesterase in mild disease, and to continue anticholinesterase in severe disease.

Leventhal, Orkin and Hirsch described a preoperative scoring system to predict the need for postoperative ventilation, specifically for patients with myasthenia gravis undergoing thymectomy (Table 18–4). Ventilation is likely to be necessary with a total score of 10–34, while the patient is expected to tolerate extubation at the end of the surgery if the total score is less than 10. These criteria are less predictive for the need for ventilatory support following the less invasive transcervical approach.

Table 18–4. Scoring system to predict the need for postoperative ventilation

Risk Factors	Points
1. Duration of myasthenia gravis > 6 years	12
2. Chronic respiratory disease other than respiratory problems associated with MG	10
3. Dose of pyridostigmine > 750 mg daily in 48 hours prior to surgery	8
4. Preoperative vital capacity < 2.9 litres (40 ml/kg)	4

2. **Intraoperative management**

   General principles

   — Opt for regional anaesthesia wherever appropriate.
   — A combined epidural and general anaesthetic technique provides good intra- and postoperative analgesia while reducing requirement for general anaesthetic agents.
   — Avoid or minimize the use of neuromuscular blocking drugs if possible.

   The respiratory depressant effects of intravenous induction agent may be accentuated in myasthenia gravis. In many patients with co-existing muscle weakness, tracheal intubation without neuromuscular blocking drugs can be accomplished with a combination of opioid, intravenous induction agent (propofol in particular) and volatile anaesthetic.

   Suxamethonium should be avoided if possible because of its unpredictable effect and propensity for phase II blocks even following a single dose. This drug may be used cautiously in cases with full stomach and potential difficult intubation, but its effect should be allowed to wear off before maintaining muscle relaxation with a non-depolarizing neuromuscular blocker.

   The initial dose of non-depolarizing neuromuscular blocker should be decreased by at least half to two-thirds. Neuromuscular function should be closely monitored by means of peripheral nerve stimulator and subsequent doses titrated accordingly. Both atracurium and cisatracurium have been used successfully in myasthenia gravis. All the predisposing factors – hypokalaemia, acidosis, hypothermia – that may impair neuromuscular function should be controlled. Neuromuscular function should be allowed to return spontaneously because the administration of anticholinesterase as reversal agents may result in cholinergic crisis and cause confusion in diagnosis when the patient presents with continued weakness.

3. **Postoperative management**

   — The patient should be admitted to ICU or HDU for further management.
   — Keep the patient intubated unless there is full recovery of muscle power and maintenance of adequate ventilation.
   — Criteria for extubation include these.
   - Good clinical recovery: the patient is conscious, able to breathe deeply and cough, demonstrates good muscle power, and is able to maintain head lift for longer than 5 seconds.
   - Full return of train of 4 ratio as demonstrated on the peripheral nerve stimulator.

  - Normal pH, PaO_2 and $PaCO_2$ in ABG analysis.
- — Effective postoperative analgesia is essential to avoid retention of secretion and atelectasis. It also enables effective chest physiotherapy and early mobilization to be carried out. Analgesic techniques include:
  - Regional analgesia if applicable: preferred technique.
  - Intravenous opioid infusion (fentanyl preferred) in ICU or HDU setting.
  - Intravenous patient-controlled analgesia.
- — Substitute oral anticholinesterase with equivalent doses of parenteral neostigmine when the patient is kept nil by mouth. Equivalent doses are:
  - pyridostigmine oral: 120 mg
  - neostigmine oral: 30 mg
  - neostigmine IV, IM or SC: 1 mg
- — Recommence oral anticholinesterase therapy once oral intake is allowed.
- — Dose requirement for anticholinesterase following thymectomy may alter significantly. The neurologist or physician should review the patient and make the necessary dose adjustments.
- — Beware of the possible occurrence of myasthenic or cholinergic crisis, with these presenting features.
  - Myasthenic crisis: inadequate dose of anticholinesterase, presenting with worsening of muscle weakness which can progress rapidly to respiratory failure necessitating urgent tracheal intubation and respiratory support.
  - Cholinergic crisis: excessive dose of anticholinesterase, presenting with similar features but is accompanied by features of parasympathetic hyperactivity (abdominal cramps, diarrhoea and blurred vision, excessive oral secretions, bradycardia).

  If the diagnosis is in doubt, differentiate by giving a small dose (2 mg) of intravenous edrophonium. Clinical improvement is seen in myasthenic crisis while the symptoms worsen in cholinergic crisis.

Myasthenic Syndrome

Eaton-Lambert syndrome, an example of myasthenic syndrome, is an immune-mediated neuromuscular junction disease that typically occurs in the setting of malignancy (pulmonary, gastric, renal or bowel). Unlike myasthenia gravis, the proximal muscle weakness improves transiently with exercise, and cranial muscle involvement is less common. Management includes treating the underlying malignancy, as effective cancer therapy is associated with neurologic improvement. Symptomatic treatment includes 3,4-diaminopyridine to promote acetylcholine release at the muscle end-plate, glucocorticoids and other immunosuppressants, and intravenous immunoglobulins. Anticholinesterase therapy is not useful.

Anaesthetic management includes these.

- There should be a high index of suspicion for patients with malignancy, especially small cell carcinoma of the lung, coming for diagnostic or therapeutic procedures under anaesthesia.
- Patients demonstrate increased sensitivity to both depolarizing and non-depolarizing neuromuscular blockers. If muscle paralysis is indicated, it is recommended that the initial dose of neuromuscular blocking drug should be one-tenth of the usual dose. Subsequent doses should be titrated with monitoring of neuromuscular blockade.
- The need for postoperative ventilatory support should be anticipated.

MUSCLE DISORDER (MYOPATHY)

Myopathies are a heterogeneous group of disorders related to abnormalities in the skeletal muscle. Two clinically important categories are muscular dystrophies (e.g., Duchenne muscular dystrophy) and dystonias (e.g., myotonic dystrophy).

Muscular dystrophies are rare, genetically determined degenerative muscle diseases. Duchenne muscular dystrophy is caused by an X-linked recessive gene. It presents with progressive weakness and wasting in childhood, leading to death from cardiac or respiratory failure in late adolescence. The patient may present for anaesthesia for correction of scoliosis, tendon release for contracture, or exploratory laparotomy for ileus. Anaesthetic concerns are as follows:

- Impairment in cardiac function with risks of life-threatening cardiac dysrhythmias may be a feature.
- Suxamethonium is contraindicated because of the risks of hyperkalaemia and malignant hyperthermia.
- The patient has significant aspiration risks because of weak laryngeal reflexes and prolonged gastric emptying times.
- Macroglossia is frequent and may pose difficulty in laryngoscopy and intubation.
- Sensitivity to non-depolarizing neuromuscular blocker is increased.
- Postoperative pulmonary complications are common, and prolonged intubation may be necessary.

Myotonic dystrophy is a multi-system disorder with progressive deterioration of skeletal, cardiac and smooth muscles. It is characterized by persistent contracture of the skeletal muscle after stimulation (myotonia), frontal baldness, cataract and intellectual impairment. Its multi-system nature affects the heart (conduction abnormalities, septal or valvular defects, cardiomyopathy), endocrine system (diabetes mellitus, hypothyroidism, adrenal insufficiency), respiratory system (respiratory insufficiency with progressive failure) and central nervous system (progressive bulbar palsy). These anaesthetic concerns should be noted.

- Myotonic crisis can be triggered by hypothermia, surgical stimulation, electrocautery and certain drugs (e.g., suxamethonium, neostigmine).
- The risk of aspiration is increased because of bulbar palsy and delayed gastric emptying.
- Suxamethonium is contraindicated because it produces exaggerated hyperkalaemic response and prolonged muscle contraction which may interfere with intubation, ventilation and surgery.
- There is a weak association with malignant hyperthermia.
- Even small doses of induction agents can produce profound cardiorespiratory depression.
- The use of general anaesthesia mandates intubation for airway protection, and prolonged intubation and mechanical ventilation may be required in the postoperative period.

FURTHER READING

1. Naguib M, Flood P, McArdle JJ, Brenner HR. Advances in neurobiology of the neuromuscular junction: Implications for the anesthesiologist. Anesthesiology 2002;96:202–31.
2. Stevens RD. Neuromuscular disorders and anesthesia. Curr Opin Anaesthesiol 2001;14:693–8.
3. Dutton RP. Anesthetic management of spinal cord injury: Clinical practice and future initiatives. Int Anesthesiol Clin 2002;40:77–93.
4. Dangor A, Lam AM. Perioperative management of patients with head and spinal cord injuries. Anesth Clin North Am 1999;17:155–70.
5. Hamby PR, Martin B. Anaesthesia for chronic spinal cord lesions. Anaesthesia 1998;53:273–89.

6. Petrozza PH. Anesthetic considerations for the patient with acute spinal cord injury. Anesth Analg 1998;Mar (supp): 85–90.
7. Fox RSR, Mulnier C. The anaesthetic management of acute spinal injury patients. Curr Anaesth Crit Care 2001;12:147–53.
8. Ford P, Nolan J. Cervical spine injury and airway management. Curr Opin Anesthesiol 2002;15:193–201.
9. Chevalley C, Spiliopoulos A, de Perrot M, Tschopp JM, Licker M. Perioperative medical management and outcome following thymectomy for myasthenia gravis. Can J Anesth 2001;48:446–51.
10. Imison AR. Anaesthesia and myotonia – an Australian experience. Anaesth Intens Care 2001;29:34–7.

Chapter 19

Anaesthesia for Patients with Diabetes Mellitus

INTRODUCTION

Diabetes mellitus is a multi-system disease. It affects every organ system either directly or indirectly as a result of microangiopathy. Glycaemic control is only one aspect in the overall management; it is just as important to treat any concomitant hypertension or nephropathy in order to prevent diabetic complications. Tight long-term control of glucose and blood pressure has been shown to improve outcome in diabetics by retarding the onset of complications and the severity of the associated target organ damage.

The same tight glycaemic control is advocated in the perioperative period. Since the signs of hypoglycaemia are masked during general anaesthesia, anaesthesiologists tend to adopt a "rather high than low" approach to glycaemic control. However, hyperglycaemia has been shown to increase the likelihood of short-term diabetic complications such as cardiovascular complications, delayed wound healing and wound infection. The development of rapid, reliable methods for blood glucose measurement has facilitated intraoperative glucose monitoring and more precise glycaemic control with appropriate insulin therapy.

CLASSIFICATION OF DIABETES MELLITUS

This classification of diabetes mellitus is proposed by American Diabetes Association (ADA) and World Health Organization (WHO).

1. Type 1 diabetes mellitus, formerly juvenile or insulin dependent diabetes mellitus (IDDM).
   — Immune-mediated, associated with idiopathic forms of pancreatic β-cell dysfunction leading to absolute insulin deficiency in genetically predisposed individuals.
   — Treatment is by administration of exogenous insulin.

2. Type 2 diabetes mellitus, formerly non-insulin dependent diabetes mellitus (NIDDM).
   — Caused by insulin resistance and/or impaired insulin secretion secondary to diverse genetic and environmental factors.
   — Treatment is multi-modal: diet, exercise, drugs that stimulate insulin secretion (e.g., sulfonylureas), drugs that increase insulin sensitivity (e.g., metformin), and exogenous insulin itself.

3. Type 3 diabetes mellitus comprises a wide range of specific types of secondary diabetes mellitus.
   — Pancreatic diseases: carcinoma, chronic pancreatitis, haemochromatosis.
   — Endocrinopathies (caused by over-production of hormones which are anti-insulin).
      - Cushing's syndrome – cortisol
      - Acromegaly – growth hormone
      - Thyrotoxicosis – thyroxine
   — Drugs and chemicals: glucocorticoids, diuretics such as frusemide.

4. Type 4 diabetes mellitus or gestational diabetes mellitus.
   — 30–50% develop a Type 2 diabetes mellitus within 10 years.

PREOPERATIVE ASSESSMENT

— Determine the type and duration of diabetes mellitus, as well as details of treatment
  - Nature, duration and compliance to treatment.
  - Adequacy of blood glucose control as shown by glycosylated haemoglobin (HbA_{1c}) level; a value of > 9% (normal 3.8–6.4%) suggests inadequate control.
  - Presence and severity of target organ involvement.

— Identify and assess severity of associated medical conditions
  - Cardiovascular system: hypertension, coronary artery disease, cerebrovascular disease, peripheral vascular disease.
  - Renal system: diabetic nephropathy.
  - Nervous system: peripheral neuropathy, autonomic neuropathy.
  - Eyes: premature cataract, diabetic retinopathy.

— Implications for anaesthetic management
  - Acute consequences of untreated or poorly treated diabetes mellitus include osmotic diuresis with dehydration, ketoacidosis or hyperosmolar non-ketotic hyperglycaemic crisis. This is a medical emergency and requires urgent resuscitation and stabilization before surgery.
  - Perioperative blood pressure control may be problematic with wide fluctuations necessitating close monitoring and treatment.
  - As a result of diabetic nephropathy, renal excretion of anaesthetic drugs and other medications may be impaired leading to prolonged pharmacological effect or overdosage.
  - Autonomic neuropathy, affecting 30–40% of diabetic patients, may give rise to delayed gastric emptying, perioperative hypothermia, postural hypotension, abnormal cardiac reflexes and silent myocardial ischaemia.
  - Thickening of soft tissues and joint immobility involving the temporomandibular joint, atlanto-occipital joint and cervical spines may render proper positioning, laryngoscopy and endotracheal intubation difficult.
  - Altered level of consciousness may occur as a result of hypoglycaemia, hyperglycaemic crises or cerebrovascular insufficiency.
  - In situations of cardiac arrest and cerebral ischaemia, diabetic patients have a worse neurological outcome compared to non-diabetics. This is probably due to presence of lactic acidosis as a result of anaerobic metabolism.

- Risk of infection is high, wound healing may be delayed in the presence of poor diabetic control, and incidence of chest infection is higher especially if the patient is obese and a smoker.

— Management of diabetic medication for major surgery
- Insulin requirement in the perioperative period tends to be altered as part of the body's stress response to surgery. This effect persists until the patient recovers from surgery; hence the nature and dose of diabetic medication may need to be adjusted accordingly.
- Type 1 diabetes mellitus:
  — Long-acting insulin (e.g., crystalline insulin zinc suspension) should be stopped and substituted with short- or intermediate-acting insulin.
- Type 2 diabetes mellitus:
  — Metformin should be stopped 2 days before major surgery as it may precipitate lactic acidosis.
  — Chlorpropamide should ideally be stopped for 3 days because its duration of action lasts for 36 hours. As this is not always possible, the patient should have frequent blood glucose monitoring to exclude hypoglycaemia.
  — A shorter-acting oral hypoglycaemic agent such as glibenclamide may be substituted, or more commonly this is replaced by conversion to insulin.

INTRAOPERATIVE MANAGEMENT

— Choice of anaesthetic
- There is no clear evidence that any one technique is superior to the other although regional anaesthetic techniques are recommended whenever suitable. However, it should be noted that central neuraxial blockade may result in profound hypotension in a patient with autonomic neuropathy. The increased incidence of peripheral neuropathies is also a consideration when choosing a regional anaesthetic technique in such patients.
- The choice of anaesthetic agents and monitoring techniques depends on the extent of surgery and the severity of systemic disease such as coronary artery disease, hypertension and nephropathy.
- Attempts should be made to attenuate the stress response to surgery since it causes release of stress hormones, catecholamines and other mediators in addition to having deleterious effects on the cardiovascular system.

- Airway management and positioning
  - Decrease in joint mobility occurs as a result of deposition of collagen in joint tissue.
  - Cervical spine immobility can make direct laryngoscopy and intubation difficult, and may necessitate an awake fibreoptic intubation.
  - There is a need for careful positioning during surgery to decrease the likelihood of musculoskeletal and neurovascular injuries.
- Intraoperative glycaemic control
  - Many diabetic patients presenting for minor surgery do not require insulin supplement.
  - Avoid large fluctuations in blood glucose level as both hypo- and hyperglycaemia are undesirable.
    - Hypoglycaemia is especially dangerous in an anaesthetized patient due to the lack of warning symptoms – sweating, restlessness, abdominal pain – and the consequences of major cerebral complications.
    - Hyperglycaemia may lead to hyperosmolarity, osmotic diuresis and dehydration.
  - Avoid rapid reduction in blood glucose concentration as severe hypokalaemia can occur in addition to hypoglycaemia.
  - Patients with poorly controlled diabetes, or those requiring large doses of insulin for satisfactory control, need to be closely monitored and the rate of insulin infusion adjusted accordingly.

PERIOPERATIVE MANAGEMENT OF DIABETES MELLITUS

- The nature and extent of therapy is tailored to the type of surgery: whether the surgery is elective or emergency; and whether it requires prolonged postoperative fasting > 24 hours (empirically termed "major" surgery) or postoperative fasting until post-nausea (empirically termed "minor" surgery).
- Early admission for stabilization is necessary for patients with poorly controlled diabetes. An endocrinologist should be consulted in the perioperative period to jointly manage patients scheduled for major surgery.
- If possible, the patient should be scheduled early in the OT list to limit the duration of preoperative fasting.
- Bedside blood glucose concentration monitoring using reagent strip and

refractometer is usually adequate. Measurement should be performed regularly and blood glucose concentration maintained between 6–10 mmol/L.

Minor Surgery

Type 1 diabetes mellitus

— Omit morning dose of insulin if blood glucose < 7 mmol/L; give half the normal dose if > 7 mmol/L.

— Measure blood glucose concentration 1 hour before surgery; at least once during surgery; postoperative 2-hourly until return to oral intake and 4-hourly thereafter.

— Recommence insulin when the patient starts oral intake.

Type 2 diabetes mellitus

— **Diet control**
  - No special treatment is necessary in the well controlled, diet-treated patient.

— **On oral hypoglycaemic agent**
  - Omit morning dose on day of surgery.
  - Measure blood glucose concentration 1 hour before surgery; at least once during surgery; postoperative 2-hourly until return to oral intake and 8-hourly thereafter.
  - Recommence oral hypoglycaemic agent when the patient starts oral intake.

Major Surgery

— Check blood glucose and potassium concentrations preoperatively.

— Omit insulin or oral hypoglycaemic agent on day of surgery.

— Begin intravenous infusion of dextrose 5% (500 ml over 4 hours), or dextrose 10% (500 ml over 8 hours) depending on fluid requirement.

— Start variable-rate insulin infusion according to sliding scale insulin regime (*vide infra*).

— Measure blood glucose concentration every 2-hourly from the start of infusion, hourly during surgery, hourly postoperatively for 4 hours then every 2-hourly.

— Recommence insulin or oral hypoglycaemic agent when the patient starts oral intake.

INSULIN INFUSION REGIMES

Various types of infusion regimes have been recommended, the most common ones being the GIK (Glucose-Insulin-Potassium) or Alberti regime, and insulin infusion according to sliding scale. The Alberti regime is simpler, does not utilize an infusion pump but offers less accurate glycaemic control.

GIK Regime (Alberti Regime)

Insulin is added to 500 ml of dextrose 10% and the solution is infused at 100 ml/hr, 10 mmol potassium chloride is added to the solution if serum potassium < 3.5 mmol/L

Blood glucose concentration (mmol/L)	Insulin added (U)
< 5	omit
5–10	10
10–15	15
>20*	20

* requires hourly review

Sliding Scale Insulin Regime

Variable-rate infusion of insulin 50 U in 50 ml 0.9% saline (concentration of insulin 1 U/ml), adjusted according to blood glucose concentration.

Blood glucose concentration (mmol/L)	Infusion rate (ml/hr)
< 5	omit
5–10	1
10–15	3
15–20	4
>20*	5

* Increase rate of infusion by 2 ml/hr if blood glucose concentration remains high, check half-hourly and adjust infusion rate accordingly.

$$\textit{Approximate guide: Insulin infusion rate} = \frac{\textit{blood glucose concentration}}{5}$$

EMERGENCY SURGERY

— This often poses a management dilemma if the surgical procedure is urgent despite poor glycaemic control. The presence of sepsis such as abscess or infected diabetic gangrene may render glycaemic control problematic.
— Such patients should be reviewed and managed by the endocrinologist. Other than insulin therapy and regular blood glucose monitoring, acidosis, dehydration and electrolyte imbalance should be corrected if present.
— Blood glucose concentration up to 15 mmol/L may be accepted for surgery provided that treatment is on-going.

FURTHER READING

1. Dierdorf SF. Anesthesia for patients with diabetes mellitus. Curr Opin Anaesthesiol 2002;15:351–7.
2. Inzucchi SE. Glycemic management of diabetics in the perioperative setting. Int Anesthesiol Clin 2002;40:77–93.
3. Sonksen P, Sonksen J. Insulin: Understanding its action in health and disease. Br J Anaesth 2000;85:69–79.
4. Owens DR, Zinman B, Bolli GB. Insulins today and beyond. Lancet 2001;358:739–46.
5. Atkinson MA, Eisenbarth GS. Type 1 diabetes: New perspectives on disease pathogenesis and treatment. Lancet 2001;358:221–9.
6. American Diabetes Association. Hyperglycemic crises in patients with diabetes mellitus. Diabetes Care 2001;24:154–61.
7. Scherpereel PA, Tavernier B. Perioperative care of diabetic patients. Eur J Anaesthesiol 2001;18:277–94.
8. McAnulty GR, Robertshaw HJ, Hall GM. Anaesthetic management of patients with diabetes mellitus. Br J Anaesth 2000;85:80–90.
9. Gu W, Pagel PS, Warltier DC, Kersten JR. Modifying cardiovascular risk in diabetes mellitus. Anesthesiology 2003;98:774–9.

Chapter 20

Endocrine Disease and Anaesthesia

INTRODUCTION

Patients with endocrine diseases often present for anaesthesia and surgery that may or may not be directly related to the disease condition. It is important to be familiar with the disease in order to provide optimal management during the perioperative period.

Endocrine disorders are commonly found in:

— Pancreas: diabetes mellitus (see Chapter 19).

— Pituitary gland: hyper- and hypopituitarism.

— Thyroid gland: hyper- and hypothyroidism.

— Parathyroid glands: hyperparathyroidism.
— Adrenal glands: Cushing's syndrome, Conn's syndrome, glucocorticoid deficiency.
— Chromaffin cells (adrenal and extra-adrenal): phaeochromocytoma.

THYROID DISEASE AND ANAESTHESIA

Enlargement of the thyroid gland may be due to a variety of conditions such as multinodular goitre, Graves' disease, Hashimoto's disease (autoimmune thyroiditis), benign thyroid nodule or carcinoma of thyroid. The patient may be clinically and biochemically euthyroid, hyperthyroid on antithyroid medication, or hypothyroid on thyroid hormone supplement.

Patients with thyroid disease can present for surgery to the thyroid gland (thyroid lobectomy, subtotal or total thyroidectomy) or surgery to the pituitary gland in the presence of a pituitary adenoma (hypophysectomy via the transphenoidal or frontal approach). They may also present for any incidental surgery unrelated to the thyroid gland.

Thyroid surgery may consist of a straightforward removal of a solitary thyroid nodule; or it may involve extensive dissection for removal of thyroid carcinoma. Longstanding retrosternal goitre may require surgery to relieve tracheal compression symptoms. This is usually approached via a standard neck incision, but occasionally a sternal split is necessary to access the retrosternal thyroid mass.

Problems in anaesthesia are three-fold.

1. **Problems pertaining to the airway**
   - Tracheal compression or deviation by an enlarged thyroid gland.
   - Infiltration by thyroid carcinoma giving rise to distorted airway anatomy, vocal cord palsies, intraluminal spread leading to obstruction anywhere from the supraglottic to bronchial level.
   - Presence of retrosternal goitre leading to lower tracheal compression or superior vena cava (SVC) obstruction.
   - Possibility of tracheomalacia as a result of longstanding compression of the trachea.

2. **Problems pertaining to the endocrine status**
   - Hyperthyroidism with risks of thyrotoxic crisis, cardiac arrhythmias, cardiac failure, impaired glucose tolerance, thyrotoxic myopathy.

— Hypothyroidism with increased sensitivity to anaesthetic agents and delayed recovery, poor tolerance to blood loss and other perioperative stresses.

3. **Problems related to the surgery**
   — Head and neck surgery with decreased accessibility to the airway during surgery.
   — Damage to the recurrent laryngeal nerve, with postoperative hoarseness or stridor.
   — Damage or accidental removal of parathyroid glands, with postoperative hypocalcaemia.
   — Risk of venous air embolism during neck dissection.
   — Haematoma leading to postoperative airway compression.
   — Hypothyroidism (late complication).

Preoperative Assessment and Preparation

1. **Thyroid gland and airway assessment**
   — Inquire about duration of thyroid enlargement.
   - Sudden increase in size suggests malignancy or haemorrhage into the gland.
   - Longstanding tracheal compression may give rise to tracheomalacia.

   — Ask specifically for presence of compressive symptoms.
   - Features of positional breathlessness, stridor or dysphagia indicate significant airway compression and should be further investigated with CT scan or MRI to delineate the extent of tracheal compression.

   — Examine the thyroid gland.
   - Note the size, consistency (hardness suggests malignancy), extent of the thyroid enlargement and the presence of bruit on auscultation.
   - Look for tracheal deviation.
   - Feel for the lower border of thyroid enlargement to rule out retrosternal extension.

   — Note the patient's range of neck movements and do a thorough airway assessment to determine ease of intubation.
   — Examine cervical X-ray (antero-posterior and lateral views) for tracheal deviation or compression.
   — If CT scan or MRI has been done on the patient, examine the films to delineate the extent of retrosternal extension and evidence of compression of the airway.

— Refer to the ENT team for assessment of vocal cord function under indirect laryngoscopy. Any preexisting vocal cord palsy should be clearly documented.

2. **Endocrine status**

— Ensure that the patient is clinically euthyroid before elective surgery.

— Exclude features of hyperthyroidism.

- Ask for history of palpitations, weight loss, heat intolerance, anxiety, muscle weakness, tremors.
- Examine for atrial fibrillation, tachycardia (awake and sleeping pulse), hyperreflexia, sweaty palms, tremors, bruit over the thyroid gland, myxoedema, myopathy, eye involvement (exophthalmos, lid lag, lid retraction).

— Exclude features of hypothyroidism.

- Ask for history of lethargy, cold intolerance, features of congestive cardiac failure.
- Examine for coarse dry skin, slow mentation, bradycardia, hypertension, hyporeflexia.

— Review the latest thyroid function test.

— Look for features suggestive of other autoimmune disorders which may be associated with Graves' disease or Hashimoto's thyroiditis, such as myasthenia gravis, adrenal insufficiency, ovarian failure.

3. **Cardiovascular system**

— Check heart rate and rhythm, look for atrial fibrillation.

— Careful cardiac assessment to rule out heart failure or ischaemic heart disease.

— Look for features of SVC obstruction such as facial plethora, raised jugular venous pressure, distended neck veins which do not alter with respiration.

4. **Current treatment**

— Review the patient's medications, assess compliance to treatment and look for side-effects of the medications.

- Antithyroid drugs: carbimazole (rarely causes agranulocytosis), or propylthiouracil (may be associated with hepatitis, thrombocytopaenia or hypoprothrombinaemia).
- β-adrenergic blockers: propranolol, atenolol.
- Lugol's iodine: this acutely inhibits release of thyroid hormones and reduces vascularity of the thyroid gland; may be administered for 7–10 days preoperatively.

    - thyroxine therapy in patients with hypothyroidism.
  - Instruct the patient to continue taking the medication on the morning of surgery.

5. **Premedication**
   - Premedication with a benzodiazepine helps to allay anxiety and apprehension before surgery.
   - Sedative premedication should be omitted in any patient with airway obstruction.
   - Prescribe an antisialogogue if fibreoptic intubation is the planned anaesthetic technique.

Anaesthetic Management

Airway management options

Based on the preoperative airway assessment, these are the airway management options.

1. No airway difficulty anticipated
   - Preoxygenation followed by intravenous induction and intubation facilitated by a non-depolarizing neuromuscular blocking drug.

2. Possible difficulty in intubation
   - Difficult airway equipment should be checked and ready for use if required.
   - Preoxygenation followed by intravenous induction, gently assist ventilation to assess possibility of ventilation via face mask.
   - If mask ventilation is adequate, proceed to intubation following muscle relaxation with suxamethonium.
   - If mask ventilation is difficult, continue with 100% oxygen and allow the patient to awaken. Consider alternative intubation techniques, e.g., fibreoptic intubation.

3. Definite intubation problem, or evidence of airway obstruction
   - Awake fibreoptic intubation
     - This is useful when there is marked displacement of the larynx or presence of co-existing features of difficult intubation.

    - A smaller sized ETT may be required in the presence of airway compression.
- — Inhalational induction with sevoflurane in 100% oxygen
    - It is useful to apply topical local anaesthetic to the upper airway prior to induction of anaesthesia.
    - Remember that stridor and decreased minute ventilation may make it difficult to attain sufficient anaesthetic depth for intubation. This can be facilitated by assisted ventilation and continuous positive airway pressure (CPAP).
    - When the patient is adequately anaesthetized, perform a gentle laryngoscopy to visualize the vocal cords. If these can be visualized, it would be safe to administer a neuromuscular blocking drug to facilitate tracheal intubation. If the cords cannot be visualized, proceed to fibreoptic intubation with the patient anaesthetized and breathing spontaneously.
- — Tracheostomy under local anaesthesia
    - This may not be a viable option in the presence of an enlarged thyroid gland or severely distorted airway anatomy.
    - This same difficulty would be encountered by cricothyrotomy should an emergency surgical airway become a necessity.
- — Ventilation through a rigid bronchoscope
    - This may be a life-saving manoeuvre when all else fails.
    - The ENT surgeon and necessary equipment must be immediately available in complex cases, particularly if mid- to lower tracheal narrowing is evident on CT scan or MRI.

Endotracheal tube (ETT)

- — The flexometallic (armoured) tube is most widely used since the possibility of kinking is less. A stylet is needed to aid insertion, and it is slightly more difficult to insert compared to ordinary polyvinyl chloride (PVC) tubes. As such PVC tubes should be available in case difficulty is encountered.
- — The ETT and its connection to the breathing system should be taped securely as this is not accessible during surgery.

Conduct of anaesthesia

- — Monitors include ECG, non-invasive BP, pulse oximetry, capnography, temperature and peripheral nerve stimulator.

— The patient is positioned supine with 15° head up tilt to aid venous drainage and reduce intraoperative blood loss. The neck is hyper-extended to provide optimal surgical exposure. Make sure that the eyes are kept closed and protected with eyepads, particularly if exophthalmos is present.
— The common anaesthetic technique is balanced anaesthesia with nitrous oxide-oxygen-volatile anaesthetic mixture, neuromuscular blocking drug, opioid and IPPV.
— Airway pressure should be closely monitored at all times. Inform the surgeon if this increases excessively during manipulation of the trachea as it may be due to obstruction distal to the ETT or the bevel of the ETT abutting on the trachea. Be alert for disconnection or accidental extubation because these mishaps may still occur despite our best efforts to secure the ETT.
— If tracheomalacia is suspected, the state and consistency of the trachea should be assessed intraoperatively after removal of the thyroid.
— The possibility of thyrotoxic crisis should always be borne in mind if signs of hypercarbia, hyperpyrexia and tachyarrhythmia are present (*vide infra*). The surgeon should be alerted and appropriate treatment instituted.

Reversal of neuromuscular blockade

— Usual criteria for reversal and extubation apply for uncomplicated cases.
— Observation of vocal cord movements under direct laryngoscopy on extubation, though advocated, may be difficult to perform in most cases.
— The patient's respiratory pattern should be closely observed in PACU.
— Consider the possibility of tracheomalacia especially in long-standing huge goitre. Options include:
- Trial of extubation with Cook™ airway exchange catheter in place; and early reintubation if postoperative stridor occurs.
- Elective tracheostomy after thyroidectomy is performed.

Possible Problems

1. **Thyrotoxic crisis or thyroid storm**

— This is a hypermetabolic state which complicates decompensated hyperthyroidism, caused by uncontrolled release of excessive thyroid hormones and associated with sensitization to endogenous and exogenous catecholamines. It can be fatal (reported mortality 20–30%) and requires urgent treatment.

— The condition is usually triggered off by a stimulus such as trauma, infection or surgery. It may present intra- or postoperatively with these clinical features.
  - Hyperpyrexia.
  - Confusion, agitation, delirium.
  - Tachyarrhythmia (sinus tachycardia, atrial fibrillation, supraventricular tachycardia), hypertension, high output cardiac failure.
  - Hyperventilation, tachypnoea, hypercarbia.
  - Vomiting, dehydration, ketosis, hyponatraemia, hypokalaemia.

— Clinical manifestations may mimic malignant hyperthermia, and dantrolene has been used with no adverse effects.

— Management: general measures
  - Airway, breathing and circulation: 100% oxygen, airway protection if necessary, hyperventilation, aggressive intravenous fluid replacement, treatment of heart failure and/or tachyarrhythmias.
  - Active cooling measures: cold intravenous fluids, cooling blankets, nasogastric or bladder lavage, antipyretics (avoid aspirin).
  - Remove or correct precipitating cause.
  - ICU admission for further management.

— Management: specific measures
  - β-adrenergic blockade: IV esmolol 0.5 mg/kg followed by further bolus doses or infusion of 50–200 μg/kg/min; or IV propranolol 0.5 mg increments to a maximum of 5 mg.
  - Antithyroid drugs: carbimazole 60–120 mg or propylthiouracil 200 mg orally or via nasogastric tube (effect is seen 1 hour later).
  - Iodides: consider potassium iodide 60 mg via nasogastric tube every 8-hourly; this should be given only after antithyroid medication has been started.
  - Corticosteroids: consider IV hydrocortisone or dexamethasone; they help to inhibit thyroid hormone production and treat relative adrenal insufficiency which often occurs concomitantly.

2. **Postoperative airway obstruction** (see Chapter 67)

— This may sometimes occur in PACU, and is an emergency which requires urgent intervention.

— Possible causes include:
  - Surgical factors: neck haematoma with tracheal compression, recurrent laryngeal nerve palsy, tracheomalacia, hypocalcaemia secondary to hypoparathyroidism.

  - Anaesthetic factors: incomplete reversal of neuromuscular blockade, central respiratory depression with hypoventilation, laryngospasm, laryngeal oedema, blood or secretions in the airway.
- — Management options depend on the severity of airway obstruction and the underlying cause. Most severe cases require immediate re-intubation because other airway management measures are often inadequate to overcome the obstruction.

3. **Postoperative hypocalcaemia**
   - — This may result from accidental removal, damage or interruption of blood supply to the parathyroid glands during neck dissection.
   - — Clinical manifestations include these.
     - Circumoral tingling, paraesthesia, cramps, carpopedal spasm.
     - Stridor secondary to laryngospasm.
     - Tetany with positive Chvostek's and Trousseau's signs.
     - Mental confusion, convulsions.
     - Prolonged QT interval, arrhythmias (especially torsades de pointes).
   - — Send blood sample for measurement of serum calcium concentration.
   - — Treat with slow intravenous injection of 10 ml of 10% calcium chloride under ECG monitoring.

4. **Myxoedema coma**
   - — This is a relatively rare complication of severe hypothyroidism and may be precipitated by infection, trauma, surgery or drugs (opioids, sedatives, β-blockers).
   - — Clinical features include:
     - Decreased level of consciousness, coma, increased sensitivity to sedatives.
     - Bradycardia, decreased cardiac output, pericardial effusion.
     - Depressed response to hypoxia and hypercarbia, respiratory muscle weakness, hypoventilation, respiratory failure.
     - Hypothermia (core temperature $< 36°C$), hypoglycaemia, hyponatraemia, cortisol deficiency.
   - — Management: general measures
     - Slow rewarming.
     - Respiratory support by means of mechanical ventilation.
     - Correction of glucose and electrolyte disturbances.
     - Remove or correct precipitating cause.

- Management: specific measures
  - Thyroid hormone replacement: IV liothyronine (T_3) 50–100 μg slowly under ECG monitoring, followed by 25 μg 8-hourly.
  - Corticosteroid: IV hydrocortisone 100 mg 6-hourly.

ANAESTHESIA FOR PARATHYROID SURGERY

Parathyroid disorders affect calcium and phosphate homeostasis. Surgery to the parathyroid glands involves neck dissection; and in cases of recurrent disease the mediastinum may need to be explored. Reliable airway control is required to allow for unrestricted tissue traction and neck dissection.

Preoperative Assessment

Hyperparathyroidism may be primary, secondary or tertiary. It leads to excessive bone resorption, renal calculi with deteriorating renal function, dehydration and electrolyte imbalance with hypercalcaemia and hypophosphataemia.

Clinical presentation of hyperparathyroidism may be subtle, being asymptomatic in 50% of the cases. Most of the clinical manifestations of hyperparathyroidism are due to hypercalcaemia. These include:

- Hypertension, ventricular arrhythmia, prolonged PR interval, shortened QT interval on ECG.
- Polyuria, polydipsia, renal calculi, renal failure, hyperchloraemic metabolic acidosis.
- Ileus, nausea and vomiting, pancreatitis, peptic ulcer disease.
- Mental changes: depression, delirium, psychosis, coma.

Hypercalcaemia can also be caused by malignancy with destructive bone metastases, such as breast carcinoma and multiple myeloma. Carcinoma of the lung may rarely release a parathyroid hormone-like substance, causing hypercalcaemia.

Hypercalcaemic crisis requires urgent treatment. This includes:

- Fluid rehydration, often in excess of 4 L/day.
- Forced saline diuresis with frusemide.
- Corticosteroids, mithramycin, and phosphate replacement.
- Dialysis for patients with renal failure.

Essential investigations include liver function test, serum calcium concentration, urea, creatinine and electrolytes and ECG.

- Correction for serum calcium concentration in cases of hypoalbuminaemia:

  (40 – measured albumin) × 0.02 + measured serum calcium
- Normal serum calcium concentration: 2.2–2.5 mmol/L (total); 0.9–1.1 mmol/L (ionized)

The corrected serum calcium concentration should be less than 3 mmol/L. An elevated serum calcium concentration together with ECG changes of hypercalcaemia and cardiovascular or renal impairment requires further treatment and deferment of surgery.

Anaesthetic Management

General anaesthesia with endotracheal intubation and controlled ventilation is the anaesthetic technique of choice, with these considerations.

- Be aware of the problems associated with neck surgery, such as reduced accessibility during surgery, risk of recurrent laryngeal nerve damage, baroreceptor stimulation and venous air embolism.
- The patient's concomitant medical conditions, in particular cardiovascular and renal disease problems, may necessitate modification of the anaesthetic technique, anaesthetic drug choices or dosages.
- The patient's intravascular volume may be inadequate and result in hypotension on induction of anaesthesia. Normal saline should be used for fluid replacement rather than Ringer's lactate solution, which contains calcium.
- Possibility of osteoporosis predisposes the patient to vertebral compression during laryngoscopy and pathological fractures during transport and positioning.
- Increased ventricular irritability secondary to hypercalcaemia may precipitate fatal arrhythmias and enhance digitalis toxicity.
- Monitoring of neuromuscular blockade is indicated as response to neuromuscular blocking drugs may be altered in the presence of hypercalcaemia.
- Hypoventilation should be avoided since acidosis increases ionized calcium and worsens the clinical condition.
- Postoperative problems are similar to that following thyroid surgery.

ANAESTHESIA AND THE ADRENAL GLAND

The adrenal cortex secretes glucocorticoids (e.g., cortisol), mineralocorticoids (e.g., aldosterone) and androgens, while the adrenal medulla secretes catecholamines (adrenaline, noradrenaline and dopamine). Both hypersecretion and hyposecretion states are encountered clinically. The patient may present for adrenalectomy or any incidental surgery unrelated to the endocrine problem.

Glucocorticoid Excess (Cushing's Syndrome)

Causes of Cushing's syndrome include:

— Exogenous administration of steroid hormones.

— Hyperfunction of adrenal cortex, such as adrenocortical adenoma.

— Ectopic secretion of adrenocorticotropic hormone (ACTH).

— Hypersecretion of ACTH by pituitary adenoma, also known as Cushing's disease.

— Malignant tumours such as oat cell carcinoma of the lung which secrete ACTH-like hormone.

Clinical manifestations

— Hypertension, fluid retention, increased total blood volume, congestive cardiac failure.

— Muscle wasting with proximal myopathy, osteoporosis, atrophic skin, easy bruising.

— Redistribution of fat with moon face, truncal obesity and "buffalo hump".

— Hypernatraemia, hypokalaemia, metabolic alkalosis, impaired glucose tolerance, increased susceptibility to infections.

— Mental changes, psychosis.

Anaesthetic considerations

— Hypertension and/or heart failure should be managed accordingly. The patient may require intraoperative CVP and/or pulmonary artery pressure monitoring.

— Hypokalaemia may result in cardiac arrhythmias, muscle weakness and postoperative respiratory embarrassment. Metabolic abnormalities should be corrected preoperatively with potassium supplement and spironolactone.

— Suitable regimen for perioperative control of blood glucose should be instituted.

— Osteoporosis requires care in positioning and transport to prevent pathological fractures while venous access may be difficult due to fragility of veins.
— Initiate steroid replacement if the adrenal glands are removed, or if the cause of Cushing's syndrome is exogenous glucocorticoids (*vide infra*).
— Beware of surgical problems such as increased blood loss during resection of vascular tumour, or unintentional penetration into the pleural cavity causing pneumothorax.

Mineralocorticoid Excess

This can be due to intrinsic hypersecretion of aldosterone by the adrenal cortex (primary hyperaldosteronism or Conn's syndrome) or as a result of stimulation of the renin-angiotensin-aldosterone system (secondary hyperaldosteronism, associated with congestive heart failure, liver cirrhosis with ascites, renal artery stenosis).

Clinical manifestations

— Hypertension, secondary to sodium retention and increased extracellular fluid volume.
— Muscle weakness or paralysis, secondary to hypokalaemia.
— Hypokalaemia, hypocalcaemia, metabolic alkalosis.
— Impaired glucose tolerance.
— Nephrogenic diabetes insipidus secondary to renal tubular damage.

Anaesthetic considerations

— Blood pressure should be controlled preoperatively, and spironolactone should be included to control hypertension and potassium loss.
— Hypertension occurs with excessive sympathetic responses during intubation. Precautions should be taken to obtund sympathetic responses during airway instrumentation.
— Potassium replacement may be needed pre- and intraoperatively because of depletion of total body potassium. However, ECG and plasma potassium concentrations are unreliable guides to potassium therapy.
— Avoid hyperventilation resulting in respiratory alkalosis; this promotes potassium

shift into the cells and worsens preexisting hypokalaemia.

— Handling of the adrenal gland during surgery can cause cardiovascular instability but this is not as marked as with phaeochromocytoma. Following tumour removal, the electrolyte abnormalities usually reverse earlier than the correction of hypertension.

Glucocorticoid Deficiency

Primary adrenal insufficiency or Addison's disease is caused by destruction of the adrenal gland resulting in both glucocorticoid and mineralocorticoid deficiency.

Secondary adrenal insufficiency is caused by inadequate ACTH secretion by the pituitary gland. Unlike primary adrenal insufficiency, fluid and electrolyte disturbances are usually absent because mineralocorticoid secretion is usually adequate in this disease.

Adrenocortical deficiency may also present acutely following sepsis, pharmacological adrenal suppression or adrenal haemorrhage. Patients who are critically ill often exhibit features of relative adrenal insufficiency. Clinical features include nausea and vomiting, postural hypotension, apathy, coma and hypoglycaemia.

Adrenal supplementation therapy

— Supplementation is based on the likelihood of adrenal suppression, the degree of surgical stress, and the cardiovascular and metabolic response to therapy.

— The optimal dosing, frequency and duration of steroid replacement therapy continue to be debated, but recent expert recommendations call for lower doses and shorter duration of therapy.

— The routine administration of conventional doses of hydrocortisone in the range of 100–300 mg irrespective of patient condition or surgical procedure should be discouraged. Deleterious effects of excessive steroid supplementation include immunosuppression, glucose intolerance, delayed wound healing, hypertension, volume overload and acute corticosteroid-induced psychosis.

The doses for steroid supplementation are now much lower than previously recommended (Table 20–1).

Table 20–1. Adrenal supplementation therapy

Status	Recommendations	
Patients currently taking steroids		
< 10 mg/day	Additional steroid cover not required	
> 10 mg/day	*Minor surgery*	IV hydrocortisone 25 mg at induction
	Intermediate surgery	Usual preoperative steroids, IV hydrocortisone 50–75 mg at induction, taper over 1–2 days to usual dose
	Major surgery	Usual preoperative steroids, IV hydrocortisone 100–150 mg at induction, taper over 1–2 days to usual dose
High dose immuno-suppression	Usual immunosuppressive doses perioperatively	
Critically ill, e.g., sepsis-induced hypotension or shock	IV hydrocortisone 50–100 mg every 6–8 hours or 0.18 mg/kg/hr as a continuous infusion + fludrocortisone 50 μg/day until the shock state has been resolved	
Patients stopped taking steroids		
< 3 months ago	Treat as if on steroids	
> 3 months ago	No perioperative steroid supplementation required	

Anaesthetic considerations

— A well-controlled case of Addison's disease undergoing surgery will require nothing more than supplementary hydrocortisone, but one should be aware that the patient may exhibit increased sensitivity to sedatives and anaesthetic agents.

— Perioperative hypotension is often attributed to adrenal insufficiency; other causes – such as hypovolaemia sepsis, myocardial depression – should be excluded and managed accordingly.

— Metabolic abnormalities in severe cases include hyponatraemia, hyperkalaemia, hypoglycaemia, hypercalcaemia and elevated urea level. These abnormalities should be corrected.

— A previously undiagnosed Addisonian crisis may be a rare cause of cardiovascular collapse during surgery and anaesthesia.

— Management of Addisonian crisis includes these measures.
  - IV hydrocortisone 200 mg stat dose, then 100–200 mg daily in divided doses until oral replacement is possible.
  - Fluid resuscitation using normal saline, guided by urine output and CVP monitoring; large volumes may be required.
  - Dextrose as necessary to correct hypoglycaemia.
  - Inotropes if hypotension persists despite the above measures.
  - Consider mineralocorticoid replacement if biochemical abnormalities persist despite treatment.
  - Treatment of underlying causes which precipitate the crisis.

ANAESTHESIA AND PHAEOCHROMOCYTOMA

Phaeochromocytoma is an uncommon tumour that secretes catecholamines (predominantly noradrenaline but sometimes adrenaline or dopamine). It develops in the chromaffin cells derived from the primitive neural crest. They are mostly, but not exclusively, found in the adrenal glands, about 10% being extra-adrenal. Phaeochromocytoma may be associated with other disorders such as neurofibromatosis, medullary thyroid carcinoma and parathyroid adenoma as manifestation of an autosomal dominant multi-glandular neoplastic syndrome termed multiple endocrine neoplasia (MEN).

Clinical Manifestations

The patient can present perioperatively with hypertension and cardiovascular instability under anaesthesia. The mortality for unrecognized phaeochromocytoma is high (up to 50%) unless the diagnosis is considered and appropriate treatment instituted.

Common presenting symptoms (5 H's) are **H**ypertension, **H**eadache, **H**yperhidrosis, **H**ypermetabolic states and **H**yperglycaemia.

Other clinical features include:

— Palpitations and tachyarrhythmias, particularly with adrenaline-secreting tumour.

— Dilated cardiomyopathy with left ventricular failure, acute pulmonary oedema, myocarditis.

— Psychiatric changes, ranging from mild anxiety to frank psychosis.

— "Phaeochromocytoma crisis"
- Hypertensive encephalopathy, neurological deficit, cortical blindness, coma.
- Impalpable peripheral pulses.
- Metabolic acidosis.

— Hypotension and high output cardiac failure may be the initial presenting features of adrenaline-secreting tumour.

Preoperative Preparation

The main objective of preoperative preparation is to control arterial pressure, heart rate and arrhythmias, and to allow blood volume to be restored to normal. Other than routine preanaesthetic assessment, the following systems need to be carefully evaluated.

1. **Cardiovascular system**

   — Thorough assessment of the cardiovascular system is essential. This involves consultation with a cardiologist or physician for echocardiography and other forms of investigations.

   — Blood pressure control is usually achieved using an α-adrenergic blocker (phenoxybenzamine, prazosin) followed by a β-adrenergic blocker (atenolol, labetalol, propranolol). Note that β-blockade should not be started first because hypertension may be exacerbated by unopposed α-mediated vasoconstriction. Avoid β-blockers in patients with limited myocardial reserve or evidence of catecholamine-induced cardiomyopathy.

— Assess adequacy of blood pressure control
  - Baseline should be BP 140/90 mmHg or less.
  - Resting heart rate should be 100/min or less.
  - Postural hypotension with compensatory tachycardia should be present.
— Assess the intravascular volume. Chronic vasoconstriction can lead to a depleted blood volume resulting in hypotension during induction of anaesthesia.
— Assess and optimize associated cardiac conditions.
— Serve the usual medication on the morning of surgery. Phenoxybenzamine, if used, should be withheld 48 hours before surgery because of its long half-life.

2. **Endocrine system**
— Excessive catecholamines give rise to increased glycogenolysis and insulin resistance; the resultant hyperglycaemia may require insulin therapy.
— Preoperative hypercalcaemia may indicate presence of hyperparathyroidism as part of MEN.

Surgery

— Adrenalectomy for phaeochromocytoma has traditionally been performed using the lateral retroperitoneal approach, though a transabdominal approach may be necessary in some patients. It is now feasible to perform laparoscopic adrenalectomy in selected patients with benign pathology of the adrenal gland, either transperitoneally or retroperitoneally.
— Open surgery is usually quicker, and haemodynamic responses during tumour manipulation, while inevitable, are usually of short duration.
— Laparoscopic excision involves a considerable learning curve; hence the operating time is significantly longer and some cases may necessitate conversion to open surgery. The patients are usually remarkably stable haemodynamically during the procedure, with risks of hypertension occurring during creation of the pneumoperitoneum and manipulation of the adrenal gland. This haemodynamic stability is enhanced in retroperitoneal laparoscopic surgery, during which only a small increase in intraabdominal pressure is produced.
— Further advantages of laparoscopic adrenalectomy include lower intraoperative blood loss, better cosmetic effect, less postoperative analgesic requirement, faster postoperative recovery and shorter hospital stay.

Anaesthetic Management

The anaesthetic management plan, extent of intraoperative monitoring and choice of postoperative analgesic technique are all influenced by the patient's medical condition as well as the surgical approach for adrenalectomy.

— Premedication
  - A heavy premedication is desirable provided that the cardiac status is satisfactory. This serves to reduce anxiety, which may increase catecholamine secretion.
  - Avoid the use of atropine as premedicant.

— Monitors include ECG, non-invasive BP, SpO_2, capnography, intraarterial BP, CVP. Consider pulmonary artery catheterization in patients with significant cardiac involvement.

— Anaesthetic technique and drugs
  - Combined thoracic epidural and general anaesthesia is the anaesthetic technique of choice for open surgery. Epidural anaesthesia is not necessary in laparoscopic surgery.
  - It is advisable to avoid drugs known to cause histamine release, such as morphine, suxamethonium, atracurium.
  - Suxamethonium should also be avoided because it may provoke catecholamine release from the tumour during the period of transient muscle fasciculation.
  - Halothane is seldom used because of its arrhythmogenicity in the presence of catecholamines. Other volatile anaesthetics – isoflurane, sevoflurane, desflurane – are preferred.
  - There are no contraindications to the use of nitrous oxide.

— Avoid hypertensive response during airway manipulation by ensuring adequate depth of anaesthesia and taking measures to attenuate sympathetic responses. However, rapid administration of the intravenous induction agent should be avoided since the resultant hypotension may stimulate catecholamine secretion from tumour cells.

— Maintain normocarbia and adequate oxygenation by adjusting the ventilatory parameters and monitoring the SpO_2, $ETCO_2$ and serial ABG analyses.

— Intensive intraoperative monitoring is essential. These problems may be encountered.

  1. **Hypertension**
     - This is often seen during airway instrumentation and when the surgeon handles the tumour.

- It can be controlled by intravenous infusion of sodium nitroprusside or other vasodilators.
- Labetalol, with its α- and β-blocking actions, has been used alone or in combination with sodium nitroprusside. Esmolol may also be used.
- Phentolamine, an α-blocker, may be used if available, but it is less satisfactory because of the problems of tachycardia and tachyphylaxis.
- Hypertensive episodes tend to be transient hence it is preferable to use antihypertensive agents with rapid onset and offset of action (e.g., sodium nitroprusside).

2. **Tachycardia**
   - β-blockers may be used with caution as they may accentuate LV dysfunction and precipitate cardiac failure in patients with cardiomyopathy.
   - Ventricular premature contractions, if frequent, can be treated with lignocaine.
   - Amiodarone may be effective in controlling catecholamine-induced supraventricular tachycardia.

3. **Hypotension**
   - The underlying cause(s) of hypotension should be elicited and appropriate treatment instituted, for example:
     - — Significant bleeding during resection of a vascular tumour: fluid resuscitation and transfusion of blood and/or blood products.
     - — Depletion of catecholamine effects after tumour resection: ensure adequate preload by maintaining CVP 10–15 mmHg.
     - — Low cardiac output: judicious use of small amounts of adrenaline, titrating to effect.
     - — Low systemic vascular resistance: consider using noradrenaline in refractory cases.
   - It is often possible to discontinue the inotrope support by the end of the surgery unless there are preexisting cardiac problems.

Postoperative Management

The patient should be transferred to ICU or HDU for further management, with particular attention to these areas.

— **Respiratory system**
  - Continue ventilatory support until the patient is warmed, conscious, haemodynamically stable, has regained good respiratory effort and is able to maintain satisfactory ABG.

— **Analgesia**
  - This may be provided by parenteral opioid or local anaesthetic-opioid infusion via the epidural route.
  - The patient may be somnolent during the first 48 hours after surgery and the dose of opioid should be titrated according to effect.

— **Cardiovascular system**
  - Continue invasive haemodynamic monitoring and treat any derangements early and aggressively.
  - Volume replacement usually continues to exceed measured losses and should be guided by CVP measurements.
  - Sustained postoperative hypertension may indicate the presence of residual tumour with incomplete surgical removal.

— **Steroid replacement**
  - This is indicated in bilateral adrenalectomy, but occasionally even patients with unilateral resection may be relatively hypoadrenal and require steroid replacement.

— **Hypoglycaemia**
  - This may occur in the early postoperative period because the action of insulin is no longer opposed by catecholamines.
  - Residual β-blockade may mask clinical signs and symptoms of hypoglycaemia; thus regular monitoring of blood glucose concentration is indicated.
  - Intravenous glucose maintenance is often necessary during the first 12–24 hours after surgery.

PITUITARY GLAND DYSFUNCTION

The pituitary gland consists of the anterior and posterior pituitary lobes, which are anatomically distinct. The anterior pituitary secretes hormones under the control of the hypothalamus. These hormones in turn exert effect on the target organs and are subjected to closely controlled negative feedback mechanism. The anterior pituitary hormones are growth hormone (GH, or somatotropin), adrenocorticotropic hormone (ACTH, or corticotropin), thyroid-stimulating hormone (TSH, or thyrotropin), follicle-stimulating hormone (FSH), luteinizing hormone (LH), and luteotropic hormone (LTH, or prolactin). The posterior pituitary gland secretes vasopressin (antidiuretic hormone, ADH) and oxytocin.

Pituitary gland dysfunction often arises from an adenoma which may be hormone-secreting, giving rise to Cushing's disease (excessive ACTH), acromegaly (excessive GH), thyrotoxicosis (excessive TSH), or hyperprolactinaemia (excessive prolactin). It can also be non-secreting but exerts effects by compression on the normal tissue and results in hypopituitarism. Panhypopituitarism can occur as a result of severe ischaemia as in the case of Sheehan syndrome. Metastatic tumour, most often from the breast or lung, also causes pituitary hypofunction.

For posterior pituitary, abnormalities in ADH secretion lead to diabetes insipidus as a result of absence of ADH, and inappropriate secretion leading to SIADH – syndrome of inappropriate ADH secretion.

Anaesthetic management for pituitary surgery is discussed in Chapter 44.

FURTHER READING

1. Farling PA. Thyroid disease. Br J Anaesth 2000;85:15–28.
2. Stathatos N, Wartofsky L. Thyrotoxic storm. J Intensive Care Med 2002;17:1–7.
3. Mihai R, Farndon JR. Parathyroid disease and calcium metabolism. Br J Anaesth 2000;85:29–43.
4. Jabbour SA. Steroids and the surgical patient. Med Clin N Am 2001;85:1311–7.
5. Nicholson G, Burrin JM, Hall GM. Peri-operative steroid supplementation. Anaesthesia 1998;53:1091–1104.
6. Coursin DB, Wood KE. Corticosteroid supplementation for adrenal insufficiency. JAMA 2002;287:236–40.
7. Winship SM, Winstanley JH, Hunter JM. Anaesthesia for Conn's syndrome. Anaesthesia 1999;54:564–74.
8. Prys–Roberts C. Phaeochromocytoma – recent progress in its management. Br J Anaesth 2000;85:44–57.
9. Atallah F, et al. Haemodynamic changes during retroperitoneoscopic adrenalectomy for phaeochromocytoma. Br J Anaesth 2001;86:731–3.

Chapter 21

Anaesthesia for Patients with Connective Tissue Disorder

INTRODUCTION

Connective tissue disorder is a mixed group of diseases which share some common characteristics.

— They are chronic inflammatory conditions affecting multiple organs.

— They are thought to be autoimmune in aetiology since various autoantibodies can be detected in the patient's serum. These antibodies are produced against the host antigens and an immune response is induced which results in tissue injury and subsequent clinical manifestations.

— The course of the disease is punctuated with episodes of acute exacerbations.

These are examples of connective tissue disorders.

— Rheumatoid arthritis
— Systemic lupus erythematosus
— Progressive systemic sclerosis
— Dermatomyositis
— Mixed connective tissue disorder

The first three conditions will be discussed in this chapter.

RHEUMATOID ARTHRITIS

This is a chronic inflammatory disorder which not only affects the peripheral joints but has widespread systemic involvement. Many of the systemic ("non-articular") manifestations of rheumatoid arthritis are thought to be secondary to deposition of immune complexes on the vessel wall, causing widespread vasculitis and inflammatory reactions. Rheumatoid factors, which are autoantibodies of IgE, IgA and IgM classes, are present together with hypergammaglobulinaemia.

Clinical Manifestations

1. **Joints**
   - Multiple joints are affected in a symmetrical fashion, with inflammation and fibrosis leading to joint destruction and deformity.
   - Although any joint may be involved, those of particular concern to the anaesthesiologist are the cervical spine, the temporomandibular and cricoarytenoid joints.
     - Cervical spine involvement includes cervical spine fusion and atlantoaxial subluxation, presenting with neck pain, limited movement, nerve root impingement or spinal cord compression.
     - Erosion of the mandibular condyle and temporal joint surface can give rise to limitation of mouth opening.
     - Inflammation and immobilization of cricoarytenoid joints may result in voice changes, hoarseness or rarely stridor secondary to glottic stenosis.
   - *All patients with rheumatoid arthritis should be assumed to have a difficult airway unless proven otherwise.*

2. **Lungs ("Rheumatoid lungs")**
   - Most common pulmonary manifestations are pleural effusions.
   - Others include rheumatoid nodules on lung parenchyma and pleural surfaces, diffuse interstitial fibrosis (Caplan's syndrome), restrictive respiratory disease with reduced chest wall compliance.

3. **Cardiovascular system**
   - Pericardial disease may occur with pericarditis, pericardial thickening or effusion which may necessitate pericardiocentesis.
   - Other cardiac conditions include endocarditis, myocarditis, inflammatory valve disease especially aortic insufficiency, left ventricular failure, conduction defects and arrhythmias.

4. **Other manifestations**
   - Kidney: renal failure, associated amyloidosis.
   - Haematological system: normocytic hypochromic anaemia, eosinophilia, thrombocytosis.
   - Peripheral neuropathy.
   - Purpura, skin ulcers.

Anaesthetic Considerations

1. **Intubation problems**
   - Instability of the cervical spine, usually in the form of atlantoaxial subluxation, may occur in 25% of patients, and excessive movement of head and neck during intubation may result in cervical cord damage.
   - Preoperative radiological examination of the neck is required; in emergency situations the patient should be assumed to have cervical spine disease and precautions taken accordingly.
   - Limitation of mouth opening may make it difficult to perform airway manoeuvres; and in conjunction with cervical spine involvement it may be virtually impossible to perform direct laryngoscopy and visualize the vocal cords.
   - In order to reduce the risk of laryngeal oedema and/or cricoarytenoid joint dislocation during intubation, the intubating process should be performed gently using an endotracheal tube which is one size smaller. Stridor and airway obstruction postextubation are possible complications which should be looked out for.

— It may be prudent to consider the option of an awake fibreoptic intubation, or, if applicable, avoid endotracheal intubation altogether by opting for regional anaesthesia or using an airway adjunct (e.g., laryngeal mask airway) under general anaesthesia.

2. **Problems of central neuraxial blockade**
   — Vertebral deformity may pose problems in optimal positioning for the block procedure and location of the intrathecal or epidural space.
   — Some anaesthesiologists consider the use of central neuraxial blockade unwise in cases of anticipated intubation difficulty. The intubating conditions would then be suboptimal if urgent intubation is required in case of failed block, excessively high block or total spinal.

3. **Other considerations**
   — A thorough systemic review should be carried out during preoperative assessment to identify the nature and severity of the disease. Anaesthetic management should be modified accordingly.
   — Take note of the patient's medications and their possible side-effects:
   - Non-steroidal antiinflammatory drugs (NSAIDs), including aspirin, may interfere with platelet function and renal function.
   - Corticosteroids, gold, methotrexate which may give rise to adrenal insufficiency, pulmonary impairment and immunosuppression.

SYSTEMIC LUPUS ERYTHEMATOSUS (SLE)

This is an autoimmune connective tissue disorder predominantly affecting females in the reproductive years. As in rheumatoid arthritis, multi-system involvement is common in SLE and the disease condition typically waxes and wanes. Stress, infection, pregnancy and certain drugs may bring about exacerbations. The course is highly variable, ranging from relatively mild and uncomplicated to major life-threatening disease.

Clinical Manifestations

The clinical manifestations of the disease are variable and depend on the severity of damage to the various organ systems.

1. **Cutaneous lesions**
   — Butterfly rash, Raynaud's disease.
   — Angioneurotic oedema.
   — Nasal and oral mucosal lesions.

2. **Musculoskeletal system**
   — Arthritis and arthralgia affecting small and large joints.

3. **Renal system**
   — SLE nephropathy in the form of glomerulonephritis: proteinuria, hypertension, nephrotic syndrome, azotaemia, renal insufficiency.
   — This is the major cause of morbidity and mortality.

4. **Haematological system**
   — Anaemia, leucopaenia, thrombocytopaenia.
   — The lupus anticoagulant is an antibody against IgG that interferes with coagulation tests and results in abnormal PTT and rarely PT.
   — Paradoxically patients are at increased risk of developing recurrent arterial or venous thromboembolism.
   — Antibodies to coagulation proteins may also be present, and both quantitative and qualitative platelet dysfunction have been reported.

5. **CNS lesions**
   — Presentations are diverse and not specific to SLE.
   — Symptoms include neurological defect, seizures, frank psychosis.

6. **Heart lesions**
   — Valvular lesions, bacterial endocarditis (Libman-Sachs), myocarditis, pericarditis.
   — Coronary artery disease secondary to vasculitis or atherosclerosis.

7. **Lung lesions**
   — Pneumonitis, fibrosing alveolitis, restrictive lung disease.
   — Pulmonary hypertension.
   — Frequent pulmonary infections.

8. **Constitutional symptoms**
   — Fever, weight loss, malaise, fatigue.

Anaesthetic Considerations

— Cardiovascular and respiratory systems need to be assessed thoroughly. Infective endocarditis prophylaxis is necessary for patients with valvular heart lesions.

— Check coagulation studies especially if regional anaesthesia is contemplated. The PT, APTT and platelet count may be abnormal. Even though the abnormal results may be interference from lupus anticoagulant and not a true bleeding disorder, it seems prudent not to perform regional anaesthesia when the test results are abnormal especially if there is concomitant thrombocytopaenia.

— The patient may be on long-term corticosteroid therapy and may have Cushingoid features. As there is a risk of adrenal suppression, perioperative steroid supplementation may be indicated.

— Grouping and cross-matching for blood may be problematic as there are irregular antibodies in the serum.

PROGRESSIVE SYSTEMIC SCLEROSIS

Progressive systemic sclerosis, also referred to as scleroderma, is a multi-system disorder characterized by fibrosis of blood vessels, skin, musculoskeletal system, and visceral organs. There is overproduction and accumulation of collagen, activation of immunologic mechanisms and increased fibroblast proliferation. There are two major forms of the disease: limited cutaneous systemic sclerosis or CREST syndrome (**C**arcinosis, **R**aynaud's phenomenon, O**E**sophageal hypomotility, **S**clerodactyly, **T**elangiectasia) and diffuse cutaneous systemic sclerosis.

Clinical Manifestations and Anaesthetic Implications

1. **Skin and musculoskeletal system**
   — Raynaud's phenomenon: usually the first presenting symptom.
   — Dermal thickening with flexion contractures, ischaemic ulcers, resorption of distal phalanges.
   — Shiny, taut, waxy-looking skin with loss of skin folds, non-pitting oedema.

- — Multiple telangiectasia on fingers, face, tongue, lips, buccal or nasal mucosa.
- — Small mouth, beaked nose.
- — Symmetric polyarthritis and joint crepitation
    - Raynaud's phenomenon: peripheral vasoconstriction.
    - Dermal thickening with joint contractures: difficult venous access, difficulties in patient positioning for surgery or nerve blocks.
    - Skin tightening, limited mouth opening, decreased neck mobility: difficult airway management.
    - Fragile skin susceptible to damage.
    - Telangiectasia in the mouth and nose: risk of trauma and bleeding during airway instrumentation.

2. **Gastrointestinal system**
    - — Thinning of oesophageal mucosa with fibrotic thickening of remaining layers.
    - — Mucosal ulceration, oesophageal dilation.
    - — Dysphagia, reflux oesophagitis, disturbances in oesophageal motility.
    - — Smooth muscle atrophy in small intestine with decreased absorption and diverticuli formation.
        - Oesophageal dilation with decreased lower oesophageal sphincter tone: risk of reflux, regurgitation and aspiration.
        - Intestinal malabsorption: decreased Vitamin K-dependent clotting factors.

3. **Cardiac involvement**
    - — Myocardial fibrosis with cardiac conduction defects, ventricular hypertrophy, diastolic dysfunction.
    - — Sclerotic coronary vessels, increased tendency for vasospasm.
    - — Pericarditis with effusion.
    - — Myocarditis with left ventricular dysfunction.
    - — All the above pose problems during anaesthetic management and increase cardiac morbidity.

4. **Respiratory involvement**
    - — Restrictive lung disease with interstitial and peribronchial fibrosis.
    - — Respiratory muscle weakness.
    - — Pulmonary hypertension secondary to smooth muscle hypertrophy in pulmonary blood vessels.

— Cor pulmonale with right ventricular failure: restrictive pulmonary disease with increased risk of hypoxaemia and postoperative respiratory insufficiency requiring postoperative ventilatory support.

5. **Renal involvement**

Nephropathy with systemic hypertension

— Decreased renal clearance of drugs.

— Problems associated with hypertension during anaesthesia.

Anaesthetic Management

— Assessment to determine severity of disease and extent of multiple organ involvement.

- Further investigations as indicated.
- Formulate plans for airway management.
- Prescribe acid aspiration prophylaxis.
- Arrange for postoperative ICU or HDU management in severe cases.

— Intraoperative management

- Maintain OT temperature above 20°C and use other means to prevent hypothermia in order to minimize peripheral vasoconstriction.
- There are no specific contraindications to the use of any type of anaesthetic.
- Consider regional anaesthesia in appropriate cases.
- Avoid or modify dose of renally excreted drugs.

SUMMARY

The clinical features and problems relevant to the anaesthesiologist are highlighted.

As in other systemic diseases with multi-organ involvement, there should be a multi-disciplinary approach involving the primary physician, cardiologist, respiratory physician, haematologist, nephrologist and physiotherapist in addition to the surgeon and the anaesthesiologist. The patient should be assessed carefully, the likely problems identified, the anaesthetic management planned in advance and the patient closely monitored during the postoperative period.

FURTHER READING

1. MacArthur A, Kleiman S. Rheumatoid cervical joint disease – a challenge to the anaesthetist. Can J Anaesth 1993;40:154–9.
2. Skues MA, Welchew EA. Anaesthesia and rheumatoid arthritis. Anaesthesia 1993;48:989–97.
3. Madan R, et al. The anaesthetist and the antiphospholipid syndrome. Anaesthesia 1997;52:72–6.
4. Roberts JG, Sabar R, Gianoli JA, Kaye AD. Progressive systemic sclerosis: Clinical manifestations and anesthetic considerations. J Clin Anesth 2002;14:474–7.

Chapter 22

Anaesthesia and Obesity

INTRODUCTION

Obesity is a complex, multi-factorial disease with metabolic, genetic, environmental and psychological components. It occurs when net energy intake exceeds net energy expenditure over a long period of time. Various indices have been used to define obesity. The common ones are:

— *Broca index*, where ideal weight is [height (cm) – 105] kg for females, and [height (cm) – 100] kg for males. An individual is said to be obese when the weight is more than 20% above the ideal weight, and morbidly obese when the weight is double the ideal weight.

— *Body mass index (BMI)* = weight (kg)/[height (m)]^2
  - normal < 25
  - overweight 26–29
  - obese 30–34
  - morbidly obese > 35

The vast majority (90–95%) is classified as simple obesity. The remaining 5–10% come under the category of obesity hypoventilation syndrome (OHS) or Pickwickian syndrome, where there is a progressive desensitization of the respiratory centre to carbon dioxide. Features of OHS include somnolence, polycythaemia, periodic respirations, cardiomegaly with biventricular hypertrophy, severe hypoxaemia, hypercarbia and pulmonary hypertension.

There is a whole host of medical and surgical conditions which are associated with obesity. Some of these are listed here.

— Respiratory system: obstructive sleep apnoea, obesity hypoventilation syndrome, restrictive respiratory disease.

— Cardiovascular system: hypertension, cardiomegaly, coronary artery disease, congestive heart failure, cerebrovascular disease, peripheral vascular disease, pulmonary hypertension, thromboembolism (deep vein thrombosis, pulmonary embolism).

— Endocrine/metabolic system: diabetes mellitus, Cushing's syndrome, hypothyroidism, hypercholesterolaemia, hypertriglyceridaemia.

— Gastrointestinal system: hiatus hernia, gallstones, fatty infiltration of liver.

— Musculoskeletal system: osteoarthritis, back pain.

ANTICIPATED PROBLEMS IN ANAESTHETIC MANAGEMENT

The obese patient may undergo any incidental surgery or obesity-related surgery such as gastroplasty or gastric bypass. The latter are usually recommended for individuals with severe obesity (BMI > 40). Anaesthetic management of the obese patient poses an interesting challenge as the anaesthesiologist may be faced with problems throughout the perioperative period. These should be anticipated and managed appropriately. These are some examples.

— The patent's concomitant medical conditions may require special attention and management.

- Airway management issues: potential difficulty in intubation and/or mask ventilation as a result of obesity-related anatomic features, such as fat face and cheeks, large tongue, excessive palatal and pharyngeal soft tissue mass, limited mouth opening, short neck, restricted neck mobility, large breasts.
- Increased gastric volume, raised intraabdominal pressure, increased incidence of hiatus hernia: risk of regurgitation and aspiration under anaesthesia.
- Increased oxygen consumption (increased metabolic requirements) with reduced functional residual capacity (airway closure, splinting of diaphragm with abdominal contents): rapid oxygen desaturation during period of apnoea.
- Restrictive lung disease, reduced chest wall compliance, splinting of diaphragm: increased work of breathing on spontaneous respiration, increased airway pressures with risk of barotraumas on IPPV.
- Practical issues: extra personnel required for transport and positioning, OT table may be unable to support the patient's weight or girth, problems with suitable monitoring equipment, presence of arthritis or reduced joint movements may cause problem in positioning, difficult venepuncture sites and indistinct landmarks for regional blocks, increased tissue trauma caused by excessive surgical retraction to achieve adequate exposure, increased operating time as a result of difficult surgery.
- Altered drug pharmacokinetics: increased volume of distribution, variable protein binding, problems with dosage adjustments, drug accumulation with relative overdose and residual effects.
- Increased risk of thromboembolic events: need for perioperative thromboprophylaxis.
- Postoperative management: requirement for effective analgesia, monitoring, oxygen therapy, chest physiotherapy and early mobilization.

PREOPERATIVE ASSESSMENT

History

- Look for features of diseases commonly associated with obesity.
- Inquire about details of sleep pattern, presence of snoring, episodes of apnoea with disturbed sleep, presence or severity of somnolence: it may be necessary to obtain this history from the sleeping partner.
- Assess the patient's psychological status.

— Review the patient's medication history and assess compliance to treatment. Besides treatment for concomitant medical conditions, the patient may be on appetite suppressants such as fenfluramine, sibutramine, orlistat. Fenfluramine has been reported to produce unacceptable side-effects such as pulmonary hypertension, and there have been case reports of sudden cardiac arrest and death under anaesthesia.

Physical Examination

— General condition: assess the presence of somnolence, hypoventilation, polycythaemia; check for possible venepuncture sites.

— Cardiovascular system: examine for cardiomegaly, heart murmurs, signs of cardiac failure; obtain BP measurement in the erect and supine position for evidence of postural hypotension.

— Respiratory system and airway: do a thorough airway assessment to rule out potential difficult intubation; observe the patient's respiratory pattern in the supine position; auscultate the lungs for breath sounds and presence of crepitations or rhonchi.

— Musculoskeletal system: check for presence of arthritis or reduced joint movements, examine the spine if central neuraxial blockade is contemplated.

Investigations

— FBC may indicate polycythaemia secondary to chronic hypoxaemia.

— Blood glucose concentration to exclude glucose intolerance.

— Urea, creatinine, electrolyte concentrations to check renal function and rule out electrolyte imbalance.

— 12-lead ECG usually reveals small ECG complexes due to thick chest wall: examine for evidence of myocardial ischaemia, ventricular hypertrophy and strain pattern, signs of cor pulmonale.

— CXR may show cardiac enlargement and features suggestive of pulmonary hypertension.

— ABG to document baseline pH, PaO_2 and $PaCO_2$; PaO_2 may be low and $PaCO_2$ raised in OHS.

— Liver function test may be abnormal because of fatty infiltration to the liver.

— Lung function test may be indicated to assess the severity of respiratory impairment.

Preoperative Preparation

— Chest physiotherapy, breathing exercises and incentive spirometry should be started preoperatively to familiarize the patient with such manoeuvres.

— The risk of thromboembolism is increased in obesity; thus an appropriate form of thromboprophylaxis should be administered in the perioperative period.

— No sedative premedication should be given for patients with OHS; oral benzodiazepine may be prescribed for the others.

— Prophylaxis against acid aspiration using antacid and H_2 receptor antagonist should be prescribed in view of increased incidence of hiatus hernia with the risk of gastro-oesophageal reflux and regurgitation.

INTRAOPERATIVE MANAGEMENT

Regional Anaesthesia

— Central neuraxial blockade is suitable for lower abdominal and lower limb surgery. Peripheral nerve blocks are suitable for peripheral surgery and procedures involving the limbs.

— Regional anaesthesia poses certain attractive advantages over general anaesthesia, as it obviates the problems of difficult airway management, pulmonary aspiration and hangover effects of GA. In certain techniques RA provides effective postoperative analgesia and minimizes the use of opioids. However, RA is not without its problems.

— Regional anaesthetic blocks may be technically difficult because of difficulty in optimally positioning the patient for the block, as well as indistinct landmarks obscured by thick subcutaneous layer.

— In view of fatty infiltration and vascular engorgement in the epidural space, the level and onset of block may be unpredictable. It is recommended that the dose of local anaesthetic for central neuraxial blockade be reduced by 20% compared to non-obese patients.

— Regional anaesthesia alone is unsuitable for upper abdominal surgery because the block should be dense enough to provide adequate anaesthesia and muscle relaxation to facilitate surgical exposure. This is likely to result in extensive sympathetic blockade with cardiovascular instability and/or respiratory embarrassment through blockade of the intercostal muscles. General anaesthesia alone or in combination with epidural anaesthesia would be a more appropriate anaesthetic option.

General Anaesthesia

Induction of anaesthesia

— It is essential to obtain a reliable intravenous access before induction of anaesthesia. Patients with difficult peripheral venous access may require central venous cannulation.

— Monitoring includes these.
  - ECG: may show small complexes because of thick chest wall.
  - Non-invasive blood pressure: wide cuff required.
  - Pulse oximetry, capnography.
  - Peripheral nerve stimulator: contact may not be good if skin electrodes are used.
  - Invasive haemodynamic monitoring, urine output, temperature monitoring in major surgery.

— Preoxygenation is absolutely essential in view of greater propensity for oxygen desaturation during apnoea. This is particularly so if there is difficulty in airway management and delay in achieving successful tracheal intubation.

— Prepare for difficult intubation by considering available options as well as back-up plans if the initial technique is unsuccessful. Equipment for difficult intubation, including airway adjuncts and equipment for emergency surgical airway, should be checked and ready for use.

— In cases where intubation is obviously difficult or impossible, an awake fibreoptic intubation should be performed. In less clear-cut cases, the patient may be anaesthetized by means of inhalational or intravenous induction, followed by assist ventilation to assess ease of ventilation by mask, and gentle laryngoscopy to assess degree of intubation difficulty. Suxamethonium may be administered to facilitate intubation if no difficulty is anticipated.

Maintenance of anaesthesia

— The preferred anaesthetic technique is balanced anaesthesia using neuromuscular blocking drug, volatile anaesthetic agent, opioid and oxygen-nitrous oxide. As spontaneous ventilation under GA frequently results in progressive hypoventilation, hypercarbia and hypoxaemia, it should only be employed if the surgery is of short duration.

— Neuromuscular blocking drugs of choice include atracurium, vecuronium and rocuronium. These are non-cumulative and are easily reversed. Dose of neuromuscular blocking drug should be adjusted according to the lean body mass and not the patient's actual weight. It is advisable to monitor the degree of neuromuscular blockade by means of peripheral nerve stimulator.

— Sevoflurane or desflurane is preferred because of their rapid onset and offset of action and low degree of biotransformation. Halothane should be avoided since the incidence of halothane hepatitis is higher in obese patients. Isoflurane may also be used.

— Calculate the initial dose of anaesthetic agents according to the patient's ideal weight (which reflects lean body mass) rather than actual body weight. Subsequent doses are determined by response to the initial dose. It is always safer to give small doses titrating to effect rather than a single large bolus dose.

Reversal of neuromuscular blockade

— The endotracheal tube should be removed only when the patient is fully awake and demonstrating adequate breathing efforts. The patient should be nursed in the semi-recumbent position in PACU. This position lessens the work of breathing by avoiding pressure on the diaphragm caused by abdominal contents.

— Be prepared for early intervention if the patient shows signs of respiratory insufficiency.

- Administer supplemental oxygen and ensure airway patency by performing head tilt and chin lift, or by means of an oro- or nasopharyngeal airway.
- Suction the pharynx to remove any secretions.
- Assist ventilation via a self-inflating bag or breathing system; or allow spontaneous ventilation via a CPAP mask.
- Prepare for immediate re-intubation if the above measures do not help and if the patient's condition deteriorates.

POSTOPERATIVE MANAGEMENT

— Proper postoperative management is no less important because significant morbidity can occur during the postoperative period.

— All patients with OHS as well as those with significant history of obstructive sleep apnoea should be managed in ICU or HDU. The patient may be extubated and observed in ICU, or electively ventilated overnight. Decision is based on the nature, length and extent of surgery, the severity of OHS and associated medical conditions.

— The patient should receive supplemental oxygen with pulse oximetry monitoring in PACU and in the ward for 24 hours. Postoperative hypoxaemia is a common finding in the obese patient particularly following thoracic and upper abdominal surgery.

— Adequate postoperative analgesia is essential. Options include:
  - Epidural analgesia by means of continuous infusion, patient-controlled epidural analgesia (PCEA) or intermittent bolus doses of local anaesthetic ± opioid.
  - Intravenous patient-controlled analgesia (PCA).
  - Small intravenous bolus doses of opioid in the immediate postoperative period.
  - Wound infiltration with local anaesthetic by the surgeon.
  - Intravenous opioid infusion in ICU or HDU.

  Conventional intermittent intramuscular bolus of opioid is less than ideal.

— Adequate analgesia enables early mobilization, which is essential to reduce the risk of deep vein thrombosis and pulmonary embolism. It also enables effective chest physiotherapy and breathing exercises to be carried out. These manoeuvres are important to prevent retention of secretions, atelectasis, chest infection and respiratory failure.

OBSTRUCTIVE SLEEP APNOEA

Sleep apnoea syndrome is a syndrome of sleep-induced hypoventilatory episodes which result in sleep disturbances and excessive daytime somnolence. Sequelae of sleep apnoea include systemic and pulmonary hypertension, congestive cardiac failure and respiratory failure with carbon dioxide retention. The cause of sleep apnoea may be central (due to intermittent loss of respiratory drive) or obstructive, or both. Obstructive sleep apnoea (OSA) occurs in 85% of patients with sleep apnoea and is characterized by repeated episodes of upper airway obstruction and hypoventilation during sleep. This topic is included here because obesity is one of the leading causes, *but by no means the only cause*, of obstructive sleep apnoea.

Clinical Manifestations

These are typical symptoms of OSA.

— Snoring, sudden arousals with choking or gasping.

— Disturbed and fragmented sleep, nocturnal sweating, enuresis.

— Morning headaches, dry throat on awakening, excessive daytime somnolence.

— Fatigue, lethargy, depression.

Diagnosis may be evident from the history of the patient. An overnight study of the sleep pattern is only necessary to determine the severity of the condition. These terms, obtained from sleep studies, are used in the description of OSA.

— **Hypopnoea:** reduced breathing by more than 50% for more than 10 seconds, as measured by changes in oro-nasal airflow or respiratory inductance plethysmography.

— **Apnoea:** a pause in ventilation occurring for 10 seconds or longer during sleep. A diagnosis of OSA is made when there are more than 5 apnoeic episodes per hour, or more than 30 apnoeic episodes occurring during both rapid eye movement (REM) and non-REM sleep over 7 hours.

— **Apnoeic index:** the average number of apnoeic episodes in one hour. An apnoeic index greater than 20 is associated with an increased overall mortality; and increased risk of morbidity and mortality during anaesthesia.

OSA is classified into various grades of severity from pulse oximetry findings.

— Grade 0: minor reductions in SpO_2 without repetitive desaturations.

— Grade 1: periods of repetitive desaturations.

— Grade 2: repetitive desaturation periods throughout sleep, but return to baseline levels with arousal.

— Grade 3: SpO_2 remains low in between apnoeic episodes, signifying hypoventilation.

OSA may be associated with these conditions.

— Obesity.

— Adenotonsillar hypertrophy.

- Nasal obstruction.
- Craniofacial skeletal abnormalities such as Pierre-Robin syndrome, Down's syndrome, acromegaly.
- Some neurological disorders and storage diseases.
- Chronic renal failure.

Management

- Measures which are of benefit include weight reduction, cessation of smoking and alcohol intake, avoidance of respiratory depressants (e.g., benzodiazepines, barbiturates) and sleeping on the side with head and shoulders raised.
- Mechanical devices such as nasopharyngeal airway, nasal CPAP, bilevel positive airway pressure (BiPAP) device may be used to overcome airway obstruction during sleep.
- Surgery such as adenotonsillectomy, uvulopalatopharyngoplasty (UPPP), lingual surgery, mandibular advancement and elevation hyoidplasty may be performed in selected patients.
- Tracheostomy may be essential and life-saving in patients with severe right heart failure, hypersomnolence and hypoxaemia.

Implications for the Anaesthesiologist

- The patient may undergo OSA-related surgical procedures outlined above or incidental surgery unrelated to the condition.
- The patient is frequently obese with medical and anaesthetic problems as outlined above.
- Associated medical conditions such as pulmonary hypertension, right heart failure, and hypoxaemia result in increased anaesthetic morbidity and mortality.
- The patient may exhibit markedly altered responses to anaesthetic drugs. Anaesthetic agents, sedatives and opioids worsen OSA by reducing pharyngeal muscle tone and increasing the likelihood of upper airway collapse. They also reduce the ventilatory response to hypoxaemia and hypercarbia.
- There is an increased risk of respiratory complications during the perioperative period, particularly following major abdominal or thoracic surgery.

Anaesthetic Management

- Regional anaesthetic technique should be employed wherever possible to retain conscious control of respiratory function and to avoid the problems of general anaesthesia.
- Omit sedative premedication in order to avoid hypoventilation and airway obstruction.
- The patient should be monitored with ECG, BP, pulse oximetry, capnography. Observe for occurrence of arrhythmias, myocardial ischaemia, oxygen desaturation, and hypercapnia.
- Intravenous induction of anaesthesia is preferable in the absence of potential difficult airway. It may be difficult to establish sufficient anaesthetic depth with inhalational induction because airway obstruction tends to occur early. An awake fibreoptic intubation is indicated if intubation is anticipated to be difficult.
- Anaesthetic agents with short duration of action and good recovery characteristics are preferred. Examples are propofol, alfentanil, sevoflurane, desflurane. Neuromuscular blocking drugs which are short to intermediate in duration of action, non-cumulative and easily reversed (e.g., mivacurium, rocuronium) are similarly preferred. The degree of neuromuscular blockade should be monitored by peripheral nerve stimulator and adequate reversal achieved before extubation.
- OSA-related surgery, with the risk of airway oedema, may worsen or precipitate airway obstruction. Extubation should be carried out only if the patient is without residual neuromuscular blockade, is fully awake with full return of protective airway reflexes and has adequate breathing effort. Consider using an airway exchange catheter (e.g., Cook™) especially if intubation has been difficult. The airway exchange catheter is inserted into the endotracheal tube before extubation. The endotracheal tube is then removed and the patient's respiration is observed with the airway exchange catheter *in situ*. Another endotracheal tube can be railroaded into the trachea through the airway exchange catheter if re-intubation is deemed necessary (see Chapter 25).
- The use of supplemental oxygen is debatable. Its beneficial effects include reduced incidence of myocardial ischaemia, improved cognitive function and reduced pulmonary artery pressures. However, it may delay detection of apnoeic episodes and reduce respiratory drive in certain patients, especially those with chronic obstructive pulmonary disease. Oxygen supplementation should be administered cautiously and titrated to the minimum required to maintain the patient's saturation

at preoperative level. The patient should be monitored closely for apnoea and desaturation.

— Management in the ICU or HDU is necessary in the immediate postoperative period, particularly in severe OSA patients who have undergone major surgery or airway surgery. A period of assisted ventilation in the ICU may be necessary if doubts exist about the patient's airway integrity or ventilatory efforts. The challenge of maintaining airway will extend well into the postoperative period, since respiratory events after surgery in OSA patients may occur at any time.

— Local anaesthetics are preferred over systemic opioids in providing postoperative analgesia. Systemic opioids, if indicated, should be used with extreme caution and the patient's respiration and saturation monitored closely.

FURTHER READING

1. Adams JP, Murphy PG. Obesity in anaesthesia and intensive care. Br J Anaesth 2000;85:91–108.
2. Benumof JL. Obstructive sleep apnea in the adult obese patient: Implications for airway management. J Clin Anesth 2001;13:144–56.
3. Loadsman JA, Hillman DR. Anaesthesia and sleep apnoea. Br J Anaesth 2001;86:254–66.
4. Tung A, Rock P. Perioperative concerns in sleep apnea. Curr Opin Anaesthesiol 2001;14:671–8.
5. Chung F, Imarengiaye C. Management of sleep apnea in adults. Can J Anesth 2002;49:R1–6.
6. den Herder C, Schmeck J, Appelboom DJK, de Vries N. Risks of general anaesthesia in people with obstructive sleep apnoea. Br Med J 2004;329:955–9.
7. Parish JM, Somers VK. Obstructive sleep apnea and cardiovascular disease. Mayo Clin Proc 2004;79:1036–46.

Chapter 23

Management of Patients with Coagulation Disorders

INTRODUCTION

Coagulation disorders may be hereditary or acquired, and the abnormalities may involve one or more components essential for normal clotting and haemostasis. The anaesthesiologist should be familiar with the pathophysiology of the disorder in order to be able to optimally manage such patients presenting for surgery and anaesthesia.

The common coagulation disorders are listed here.

— **Hereditary**
- Haemophilia A (factor VIII deficiency, classic haemophilia).
- Haemophilia B (factor IX deficiency, Christmas disease).
- von Willebrand's disease.

- Others: afibrinogenaemia, deficiencies in factors V, XII or XIII, hereditary haemorrhagic telangiectasis, antithrombin III deficiency, protein C deficiency (the last two give rise to hypercoagulable states).

— **Acquired**

- Perioperative anticoagulation.
- Intraoperative coagulopathies secondary to massive transfusion, dilutional thrombocytopaenia.
- Disseminated intravascular coagulation (DIC).
- Drug-induced haemorrhage, such as heparin or warfarin overdose.
- Drug-induced platelet dysfunction: aspirin, non-steroidal antiinflammatory drugs (NSAIDs).

PREOPERATIVE EVALUATION

This includes a detailed history (including drug history), physical examination and appropriate laboratory tests to quantify the coagulation problems. Careful exclusion of coagulation defects before the induction of anaesthesia facilitates the differential diagnosis of intraoperative bleeding. It must be remembered that some patients with congenital coagulation disorders may remain asymptomatic until challenged by trauma or surgery.

Clinical evaluation should include these details.

— Elicit the age of onset and symptoms of coagulation disorder, such as easy bruising, gum bleeding, epistaxis, abnormal bleeding from cuts and abrasions, menorrhagia, gastrointestinal bleeding.

— Obtain a family history of bleeding disorders. Note that a negative history does not rule out diagnosis because of the hereditary patterns, e.g., sex-linked recessive in haemophilia, autosomal dominant with variable penetrance in von Willebrand's disease.

— Determine haemostatic responses to previous procedures such as tonsillectomy, dental extraction, childbirth; whether these were associated with excessive bleeding and need for blood transfusion.

— Obtain a detailed drug history. Medications include aspirin, NSAIDs, oral anticoagulants, corticosteroids, desmopressin (DDAVP) in haemophilia or von Willebrand's disease.

— Assess the presence or severity of associated medical conditions.

— Examine the patient for pallor and evidence of abnormal bleeding such as petechiae, bruises, ecchymoses, or haemarthrosis.

Laboratory investigations (Table 23–1).

— The tests listed are useful when clinical evaluation suggests the possibility of coagulation disorders and in situations where coagulation may be altered (e.g., drugs affecting haemostasis, significant liver or renal disease, liver transplantation, cardiac or aortic surgery when the patient is on cardiopulmonary bypass). The value of such tests in asymptomatic patients is debatable.

— Due to their variability and unreliability, bleeding time and clotting time are no longer recommended as screening tests.

— Specific tests are required in specific cases, e.g., specific clotting factor activity assay, thromboelastography.

— Tests on the extrinsic pathway of the coagulation cascade are required for patients on oral anticoagulants. This is reflected in the prothrombin time (PT) or international normalized ratio (INR). The INR is a unit of measure that allows comparisons between PT results obtained from different laboratories which may utilize thromboplastins of varying international sensitivity index (ISI) values. While the PT ratio is influenced by the ISI value, this is not so for INR, which remains constant.

— When the patient is treated with heparin, the partial thromboplastin time, or more commonly the APTT, needs to be checked. In this case the intrinsic pathway of the coagulation cascade is tested.

Table 23–1. Screening tests for coagulation disorders

Test	Purpose
Full blood count (FBC)	Check for anaemia, thrombocytopaenia
Prothrombin time (PT)	Test of extrinsic pathway of coagulation cascade: deficiency of factors I, II, V, VII and X Treatment with warfarin
Activated partial thromboplastin time (APTT)	Test of intrinsic pathway of coagulation cascade: deficiency of coagulation factors, especially factors VIII and IX Treatment with heparin
Fibrinogen concentration	Hypofibrinogenaemia or dysfibrinogenaemia Treatment with heparin

Preoperative preparation and management is individualized based on the specific coagulation disorder. The correlation between the clotting factor and platelet concentrations with bleeding tendency is shown in Table 23–2. Specific blood products (clotting factors, platelets) should be transfused and the levels re-checked before surgery. More blood and blood products should be reserved for the scheduled surgery.

Table 23–2. Correlation of deficiency with bleeding tendency

Value	Clinical Implications
Factor VIII, Factor IX (normal 0.5–1.5)*	
< 0.02*	Frequent spontaneous bleeding into joints, muscles and internal organs
0.02–0.05*	Some spontaneous bleeds, bleeding after minor trauma
> 0.05*	Bleeding only after significant trauma or surgery
**can be expressed as decimal or as percentage*	
Platelet count (normal 150,000–400,000/μl)	
< 20,000	Spontaneous bleeding, including intracerebral bleed, may occur
50,000	Minimal level for surgery or invasive procedures
> 100,000	Safe for surgery and regional anaesthesia

ANAESTHETIC MANAGEMENT: GENERAL GUIDELINES

— Avoid intramuscular injection and prescribe oral premedication instead. Anticholinergic drugs, if indicated, can be given intravenously before induction of anaesthesia.

— Regional anaesthesia, in particular central neuraxial blockade, is not advisable in patients with known coagulation disorders. However, individual nerve blocks have been successfully performed in these patients.

— Invasive monitors such as arterial cannulation, central venous or pulmonary artery catheterization should be undertaken only if benefits derived from such monitors outweigh the potential risks of haematoma and uncontrolled bleeding.

— Tracheal intubation is not contraindicated but nasal intubation should be avoided wherever possible. Endotracheal tubes should be well lubricated and care must be taken to be extremely gentle during airway manipulation.

— Universal precaution should be adopted in view of possibility of transfusion-transmitted infections such as hepatitis, human immunodeficiency virus (HIV) in patients who have received multiple transfusions.

— Closely monitor the patent's haemodynamic status and intraoperative blood loss. Be prepared to transfuse blood and blood products if indicated. More blood units may be required if excessive intraoperative bleeding occurs; close communication with the Blood Bank is essential.

— Consider the use of intravenous patient-controlled analgesia for postoperative analgesia. Avoid intramuscular injections of opioids.

DISSEMINATED INTRAVASCULAR COAGULATION

This is a syndrome complex which arises from a wide variety of clinical conditions including sepsis, trauma, shock, massive transfusion, obstetric complications (amniotic fluid embolism, abruptio placentae, eclampsia), immunologic disorders (allergic reactions, haemolytic transfusion reactions, transplant rejection) and neoplasms. In DIC, there is widespread systemic activation of coagulation, which results in intravascular fibrin formation, thrombosis and occlusion of small vessels. In the meantime severe haemorrhage occurs as a result of consumption of clotting factors and platelets (hence the name "consumptive coagulopathy").

Table 23–3 lists the derangements in laboratory parameters seen in acute DIC.

Table 23–3. Commonly used laboratory tests in acute DIC

Parameter	Result
D-dimer	Elevated, specific for fibrin degradation
Fibrinogen degradation products (FDP)	Elevated due to fibrinolysis
Antithrombin (AT)	Decreased by utilization and inactivation of thrombin and factor Xa
Platelet count	Decreased with consumptive coagulopathy
Fibrinogen	May be normal; decreased only in severe cases of DIC
Partial thromboplastin time (PTT) Prothrombin time (PT)	Prolonged, but very low specificity for DIC

Management of DIC is largely supportive with identification and treatment of the underlying triggering event. Fluid replacement and transfusion of blood components (fresh frozen plasma, platelets and cryoprecipitate – the so-called "DIC regime") are indicated for patients with active bleeding and invasive procedures. The use of heparin for treatment of thrombosis in DIC is controversial, and most physicians are hesitant to use an anticoagulant in the setting of active haemorrhage.

PATIENTS ON ORAL ANTICOAGULANT THERAPY

Management of patients on oral anticoagulant therapy presenting for surgery entails a difficult balance between minimizing the risks of bleeding and those of recurrent thromboembolism. Important factors to consider include:

- Anticoagulation: indication for anticoagulant therapy, nature of anticoagulant drug, degree of anticoagulation required.
- Surgery: urgency, nature and site of the surgical procedure, anticipated difficulty or surgical complications, adequacy of postoperative haemostasis or ability to drain the surgical field.
- Others: presence of additional thromboembolic risk factors such as liver disease, thrombocytopaenia or the use of aspirin or NSAIDs, clinical consequences of a thromboembolic event.

Indications for Anticoagulation

The indication for long-term anticoagulant therapy in a patient takes into consideration the many variables that influence the risks of thromboembolism and of bleeding in a given individual. For a patient with valvular disease, such variables include the patient's age, the specific valve lesion, the heart rhythm, the duration of the disease, a history of thromboembolism, patient's attitude and lifestyle, associated diseases and medications.

- **Strong/Mandatory**
  - Mechanical prosthetic heart valve.
  - Systemic embolism due to heart disease or chronic atrial fibrillation.
  - Recurrent or recent (< 6 weeks) venous thrombosis or pulmonary embolism.

  Therapy needs to be continued pre- and postoperatively.

- **Optional**
  - After myocardial infarction.
  - Cerebrovascular disease.
  - Venous thrombosis or pulmonary embolism which is neither recurrent or recent.

  Review the indication for anticoagulation – this may be a good time to decide whether the treatment should be resumed postoperatively.

For a patient with a prosthetic heart valve, the location as well as the type of valve should be taken into consideration. The risk of thromboembolism is higher in the first-generation ball-cage or tilting-disc mechanical valves compared to the newer bioprosthetic or tissue valves. Additional risk factors include the valve in mitral position, presence of atrial fibrillation, left atrial enlargement, endocardial damage from rheumatic valve disease, low LV ejection fraction, old age and prior embolic event or hypercoagulable state. The recommended INR for mechanical heart valves is in the range of 2.5–3.0. For patients fitted with bioprosthetic valves, the period of greatest risk of thromboembolism is within the first 3 months after implantation, during which they should be treated with warfarin with a target INR of 2.5. After this time, treatment with aspirin alone is adequate for patients with no other co-existing risk factors.

Perioperative Anticoagulation Management

1. **Preoperative management**
   - Withhold antithrombotic drugs.
     - Stop warfarin 5 days before surgery for target INR 2.0–3.0; or 6 days before surgery for target INR 2.5–3.0.
     - Stop antiplatelet drugs ticlopidine and clopidogrel 7–10 days before surgery.
     - No specific precaution for low-dose aspirin therapy (some advocate to stop 7 days before surgery).
   - Monitor INR.
     - Repeat INR measurements on the day warfarin therapy is stopped, on the day before surgery and more often if necessary.
     - Maintain INR at 1.5 before surgery.
     - Consider administering low-dose Vitamin K 1–2 mg if INR remains > 1.5.
   - Start alternative anticoagulant therapy, either with low molecular weight heparin (LMWH), or standard heparin bolus or infusion.
     - LMWH: start LMWH therapy 2 days after warfarin is stopped; administer last dose of LMWH 20–24 hours before surgery.
     - Heparin infusion (if indication for anticoagulants is mandatory): start heparin therapy in full dose (1,000 U/hr by continuous infusion) before surgery; discontinue 4 hours before the procedure; adjust heparin dose to maintain APTT ratio 1.5–2.5.
     - Heparin bolus (if indication for anticoagulants is optional): start SC heparin, 5,000 U 8–12 hourly; adjust APTT ratio to 1.5.
   - GXM blood, FFP and/or cryoprecipitate in reserve; the actual quantity depends on the nature of surgery.

2. **Intraoperative management**
   - If excessive intraoperative bleeding occurs, administer Vitamin K 10 mg IV slowly; transfuse blood, FFP and/or cryoprecipitate as required.

— The surgeon should ensure proper haemostasis or consider inserting surgical drains before closure.

3. **Postoperative management**
   — Resumption of heparin.
   - Decision is based on adequacy of haemostasis and bleeding risk associated with surgery, and management should be in consultation with the surgeon.
   - If bleeding risk is high, withhold heparin until 24–48 hours after surgery.
   - If bleeding risk is low or moderate, resume low-dose heparin (e.g., SC enoxaparin 40 mg daily, or SC dalteparin 5,000 IU) on the evening of surgery.
   - Increase to full-dose heparin (e.g., SC enoxaparin 1 mg/kg twice daily, SC dalteparin 100 IU/kg twice daily) 48–72 hours after surgery.

   — Resumption of warfarin.
   - Resume warfarin therapy when the patient starts oral intake.
   - Allow 4–5 days of overlap before taking off heparin.
   - Ensure that INR is back within therapeutic range.

4. **Management of anticoagulation therapy in emergency surgery**
   — Minor surgery.
   - Continue warfarin therapy unchanged and check INR if time permits.
   - If excessive bleeding occurs, give Vitamin K; transfuse FFP and cryoprecipitate.

   — Major surgery:
   - Stop warfarin and measure INR if time allows.
   - Administer Vitamin K 10 mg IV slowly.
   - If surgery is scheduled in less than 4–6 hours, give clotting factor replacement.
   - GXM blood and FFP in reserve.
   - Begin heparin therapy as outlined above.
   - If excessive bleeding occurs, repeat Vitamin K; transfuse FFP and cryoprecipitate.
   - The use of activated recombinant factor VII has been reported in warfarin-treated patients but its precise role in the context of prior anticoagulation therapy is as yet undefined.

FURTHER READING

1. Bombeli T, Spahn DR. Updates in perioperative coagulation: Physiology and management of thromboembolism and haemorrhage. Br J Anaesth 2004;93:275–87.
2. Senno SL, Pechet L, Bick RL. Disseminated intravascular coagulopathy (DIC): Pathophysiology, laboratory diagnosis, and management. Intensive Care Med 2000;15:144–58.
3. Douketis JD. Perioperative anticoagulation management in patients who are receiving oral anticoagulation therapy: A practical guide for clinicians. Thrombosis Research 2003;108:3–13.
4. Tiede DJ, Nishimura RA, Gastineau DA, Mullany CJ, et al. Modern management of prosthetic valve anticoagulation. Mayo Clin Proc 1998;73:665–80.
5. Salem DN, et al. Antithrombotic therapy in valvular heart disease – native and prosthetic: The Seventh ACCP Conference on Antithrombotic and Thrombolytic Therapy. Chest 2004;126:457S–482S.

Chapter 24

Prophylaxis Against Venous Thromboembolism

INTRODUCTION

Pulmonary embolism is a relatively rare cause of death in the general population. However, several perioperative factors contribute to the Virchow's triad – venous stasis, abnormal coagulation and intimal damage of blood vessels – which predisposes to venous thromboembolism. In the absence of prophylactic measures, the reported incidence of postoperative fatal pulmonary embolism ranges from 0.1% to 5%.

Thromboprophylaxis, or DVT prophylaxis as it is more commonly known, encompasses a series of management strategies aimed at reducing the occurrence of thromboembolic phenomena. It should be remembered that while prophylaxis against potentially fatal pulmonary emboli is the main goal, prophylaxis to prevent late sequelae of extensive deep vein thrombosis – swelling of the legs, varicose veins, ulceration and other trophic changes – are also important considerations.

These are some of the terms used to describe this group of disorders.

— Venous thromboembolism (VTE): a broad term that refers to all aspects of thrombosis and embolism that occur in the venous system.
— Deep venous thrombosis (DVT): thrombosis within the deep limb veins.
— Pulmonary embolism (PE): embolism to the pulmonary vasculature of any substance such as blood clots, gas, fat, amniotic fluid.
— Pulmonary thromboembolism (PTE): embolism to the pulmonary vasculature of blood clots or thrombi, usually (80–90% of cases) from the proximal deep veins of the lower limbs and pelvic veins.

RISK FACTORS

See Table 24–1. These factors predispose the patient to perioperative thromboembolism.

— **Patient factors**
  - Age > 40 years (risk increases with age).
  - Morbid obesity.
  - Presence of varicose veins.
  - Prolonged immobilization.
  - Previous history of thromboembolism.
  - Pregnancy, puerperium, use of oestrogen-containing oral contraceptive pills (OCP).

— **Surgical factors**
  - Extensive surgery lasting > 60 minutes.
  - Pelvic or abdominal surgery for malignancy.
  - Major orthopaedic lower limb surgery especially hip and knee replacements.

— **Disease conditions**
  - Neoplasm, especially abdominal or pelvic malignancy.
  - Trauma, especially spinal cord injury and lower limb fractures.
  - Cardiac disease: myocardial infarction, congestive heart failure.
  - Stroke and lower limb paralysis.
  - Haematological conditions: polycythaemia, leukaemia, paraproteinaemia (e.g., multiple myeloma).
  - Hypercoagulable states: antithrombin III deficiency, protein C and protein S deficiency, thrombophilia, antiphospholipid syndrome (especially during pregnancy) and other rare syndromes.

Table 24–1. Risk of postoperative venous thromboembolism

Risk Category	Calf Vein Thrombosis	Proximal Vein Thrombosis	Symptomatic Pulmonary Embolism	Fatal Pulmonary Embolism
High Risk Major surgery in patients > 40 years with prior history of DVT or PE Extensive pelvic or abdominal surgery for malignant disease Major orthopaedic surgery, major fractures, multiple trauma	40–80%	10–20%	5–10%	1–5%
Moderate Risk Major surgery in patients > 40 years lasting > 60 minutes	10–40%	2–10%	1–8%	0.1–0.7%
Low Risk Minor surgery < 60 minutes in patients < 40 years with no additional risk factors	< 10%	< 1%	0.2%	< 0.01%

The combined oestrogen-progesterone contraceptive pill (combined OCP) is recognized to be associated with an increase in thrombotic complications, while progesterone-only preparations do not predispose to DVT. Postmenopausal hormone replacement regimens contain much less oestrogen than the contraceptive pills and do not increase the risk of DVT.

In the absence of additional risk factors, there is insufficient evidence to support routine cessation of combined OCP in such patients. No further prophylaxis is required in healthy women undergoing minor procedures. On the other hand, if the patient has additional risk factor(s), it is advisable to stop the pill before the scheduled surgery and advise her on alternative means of contraception. The patient should receive perioperative DVT prophylaxis according to guidelines.

METHODS OF DVT PROPHYLAXIS

There are three broad methods to prevent postoperative thromboembolism.

— **Pharmacological**
  - Heparin: unfractionated or "standard" heparin (SH), low molecular weight heparin (LMWH).
  - Oral anticoagulants such as warfarin.
  - Dextran: dextran 40, dextran 70.
  - Others: antiplatelet agents, antithrombotic agents.

— **Mechanical**
  - Graduated compression stockings.
  - Intermittent pneumatic compression device.
  - Electrical calf stimulation.
  - Active and passive leg exercises.
  - Early mobilization and ambulation.

— **Anaesthetic technique**
  - Regional anaesthesia, specifically central neuraxial blockade.

Heparin

— Heparin is a highly anionic polysaccharide produced by the mast cells of animals, usually derived from bovine lung and bovine or porcine intestine.

— It activates plasma antithrombin III that in turn blocks the enzymatic activity of the activated clotting factors (primarily Xa, but also IIa, IXa, XIa, XIIa and plasmin).

Standard heparin

— This is a mixture of linear polysaccharide molecules of variable chain lengths and molecular weights (5,000–36,000 Daltons), with a mean molecular weight of 12,000–15,000.

— The most widely used regime is low-dose SC heparin 5,000 U 8–12 hourly.
— Prophylaxis with SH is simple and effective, but suffers from these.
  • Large interpatient variability in anticoagulant response due to differences in bioavailability and protein binding.
  • Increase in haemorrhagic complications, such as wound haematoma, after surgery.
  • Risk of heparin-induced thrombocytopaenic syndrome (HITS) in 3% of patients.
  • Risk of osteoporosis.
— It is not recommended in surgical procedures (e.g., ophthalmic surgery, neurosurgery) where control of haemostasis is vital.

Low molecular weight heparin

— This is prepared by chemical or enzymatic depolymerization of heparin molecules. The average molecular weight of the LMWH is in the range of 4,000–6,500 Daltons.
— Compared with SH, LMWH has:
  • Greater antithrombotic potency.
  • Longer plasma half-life (4–6 hours compared with ½–1 hour in SH), further prolonged in patients with renal failure.
  • Longer duration of action; hence longer dosing interval (once daily dose is acceptable).
  • Greater than 90% bioavailability after SC injection.
  • Predictable and reproducible anticoagulant response; hence requires no laboratory testing.
  • Residual anticoagulant effect only partially reversed by protamine.
  • Less immunogenic, with lower incidence of HITS and fewer bleeding complications.
— Recommended dose: SC enoxaparin 20–40 mg daily, or SC dalteparin 2,500 U daily.
— Antiplatelet or anticoagulant medications administered in combination with LMWH may increase the risk of haemorrhage.

Dextran

— These are colloid solutions comprising glucose polymers with mean molecular weights of 40,000 (Dextran 40) or 70,000 (Dextran 70).
— They cause a relative haemodilution, reduce platelet aggregation, improve blood flow and facilitate clot breakdown by increasing fibrinolysis. As a result, Dextran

40 is frequently used in microvascular surgery to promote microcirculation and improve graft survival.

— Dextran 70 shows limited efficacy in prevention of DVT following general surgery but appears more effective following hip surgery.
— Problems of dextran include cost, fluid overload, risk of allergic reactions and possibility of precipitating acute renal failure.

Mechanical Methods

Elastic compression stockings are used in low risk cases, while electrical calf stimulation and intermittent pneumatic leg compression are used in moderate to high risk cases. Regardless of the risks, all patients would benefit from early ambulation and leg exercises.

The mechanical methods have an advantage over anticoagulants since they are not associated with an increased risk of intra- or postoperative haemorrhage. They are useful in surgical procedures (ophthalmic surgery, neurosurgery) where anticoagulants are contraindicated.

ANTICOAGULATION AND REGIONAL ANAESTHESIA

Compared to general anaesthesia, regional anaesthesia is associated with a reduction in the incidence of DVT and pulmonary embolism in patients undergoing total hip or knee replacements. Mechanisms postulated to explain the beneficial effects of regional anaesthesia include these.

— Sympathetic blockade with reduction in vascular resistance maximizes venous blood flow and prevents venous stasis.
— Improved flow characteristics due to reduced blood viscosity as a result of haemodilution from fluid preloading.
— Inhibition of platelet aggregation.
— Facilitation of earlier and pain-free mobilization in the postoperative period.

However, the practice of regional anaesthesia in patients receiving anticoagulation remains an area of controversy. Various guidelines and recommendations have been proposed by different anaesthetic organizations. Frequent updates are required as newer anticoagulant therapies are advocated and anticoagulant drugs are introduced into the market.

In patients at risk, single-shot spinal techniques without catheter or alternative regional techniques, such as peripheral nerve blocks, should be considered. Table 24–2 summarizes the safety precautions when using central neuraxial blockade in the presence of anticoagulants.

Table 24–2. Safety precautions for central neuraxial blockade in the presence of anticoagulants

Prophylactic Measure	Safety Precautions
Standard heparin (SH)	Perform block before first dose or at least 4 hours after last dose.
Low molecular weight heparin	Perform block before first dose or at least 10–12 hours after last dose.
Antiplatelet drug ▪ Aspirin and other non-steroidal antiinflammatory drugs (NSAIDs) ▪ Ticlopidine, clopidogrel	No specific precaution for low dose aspirin therapy (30–300 mg daily) or NSAIDs. Ticlopidine, clopidogrel: site block before first dose or 7–10 days after last dose.
Preoperative therapeutic anticoagulation or coagulopathy	Block absolutely contraindicated.
Intraoperative anticoagulation	Delay heparinization for 1 hour after insertion of block. Use smallest dose of heparin needed for the therapeutic goal.
Postoperative anticoagulation	Removal of epidural catheter ▪ For SH: at least 2–4 hours after the last dose, and 1 hour before the next dose. ▪ For LMWH: at least 12 hours after the last dose, and 2 hours before the next dose.

Further recommendations include these.

— Care should be taken to minimize trauma during performance of the central neuraxial block. Adopt a midline approach and use fine pencil-point spinal needle

(26G or smaller) for subarachnoid block. Do not insert the epidural catheter further than 3–4 cm into the epidural space to minimize the risk of inadvertent vascular trauma.

— If the neuraxial block is technically difficult or if bleeding occurs during epidural needle or catheter insertion, the procedure should be abandoned and an alternative anaesthetic technique utilized. Although controversial, appearance of blood in the needle and/or catheter does not mandate cancellation of the planned surgery. Frequent postoperative monitoring of the neurologic status is important, and further anticoagulation should be withheld for 6 hours (heparin) or 24 hours (LMWH).

— Short-acting local anaesthetic should be used for surgery to allow assessment of neurologic status in the immediate postoperative period.

— For postoperative analgesia, use opioid-only solutions (e.g., pethidine) or dilute local anaesthetic with opioid solutions (e.g., 0.1% ropivacaine with fentanyl) so as not to mask signs and symptoms of spinal cord or nerve root compression.

— Monitor the patient closely and regularly for neurologic sequelae. A high degree of suspicion is required. Suspect spinal haematoma in any patient with new onset of back pain or of neurological deficits, such as motor weakness progressing to flaccid paralysis, numbness, and bowel or bladder dysfunction. Note that clinical symptoms may develop at any moment with an indwelling epidural catheter and up to several days after its removal.

— Early investigation and urgent surgical evacuation of haematoma by means of decompressive laminectomy is important, as recovery is unlikely if surgery is delayed for more than 8–12 hours from the onset of initial symptoms.

Before the introduction and widespread usage of LMWH, the reported incidence of clinically significant spinal haematoma in patients undergoing central neuraxial blockade appeared to be low in both normal patients and those receiving anticoagulant DVT prophylaxis. Cases of spontaneous spinal haematoma unrelated to central neuraxial blockade have also been reported. Until 1994, the rare cases of epidural haematoma following a spinal or epidural anaesthetic had identifiable causes – either a positive history of traumatic or technically difficult blocks, or some form of perioperative anticoagulant treatment received by the patient.

Following the introduction of LMWH into clinical practice, case reports of spinal haematoma following LMWH have appeared in the literature at disconcertingly regular intervals. This is especially so in the United States, where the doses of LMWH are comparatively larger and dose intervals shorter. This was attributed in part to the failure to understand the pharmacological differences between standard heparin and LMWH, specifically the longer duration of action of LMWH and the need to time the insertion and removal of epidural catheters according to recommendations. Even though the incidence of spinal haematoma has since reduced after the European dosage recommendations were adopted, it remains an important problem and a clinical dilemma for the anaesthesiologist.

Herbal medications, for example garlic, gingko or ginseng, may be associated with increased perioperative bleeding especially when combined with other medications that inhibit platelet aggregation. Even though the use of herbal medications alone does not create a level of risk that will interfere with the performance of neuraxial blocks, one should be aware of their potential effects on haemostasis.

One should also remember that the margin of safety decreases in elderly or debilitated patients, those with liver disease or on a combination of anticoagulant drugs. The decision to perform central neuraxial blockade and the timing of catheter removal in such patients should be made on an individual basis, weighing the risk of spinal haematoma against the benefits of regional anaesthesia for each particular patient.

PULMONARY THROMBOEMBOLISM

Approximately 75% of patients who present with clinically suspected venous thrombosis or pulmonary embolism do not have these conditions. Objective testing is necessary when either is suspected, because clinical diagnosis alone is inaccurate, and consequences of misdiagnosis are serious. Failure to diagnose pulmonary embolism is associated with high mortality, while incorrect diagnosis subjects the patient to the risks of unnecessary anticoagulant therapy. Tests available for DVT are compression ultrasonography of the femoral and popliteal veins and contrast venography, while radionuclide lung imaging (ventilation-perfusion scan), contrast-enhanced spiral CT and pulmonary angiography are tests for diagnosis of pulmonary thromboembolism (PTE).

PTE may present to the anaesthesiologist as a catastrophic event in the intra- or postoperative period. At the other end of the spectrum, symptoms of minor PTE are usually subtle, non-specific and self-limiting, and some cases may even pass undiagnosed. The manifestation of symptoms depends on a variety of factors, including the degree of thrombosis, the presence and degree of collateral vessels and the severity of inflammation.

Clinical Manifestations

Presentation may be that of:

— Uncomplicated embolus with dyspnoea.

— Pulmonary infarction syndrome (pleuritic pain and/or haemoptysis).

— Circulatory collapse or syncope.

Signs and symptoms

— **Common (> 50% cases)**
- Apprehension.
- Dyspnoea, tachypnoea, cough, rales.
- Tachycardia, chest pain (pleuritic or angina-like), loud pulmonic heart sound.

— **Less common (10–40% cases)**
- Haemoptysis, low grade fever, cyanosis.
- Diaphoresis, syncope, altered mental status.
- Signs of elevated CVP, clinical DVT.

— **Rare (< 10% cases)**
- Wheezing, abdominal pain.
- Disseminated intravascular coagulation.

Investigations

— **ABG**
- This typically shows hypoxaemia and/or hypocarbia.
- However, a normal PaO_2 in ABG does not rule out diagnosis of PTE.

— **ECG**
- ECG is normal in 30% of patients with PTE.
- Changes include ST-T wave abnormalities and rhythm disturbance in the form of atrial or ventricular ectopic beats, and atrial tachycardia.
- Changes in the right heart with right atrial strain, right bundle branch block and axis deviation give rise to the classical picture of $S_1 Q_3 T_3$ (S wave in lead I, Q wave and inverted T wave in lead III).

— **CXR**
- Changes are non-specific; atelectasis and pulmonary parenchymal abnormality are most common.
- Others include elevation of hemidiaphragm, pleural effusion, "knuckle sign" (pulmonary artery tapers abruptly) and pulmonary infarction.

- **Plasma D-dimer**
  - These are generated when fibrin is degraded by the endogenous fibrinolytic system.
  - Elevated levels of plasma D-dimer may suggest presence of PTE but these are not specific to PTE alone. However, a negative D-dimer assay usually means the diagnosis of PTE can be excluded.
- **Ventilation-perfusion scan**
  - V/Q scan is the most useful non-invasive method for diagnosis of PTE; a normal perfusion scan excludes the diagnosis and further tests are unnecessary.
  - However, V/Q scans are less likely to be helpful in patients with COPD, cardiorespiratory disease or history of pulmonary embolism.
- **Helical ("spiral") CT scan:**
  - It allows for direct visualization of emboli within the pulmonary artery, as well as any abnormalities in the parenchyma that may provide a different aetiology for the patient's symptoms.
  - Sensitivity with helical CT scanning ranges between 57% and 100%, while specificity ranges between 78% and 100%.
- **Pulmonary angiography**
  - This is regarded as the "gold standard" for the diagnosis of PTE but is invasive, difficult to perform and interpret, and associated with a mortality rate of 0.5%.
  - Angiography should be employed only in patients where the diagnosis cannot be established by less invasive means.

Management

Management options are based on whether the patient is haemodynamically stable and whether systemic anticoagulation is advisable. There are also supportive measures in addition to specific therapy, listed below.

1. **Supportive measures**
   - Oxygen therapy and ventilatory support.
   - Volume resuscitation.
   - Use of vasoactive drugs: inotropes (dopamine, dobutamine), vasodilators (hydralazine) as indicated.

2. **Specific therapy**
   a. Haemodynamically stable patients
      — Standard heparin
         - This is the standard treatment for hemodynamically stable patient with venous thromboembolism.
         - It is administered in the form of continuous intravenous infusion but requires frequent laboratory monitoring and dose titration.
      — Oral anticoagulant: warfarin
         - Warfarin is administered in conjunction with heparin with a 48-hour overlap, as it takes 3–5 days for the antithrombotic effect to work.
      — Fondaparinux
         - This is a synthetic antithrombotic agent with specific anti-Factor Xa activity.
         - It is administered in a fixed dose, once daily SC injection, and requires less frequent laboratory monitoring compared to standard heparin.
      — Low molecular weight heparin
         - LMWH is given subcutaneously in either a weight-based formula (for treatment) or a fixed dose (for prophylaxis).
         - It has the benefit of not requiring laboratory monitoring, and in many studies LMWH has been shown to be superior to standard heparin in terms of bleeding complications.

   b. Haemodynamically unstable patients
      — Thrombolytic therapy
         - This therapy, using streptokinase or recombinant tissue plasminogen activator (rtPA), is indicated for haemodynamically unstable patients with acute PTE.
         - The major limitation of thrombolytic treatment is an increased risk and incidence of severe bleeding compared with heparin.
         - Some data show a decrease in recurrent pulmonary embolism in rtPA patients compared with heparin-alone patients.
      — Surgical measures
         - These are used for haemodynamically unstable patients with contraindications for thrombolysis.
         - These include pulmonary embolectomy with cardiopulmonary bypass, transvenous catheter embolectomy, or placement of inferior vena cava filter.

FURTHER READING

1. Hyers TM. Management of venous thromboembolism: Past, present, and future. Arch Intern Med 2003;163:759–68.
2. Whittle J, Johnson P, Localio AR. Anticoagulation therapy in patients with venous thromboembolic disease. J Gen Int Med 1998;13:373–8.
3. Wheatley T, Veitch PS. Recent advances in prophylaxis against deep vein thrombosis. Br J Anaesth 1997;78:118–20.
4. Walker CPR, Royston D. Thrombin generation and its inhibition: A review of the scientific basis and mechanism of action of anticoagulant therapies. Br J Anaesth 2002;88:848–63.
5. Horlocker TT, Heit JA. Low molecular weight heparin: Pharmacology, perioperative prophylaxis regimen, and guidelines for regional anesthetic management. Anesth Analg 1997;85:874–85.
6. White RH. Low-molecular-weight heparins: Are they all the same? Br J Haem 2003;121:12–20.
7. Horlocker TT, et al. Regional anesthesia in the anticoagulated patient: Defining the risks. Reg Anesth Pain Med 2003;28:172–97.
8. Tryba M. European practice guidelines: Thromboembolism prophylaxis and regional anesthesia. Reg Anesth Pain Med 1998;23:178–82.
9. Litz RJ, Hubler M, Kock T, Albrecht M. Spinal-epidural hematoma following epidural anesthesia in the presence of antiplatelet and heparin therapy. Anesthesiology 2001;95:1031–3.
10. Goldhaber SZ. Pulmonary embolism. N Engl J Med 1998;339:93–104.

Chapter 25

Difficult Airway Management

INTRODUCTION

The incidence of failed intubation is reported in the literature to be 1:2,230 (0.05%) in surgical patients, and range from 1:750 to 1:280 (0.13% to 0.35%) in obstetric patients. Airway management is fundamental to safe anaesthetic practice, since difficult or failed intubation may result in hypoxia, aspiration or trauma, leading to major morbidity or even mortality. During the preoperative assessment, it is important to identify patients who may pose problems in airway management. A planned anaesthetic approach, with different anaesthetic options available, is always better than crisis management involving difficult or failed intubation. The anaesthesiologist should also learn to deal with emergency situations where unexpected difficulties in airway management occur.

TERMINOLOGY

Difficulty in airway management may be encountered in various stages and one should be precise about the aspect in which the difficulty occurs. These are definitions suggested by the American Society of Anesthesiologists (ASA) Task Force on Management of the Difficult Airway.

- **Difficult airway** is said to occur *"when one experiences difficulty with mask ventilation, difficulty with tracheal intubation, or both."*
- **Difficult mask ventilation** is said to occur *"when it is not possible for the unassisted anaesthesiologist to maintain the $SpO_2 > 90\%$ using 100% oxygen and positive pressure mask ventilation in a patient."*
- **Difficult laryngoscopy** is said to occur *"when it is not possible to visualize any portion of the vocal cords with conventional laryngoscopy."*
- **Difficult endotracheal intubation** is said to occur *"when proper insertion of the tracheal tube with conventional laryngoscopy requires more than 3 attempts or more than 10 minutes."* A more comprehensive but cumbersome definition would be, *"when an experienced laryngoscopist, using direct laryngoscopy, requires a) more than 2 attempts with the same blade; or b) a change in the blade or an adjunct to a direct laryngoscope (i.e., bougie); or c) use of an alternative device or technique following failed intubation with direct laryngoscopy."*

PREOPERATIVE ASSESSMENT

History

- Detailed history is needed to identify the patient at risk. Conditions that may be associated with difficult airway include:
  - Obesity.
  - Pregnancy and labour: increased risk of laryngeal oedema in preeclampsia and parturient with prolonged second stage of labour.
  - Anatomical abnormalities: micrognathia, macroglossia, congenital syndromes (e.g., Pierre-Robin, Treacher-Collins), burns contracture involving the head and neck.

  - Evidence of upper airway obstruction: tumour or oedema involving the upper airway, large goitre, acute epiglottitis, maxillofacial trauma, airway burns.
  - Cervical spine problems: fracture-dislocation or subluxation of cervical spine, rheumatoid arthritis, ankylosing spondylitis.
- It is important to elicit any significant past history, such as history of radiotherapy to the head and neck region especially the oral cavity, or known history of difficult intubation during previous anaesthetics. Examine past anaesthesia records if available to look for cause(s) of difficult intubation and means to overcome these problem(s).

Physical Examination

- **Body weight and general status**
  - Expect difficulty in obese patients (body weight > 90 kg or > 20% above ideal weight) and pregnant ladies particularly those in third trimester of pregnancy.
- **Inspection in anterior and lateral views**
  - Inspect the facial features for bony or soft tissue abnormalities, such as small receding chin, mandibular or maxillary fractures, tumours and oedema.
  - Examine the neck for swelling, goitre, scarring, tracheal deviation, position of the thyroid cartilage.
  - Note the pattern of respiration for presence of stridor, tachypnoea, respiratory distress or paradoxical respiration.
- **Mouth opening**
  - Ask the patient to open mouth as wide as possible and note the modified Mallampati classification (*vide infra*).
  - Assess the degree of mouth opening and mobility of temporomandibular joints by measuring the inter-incisor gap; expect difficulty in laryngoscopy if it is less than 3 cm.
  - Examine for intraoral tumours if present, noting the size, location and friability of the tumour.
  - Assess the state of dentition for protruding incisors, loose or missing teeth, and evidence of orthodontic work with caps, crowns or dentures.
  - Ask the patient to protrude the mandible and look at the position of the lower teeth in relation to the upper teeth. Expect difficulty if the lower incisors cannot be protruded anterior to the upper incisors.

— **Neck movement**

- Assess cervical mobility by putting the patient through the full range of neck movements: flexion, extension and rotation.
- Exclude the possibility of cervical spondylosis by asking about complaints of pain in the neck, or radicular pain and/or neurological symptoms in the arms. The patient may also complain about giddiness while adopting certain neck positions, indicating vertebro-basilar artery insufficiency. Such conditions would necessitate extra care in positioning the head and neck for laryngoscopy and intubation under anaesthesia.
- Measure the thyromental distance: distance from the tip of the thyroid cartilage to the tip of the mandible on full neck extension. This should be greater than 6.5 cm. Expect difficulty if it is less than 6 cm. This estimates the potential space into which the tongue can be displaced on laryngoscopy.
- Another parameter is the sternomental distance: the distance from the upper border of the manubrium to the tip of the mandible with the neck fully extended. This should be greater than 12.5 cm. Expect difficulty if it is less than 12 cm.

— **Indirect laryngoscopy findings**

- These are relevant especially in patients with laryngeal tumour or thyroid enlargement scheduled for thyroid surgery, as they provide information regarding the size and location of laryngeal tumours and function of recurrent laryngeal nerves.

— **Radiological examinations**

- Many parameters have been described in the literature but most of them are neither practical nor useful clinically.
- Cervical X-ray is the most common and useful test. Look for fracture-dislocation of cervical spines, soft tissue shadows, and tracheal compression or deviation. Flexion/extension views give additional information about stability of the odontoid process and the mobility of the occipito-atlanto-axial complex.
- Other parameters – alveolar-mental distance, atlanto-axial distance, anterior depth of the mandible, ratio of mandibular length to posterior depth – are suggested in the literature but are not commonly used.
- In patients with partially obstructed airway, CT scan and MRI are useful to delineate the site, size and extent of the obstructing lesion, the dimensions of the trachea and evidence of compression or tumour infiltration into the tracheal wall.

Modified Mallampati Classification (Figure 25–1)

Mallampati reported a correlation between the visibility of oropharyngeal structures and the degree of difficulty of glottic exposure on direct laryngoscopy. Three oropharyngeal classes were proposed in the original classification. Samsoon and Young added a fourth class and observed that patients in whom laryngoscopy was difficult belonged predominantly to Class III and IV.

The classification is as follows:

Class I: Soft palate, uvula, tonsillar pillars visible.
Class II: Soft palate, uvula visible; tonsillar pillars not visible.
Class III: Only soft palate visible.
Class IV: No pharyngeal structures except hard palate visible.

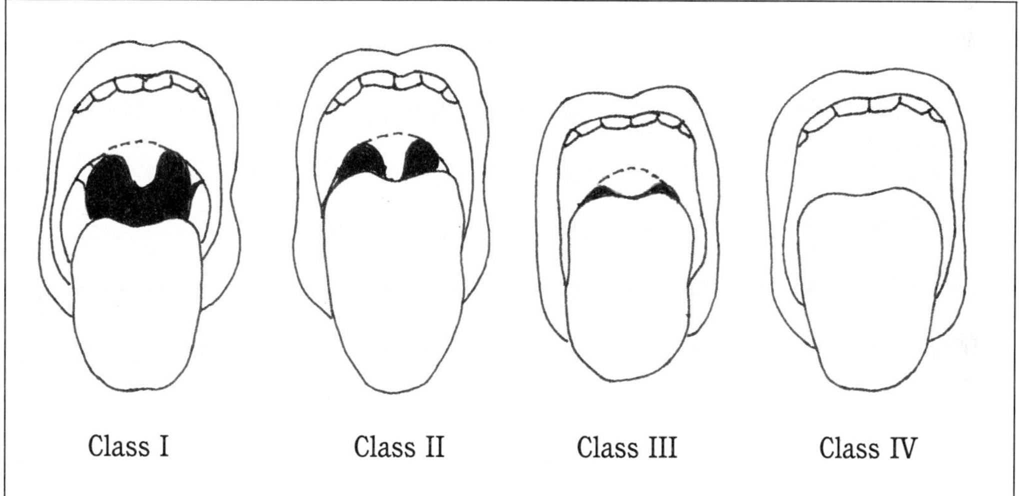

Figure 25–1. Modified Mallampati classification

The test is performed at the patient's bedside with the patient sitting up and the observer at eye level. The patient is asked to open the mouth fully and protrude the tongue as much as possible. Visualization and identification of pharyngeal structures is made *without phonation.*

The Mallampati test is subject to inter-observer variability and in prospective analyses has only achieved moderate sensitivity and specificity. This can be improved by inclusion of other risk criteria during airway assessment.

Wilson Risk-Sum

This is another scoring system, devised by Wilson *et al* in 1988, based on various parameters obtained during preoperative assessment (Table 25–1). This scoring system, although not as widely practiced as Mallampati classification, includes a wider range of parameters that may contribute to a difficult airway.

In this system, a score of ≥ 2 predicts 75% of difficult intubations but with a large number of false positives; a score of ≥ 4 reduces the number of false positives but at the cost of missing some difficult intubations.

Table 25–1. Wilson Risk-Sum

Risk Factor	Level	Point
Weight	< 90 kg 90–110 kg >110 kg	0 1 2
Head and neck movement	> 90° about 90° < 90°	0 1 2
Jaw movement	*IG ≥ 5 cm, **SLux > 0 *IG < 5 cm, **SLux = 0 *IG < 5 cm, **SLux < 0	0 1 2
Receding mandible	Normal Moderate Severe	0 1 2
Buck teeth	Normal Moderate Severe	0 1 2

* IG is Inter-incisor gap, the distance between upper and lower incisors measured with the mouth fully open.

** SLux is Subluxation, the maximal forward protrusion of the lower incisors beyond the upper incisors, where SLux > 0 means the lower incisors can be protruded anterior to the upper incisors; SLux = 0 means both are "edge to edge" and SLux < 0 means the lower incisors cannot be brought "edge to edge".

Cormack and Lehane Classification (Figure 25–2)

This system of grading is based on actual views of the glottic structures on direct laryngoscopy. It was initially proposed for the obstetric patient but is now widely used for both obstetric and non-obstetric intubations.

Grade I: Visualization of the entire laryngeal aperture
Grade II: Visualization of the posterior portion of the laryngeal aperture
Grade III: Visualization of the tip of the epiglottis
Grade IV: Visualization of the soft palate only

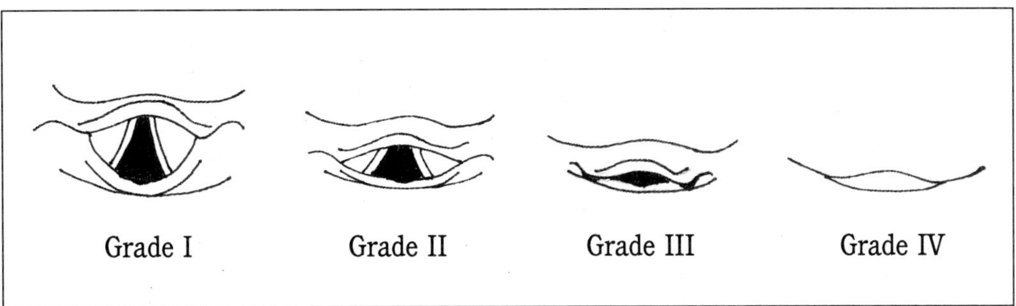

Figure 25–2. Cormack and Lehane classification

In Grades III and IV, intubation is considered to be difficult and other manoeuvres may be needed for the trachea to be successfully intubated.

MANAGEMENT OF KNOWN DIFFICULT AIRWAY

— When a patient with potentially difficult airway is identified, inform your senior colleague and discuss options available for the patient.
— Options other than general anaesthesia with tracheal intubation should be considered. For example:
  - Regional anaesthesia depending on the site and extent of surgery.
  - Local anaesthesia and/or sedation.
  - General anaesthesia with spontaneous respiration via face mask or laryngeal mask airway.

— However, this does not solve the problem of the difficult airway altogether. Complications or failure of regional anaesthesia could necessitate an urgent induction of general anaesthesia and intubation under suboptimal conditions. The same predicament applies in the event of inability to maintain an adequate airway by non-intubation methods.

— Ensure empty stomach and decreased gastric acidity to avoid problems of regurgitation and aspiration of gastric contents. This is achieved by implementation of fasting guidelines, use of antacids and H_2 receptor antagonist. Premedication should be omitted in the presence of potential upper airway obstruction; otherwise a light premedication with oral benzodiazepine can be prescribed.

— Inform the surgeon about the potential airway problem; the option of tracheostomy under local anaesthesia may be appropriate in some cases, e.g., oral or laryngeal tumour for excision and/or neck dissection.

— Difficult intubation equipment should be checked to make sure that they are in good working order. For practical purposes, a difficult intubation trolley should be set up in each OT complex with the following items included in the trolley:
  - Laryngoscopes of different types and blade sizes.
  - Endotracheal tubes of various types and sizes.
  - Stylets and gum elastic bougie.
  - Airway adjuncts such as laryngeal mask airway (LMA) of various sizes, intubating LMA, LMA ProSeal™, Trachlight™, oesophageal-tracheal Combitube, laryngeal tube.
  - Fibreoptic laryngoscope and its accessories.
  - Invasive means of establishing airway: cricothyrotomy or minitracheostomy sets, setup for transtracheal jet ventilation.

— Preoxygenation with 100% oxygen for 3–5 minutes prior to induction of anaesthesia should be carried out in all patients with potential airway problems. Establish monitors consisting of ECG, BP, pulse oximetry, capnography and others according to the nature of the surgery.

— Ensure that the intubating conditions are optimal.
  - Position the pillow to allow neck flexion to chest and head extension on neck – the "sniffing the morning air" position. This aligns the three anatomic axes – oral, pharyngeal and laryngeal – to allow successful exposure of the glottic opening during direct laryngoscopy.
  - External laryngeal pressure applied by the anaesthetic assistant during laryngoscopy may aid in visualization of vocal cords. Backward, upward,

rightward pressure should be exerted on the thyroid cartilage – the so-called "BURP" manoeuvre.
  - If the patient's breasts are pendulous, it may be necessary to retract them to facilitate laryngoscopy; or use a short laryngoscope handle which does not abut on the breasts.

— Consider using alternative laryngoscope blade or handle.
  - McCoy blade to retract the epiglottis.
  - Straight blade in a patient with receding chin, prominent incisors or if the epiglottis is long and floppy.
  - Short handle in a patient with short neck and pendulous breasts.

Management Options

1. **Intravenous induction**

   This is attempted when minimal difficulty is anticipated. It should not be used if there is any doubt about adequacy of ventilation via face mask and in the presence of upper airway obstruction.
   — Preoxygenate with 100% oxygen for 3–5 minutes.
   — Give a small titrating dose of intravenous induction agent.
   — Test-ventilate via the face mask after the patient loses consciousness to assess whether assisted ventilation is possible.
   — Do a gentle laryngoscopy in an attempt to visualize the vocal cords and assess difficulty in intubation.
   — If adequate ventilation is achieved and the vocal cords can be visualized, suxamethonium can then be administered and intubation attempted.
   — If attempts at intubation are not successful, maintain ventilation via the face mask until effect of suxamethonium wears off. Consider other airway options.

2. **Inhalational induction**
   — It is important that spontaneous ventilation is maintained in cases of upper airway obstruction because the airway may become totally obstructed on muscle paralysis.
   — Topical anaesthesia of the airway prior to induction of anaesthesia reduces the risk of laryngospasm and increases the success rate by reducing airway reflexes.

- Sevoflurane is the preferred volatile anaesthetic for inhalational induction because it is non-pungent, has a rapid onset/offset of action and does not provoke breath-holding, coughing and laryngospasm.
- It is delivered in 100% oxygen or oxygen-air mixture depending on the patient's general condition and oxygen saturation.
- Induction time may be prolonged in patients with upper airway obstruction because of low alveolar minute ventilation. This can be hastened by assist ventilation and applying continuous positive airway pressure (CPAP).
- Intubation is attempted when the patient is adequately anaesthetized.

3. **Blind nasotracheal intubation**
   - Intubation is attempted under sedation or inhalational induction, with preservation of spontaneous ventilation. Prior topical anaesthesia and vasoconstriction are useful to reduce sympathetic responses and bleeding risks.
   - A nasotracheal tube is inserted through the more patent nostril and directed towards the glottis by listening for maximal breath sounds, by observing fogging of the ETT or by capnography tracing.
   - Intubation is blind and is facilitated by flexing the patient's neck and exerting external laryngeal pressure during the manoeuvre.

4. **Fibreoptic laryngoscopy**
   - This is attempted under topical anaesthesia either while the patient is awake, or anaesthetized and breathing spontaneously.
   - This is an elective, planned procedure. It is almost always futile to attempt a fibreoptic laryngoscopy after failed attempts at intubation, when blood and secretions from repeated intubation attempts often obscure the view through the scope. Similarly, fibreoptic intubation is difficult in maxillofacial trauma where there is significant blood and secretion in the oropharynx.

5. **Other manoeuvres**
   - These include retrograde intubation, intubation through the intubating LMA (ILMA), and use of a lighted stylet intubation device called Trachlight™.
   - These techniques are useful in experienced hands but are not suitable for untrained practitioners under emergency situations.

6. **Tracheostomy**
   - If intubation is deemed not possible or all the above options are unsuitable,

the option of tracheostomy under local anaesthesia should be considered. This should be discussed with the surgeon and explained to the patient to obtain consent for the procedure.

Airway Adjuncts

1. **Classic LMA**
   - This invaluable device, invented by Brain, is widely used in routine anaesthesia as well as difficult airway situations particularly in the "cannot intubate, cannot ventilate" scenario.
   - Even though it can also be used as a conduit for tracheal intubation, this role has been superseded by intubating LMA which is designed specifically for this purpose.
   - Concerns about adequate protection of the airway against regurgitation remain; the use of LMA ProSeal™ is yet another advance made towards the modifications of the classic LMA.

2. **Intubating LMA or LMA Fastrach™**
   - This device is a modification of the classic LMA and is designed to increase the success rate of guiding the ETT into the trachea through the LMA.
   - The shape of the device is designed such that it is possible to perform single-handed insertion from any position without moving the patient's head and neck from a neutral position.
   - It comprises a rigid anatomically curved airway tube fitted with a rigid handle. Its diameter is wide enough to accept a cuffed 8 mm ETT through it.
   - An epiglottic elevator bar in the mask aperture, replacing the slits in the standard device, is designed to elevate the epiglottis when an ETT is passed through the aperture.
   - The LMA CTrach™ system is modified from the LMA Fastrach™. Using integrated fibreoptics and a portable viewer, it is possible to obtain real-time visualization of the ETT passing through the vocal cords during intubation.

3. **LMA ProSeal™**
   - This is yet another modified LMA which incorporates an oesophageal drain tube placed adjacent to the airway tube, separating the alimentary and respiratory tracts.

— The drain tube has its opening at the upper oesophageal sphincter to permit escape of gastric fluids. It prevents inadvertent gastric insufflation and poses no problems for IPPV to be used as part of the anaesthetic technique. A nasogastric tube can be passed down the drain tube to decompress the stomach and reduce the risk of regurgitation.
— The modified cuff has a pharyngeal component and forms a more effective seal compared to the classic LMA.
— A built-in bite-block is incorporated near the proximal end of the LMA.
— With practice, the success rate of insertion is comparable to that of the classic LMA.

4. **Oesophageal-tracheal Combitube (ETC)**
   — This is a double-lumen tube that allows ventilation and oxygenation in both the tracheal and oesophageal positions.
   — The tube is inserted either blindly or under direct laryngoscopy. The insertion technique can be easily learned by paramedics in the prehospital scenario.
   — The patient's head remains in the neutral position during insertion, hence it is suitable for use in cervical spine injury. Insertion of ETC can be facilitated by displacing the mandible anteriorly.
   — It has been used successfully as a means to achieve airway control during CPR, in the ICU, and under general anaesthesia both electively and under failed intubation conditions.

5. **Cuffed oropharyngeal airway (COPA)**
   — This is a modified Guedel oropharyngeal airway with an inflatable distal cuff and a proximal 15-mm connector for attachment to the anaesthetic breathing system.
   — The cuff, when inflated, displaces the base of the patient's tongue anteriorly, forms an airtight seal with the pharynx, and elevates the epiglottis from the posterior pharyngeal wall to provide a clear airway.
   — Clinical experience with the COPA is limited. Insertion is easy but additional manipulations to maintain airway patency are often necessary during maintenance of anaesthesia.

6. **Laryngeal tube (LT)**
   — This is a closed-ended S-shaped silicone tube designed for blind insertion into the oesophagus.

- It has 2 high-volume low-pressure cuffs inflated through a single port: a large pharyngeal cuff in the middle part of the tube and a smaller oesophageal cuff at the end of the tube.
- The pharyngeal cuff stabilizes the tube and prevents air leak from the mouth and nose; the oesophageal cuff occludes the oesophageal lumen and protects against regurgitation and aspiration of gastric contents.
- Ventilation occurs through a ventilation outlet between the two cuffs in the anterior aspect of the laryngeal tube. This corresponds to the level of the larynx when properly inserted and optimally positioned, and enables unimpaired ventilation into the trachea.
- A modified version of LT, known as LTS-2, incorporates an oesophageal drain which allows gastric drainage and decompression.

Intubation Aids

1. **McCoy laryngoscope blade**
   - The tip of this blade is movable or "articulating", improving glottic visualization by retracting the epiglottis.
   - Improvement in view can be seen in Grades II and III of Cormack and Lehane classification, while none is possible in Grade IV.

2. **Gum elastic bougie**
   - This 60-cm-long introducer has an angled tip and is flexible and malleable. It is passed blindly into the trachea when the glottic opening is not visible (Cormack and Lehane Grade IV), or inserted posterior to the epiglottis under direct laryngoscopy (Cormack and Lehane Grade III).
   - The bougie is advanced with the angled tip pointing anteriorly. It should be kept anterior to avoid entering the oesophagus, and in the midline to avoid hitting the pyriform fossae on either side.
   - Clicks may be felt when the bougie is passed into the trachea – these are caused by the tip of the bougie hitting the tracheal cartilages. Alternatively, a slight resistance is sensed as the bougie is held up in the bronchial tree, or the patient, if not fully paralyzed, may cough as the trachea is stimulated by the bougie.
   - An ETT is then "railroaded" over it into the trachea. This is facilitated by rotating the ETT 90° anticlockwise to orientate the bevel posteriorly thereby avoiding the right arytenoids. Use a smaller ETT if this is not successful.

3. **Lightwand or Trachlight™**
   - This is light-guided intubation using the principle of transillumination.
   - When the tip of the lightwand enters the glottic opening, a well-defined glow is visualized in the anterior neck, just below the thyroid prominence. No transillumination is observed if the lightwand is placed in the oesophagus.
   - This technique is useful in patients with limited mouth opening, hypoplastic mandible, large tongue, prominent upper incisors or restricted cervical spine movement.
   - It is not suitable in cases with tumour, polyps, infection (e.g., epiglottitis, retropharyngeal abscess), trauma or suspected foreign body in the upper airway. It is also difficult in patients in whom transillumination of the anterior neck may not be adequate (e.g., obese patient, large goitre).

4. **Indirect fibreoptic laryngoscopes**
   - Conventional direct laryngoscopy requires adequate mouth opening, flexion of the cervical spine and extension of the atlanto-occipital joint to achieve optimal position for visualization of the vocal cords. Positioning in this manner may be impossible or contraindicated in certain conditions. Indirect fibreoptic laryngoscopes have been designed for this purpose.
   - Many types of such laryngoscopes are available in the market, such as the Bullard laryngoscope, the UpsherScope, the WuScope and the Augustine Scope. They have their own unique characteristics but also share several features in common – an anatomically-shaped laryngoscope blade, fibreoptic bundles and a light source.
   - The anaesthesiologist should be familiar with whatever device is available in his/her institution before using it in an emergency difficult intubation situation.

Surgical Airway

A surgical airway is an emergency airway established transcutaneously when attempts at mask ventilation or intubation (transoral or transnasal) have failed. Examples are cricothyrotomy and tracheostomy. The anaesthesiologist should be familiar with the procedure in case emergency surgical airway access becomes a necessity in the failed intubation scenario. There are two types of cricothyrotomy.

1. **Needle cricothyrotomy**
   - This can be achieved by using either a large bore (12–14G) intravenous cannula or one of the commercially available cricothyrotomy devices.
   - The cricothyroid membrane is punctured and the tracheal lumen entered. The cannula is connected to the breathing system, resuscitation bag or jet ventilation device, via the barrel of a 2-ml syringe and the connector of a 7.5-mm endotracheal tube.
   - Two types of oxygen delivery systems can be used once access has been achieved.
     - Low-flow system: the patient is manually ventilated via the resuscitation bag or breathing system. Ventilation is seriously impeded since airway resistance is high with gas flows through the narrow cannula. This technique is only a temporary measure until more efficient forms of oxygenation and ventilation become available.
     - High-pressure system: the cannula is connected to a jet injector which delivers oxygen from the wall outlet or oxygen tank. Jet insufflation is performed at 8–10 breaths/min with inspiratory duration of 1 second. This is a much more efficient system, and its components should be included in the difficult intubation trolley.
   - Allow expiration to occur between inflations to prevent air trapping and barotrauma. If the patient is unable to expire because of glottic obstruction, a second cannula should be inserted (for low-flow system) or a stopcock incorporated into the circuit (for high-pressure system) to allow passive expiration.
   - The commercially available cricothyrotomy sets overcome the problem of small-diameter, thin-walled intravenous cannulae by using cannulae which are larger (3.5–7.2 mm internal diameter) and more rigid. The differences between these sets lie in the method of insertion and the rigidity of the cannula walls: Seldinger guide wire technique, insertion of rigid metal cannula over a needle or a single-puncture technique with a plastic cannula housed over a curved needle. The anaesthesiologist should be familiar with whichever system is available in the OT.

2. **Surgical cricothyrotomy**
   - A transverse skin incision is made and blunt dissection performed to the level of the cricothyroid membrane. A transverse incision is made through the inferior third of the membrane and an endotracheal tube inserted into the tracheal lumen.

Complications of cricothyrotomy include inability to cannulate the airway, haemorrhage, aspiration, perforation through the tracheal wall resulting in subcutaneous or mediastinal emphysema, pneumothorax, laryngeal damage, hoarseness of voice due to superior laryngeal nerve damage and subglottic stenosis. However, it is a life-saving procedure and should not be withheld in view of these potential complications.

Tracheostomy (surgical or percutaneous) is seldom performed as an emergency procedure in failed intubation. Cricothyrotomy takes a shorter time to perform and hence is more appropriate in emergency situations. Exceptions include small children (< 6 years) and distorted laryngeal anatomy where the use of cricothyrotomy is contraindicated.

MANAGEMENT OF FAILED INTUBATION

Guidelines for management of the difficult airway and failed intubation have been published by various organizations and national societies, the most widely adopted one being the ASA Difficult Airway Algorithm. Another set of guidelines for management of the unanticipated difficult intubation was published by the Difficult Airway Society (DAS) in the UK in 2004. It is advisable for the anaesthesiologist to study these guidelines closely, device his/her own flow-chart if necessary and commit this to memory, so that in the event of failed intubation the management steps to be followed would be clear and succinct.

The main aims of the management steps in any algorithm are to maintain oxygenation and ventilation, and to prevent pulmonary aspiration. It should be remembered that patients do not die or suffer hypoxic brain damage from failure to intubate, but from failure to achieve adequate oxygenation and ventilation. As such it would be a folly to make repeated attempts at intubation without resorting to alternative plans of management. The patient's haemodynamic status and oxygen saturation must be monitored at all times, while capnography is extremely useful for confirming tracheal placement of the ETT.

Figure 25–3 depicts management of failed intubation in a patient with no aspiration risks. A similar scenario in a patient with full stomach, typically a pregnant patient scheduled for caesarean section under general anaesthesia, is outlined in Figure 34–1 in Chapter 34.

Multiple and prolonged intubation attempts by the same anaesthesiologist are self-defeating; success rate does not increase beyond the second "good" attempt while risks of trauma, laryngeal oedema, desaturation and aspiration increase proportionately. It is not justifiable to attempt more than 4 times unless intubation is taken over by another, more experienced colleague. Similarly, subsequent insertions of LMA or ILMA should be limited to 2 before moving on to the next step of the algorithm.

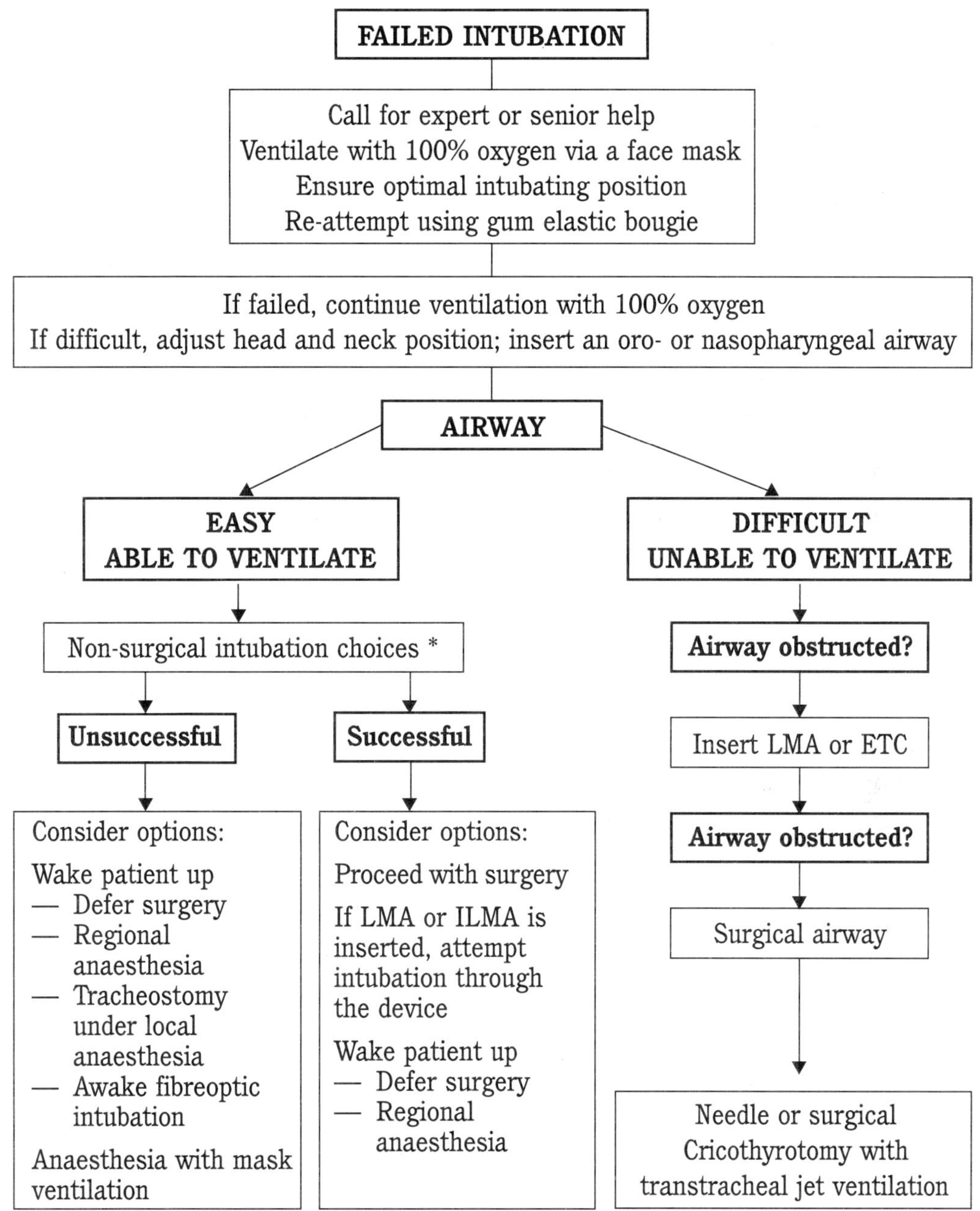

* *Non-surgical intubation choices* include laryngoscopy with alternative laryngoscope blades or indirect fibreoptic laryngoscope, LMA or intubating LMA, ETC, laryngeal tube, Trachlight™, LMA ProSeal™.

Figure 25–3. Algorithm for unrecognized difficult airway

EXTUBATION OF THE DIFFICULT AIRWAY

— Management of the difficult airway does not end with successful tracheal intubation. Equal emphasis should be placed on management strategies for safe and successful extubation.

— It is not advisable to extubate the patient "deep" in the context of difficult airway because of the risks of hypoventilation and airway obstruction. The possibility of airway oedema after repeated attempts at intubation should always be borne in mind. The patient should be fully conscious and able to demonstrate adequate breathing efforts prior to extubation. It is always safer to err on the side of caution and leave the ETT *in situ* if any doubt exists regarding patient's respiratory efforts or airway patency postextubation.

— Devices such as airway exchange catheters are useful in such situations. One of the commonest devices is the Cook™ airway exchange catheter. This is a semi-rigid radio-opaque polyurethane catheter through which oxygen can be insufflated and end-tidal CO_2 can be intermittently measured. The proximal end of the catheter is fitted with a 15-mm connector for connection to the breathing system or self-inflating bag, and a Luer-Lok connector for jet ventilation. There are distance markings on the catheter to allow proper depth determination.

— Recommended technique for extubation
  - Turn off all inhalational anaesthetic agents. Reverse neuromuscular blockade if applicable. Administer 100% oxygen and suction the oropharynx to clear secretion and blood.
  - When the patient is ready for extubation, deflate the ETT cuff and check for air leaks around the ETT: this excludes the presence of significant laryngeal oedema.
  - Insert an airway exchange catheter through the ETT to a predetermined depth.
  - Remove the ETT and leave the catheter in place.
  - Insufflate oxygen through the catheter and closely observe the patient for signs of respiratory distress.
  - Remove the exchange catheter after 30–60 minutes if no airway obstruction appears.
  - Insert an ETT by "railroading" down the exchange catheter if the need for re-intubation arises.

— Clearly document the problem in the patient's case notes and the anaesthesia record, stating the nature of difficulty encountered during intubation and methods used to overcome it.
— The anaesthesiologist should make it a point to visit the patient postoperatively. During the postoperative visit, one should look for any sequelae from intubation attempts (sore throat, trauma to the airway structures), inform the patient and elaborate on the difficulty in intubation encountered, and emphasize the need for the patient to alert his/her future anaesthesiologist regarding the problem.

SUMMARY

These are some of the pitfalls that result in increased morbidity or mortality. These should be avoided in order to ensure favourable patient outcome.

— Inadequate preoperative assessment of the airway.
— Inappropriate anaesthetic technique.
— Inexperience, lack of training or supervision, fatigue of the anaesthesiologist.
— Lack of skilled and dedicated anaesthetic assistance.
— Persistent attempts at intubation without providing oxygenation.
— Failure to recognize oesophageal intubation.
— Failure to follow a failed intubation protocol.
— Failure to recognize cyanosis in dark-skinned patients.

These are measures to overcome the above problems.

— Careful preoperative airway assessment and preoxygenation for patient considered at risk. Ensure availability of difficult airway equipment.
— Be familiar with failed intubation protocol and be ready to implement it early. Anaesthetic airway simulator may have an important role in education and training.
— Aim to be competent in fibreoptic intubation and other airway management techniques. Practice on airway mannequins and patients with normal airway anatomy to gain experience and confidence in using the device.
— Ensure that equipment for emergency surgical airway and trans-tracheal ventilation is immediately available should the need arise.

FURTHER READING

1. Practice guidelines for management of the difficult airway: An updated report by the American Society of Anesthesiologists Task Force on Management of the Difficult Airway. Anesthesiology 2003;98:1269–77.
2. Charters P, O'Sullivan E. The 'dedicated airway': A review of the concept and an update of current practice. Anaesthesia 1999;54:778–86.
3. Henderson JJ, Popat MT, Latto IP, Pearce AC. Difficult Airway Society guidelines for management of the unanticipated difficult intubation. Anaesthesia 2004;59:675–94.
4. Crosby E, Cooper RM, Douglas MJ, Doyle DJ, et al. The unanticipated difficult airway with recommendations for management. Can J Anaesth 1998;45:757–76.
5. Agro F, Hung OR, Cataldo R, et al. Lightwand intubation using the Trachlight™: A brief review of current knowledge. Can J Anaesth 2001;48:592–9.
6. Davis L, Cook-Sather SD, Schreiner MS. Lighted stylet tracheal intubation: A review. Anesth Analg 2000;90:745–56.
7. Benumof JL. Laryngeal mask airway and the ASA difficult airway algorithm. Anesthesiology 1996;84:86–99.
8. Brimacombe J, Brain AIJ, Berry A. *The Laryngeal Mask Airway Instruction Manual*, Third Edition. Henley-on-Thames, UK, Intavent Research Limited, 1996.
9. Caponas G. Intubating laryngeal mask airway. Anaesth Intens Care 2002;30:551–69.
10. Brain AIJ, Verghese C, Strube PJ. The LMA "ProSeal" – A laryngeal mask with an oesophageal vent. Br J Anaesth 2000;84:650–4.
11. Gaitini LA, Varda SJ, Mostafa S, Yanovski B, et al. The Combitube in elective surgery: A report of 200 cases. Anesthesiology 2001;94:79–82.
12. Uezono S, Goto T, Nakata Y, et al. The cuffed oropharyngeal airway, a novel adjunct to the management of difficult airways. Anesthesiology 1998;88:1677–9.
13. Dörges V, Ocker H, Wenzel V, Schmucker P. The laryngeal tube: A new simple airway device. Anesth Analg 2000;90:1220–2.
14. Benumof JL. Airway exchange catheters for safe extubation: The clinical and scientific details that make the concept work. Chest 1997;111:1483–6.

Chapter 26

Anaesthesia for the Trauma Patient

INTRODUCTION

Trauma is the leading cause of death in the younger population and occurs mainly as a result of road traffic accidents. Nearly half of the deaths are immediate due to massive injury to major vessels or vital organs, namely the heart, brain or spinal cord. Approximately a third of the patients succumb after a brief period (the so-called "golden hour") as a result of potentially treatable conditions such as hypoventilation, haemorrhage, haemo-pneumothorax, cardiac tamponade or an expanding intracranial mass. Factors important in reducing mortality include accident prevention, prehospital stabilization, rapid transport, early resuscitation, timely operative intervention and postoperative care and rehabilitation.

In view of the need for immediate management to reduce mortality due to trauma, the American College of Surgeons established the Advanced Trauma Life Support (ATLS) programme to provide comprehensive and structured care for the trauma patient. Another similar programme is the Early Management of Severe Trauma (EMST) programme in Australia and New Zealand. The initial management is considered in 4 phases – primary survey, resuscitation, secondary survey and definitive care. The first 2 often occur concurrently while secondary survey will commence after the patient has been adequately resuscitated.

As anaesthesiologists, we are a part of the trauma team and are frequently called to resuscitate patients in the Accident and Emergency (A&E) Department. Our expertise in airway management, intravenous cannulation and volume resuscitation are skills which are useful in the A&E. Some of these patients may require monitored sedation while undergoing radiological examination, or may require anaesthetic for emergency surgery, and they may be admitted to ICU for postoperative management.

PROBLEMS ASSOCIATED WITH THE TRAUMA PATIENT

These problems should be anticipated and addressed.

- The sustained injuries may be life-threatening, multiple or occult.
- Adequacy of airway, breathing, circulation may be compromised, requiring active, urgent and on-going resuscitation.
- The patient may be intoxicated, restless, comatose or in shock. It may not be possible to obtain a detailed history on the patient's premorbid health status or circumstances surrounding the trauma.
- The patient's status in terms of transmissible infection (HIV or hepatitis) is unknown, hence the need for universal precaution during resuscitation.
- There may be inadequate time to prepare the patient for anaesthesia.
- There is a definite risk of full stomach leading to vomiting, regurgitation and aspiration of gastric contents during anaesthesia.

BASIC MANAGEMENT PRINCIPLES

Primary Survey and Resuscitation: ABC's of Resuscitation

- **Airway with cervical spine control**
  - Ensure a clear airway and ability to maintain adequate oxygenation.

- Watch for signs of airway obstruction, such as stridor, respiratory distress, cyanosis.
- Assume cervical injury in all patients with head and maxillofacial injuries unless proven otherwise.
- Provide oxygen supplementation with SpO_2 monitoring.
- Assess the need for immediate intubation.

— **Breathing**
- Look out for inadequate breathing efforts – tachypnoea, abnormal pattern of respiration, use of accessory muscles of respiration, cyanosis, mental confusion – and intervene early.
- Rule out serious life-threatening chest injuries such as tension pneumothorax, cardiac tamponade, significant pneumo-haemothorax, disruption of tracheobronchial tree.

— **Circulation and haemorrhage control**
- Watch out for signs of shock, such as cold clammy peripheries, poor capillary return, pallor, thready small volume pulse, hypotension.
- Control major external haemorrhage with direct pressure.
- Insert large bore intravenous cannulae and rapidly infuse fluids to correct hypovolaemia.
- Send blood samples for GXM and laboratory investigations.

— **Disability: rapid neurologic assessment**
- Perform a quick neurological evaluation by assessing the pupil size and reaction to light, Glasgow Coma Scale (GCS) score, movement of limbs spontaneously or in response to stimulus.

— **Exposure**
- Completely undress the patient for a thorough survey of other injuries, and then cover with warm blankets to prevent hypothermia.

Exclude life-threatening conditions under primary survey.

— Tension pneumothorax.

— Upper airway obstruction.

— Cardiac tamponade.

— Massive bleeding from ruptured major vessels.

Oxygen Therapy

— Oxygen therapy should be instituted for patients in shock and those with multiple trauma, chest and head injuries.

— Oxygen may be administered by means of nasal catheter, clear Hudson® mask, Ventimask® or high-flow mask with reservoir, as indicated by clinical condition, pulse oximetry and ABG results.

— These conditions require urgent intubation.
  - Upper airway obstruction with ventilatory insufficiency.
  - Severe lung contusion with signs of hypoxaemia; haemo- or pneumothorax needs urgent chest drain insertion.
  - Severe head injury with GCS < 9.
  - Inability to protect the airway, or active bleeding in the oral cavity with risk of aspiration.
  - Shock of any nature requiring cardiopulmonary resuscitation.

Blood and Fluids

— Insert large bore intravenous cannulae and infuse crystalloid and/or colloid solutions while waiting for blood to be available.

— Send blood for emergency GXM and laboratory investigations.

— Use Group O negative blood in dire emergencies.

— Check ABG for patients with respiratory distress and chest injuries.

— Insert central venous catheter and urinary catheter to assess adequacy of fluid resuscitation.

— There has been a rethink about the concept of aggressive fluid resuscitation in trauma, due to its adverse effects on haemostatic mechanisms that may result in exacerbation of blood loss. Two strategies in trauma resuscitation have been proposed: delayed resuscitation, where fluid is withheld until haemostasis is definitively achieved; and permissive hypotension, when fluid is administered but the end-point for resuscitation is lower than normotension. In practical terms, it means giving fluids in small aliquots to achieve a systolic BP of 80–90 mmHg, a value deemed sufficient to maintain vital organ perfusion in an adult. This end-point may have to be raised in ill patients with preexisting cardiorespiratory or cerebrovascular diseases.

Secondary Survey and Definitive Care

It is easy to miss occult injuries; hence, it is important to evaluate the various systems in an organized manner.

a. **Head**
   - Assess the patient's conscious level and evaluate according to the GCS score.
   - Inspect and palpate the scalp for lacerations, haematoma or depressed skull fractures.
   - Check for signs of basal skull fracture. Inspect the nose and ears for blood or cerebrospinal fluid.
   - Assess severity of maxillofacial injury, extent of active bleeding into the airway and identify potential difficulty in intubation.
   - Ask for an urgent CT scan if head injury is suspected, or in the presence of deteriorating conscious level, coma after resuscitation, confusion and focal neurological signs.
   - Patients with low GCS (< 9) and unable to protect the airway should be intubated, particularly in the presence of concomitant chest injuries.

b. **Spine**
   - Assume cervical injury in all patients with head and neck injuries unless it has been actively excluded. If the patient is conscious, ask specifically for pain in the neck and examine for local bruising or tenderness. Do a quick neurological examination of the upper and lower limbs.
   - Use a cervical collar if there is any doubt regarding cervical injury. Take care during transport of the patient to ensure that the head and neck are not subject to jerks or sudden movements.
   - Send for X-rays of the cervical spines. All the cervical spines (C1–C7) should be examined. It is easy to miss out abnormalities in the lower cervical spines if the view is obscured by the shoulders.
   - Injury to the rest of the spine should be excluded. The patient should be log-rolled to the lateral position so that a thorough inspection and palpation of the whole length of the spine can be carried out.
   - High-level spinal cord injury often results in spinal shock with loss of sympathetic tone and myocardial dysfunction. The resultant hypotension and bradycardia may be persistent and difficult to treat (see Chapter 18).

c. **Chest**

- The following conditions should be ruled out: pulmonary contusion, myocardial injury and/or cardiac tamponade, traumatic rupture of the aorta, ruptured diaphragm, oesophageal rupture and disruption of the tracheobronchial tree.
- These conditions should be diagnosed clinically and treatment of life-threatening conditions instituted immediately rather than waiting for radiological confirmation.

d. **Abdomen**

- Examine the abdomen for laceration, bruising, distension and tenderness.
- Look for injury to any of the intraabdominal structures as well as the kidneys, and determine whether there is a need for urgent laparotomy.
- When the clinical signs are equivocal, a diagnostic peritoneal lavage may be of value to detect the presence of haemoperitoneum indicative of intra-abdominal injury.
- Other investigations include ultrasound and CT scan of the abdomen but these may not be practical in emergency situations.

e. **Pelvis**

- Pelvic fractures and injury to the pelvic structures are difficult to diagnose clinically, as the signs may be variable and bleeding may be massive but concealed within the pelvis.
- The possibility of a pelvic injury should be entertained in a pale and hypotensive patient with no obvious source of bleeding, as blood loss is often occult.
- The patient with bladder and/or urethral damage may present with haematuria or extravasation of urine.
- Antero-posterior view of the pelvic X-ray may indicate widening (diastasis) of the symphysis pubis of greater than 2 cm, or vertical displacement of one side of the pelvis, or evidence of fractures to the pelvic bones.

f. **Extremities**

- Examine for fractures and damage to peripheral nerve, tendon or blood vessel. Feel for peripheral pulses. Look out for compartment syndrome especially in tibial and forearm fractures.
- Urgent surgery is required if there is arterial injury compromising limb perfusion or development of compartment syndrome.

ANAESTHETIC MANAGEMENT

- Preoperative evaluation and resuscitation are as outlined above. It is important to identify the nature and severity of injuries in the multi-trauma patient so that appropriate treatment may be given to each.
- Obtain consent from the patient or next-of-kin if available. Under life-threatening circumstances, consent from consultants of two units managing the patient would suffice as it would be impractical to delay definitive treatment for the purpose of obtaining a written consent.
- Send blood samples for emergency GXM for blood and plasma in cases likely to have substantial intraoperative bleeding and require massive transfusion.
- Monitors include ECG, BP, pulse oximetry, capnography, CVP, urine output, temperature and peripheral nerve stimulator. The type and extent of monitoring depends on the general condition of the patient, the extent and severity of the injury, and the nature and urgency of surgery.
- Active steps should be taken to minimize perioperative hypothermia (see Chapter 6).
- Patients with severe trauma in shock and with decreased level of consciousness may require nothing more than 100% oxygen, neuromuscular blocking drug and small doses of volatile anaesthetics and/or opioid. However, the incidence of awareness under anaesthesia is known to be higher in such situations, and the depth of anaesthesia should be increased at the first opportunity.
- *No single anaesthetic agent or technique has proved to be superior to others.* The choice depends on the clinical condition of the patient – the haemodynamic, respiratory and neurological status in particular – and the site, duration and complexity of surgery.

General Anaesthesia

- Identify potential airway problems during preoperative assessment and consider various options of anaesthetic induction if problems are anticipated.
- Preoxygenate the patient with 100% oxygen for 3–5 minutes. In extremely ermergent situation, place the face mask firmly over the patient's face and instruct the patient to take 4 vital capacity breaths before induction of anaesthesia.
- Use rapid sequence induction and intubation. Instruct the anaesthetic assistant to apply cricoid pressure when the patient loses consciousness and maintain the cricoid pressure until the trachea is successfully intubated, the ETT cuff is inflated and its correct placement is confirmed by auscultation and capnography.

— Intravenous induction agents that may be used include thiopentone and propofol in normotensive patients. Ketamine is suitable in hypotension or hypovolaemia because it stimulates the sympathetic nervous system and maintains blood pressure.
— Use suxamethonium for intubation unless contraindicated. Maintain neuromuscular blockade with a non-depolarizing neuromuscular blocking drug.
— Avoid nitrous oxide in patients who are hypotensive, hypovolaemic or hypoxaemic; use 100% oxygen or oxygen-air mixture instead. This avoids the myocardial depressant effect of nitrous oxide and ensures that adequate FiO_2 is delivered to the patient.
— Supplement anaesthesia with volatile anaesthetic and opioids as appropriate.
— Continue volume resuscitation during surgery, replace blood loss and obtain more intravenous access if necessary.
— Utilize autologous blood transfusion by means of intraoperative cell salvage in suitable cases, e.g., ruptured abdominal aortic aneurysm, extensive liver surgery.
— Beware of complications of massive transfusion, such as dilutional thrombocytopaenia, disseminated intravascular coagulation, acid-base and electrolyte imbalance, and manage them accordingly.
— FBC with haematocrit, ABG, electrolyte concentrations should be frequently analyzed. Send blood samples to check coagulation profile if coagulopathy is suspected.
— Emergence from anaesthesia and reversal of neuromuscular blockade at the end of the surgery is carried out in the usual manner.
— Consider ICU admission in these cases.
  - Severe head injury for cerebral resuscitation.
  - Severe chest injury with flail chest, lung contusion, haemo- or pneumothorax.
  - Evidence of aspiration pneumonia.
  - Multi-system trauma requiring ventilatory support.
  - Old, ill ASA III–V patients.
  - Unstable haemodynamics requiring inotrope support.
  - Massive transfusion with evidence of disseminated intravascular coagulation.

FAT EMBOLISM SYNDROME

— This topic is included in this chapter because the syndrome may be associated with trauma to the long bones in particular. Fat embolism syndrome can also result from other surgical and medical conditions.

— One should differentiate between fat embolism and fat embolism syndrome.
  - Fat embolism (FE) is fat within the circulatory system, which can produce embolic phenomena, with or without clinical sequelae.
  - Fat embolism syndrome (FES) is fat in the circulatory system associated with an identifiable clinical pattern of respiratory, haematological, neurological and cutaneous symptoms and signs. These are listed in Table 26–1.

— The incidence of the clinical syndrome is low (< 1% in retrospective reviews) even though the embolization of marrow fat appears to be an almost inevitable consequence of long bone fractures.

— Many therapeutic interventions and prophylactic strategies have been tried with varying success. Current treatment is supportive and the condition is usually associated with a good outcome.

— The cornerstone of treatment is prevention of the stress response, hypovolaemia and hypoxia. Operative stabilization of fractures should be carried out within 24 hours in the absence of chest trauma.

— The most common manifestation of FES is pulmonary dysfunction. The routine use of pulse oximetry may detect hypoxaemia early and allow prompt correction by oxygen therapy.

Table 26–1. Features of fat embolism syndrome

Major Criteria	Petechial rash Respiratory features: tachypnoea, dyspnoea, bilateral inspiratory crepitations, haemoptysis, bilateral diffuse patchy shadowing on chest X-ray Neurological signs: confusion, drowsiness, coma
Minor Criteria	Tachycardia > 120/min Pyrexia > 39.4°C Retinal changes: fat or petechiae Jaundice Renal changes: anuria or oliguria
Laboratory Features	Thrombocytopenia > 50% decrease on admission value Sudden decrease in haemoglobin level > 20% of admission value High erythrocyte sedimentation rate > 71 mm/hr Fat macroglobulaemia

FURTHER READING

1. Johnstone RE, Graf DF. Acute trauma with multiple injuries. Curr Opin Anaesthesiol 2001;14:211–5.
2. Peerless JR. Fluid management of the trauma patient. Curr Opin Anaesthesiol 2001;14:221–5.
3. Revell M, Greaves I, Porter K. Endpoints for fluid resuscitation in hemorrhagic shock. J Trauma 2003;54:S63–7.
4. Stainsby D, MacLennan S, Hamilton PJ. Management of massive blood loss: A template guideline. Br J Anaesth 2000;85:487–91.
5. Morris CGT, McCoy E. Clearing the cervical spine in unconscious polytrauma victims, balancing risks and effective screening. Anaesthesia 2004;59:464–82.
6. Smith CE, DeJoy SJ. New equipment and techniques for airway management in trauma. Curr Opin Anaesthesiol 2001;14:197–209.
7. Karmakar MK, Ho AMH. Acute pain management of patients with multiple fractured ribs. J Trauma 2003;54:615–25.
8. Mellor A, Soni N. Fat embolism. Anaesthesia 2001;56:145–54.

Chapter 27

Anaesthesia for Patients with Thermal Injury

INTRODUCTION

Thermal injuries continue to cause many complications and deaths. Although recent advances in burn resuscitation and critical care have resulted in improved outcome and survival rates after major burns, management of these patients remains challenging to all involved in their care. The improved survival rates have been attributed to the development of the multi-disciplinary burn team, an early aggressive surgical approach to major burns, and better understanding of the pathophysiologic nature of thermal injuries.

Agents that cause thermal injury include flame or fire in open or enclosed space, hot liquid, chemical (including explosives), electric current, radiation, and frostbite in cold countries. One should note that patients involved in fires in enclosed spaces may present with inhalation of carbon monoxide and other toxic fumes; and electrical burns are usually more serious than superficial inspection would suggest because of underlying tissue damage.

The anaesthesiologist may encounter such patients at various stages of the hospital stay.

— Initial assessment and resuscitation, including emergency airway management.
— ICU or HDU management for major burns.
— Anaesthesia for escharotomy, desloughing and skin grafting; emergency surgery for associated injuries; and later for release of burn contractures.
— Acute pain management, including analgesia for change of burn dressing especially in paediatric patients.

CLASSIFICATION

The degree of thermal injury is assessed according to the depth of skin destroyed, the extent of the body surface area involved and the presence or absence of an inhalational injury.

1. **Depth of skin destroyed**

   The classification shown in Table 27–1 is frequently used.

2. **Percentage of body surface area involved**

   The commonly employed formula is Wallace "Rule of Nines" for adults, in which the body surface area (BSA) is divided into areas of 9% or multiples of 9%.

   — Entire head and neck: 9%
   — Anterior surface of trunk: 18%
   — Posterior surface of trunk: 18%
   — Entire upper limb: 9%
   — Entire lower limb: 18%
   — Perineum: 1%

   Surface area of one side of the patient's hand represents 1% of BSA.

   Estimation of percentage of burns in children is different because of differences in proportional size of the head, water content per kilogram, fluid requirements and sensitivity to fluid deficit. However, even a modified version appears to underestimate the extent of burn injury in children.

Table 27–1. Classification of burn depth

Classification	Burn Depth	Outcome
Superficial First degree	Confined to epidermis	Heals spontaneously
Partial thickness Second degree		
▪ Superficial dermal burn	Epidermis and upper dermis	Heals spontaneously
▪ Deep dermal burn	Epidermis and deep dermis	Requires excision and grafting for rapid return of function
Full thickness Third degree	Destruction of epidermis and dermis	Wound excision and grafting required; some limitation of function and scar formation
Fourth degree	Muscle, fascia, bone	Complete excision required, limited function

According to the American Burn Association Injury Severity Grading System, burns are considered to be major if there are:

— Full thickness burns > 10% BSA.

— Partial thickness burns > 25% BSA in adults, or > 20% BSA at extremes of age.

— Burns involving the face, eyes, ears, hands, feet, genitalia or perineum.

— Inhalational, chemical or electrical burns including lightning injury.

— Burns in patients with serious preexisting medical disorders.

Such patients should be managed in hospitals, preferably in centres with dedicated facilities for the treatment of major burns.

INITIAL ASSESSMENT AND RESUSCITATION

1. **Airway**
   - Airway assessment includes evaluation of preexisting airway abnormality, current airway injury and signs of airway obstruction.
   - Look for signs of inhalational injury and upper airway obstruction.
     - Facial and airway oedema.
     - Singeing of nasal hair or eyebrows.
     - Soot in sputum or in the oropharynx.
     - Burns to face and neck.
     - Stridor, hoarseness of voice, dysphagia.
     - Respiratory distress.

     Note that the absence of a facial burn does not rule out a significant upper airway injury.
   - *Intervene early rather than late*, since airway oedema often develops and complicates airway management.
   - If time permits, endotracheal intubation should be performed under optimal conditions in OT or ICU where monitoring, equipment and personnel are adequate. However, intubation should not be delayed if the patient's condition warrants immediate intervention since airway obstruction can be severe and life-threatening.
   - Intubation can be performed under inhalational anaesthesia or by means of awake fibreoptic laryngoscopy.
   - Prepare for difficult intubation with equipment and airway adjuncts checked and ready for use. Smaller sized endotracheal tubes may be required.
   - Suxamethonium is not contraindicated in the initial period of resuscitation when the hyperkalaemic response has not set in. However, its use may not be advisable in upper airway obstruction and potential difficult intubation.
   - Establishment of a surgical airway – needle or surgical cricothyrotomy, or tracheostomy – may be indicated if the upper airway anatomy is badly distorted and endotracheal intubation is not possible. This should be considered as a last resort since surgical airway is associated with high incidence of complications.

2. **Breathing**
   - Look for features of respiratory distress, such as tachypnoea, shallow respiration, paradoxical respiration, wheezing or cyanosis.

— Look for signs of carbon monoxide poisoning particularly in a patient with history of burns within an enclosed space. Clinical features depend on the degree of exposure and reflect the effects of carbon monoxide in reducing oxygen carrying capacity of blood and causing tissue hypoxia. Symptoms include these.
  - Headaches, tinnitus, mild confusion (carboxyhaemoglobin, COHb < 20%).
  - Lethargy, drowsiness, nausea and vomiting, disorientation (COHb 20–40%).
  - Severe neurologic disturbance, hallucinations, seizure, coma (COHb 40–60%)
  - Death may occur when COHb exceeds 60%.

  Note that PaO_2 and SaO_2 may be normal in carbon monoxide poisoning.

— Administer oxygen via high-flow mask or endotracheal tube.

— The patient may develop acute pulmonary oedema secondary to decreased plasma oncotic pressure and increased pulmonary capillary permeability. This may occur in the absence of a direct lung injury.

— Respiratory failure can result from smoke inhalation injury, infection and acute respiratory distress syndrome (ARDS).

3. **Circulation**

— Besides fluid loss from the burned area to the environment, there is a large fluid shift from the plasma volume to the interstitial space secondary to increased membrane permeability. The intravascular volume may be depleted despite the presence of peripheral oedema.

— Look for signs of hypovolaemic shock, in the form of disturbed sensorium, cold clammy peripheries, weak, rapid, thready pulse, hypotension, oliguria or anuria.

— Fluid resuscitation should be started early. Intravenous access may be difficult if the usual venepuncture sites are involved in the burned area.

— Insert central venous catheter and urinary catheter to monitor fluid resuscitation. The site for central venous access may be limited by the location and extent of burns.

— Inotropes and vasopressors may be needed if blood pressure remains low when the volume status is normal or near-normal.

4. **Fluid resuscitation**

— Various regimens have been proposed as guidelines for fluid resuscitation (see Table 27–2).

Table 27–2. Fluid resuscitation for adults with major burns

Regimen	Intravenous Solution	Amount
Crystalloid regimens		
Parkland	Ringer's lactate	4 ml/kg/% BSA
Modified Brooke	Ringer's lactate	2 ml/kg/% BSA
Colloid regimens		
Evans	Normal saline	1 ml/kg/% BSA
	Colloid	1 ml/kg/% BSA
	5% dextrose	2,000 ml/24 hours
Brooke	Ringer's lactate	1.5 ml/kg/% BSA
	Colloid	0.5 ml/kg/% BSA
	5% dextrose	2,000 ml/24 hours

— The usual practice is to use predominantly crystalloid solutions in first 24 hours at 2–4 ml/kg/% BSA and add on colloids after 24 hours as capillary integrity is expected to return to normal after 24–48 hours. Administer half the calculated amount of resuscitation fluid in the first 8 hours and the rest over the next 16 hours.

— Gelatins and synthetic colloids are useful in haemodynamically unstable patients with major burns. Recent work tends to favour earlier introduction of colloids after the first 6 hours.

— Ringer's lactate remains the preferred crystalloid solution for resuscitation. However, only 20–30% of the crystalloid administered remains within the vascular system after an hour.

— Glucose-containing solutions should not be used unless specifically indicated. They are associated with adverse cardiovascular and neurological outcomes following cardiac arrest and cerebral ischaemia.

— Results following the use of hypertonic saline as well as albumin solutions have been disappointing.

— Fluid requirements are greater if resuscitation has been delayed, in children with large burns, and in patients with smoke inhalation.

— Children require special care as published formulae may underestimate their fluid requirements. This is especially so in small patients (< 10 kg) and in those with extensive burns (> 40% BSA).

— Adequacy of resuscitation is traditionally monitored by urine output and vital signs. In most patients the hourly urine output (0.5 ml/kg/hr in adults and 1.0 ml/kg/hr in children < 25 kg) is a reasonable indicator of organ perfusion and the principal guide to fluid therapy. Invasive haemodynamic monitoring may be indicated in selected patients with major burns who do not respond as expected to fluid resuscitation.
— Dangers of overresuscitation include tissue oedema, pulmonary oedema, cardiac failure, a need for fasciotomy and the abdominal compartment syndrome.

5. **Associated injuries**
   — A careful and systematic secondary survey is important to exclude injuries which may not be obvious initially.

SUBSEQUENT MANAGEMENT

Following initial resuscitation, these measures are no less important.

1. **Pain relief**
   — Partial thickness burn is painful and some form of analgesia is necessary
   — Treatment options include morphine in the form of intravenous bolus doses, continuous infusion or patient-controlled analgesia (PCA).
   — The intravenous route is preferred since absorption from other routes may be erratic and unreliable.

2. **Stress ulcer prophylaxis**
   — Use H_2 receptor antagonist (such as ranitidine) or sucralfate to prevent stress ulcer formation.
   — Establish early enteral feeding.

3. **Temperature control**
   — Take measures to prevent heat loss initially because insulation provided by the skin covering is lost and the patient may become hypothermic.
   — Fever usually develops a few days later due to the hypermetabolic state or concurrent infection.

4. **Infection control**
   - Measures for early prevention of sepsis is necessary. These include:
     - Barrier nursing in separate room with good ventilation.
     - Topical dressing with 1% silver sulphadiazine cream.
     - Frequent change of dressing.
   - The systemic antibiotics used depend on culture and sensitivity results.
   - Prognosis worsens in patients with overwhelming sepsis and multi-organ failure.

5. **Electrolyte and acid-base balance**
   - Electrolyte and acid-base disturbances are common following the initial resuscitation phase, for example:
     - Hypernatraemia due to salt loading and inadequate replacement of insensible fluid losses.
     - Hyperkalaemia due to tissue and red cell destruction.
     - Hypocalcaemia due to albumin depletion.
     - Acidosis, either respiratory, or metabolic, or both.
   - These abnormalities should be corrected and then reassessed as appropriate.

6. **Nutritional support**
   - A hypermetabolic state develops in proportion to the severity of burn injury.
   - Early feeding decreases muscle catabolism and should be started soon after initial resuscitation.
   - Oral and enteral feeding also helps to maintain intestinal barrier function, thus preventing bacterial and fungal translocation.
   - Consider total parenteral nutrition if oral or enteral feeding is not possible or not tolerated.

7. **Liver and kidneys**
   - Hypoalbuminaemia is common in severe cases.
   - Liver failure may develop as part of multi-organ failure secondary to sepsis.
   - Watch for acute renal failure.
     - Early renal dysfunction is usually associated with delay in initial resuscitation.
     - Subsequent renal dysfunction may be secondary to sepsis as part of multi-organ dysfunction.

- Mortality rate remains high (approaching 90%) despite advances in renal replacement therapies.

8. **Haematological system**
   - Initial haemoconcentration is observed as the skin barrier is breached allowing loss of fluids.
   - Anaemia and thrombocytopaenia are common following major burns.
   - Both thrombotic and fibrinolytic systems are activated, and disseminated intravascular coagulation may be a feature especially when sepsis intervenes.

ANAESTHETIC MANAGEMENT

The anaesthesiologist may be requested to provide analgesia for the change of dressing especially in young children. This is usually carried out in the treatment room in the ward unless the wound is extensive and necessitates desloughing in the OT.

If the patient is on some form of opioid analgesic, an additional dose may be administered in anticipation of the procedure. Alternatively, a small dose of IV ketamine (1 mg/kg) may be used for its good analgesic effect. The patient's heart rate, blood pressure and respiration should be closely monitored both during and after the procedure. Oxygen and airway equipment should be available in case airway intervention becomes necessary.

The early elimination of burned tissue is shown to reduce morbidity and mortality. Escharotomy is performed to excise the coagulated dead skin of a full thickness burn ("eschar") and incision is made down to the subcutaneous tissue. The most widely used approach involves an initial 48-hour period of patient stabilization, followed by excision and grafting of the burn wound. The patient may require repeated anaesthesia within short periods of time until the staged surgical procedures are completed.

The anaesthesiologist is faced with these problems.

- Difficult airway management if the patient's airway is compromised.
- Problems with oxygenation and ventilation in patients with profound respiratory injury.
- Inadequate resuscitation prior to anaesthesia for emergency procedures.
- Difficulty in establishing vascular access and monitors.
- Hyperkalaemic response to suxamethonium (after 48–72 hours following injury).

- Resistance to non-depolarizing neuromuscular blocking drugs.
- Often significant intraoperative blood and plasma loss.
- Patient positioning depending on location of burn and skin graft sites.
- Maintenance of perioperative normothermia.
- Management of intra- and postoperative analgesia.

Preoperative Management

It is important to fully assess the patient's current cardiorespiratory status to individualize anaesthetic management. The site and extent of the proposed surgical procedure should be discussed with the surgeon as this information has a direct bearing on the anaesthetic technique, extent of monitoring and requirements for blood and blood products.

Steps taken in preoperative preparation include:

- Review of the latest investigation results.
- Request for blood and blood products. The precise amount depends on the extent of the procedure and the patient's preoperative status.
- Review of the patient's current analgesic requirements and plan for postoperative analgesia.

Minimize the fasting period before surgery in order to minimize disruption to achieving adequate caloric intake. Tracheally intubated patients receiving enteral feeding do not require preoperative fasting.

Intraoperative Management

- Prepare for difficult intubation if the head and neck region is involved. The presence of facial burns may pose problems in achieving adequate seal during ventilation via face mask. Oedema, scarring or contracture may limit mouth opening and neck mobility.
- Take steps to prevent hypothermia by using forced-air warming device, warming mattress, warmed intravenous fluids and humidifier in the breathing system. Consider increasing ambient OT temperature.
- Monitors include ECG, BP, pulse oximetry, capnography, CVP, urine output, temperature. These may be difficult to establish in the presence of burns.

— Choice of anaesthetic agent: the pharmacokinetics of drugs are markedly affected by the hypermetabolic state, and dosages may need to be modified accordingly.
  - Intravenous induction agent: ketamine has good analgesic properties and maintains blood pressure in hypovolaemic patients. However, it is associated with increased bronchial secretions and has poor recovery characteristics with long hangover effect. Propofol enables rapid and clear-headed recovery but does not possess analgesic effect and tends to cause hypotension if administered rapidly.
  - Volatile anaesthetic: isoflurane, sevoflurane or desflurane is preferred over halothane as the patient may be coming for repeated anaesthesia within short time intervals.
  - Neuromuscular blocking drugs: avoid the use of suxamethonium after 72 hours because of the dangers of hyperkalaemic response. This response may persist until 6 months to 2 years post-burn. There is an increased requirement for non-depolarizing neuro-muscular blockers especially in burns > 30% BSA. These patients require larger doses and shorter dosing intervals.

— Ensure that the endotracheal tube is in place after any change of position.

— Provide adequate analgesia using intravenous fentanyl, morphine or pethidine. Dose requirements may be higher as a result of increased metabolism or tolerance.

— Close monitoring of haemodynamic status is required.

— Rapid infusion devices of large volumes of warmed fluids, blood or blood products may be needed.

— Replace blood loss early: this is often significant but may be difficult to estimate.

— There should be close communication between surgeon and anaesthesiologist; the surgeon should limit the extent of the surgery if the patient is haemodynamically unstable.

Postoperative Management

Attention should be paid to these aspects.

— Oxygen therapy.

— Analgesia.

— Temperature control: radiant heater, warm blankets to prevent shivering.

— Fluid and blood transfusion.
— Close monitoring of cardiovascular and respiratory systems.
— Repeat laboratory investigations if indicated.

Subsequent Anaesthesia

The patient may present a few months or years later for release of burn contractures. Anaesthetic management is usually straightforward unless the head and neck region is involved. Awake fibreoptic intubation may be necessary for release of burn contracture at the neck. Alternatively, laryngeal mask airway has been used for the initial stage of surgery, with subsequent conversion to endotracheal tube when the neck contracture is released.

FURTHER READING

1. MacLennan N, Heimbach DM, Cullen BF. Anesthesia for major thermal injury. Anesthesiology 1998;89:749–70.
2. Berger MM, Bernath MA, Chiolero RL. Resuscitation, anaesthesia and analgesia of the burned patient. Curr Opin Anaesthesiol 2001;14:431–5.
3. Yowler CJ. Recent advances in burn care. Curr Opin Anaesthesiol 2001;14:251–5.
4. Marko P, Layon AJ, Caruso L, Mozingo DW, Gabrielli A. Burn injuries. Curr Opin Anaesthesiol 2003;16:183–91.
5. Ernst A, Zibrak JD. Carbon monoxide poisoning, N Engl J Med 1998;339:1603–7.
6. Monafo WW. Initial management of burns. N Engl J Med 1996;335:1581–6.
7. Abdi S, Zhou Y. Management of pain after burn injury. Curr Opin Anaesthesiol 2002;15:563–7.

Chapter 28

Paediatric and Neonatal Anaesthesia

Felicia Lim and C.Y. Lee

INTRODUCTION

Patients managed under the category of paediatric anaesthesia range from premature neonates, full term neonates, infants, children to adolescents. The paediatric patient should not be regarded as a "little adult" because the physiological, pharmacological, behavioural and psychological responses are quite distinct from those of the adult, particularly in the first few years of life. The margin of error in managing such a young patient can be extremely small since the body reserves are limited and the organ systems are not fully developed.

APPLIED PHYSIOLOGY OF THE NEONATE

Airway Considerations

— Neonates and infants are obligate nose breathers. Their nasal passages are narrow. Anything that causes obstruction of the nasopharynx will greatly compromise ventilation.

— Infants have relatively large tongues which may obstruct the airway during mask ventilation and interfere with laryngoscopy and intubation.

— The glottis is located more anteriorly and higher than adults. It is at C3 level in the premature infant, at C4 level in children aged 1–4 years instead of C5–6 in adults.

— The large, floppy and U-shaped epiglottis can make visualization of the glottis during intubation difficult.

— The narrowest part of the airway is at the cricoid ring with an approximate area of 14 mm^2. A mere 1 mm thickness of oedema will reduce this area by 65%.

— The trachea is 6 mm in diameter, 4 cm in length. Do not pass the endotracheal tube more than 3 cm beyond the vocal cords since this increases the likelihood of endobronchial intubation.

— Extension of the head does not facilitate intubation; it may even obstruct the airway. External laryngeal pressure may facilitate intubation by bringing the anterior larynx into view.

— Some congenital abnormalities may be associated with difficult intubation, e.g., Pierre-Robin syndrome, Treacher-Collins syndrome, cystic hygroma, congenital subglottic stenosis.

Respiratory System

- Preterm babies and neonates have low amount of Type 1 respiratory muscle that are important for sustaining activity, and thus are more susceptible to fatigue.
- Respiration is diaphragmatic. The ribs are more horizontal and tend to lie in a position of inspiration (lack of bucket handle advantage). Respiration is easily hampered by intrathoracic or abdominal distension.
- Respiratory rate of a neonate is 35–40/min, 2–3 times that of an adult; oxygen consumption in the neonate (6.9 ml/kg/min) is also about twice that in adult (3.3 ml/kg/min).
- The closing volume is relatively large and encroaches on the normal tidal volume; this predisposes to airway closure and atelectasis. The apnoeic child can become cyanosed in a few seconds.
- The preterm baby is more prone to periodic breathing and apnoeic spells because the respiratory centre may be immature. Sensitivity to central depressant drugs is increased while response to hypercarbia is decreased.

Cardiovascular System

- The resting cardiac output is large and the circulation time is fast, reflecting on high oxygen consumption.
- Parasympathetic innervation of the heart is complete but sympathetic innervation is lacking, thus predisposing the neonates to bradycardia. This has a deleterious effect on the heart as cardiac output is dependent on the heart rate rather than the stroke volume.
- Heart rate in neonates is about 120–140/min and decreases with age, while blood pressure in neonates is about 60/35 mmHg and increases with age.
- The right ventricular wall is as thick as that of the left ventricle. There is relative right ventricular dominance as shown on ECG.
- The baroreceptor and chemoreceptor reflexes are less active. There is little effective vasoconstriction because of a small peripheral vascular bed.
- Circulatory adaptation at birth is dependent on establishment of respiration. Reversal to fetal shunting situation may occur in respiratory insufficiency, hypoxia, hypercarbia or acidosis, resulting in persistent fetal circulation.

Temperature Control

— Neonates and infants are more prone to hypothermia during anaesthesia because of:
  - Large body surface area/weight ratio (2–2.5 times greater than adults) resulting in greater heat loss by radiation, evaporation, convection and conduction.
  - Less insulating subcutaneous tissue.
  - Immature heat-regulating mechanism especially in the preterm baby.
  - Absence of shivering in neonates, with the mechanism of heat production limited to non-shivering thermogenesis through brown fat metabolism; this metabolism is inhibited under anaesthesia.
  - Exposure to cold ambient air, irrigating fluid, intravenous fluids and dry anaesthetic gases.

— Hypothermia is the principal cause of postoperative apnoea and circulatory failure.

— A hypothermic patient may become acidotic and apnoeic, may have delayed awakening from anaesthesia and a delayed recovery of neuromuscular function following neuromuscular blockade.

Other Considerations

1. Hepatorenal system
   — Immature liver and kidneys may result in impairment of drug metabolism and excretion.
   — Low glycogen stores increase risk of hypoglycaemia following prolonged fasting.

2. Haematology
   — The haematocrit is 60%, haemoglobin is 18–19 g/dl in neonates.
   — More than 70% of the haemoglobin consists of Haemoglobin F (HbF), which has a higher affinity for oxygen and results in less unloading (hence availability of oxygen) at tissue level.
   — Haematocrit decreases to about 30% in 3rd month of life before rising to 35% by 6 months.
   — Total blood volume varies with age: preterm babies 90–100 ml/kg, neonates 80–90 ml/kg, infants 70–80 ml/kg.

3. Fluid and electrolytes
   — The neonate is prone to dehydration; hence prolonged fasting should be avoided.
   — Intravenous fluid should be administered according to maintenance requirement (*vide infra*) if fasting is unavoidably prolonged.

PREOPERATIVE ASSESSMENT

A preoperative visit is important for the anaesthesiologist to get acquainted with the patient and his/her family. An established physician-patient relationship will go a long way towards reassuring the frightened child and anxious parents. It gives the opportunity for the anaesthesiologist to explain the planned anaesthetic procedure to the parents – the preoperative fasting, method of induction of anaesthesia and postoperative pain management.

Clinical Evaluation

This is similar to that of adults. In addition these features are of particular relevance.

— History
- Birth history for a child less than 6 months of age: gestational age, birth weight, maternal health during pregnancy, events during labour and delivery (including Apgar scores), neonatal hospitalization.
- Developmental milestones.
- Feeding pattern.
- Recent history of respiratory tract infection (RTI), croup or asthmatic episodes.

— Physical examination
- General appearance, height, weight and general build.
- Congenital anomalies.
- Evidence of RTI.
- Potential intubation problems.
- Potential sites for venepuncture (mark out the site for application of EMLA cream if intravenous induction is planned).

The Child with RTI (See Chapter 15)

This frequently-encountered problem often poses a management dilemma. Anaesthetic complications for such patients include laryngospasm, bronchospasm, stridor, breath-holding or obstruction of airway by secretion. The incidence of perioperative respiratory complications is 2–7 times greater in the presence of RTI, and 11 times more if the trachea had been intubated.

Recommendations for anaesthesia depend on the patient's condition and the nature of surgery.

— Mild infection
  - On examination: no fever, small amounts of clear nasal discharge, mild cough, active child.
  - Can be anaesthetized for minor surgical procedure without intubation.

— Active infection
  - On examination: fever, recent onset of purulent nasal discharge, cough, ill-looking child.
  - May represent a prodrome of a more serious or infectious illness such as chickenpox, measles.
  - Surgery should be deferred for at least 2 weeks.

— Emergency surgery
  - Minimal interference technique: no airway manipulation, use face mask or laryngeal mask airway if appropriate.
  - Maximal support technique when intubation is required: preoperative nebulizer, controlled ventilation, oropharyngeal and tracheal suction if indicated, post-operative oxygen therapy.

Laboratory Investigations

These are tailored to the physical condition of the child and the nature of the surgery. The value of routine tests is questionable when the surgical procedures are minor and do not involve significant blood loss.

Preoperative Fasting (See Chapter 3)

It is now established that drinking clear fluid up to 2 hours before surgery does not increase the residual gastric volume. More liberal use of clear fluid in the immediate preoperative period may decrease the incidence of preoperative dehydration and possible hypotension during induction of anaesthesia, prevent hypoglycaemia and result in a less agitated child with happier parents.

Fasting guidelines for children (hours of fasting)

— Clear fluid: 2 hours
— Breast milk: 3–4 hours
— Infant formula/cow's milk: 4–6 hours
— Solid: 6–8 hours

Premedication (See Chapter 3)

Premedicant drugs are prescribed with the objectives of relieving the patient's anxiety and providing tranquility before surgery. The appropriate premedication is selected on the basis of the child's age, weight, emotional maturity, personality, anxiety level, degree of co-operation, physiological and psychological status. The ideal premedication for infants and children should be safe and easy to administer in a formulation that is acceptable to children (no intramuscular injection). It should have minimal side-effects and should be efficacious to achieve short-term sedation to facilitate a smooth separation from parents and a smooth anaesthetic induction.

These drugs are commonly used for premedication.

— Midazolam: 0.5–0.7 mg/kg
— Diazepam: 0.2 mg/kg
— Trimeperazine: 3 mg/kg

ANAESTHETIC EQUIPMENT

Check that the anaesthetic equipment is available and in good working condition before commencement of anaesthesia.

Airway Equipment

— Face masks of different sizes: either Randell-Baker-Soucek masks which have minimal dead space or clear plastic masks with inflated cushioned rims. Some are impregnated with scent to increase patient acceptance of the mask.

— Oropharyngeal airways: the appropriate length is equal to the distance from the corner of the mouth to the angle of the jaw.

— Laryngoscopes: a straight blade is suitable for use in neonates and infants (to lift up the epiglottis) and a curved blade for older children.

— Approximate sizes of endotracheal tubes according to age, expressed according to internal diameters in millimetres.
  - Premature: 2.5–3
  - Neonates: 3–3.5
  - 6 months: 3.5–4
  - 1–2 years: 4–4.5
  - > 2 years: $\frac{\text{age (yr)}}{4} + 4$

— Always prepare endotracheal tubes one size larger and one size smaller. Ideal size will allow a small air leak at 20 cmH_2O peak inflation pressure. Uncuffed tubes should be used for children below 8 years old.

— Stylets for endotracheal tubes should be available in appropriate lengths and sizes.

— Paediatric sized Yaunkeur suction tip as well as soft suction catheters of various sizes should also be available.

— Appropriate sizes of laryngeal mask airway according to body weight.
  - Neonates and infants up to 5 kg: 1
  - Infants 5–10 kg: 1.5
  - 10 to 20 kg: 2
  - 20 to 30 kg: 2.5
  - > 30 kg: 3

Breathing System and Ventilator

— Jackson Rees' modification of Ayres' T-piece can be used for children up to 20 kg. Include a humidifier circuit especially for long cases and small babies. Scavenging used to be a problem but newer versions of the T-piece incorporate a closed bag with an expiratory valve and scavenging attachment.

— Adult breathing system is usually recommended for older children > 20 kg. However, the circle system using 15 mm flexible lightweight plastic tubes can be used for infants and small children > 5 kg. A smaller reservoir bag of 800–1,000 ml capacity is used.

— Ventilator for smaller children < 20 kg should be able to deliver small tidal volumes, high respiratory rates, variable inspiratory flow rates and different I:E ratios. Pressure-controlled ventilation is commonly used in paediatric patients.

Monitoring Devices

These should include accessories which are suitable for use in babies and small children.

— Appropriate-sized blood pressure cuff.

— Small ECG electrodes.

— Appropriate-sized pulse oximetry probes.

— Paediatric-sized temperature probes.

— Paediatric-sized central venous catheter for CVP monitoring.

Temperature Control (See Chapter 6)

These measures are taken to reduce intraoperative heat loss.

— Increase OT temperature to 24°C for neonates and small infants and 22°C for older children.

— Use warming mattress on OT table and paediatric-sized forced-air warming device on the patient.

— Place small babies inside incubators during transport and at PACU.

— Use overhead radiant heater during anaesthetic induction and emergence.

— Avoid unnecessary exposure by covering unoperated parts and wrapping extremities with cotton wool.

— Cover the head with a cap since this constitutes a large proportion of body surface area.

— Use humidifier or heat and moisture exchanger (HME) to warm and humidify anaesthetic gases.

— Prewarm intravenous fluids, blood and blood products.

— Use warmed packs and irrigation fluids during surgery.

ANAESTHETIC MANAGEMENT

Preparation

Check all anaesthetic equipment and ensure that the appropriate-sized equipment is available. Prepare anaesthetic drugs. Dilute the drugs or draw up in 1 ml "insulin syringe" if available. Clearly label the name of drug and its dilution on the syringe. It is mandatory to have atropine diluted and drawn up in a syringe for immediate treatment of bradyarrhythmias.

Induction of Anaesthesia

This should allow a smooth transition from the awake to the unconscious state with minimal physiological and psychological disturbance. Induction may be an extremely stressful and critical period for the anaesthesiologist as problems such as laryngospasm and bradycardia can occur.

Prior to induction, confirmation should be made on the patient's identification, fasting period and consent for the procedure. The patient's weight is important as drugs are calculated based on body weight. A useful formula to estimate the patient's weight in kilogram is [2 × age (years) + 8].

Where possible, apply monitoring equipment before induction of anaesthesia without unduly upsetting the child. Pulse oximetry is the absolute minimum, but for a sick child additional monitoring should be applied prior to induction.

Parental presence at induction is desirable to allay the child's anxiety and enhance co-operation with the anaesthesiologist. Parents must be counselled beforehand about what to expect during induction and how they can be of help. It would be advisable for parents who are extremely anxious or distressed not to be with the child during induction.

Inhalational induction is used in most infants less than 6 months of age, when the child is already asleep after premedication, and when intravenous access is not available. Both halothane and sevoflurane are suitable for inhalational induction as both agents are non-pungent and are well tolerated by the patient. Sevoflurane is the preferred agent because it has a rapid onset and offset of action with less cardiovascular depression than halothane. Enflurane and isoflurane are less suitable as they tend to produce airway irritation because of their pungency.

Intravenous induction is suitable in older children where insertion of intravenous cannula may be facilitated with the use of EMLA cream, those with preexisting intravenous access, and patients with full stomach as part of a rapid sequence induction technique. Thiopentone is the most commonly used intravenous induction agent. The recommended induction dose for healthy unpremedicated children is 5–6 mg/kg; this should be reduced in neonates and severely ill patients. Propofol can also be used for children at a higher induction dose (3–4 mg/kg) than adults. Pain during injection can be minimized by mixing with 1% lignocaine (1 ml/10 ml).

Intubation may be carried out after administration of a neuromuscular blocking drug or under deep inhalational anaesthesia. Awake intubation is not recommended because of the risk of intraventricular haemorrhage. If suxamethonium is used to aid intubation, atropine should be administered to prevent bradycardia especially in neonates and infants.

In neonates and infants, the occiput is large and tends to result in overflexion of the neck. Optimal position for intubation is achieved without a pillow under the head and with the shoulder elevated by using a rolled towel. The same intubating position for adult patients, namely flexion at the neck and extension at the atlanto-occipital joint, can be adopted for older children.

The endotracheal tube (ETT) should not be forced into the trachea if resistance is encountered during intubation. Another tube one size smaller should be used. ETT with the correct size should allow a small air leak during inspiration. Fasten the ETT securely after checking for correct placement. Insert a moist pharyngeal pack but remember to remove this at the end of the surgery.

Maintenance of Anaesthesia

Neonates and infants less than 6 months are poor candidates for anaesthesia with spontaneous ventilation because of poor respiratory mechanics. They are usually intubated and their ventilation controlled or assisted with IPPV.

The anaesthetic gas mixture depends on the condition of the patient and the nature of surgery.

- 100% oxygen if the baby is ill or hypoxic.
- Oxygen-air mixture in conditions where the use of nitrous oxide is undesirable, e.g., diaphragmatic hernia, gastroschisis or omphalocele, tracheo-oesophageal fistula, intestinal obstruction.
- Oxygen-nitrous oxide mixture if there is no contraindication to the use of nitrous oxide.

The anaesthetic gas mixture is supplemented with volatile anaesthetic and opioid.

Remember that both hypoxia and hyperoxia are harmful especially in the preterm baby.

Intraoperative Analgesia

Where appropriate, various modes of analgesia should be employed intraoperatively to enhance their synergistic effects with one another. Examples of analgesic modalities include:

— Intravenous opioid, typically fentanyl at induction.

— Rectal suppositories of paracetamol or diclofenac.

— Regional anaesthesia by means of caudal, epidural, nerve blocks or subcutaneous infiltration of incision site.

For major surgery, means of extending intraoperative analgesia to the postoperative period should be provided and the patient managed by the Acute Pain Service (APS) team.

Fluid Management (See Chapter 4)

There are three aspects to consider: preoperative deficit, maintenance requirement and on-going losses.

Fluid requirements for neonates:

— Day 1 of life: 60 ml/kg/day

— Day 2 of life: 90 ml/kg/day

— Day 3 of life: 120 ml/kg/day

— Day 4 and thereafter: 150 ml/kg/day

Rule of thumb for older children, based on fluid requirement of approximately 100 ml/kg/day:

— < 10 kg: 4 ml/kg/hr

— 10–20 kg: 40 ml/hr + 2 ml/kg/hr for each kilogram above 10 kg

— > 20 kg: 60 ml/hr + 1 ml/kg/hr for each kilogram above 20 kg

Calculate for:

— *Maintenance requirement* as shown above.

— *Deficit*, equal to the hourly requirement multiplied by the number of hours of fasting; replace ½ deficit in the first hour, ¼ deficit in the second hour and ¼ deficit in the third hour.
— *On-going losses*, consisting mainly of blood loss and evaporative losses.
  - Blood loss from the surgical field may be difficult to estimate, particularly in small children or when irrigation fluids are used intraoperatively.
  - Evaporative losses from the exposed surgical field may need to be replaced according to the extent of exposure.

Remember that these are only guidelines to aid in calculating the amount of intravenous fluids required. The child's clinical parameters should be closely monitored to see if the fluid therapy is appropriate.

Various types of intravenous fluids can be used for maintenance and replacement. Maintenance fluids consist of 10% dextrose on the first day of life, and 0.18% saline in 10% dextrose from second day onwards. Replacement fluids include Ringer's lactate, normal saline and colloids solution such as Gelafundin®. Blood and blood products should be transfused when indicated.

Blood Transfusion

Blood volume is approximately 90–100 ml/kg in a preterm baby, 80–90 ml/kg in a neonate and 70–80 ml/kg in an infant. Blood transfusion is imperative when the estimated blood loss is more than 15% of the total blood volume.

Decision to transfuse also depends on:

— Clinical signs: heart rate, blood pressure, pallor, CVP if present.
— Preoperative haemoglobin and general status of the patient.
— Nature of surgery.
— Amount and speed of blood loss.
— Likelihood of further losses.

POSTOPERATIVE MANAGEMENT

At the end of surgical procedure, it is essential to keep the patient warm by using an overhead radiant heater or a forced-air warming device. Neuromuscular blockade should be reversed only when the patient is not hypothermic and has shown signs of return of neuromuscular function. Remove the pharyngeal pack (if inserted) and suction the pharynx before extubation. Facilities for re-intubation should be available.

Extubation can be performed either awake or deep.

— In awake extubation, the child is fully awake, moving all limbs, able to open eyes and has adequate respiration. The ETT is withdrawn as the reservoir bag is squeezed so that the patient coughs the moment the tube leaves the trachea.

— In deep extubation, volatile anaesthetic is continued in 100% oxygen and following pharyngeal suction, extubation is done with the child in the lateral position. Deep extubation is carried out in order to minimize coughing on the ETT which is undesirable after certain surgical procedures (e.g., neurosurgery and ophthalmic surgery), or to avoid bronchospasm (e.g., in asthmatic patients). Complications of this technique include airway obstruction, laryngospasm and aspiration.

Observe the child in the PACU. Usual discharge criteria apply.

ICU management and/or ventilation would be indicated in:

— Ill, small, premature babies.

— Specific conditions such as tracheo-oesophageal fistula, diaphragmatic hernia, gastroschisis.

— Respiratory problems such as aspiration, infection.

— Intraoperative complications such as cardiovascular instability, massive blood loss, hypoxaemia.

— Protracted major surgery.

PAEDIATRIC ACUTE PAIN MANAGEMENT

General Principles

— Analgesic dose for the paediatric patient should be calculated on a mg/kg basis.

— Children *do not* like intramuscular injections, which are also unpredictable and largely ineffective in terms of absorption and drug action.

— Pain is best prevented rather than treated. Analgesic requirement is lower if children are allowed to emerge from anaesthesia comfortable and pain-free, or are pretreated before painful procedures.

— Severe pain is best treated with continuous methods of analgesic administration in the form of intravenous or epidural infusion, or patient-controlled analgesia (PCA) where appropriate.

— Neonates and some ex-premature infants may be sensitive to opioids. If opioid analgesic is required, these patients should be closely monitored in HDU or ICU.

— Postoperative pain management should be planned before the surgery. Suitable patients should be identified and some techniques (e.g., PCA) should be explained to the patient and parents during the preoperative visit.

— Assessment of pain and adequacy of therapy in infants and small children may be difficult.

Common Methods of Analgesia

1. **Paracetamol**
   - A simple analgesic and antipyretic drug which is useful for all types of mild pain.
   - Dosage: 15–20 mg/kg 4-hourly (oral), 20–30 mg/kg 6-hourly (rectal); do not exceed 80 mg/kg or 4 g/24 hr.

2. **Diclofenac sodium**
   - A non-steroidal antiinflammatory drug effective for moderate to severe pain.
   - Dosage: 0.5–1 mg/kg 8-hourly oral or rectal.

3. **Intravenous opioid infusion**
   - Parenteral morphine or pethidine is used to treat moderate to severe pain following major surgery.
   - This method is contraindicated in patients with history of apnoea, airway obstruction or intracranial hypertension.

   Preparation of solution for infusion
   - 0.5 mg/kg of morphine or 5 mg/kg of pethidine, make up to 50 ml with normal saline.
   - 1 ml of solution contains 10 μg/kg of morphine or 100 μg/kg of pethidine respectively.

Prior to commencement of the infusion, the patient should be made comfortable with intravenous bolus doses (2–3 ml) of the same opioid. Infusion rate depends on the age of the patient:

— Neonates: 0.5–0.7 ml/hr, maximum rate 1 ml/hr
— Infants 1–3 months: 1 ml/hr, maximum rate 2 ml/hr
— Infants > 3 months and older children: 1–2 ml/hr, maximum rate 4 ml/hr

Adjust infusion rate according to the degree of analgesia and sedation of the patient.

Bolus doses

— In order to reduce "incident pain" such as chest or abdominal drain removal, physiotherapy and wound dressing, a bolus dose should be given 10–15 minutes prior to the anticipated painful procedure.
— If pain relief is inadequate, a bolus dose should be administered and titrated until the patient is comfortable. This is followed by increasing the infusion rate by 0.5–1 ml/hr.

4. **Patient-controlled analgesia (PCA)**

— This technique is useful in older children who can be instructed to "press a button when it hurts".
— Ensure that the patient is relatively pain-free before commencement of PCA; administer bolus doses of analgesic if necessary.

Preparation of solution for infusion

— 0.5 mg/kg of morphine made up to 50 ml with normal saline.
— 1 ml of the solution contains 10 μg/kg of morphine.

PCA settings

— Bolus dose: 10 μg/kg (1 ml)
— Lockout interval: 5 minutes
— Background infusion: 10 μg/kg/hr (1 ml/hr)

5. **Regional analgesia**

Analgesia involving the use of local anaesthetics includes these.

— Local wound infiltration: maximum dose of 0.25% bupivacaine is 1 ml/kg.
— Nerve block: ilioinguinal block for herniotomy, penile block for circumcision.
— Epidural analgesia: caudal, lumbar or thoracic epidural.

Epidural analgesia is contraindicated in these situations.

- — Head injury or increased intracranial pressure
- — Coagulopathy.
- — Local or systemic infection.
- — Progressive neurological deficit.

Preparation of solution for continuous epidural analgesia

- — **Neonates**: bupivacaine 0.1%
  Dilute 10 ml of 0.5% bupivacaine in normal saline to make up to 50 ml.
- — **Infants**: bupivacaine 0.1% + fentanyl 1 µg/ml
  Dilute 10 ml of 0.5% bupivacaine and 50 µg fentanyl in normal saline to make up to 50 ml.
- — **Children > 1 year old**: bupivacaine 0.1% + fentanyl 2 µg/ml
  Dilute 10 ml of 0.5% bupivacaine and 100 µg of fentanyl in normal saline to make up to 50 ml.

Ensure that the patient is comfortable before starting the epidural infusion, administer a bolus dose of 0.5 ml/kg of the solution if necessary. Epidural infusion can then be started at a rate of 0.2 ml/kg/hr. If analgesia is inadequate, a bolus dose of 0.5 ml/kg should be given, followed by increasing the rate of infusion by 0.05–0.1 ml/kg/hr. Do not exceed an infusion rate of 0.4 ml/kg/hr.

Objective Pain Score

This scoring system, shown in Table 28–1, is used to assess adequacy of pain relief in babies and small children who cannot vocalize their pain. In older children, pain score similar to that utilized in adult APS can be used. Pan relief in a patient with a total score of 3 is considered to be inadequate, and measures should be taken to provide analgesia in the appropriate manner.

Table 28–1. Objective pain score

Observation	Criteria	Score
Blood pressure change	< 10% from preoperative reading 10–20% from preoperative reading 20–30% from preoperative reading	0 1 2
Crying	Not crying Crying but responds to TLC * Crying, not responding to TLC *	0 1 2
Moving	None Restless Thrashing	0 1 2
Agitation	Asleep or calm Mild Hysterical	0 1 2
Posture	No special posture Splinting, rigid, flexed Splinting and holding incision	0 1 2
Verbal evaluation or body language	Asleep or states no pain Mild pain (cannot localize) Moderate pain (can localize verbally or pointing)	0 1 2

* TLC = tender loving care.

ANAESTHESIA FOR THE "EX-PREMIE"

The term""ex-premie" refers to a former preterm infant. Besides having the problems of paediatric anaesthesia discussed above, such infants are also at risk of developing apnoea postoperatively.

Post-conceptual age refers to the infant's age calculated from the time of conception. For example, a 2-month-old infant born at 34 weeks of pregnancy has a post-conceptual age of (2 x 4) + 34 = 42 weeks. This is important since it correlates with the incidence of postoperative apnoea: approximately 26% of infants less than 44 weeks post-conceptual age develop postoperative apnoea.

Preoperative Assessment

The anaesthesiologist should pay particular attention to these factors.

- Post-conceptual age.
- Prenatal history, in particular history of ventilation or development of idiopathic respiratory distress syndrome (IRDS, also known as hyaline membrane disease).
- Presence of serious co-existing disease such as bronchopulmonary dysplasia, neurological disease, other systemic diseases.
- Weight gain, nutrition, developmental milestones.
- History of preoperative apnoea.
- Congenital anomalies, particularly those involving the airway and cardiovascular system.
- Oxygen dependence: whether the patient is ventilator dependent or requires supplemental oxygen to maintain adequate oxygen saturation.

Anaesthetic Management

- Where appropriate, the anaesthetic technique of choice is general anaesthesia supplemented by nerve blocks using local anaesthetics. This reduces the use of sedative medications for postoperative pain relief which may increase the risk of postoperative apnoea.
- Spinal anaesthesia without supplemental intravenous or inhalational sedation is thought to eliminate the possibility of inducing apnoea or bradycardia. However, there have been case reports of "ex-premies" who developed episodes of apnoea and bradycardia which persisted until the spinal anaesthesia had dissipated. Hence the use of spinal anaesthesia does *not* obviate the need for postoperative respiratory monitoring.

Postoperative Management

- The patient should be admitted to ICU or HDU for close observation.
- Respiratory monitoring consists of clinical parameters (the respiratory rate in particular), pulse oximetry and apnoea alarm.

Recommendations

- Delay elective surgery until the infant is at least 52 weeks postconception.
- Healthy infants older than 60 weeks postconception can be anaesthetized for minor surgical procedures on a day-care basis, but should be monitored for at least 2 hours postoperatively. These are infants with no past history of apnoea, bronchopulmonary dysplasia or ventilation during the neonatal period.
- Infants between 44–60 weeks postconception should be monitored for at least 12 hours postoperatively especially if the postnatal period has been stormy.
- Infants less than 44 weeks postconception should be monitored for at least 24 hours postoperatively.
- Apnoea monitoring should be continued until the infant is apnoea-free for ≥12 hours.
- *It is better to err on the side of caution!*

SPECIFIC CONDITIONS

Surgical procedures for neonates are usually urgent in nature. Examples of such surgical conditions include tracheo-oesophageal fistula (TOF), congenital diaphragmatic hernia, omphalocele/gastroschisis and necrotizing enterocolitis (NEC). However, except for rare situations of dire emergencies, there is usually time for quick preoperative assessment, resuscitation and stabilization before surgery.

Preoperative preparation includes these measures.

- Preoperative assessment and/or resuscitation.
- Review of investigation results: FBC, blood glucose concentration, urea and electrolyte concentrations, coagulation screen, CXR or abdominal X-ray if indicated.
- Arrangement for GXM blood and plasma if indicated.
- Explanation to the parents on the planned anaesthetic procedure: inform them about anaesthetic risks if the baby is ill or when significant anaesthetic risk is involved.
- Arrangement for ICU bed if postoperative ICU management is needed.

Premedication is usually omitted. The baby should be transported to the OT in an incubator.

These conditions are described.

- Congenital diaphragmatic hernia
- Tracheo-oesophageal fistula
- Omphalocele/gastroschisis
- Congenital pyloric stenosis

Congenital Diaphragmatic Hernia

The incidence of congenital diaphragmatic hernia is estimated at 1:4,000. Majority of the cases (85%) herniate through the foramen of Bochdalek (left-sided). The condition may be associated with congenital heart disease, hypoplastic lung and/or gut malrotation.

Presentation and diagnosis

- Cyanosis, respiratory distress.
- Scaphoid abdomen with barrelling of the chest.
- Apparent dextrocardia (if herniation is left-sided) with cardio-respiratory failure.
- Diminished or absent breath sounds with hyperresonance on the affected side.
- Increasing respiratory distress due to gaseous distension of the gut leading to further mediastinal shift or pulmonary aspiration.
- Radiological confirmation with evidence of abdominal contents in the thorax.

The earlier the signs become obvious, the poorer the prognosis will be.

Initial resuscitation

- The baby needs to be stabilized first before surgery: medical stabilization with delayed repair may improve survival.
- Insert a nasogastric tube to decompress the stomach and prevent further gastric distension.
- If the baby presents with respiratory distress and hypoxia, intubation and ventilation should be instituted immediately. Avoid intermittent positive pressure ventilation (IPPV) by face mask as this inflates the stomach and intestines further, increasing mediastinal displacement. Ventilate with high respiratory rate and low airway pressure to avoid barotrauma.

— Correct hypothermia, acidosis, hypoglycaemia if present.

— Arterial desaturation as a result of right to left shunt (fetal circulation) may occur. Hyperventilation, tolazoline, nitric oxide and extracorporeal membrane oxygenation (ECMO) may be used to improve the status of the baby before surgical repair.

Anaesthetic management

— During the surgery, the hernia is reduced through an abdominal incision and the defect is repaired either by primary closure or by using a patch.

— Monitoring includes ECG, intraarterial BP, pulse oximetry, capnography and temperature. ABG should be checked intermittently and any abnormalities corrected.

— Nitrous oxide should be avoided to prevent further gut distension. Use oxygen-air mixture or 100% oxygen with volatile anaesthetic depending on the pulmonary status and oxygen saturation.

— There may be problems with ventilation or oxygenation because of reduced lung compliance or hypoplastic lung on the affected side.

— Manually ventilate to ensure that inflating pressures are kept below 25–30 cmH_2O. Suspect pneumothorax on the contralateral side if there is a sudden deterioration in the patient's condition.

— No attempt should be made to expand the ipsilateral lung at the end of surgery as this will invariably cause a pneumothorax to the hypoplastic lung.

— Abdominal closure may be difficult with the increase in abdominal contents especially if there is gas in the gut. Provide adequate muscle relaxation to facilitate surgery.

— After the abdominal contents have been reduced, check for diaphragmatic splinting or inferior vena cava (IVC) compression manifested as increased airway pressure and lower limb venous congestion respectively.

Postoperative care

— Unless the hernia is exceptionally small, most babies are left intubated and transferred to ICU for further management.

— Ventilate with peak inspiratory pressure < 30 cmH_2O and high frequency to produce $PaCO_2$ 35–40 mmHg, and adjust FiO_2 to produce SaO_2 95% or PaO_2 70–80 mmHg. Avoid hypoxaemia, maintain normocarbia and aggressively correct acidosis if it occurs.

- Commence opioid infusion for analgesia and sedation. In selected cases maintenance of neuromuscular blockade may be required to improve respiratory mechanics.
- There may be an initial "honeymoon period" of good oxygenation after surgery, followed by deterioration due to increasing right to left shunt with pulmonary hypertension.
- Watch for possible complications such as pulmonary hypertension, pneumothorax, persistent hypoxaemia. Treatment options available for persistent pulmonary hypertension include pulmonary vasodilators (e.g., tolazoline, low-dose dobutamine) which reduce both systemic and pulmonary pressures, inhaled nitric oxide and ECMO.

Tracheo-Oesophageal Fistula (TOF)

Tracheo-oesophageal fistula is a congenital malformation of the distal trachea and oesophagus. It occurs in 1 in 3,000 live births, and in 30–40% cases there are associated congenital abnormalities, such as

- Congenital heart defects: VSD, ASD, Tetralogy of Fallot ("double TOF"), patent ductus arteriosus, coarctation of aorta.
- Skeletal defects: hemivertebrae, absent radius.
- Gastrointestinal abnormalities: atresia, imperforate anus.
- Renal anomalies.
- Vater syndrome: vertebral (or VSD), anal, tracheal, oesophageal, renal (radial) anomalies.
- Tracheomalacia.

Six different types of oesophageal atresia with or without fistula have been described. The commonest anomaly (85%) has a blind upper oesophageal pouch and a fistula from near the carina to the lower oesophagus.

Clinical features

- History of polyhydramnios during pregnancy.
- Failure to pass a nasogastric tube into the stomach (X-ray taken with the nasogastric tube *in situ* will show it coils up in the upper pouch).
- Excessive pharyngeal secretion.

— Choking, coughing and/or cyanosis during first feeding (3Cs of oesophageal atresia).
— A plain X-ray of the chest and abdomen will demonstrate air in the stomach if there is a fistula between the tracheobronchial tree and lower oesophagus.

Preoperative management

— Initial management aims to prevent further aspiration, treat any pneumonia present, diagnose co-existing abnormalities and optimize the general condition of the baby.
— Stabilize the baby in terms of hydration, acid-base and electrolyte status, glucose, and temperature.
— Treat aspiration pneumonia, if present, with antibiotics and physiotherapy.
— Nurse the baby in the semi-upright position.
— Insert Replogle tube (a double lumen sump tube) to the upper pouch. This is to prevent dilatation of the oesophageal pouch and spill-over of secretions to the lungs. Continuous low pressure is applied to one lumen, and the second lumen entrains air thus preventing the tube from becoming stuck to the wall of the pouch.

Surgical procedure

— While surgical repair of a TOF is not done emergently as a life-saving procedure, it is best performed as soon as the general condition of the baby permits in order to minimize further pulmonary aspiration.
— The repair is done via an extrapleural approach with the baby in the left lateral decubitus position.
— The surgical procedure depends on the distance between upper and lower portions of the oesophagus. Options include primary anastomosis and closure, or a feeding gastrostomy and cervical oesophagostomy until definitive surgery is done later.

Anaesthetic management

— Suction the Replogle tube before induction of anaesthesia.
— Options for induction and intubation.
  - Inhalational induction using oxygen with sevoflurane or halothane, intubation under deep anaesthesia.
  - Intravenous or inhalational induction, with intubation facilitated by using a neuromuscular blocking drug.

Awake intubation is not recommended as intubation in a struggling child poses more risks.

Whichever method is used, atropine should be given before intubation to avoid bradycardia. Ventilation should be gently assisted to avoid high peak inspiratory airway pressure.

— Proper placement of ETT in relation to the fistula is very important. The tip of the ETT should be beyond the fistula and above the carina to ensure adequate ventilation and oxygenation. If the placement is suboptimal, ventilation will preferentially go to the stomach with subsequent hypoventilation and hypoxaemia.
— The fistula is usually situated at the posterior wall of the trachea just proximal to the carina. To ensure that the tip is beyond the fistula, advance the ETT past the carina to a main bronchus and then withdraw until there are bilateral breath sounds and equal chest expansion.
— In most cases, the lungs can be adequately inflated without gastric distension. It is extremely rare to intubate the fistula although this has been described. If a significant amount of gas is passing through the fistula, reposition the ETT by turning it so that the bevel of the tube faces anteriorly and the longer edge of the bevel occludes the fistula. A normal capnography tracing, good bilateral breath sounds, absence of breath sounds over abdomen are usual signs for normal ETT placement.
— The left lung should be adequately ventilated because the right lung will be partially collapsed during the right thoracotomy.
— Position for surgery: left lateral position with right arm abducted and strapped above the head. Recheck position of the endotracheal tube after positioning.
— Spontaneous versus controlled ventilation
  - It used to be taught that ventilation should be spontaneous until the surgeon has clamped and ligated the fistula in order to minimize gas flow through the fistula.
  - However, it is difficult for a neonate to maintain spontaneous ventilation in a lateral position for thoracotomy without significant hypoventilation, hypoxaemia and hypotension.
  - Gentle assisted or controlled ventilation with high rates and low peak pressure is now the preferred technique.
— Surgical retraction during thoracotomy may compress the lung and trachea, causing an increase in the airway pressure and making ventilation more difficult.

— Manually ventilate the lungs to detect and compensate for changes due to compression. It may be necessary for the surgeon to pause and allow temporary reinflation of the lungs to improve ventilation and oxygenation. Constant communication with the surgeon is crucial for maintaining adequate ventilation.

— Maintain anaesthesia with 100% oxygen or oxygen-air mixture, sevoflurane and neuromuscular blocking drug. Avoid nitrous oxide since this may increase gastric distension and cause diaphragmatic splinting. Do not increase the inspired oxygen fraction above that necessary to prevent hypoxaemia especially in preterm babies at risk of retinopathy of prematurity.

— Analgesia can be provided by fentanyl 1–2 μg/kg; more generous doses can be given if postoperative ventilation is planned. An epidural catheter threaded up to the thoracic region from a lumbar or caudal approach can be used to provide intra- and postoperative analgesia.

Postoperative care

— Postoperative ICU management is essential.

— Babies with no aspiration pneumonia who are awake, moving vigorously with no residual effects of neuromuscular blockade are safe to be extubated.

— Babies with aspiration pneumonia, low birth weight, symptomatic heart disease or tight oesophageal anastomosis will benefit from a period of postoperative ventilation.

— Postoperative complications include leakage from anastomotic site, pneumothorax, pneumonia and tracheomalacia at the site of fistula. Prolonged ventilatory support may be needed in these patients.

Omphalocele/Gastroschisis

Omphalocele (or *exomphalos*) refers to protrusion of abdominal contents in a thin walled sac composed of amnion and peritoneum. *Gastroschisis* refers to protrusion of abdominal contents through a defect close to the base of umbilicus; no sac is present to cover the abdominal contents, hence the contents may be thickened, matted together or oedematous.

Preoperative management

— The baby should be nursed in the incubator to prevent hypothermia.

- The protruded abdominal contents should be covered with sterile dressing to reduce heat and fluid loss due to evaporation and to reduce risk of infection.
- Correct fluid, acid base, electrolyte and glucose abnormalities.

Anaesthetic management

- Prepare drugs and equipment as outlined.
- Suction the nasogastric tube before induction of anaesthesia.
- Anaesthesia with intubation and neuromuscular blockade is required.
- Closely monitor the blood and fluid losses. Blood and/or plasma transfusion may be indicated.
- Surgical options depend on the amount and size of extruded abdominal contents. Primary closure is done if the defect is small. Otherwise the defect is covered with a silastic pouch and secondary closure is performed at a later date.
- The abdominal contents cause an increase in intraabdominal pressure which may cause problems if excessive. The anaesthesiologist should recognize these problems, alert the surgeon and take steps to correct them as soon as possible. Problems include:
    - Diaphragmatic splinting with ventilation difficulties.
    - IVC compression resulting in a decrease in venous return, bradycardia and hypotension.
    - Compression of lower limb vessels, with congestion and mottling to lower limbs.
    - Compression of renal vessels, with reduction in urine output.

Postoperative care

- Most babies require elective ventilation unless the defect is very small and primary closure is achieved with no difficulty.
- For babies with silastic pouch and planned delayed closure, ventilation with sedation, analgesia and muscle relaxation is required.

Congenital Pyloric Stenosis

The incidence of congenital pyloric stenosis is estimated at 1:300–400 live births, of whom 85% affected infants are male and 40–60% of them are firstborns. There is a gross thickening of the circular muscle of the pylorus which causes an increasing degree of gastric outlet obstruction leading to persistent vomiting. Dehydration and metabolic derangement may develop.

Clinical features

- Projectile vomiting of bile-free vomitus.
- Visible peristalsis in the left upper quadrant from left to right especially after feeds (not a reliable sign).
- A mass just to the right of umbilicus may be palpable.
- Dehydration: may range from mild dehydration to severe hypovolaemia.
- Metabolic alkalosis with hyponatraemia, hypochloraemia, hypokalaemia and paradoxical aciduria.

Preoperative management

- Note that congenital pyloric stenosis is not a surgical emergency. Dehydration and metabolic derangements should be corrected before surgery.
- Keep the baby nil orally and insert nasogastric tube to empty the gastric contents.
- Correct fluid and electrolyte imbalance in this manner.
  - Mild to moderate dehydration (fluid loss 5–10% of body weight): replace deficit over 24 hours (half the deficit over the first 8 hours, ¼ deficit over the next 8 hours and the remaining ¼ the following 8 hours).
  - Severe dehydration (fluid loss > 15% of body weight): the patient is in impending shock. Resuscitate with rapid infusion of 10–20 ml/kg of normal saline or Ringer's lactate. Once circulation is restored and urine output established, replace remaining deficit over 24–48 hours.
  - Use normal saline or Ringer's lactate for replacement and correction of electrolyte abnormality. Add potassium supplement, if indicated, when urine output is established.
  - Maintenance fluid of 0.18% saline in 5% dextrose should also be given.
- Surgery is delayed until the infant's clinical condition improves.
- Biochemical values to aim for: arterial pH < 7.5, serum sodium concentration > 132 mmol/L, serum chloride concentration > 90 mmol/L, serum potassium concentration > 3.2 mmol/L, and standard bicarbonate < 30 mmol/L.

Anaesthetic management

- Take precaution to prevent gastric aspiration during induction of and emergence from anaesthesia.
  - Apply suction to the nasogastric tube.
  - Preoxygenation followed by rapid sequence induction with thiopentone, cricoid pressure, suxamethonium and endotracheal intubation.
  - Remove the endotracheal tube when the patient is awake at the end of the surgery.
- Maintain anaesthesia with nitrous oxide-oxygen, isoflurane or sevoflurane and muscle relaxation using non-depolarizing neuromuscular blocking drug.
- The surgical procedure involves delivering the pylorus and splitting the pylorus muscle longitudinally down to the mucosa. It is important to ensure adequate pain relief and depth of anaesthesia so that the child does not cough or strain at the time of muscle splitting to avoid cutting the mucosal layer, as postoperative morbidity is increased if this is incised.
- Postoperative pain relief can be provided by subcutaneous wound infiltration with local anaesthetic and oral or rectal paracetamol.

FURTHER READING

1. Leelanukrom R, Cunliffe M. Intraoperative fluid and glucose management in children. Paed Anaesth 2000;10:353–9.
2. Anderson BJ, Meakin GH. Scaling for size: Some implications for paediatric anaesthesia dosing. Paed Anaesth 2002;12:205–19.
3. James I. Cuffed tubes in children (Editorial). Paed Anaesth 2001;11:259–63.
4. Hatch DJ. New inhalation agents in paediatric anaesthesia. Br J Anaesth 1999;83:42–9.
5. Tobias JD. Spinal anaesthesia in infants and children. Paed Anaesth 2000;10:5–16.
6. Tobias JD. Brachial plexus anaesthesia in children. Paed Anaesth 2001;11:265–75.
7. Krane EJ, Haberkern CM, Jacobson LE. Postoperative apnea, bradycardia and oxygen desaturation in formerly premature infants. Prospective comparison of spinal and general anesthesia. Anesth Analg 1995;80:7–13.
8. Baines D. Postoperative nausea and vomiting in children. Paed Anaesth 1996;6:7–14.

Chapter 29
Anaesthesia for the Pregnant Surgical Patient

INTRODUCTION

It is estimated that between 1.6% and 2.2% of pregnant women require a surgical procedure at some time during gestation. These include emergency surgery as well as pregnancy-related surgery, such as dilatation and curettage for abortion, hysterotomy, and cervical cerclage procedures for cervical incompetence.

The particular hazards of anaesthesia during pregnancy are related to the physiological changes in the mother and possible adverse effects on the foetus. Optimal anaesthetic management should, therefore, ensure both maternal safety and foetal well-being.

There are several important distinctions between anaesthesia for surgery during pregnancy and obstetric analgesia and anaesthesia for labour and delivery. For example:

- Anaesthesia for surgery during pregnancy aims to inhibit uterine activity in order to prevent spontaneous abortion or preterm labour, whereas obstetric analgesia aims to avoid inhibition of uterine activity which would interfere with the course of labour.
- Central nervous system depression in the foetus is well tolerated in anaesthesia for surgery during pregnancy since the centrally depressant drugs can be excreted back to the mother for disposition, whereas the risk of neonatal depression is a concern in anaesthesia for labour and delivery.
- In surgical anaesthesia the potential teratogenic effects of anaesthetic agents is a cause for concern, but this is not a problem in anaesthesia for labour and delivery.

PHYSIOLOGICAL CHANGES DURING PREGNANCY

In general, changes in the early stages of pregnancy are due to hormonal alterations, while mechanical effects of the gravid uterus tend to predominate during the third trimester. A few pertinent points will be emphasized here.

- **Cardiovascular system**
  - Increases in cardiac output, stroke volume, heart rate.
  - Redistribution of cardiac output with increased flow to placenta, uterus, skin, kidneys and mammary glands.
  - Decrease in systemic vascular resistance because of relaxation of vascular smooth muscles.

  Aorto-caval compression may occur in the supine position even without evidence of maternal hypotension.
- **Respiratory system**
  - Capillary venous engorgement of nasal mucosa, oropharynx and respiratory tract may increase risk of trauma during airway manipulation.
  - Increased incidence of difficult and failed intubation due to various factors such as weight gain, breast engorgement, altered airway anatomy, laryngeal oedema.
  - Increased alveolar ventilation with mean $PaCO_2$ of 32 mmHg compared to 40 mmHg in non-pregnant state.
  - Decrease in functional residual capacity by 20% from the second trimester onwards.
  - Increase in basal metabolic rate and oxygen consumption

  Oxygen reserves are diminished and hypoxaemia develops rapidly during apnoea or hypoventilation, or if airway problems occur under anaesthesia.

— **Haematological system**
  - Relative haemodilution due to a greater increase in plasma volume (by 40%) relative to red blood cell volume (by 20%).
  - Increase in blood clotting activity causes the blood to be hypercoagulable, increasing risks of thromboembolism.

— **Gastrointestinal system**
  - Increase in gastric volume and acidity.
  - Decrease in lower oesophageal sphincter tone.
  - Decrease in gastric and intestinal motility.
  - Decrease in rate of gastric emptying, more so following trauma or administration of parenteral opioids.
  - Mechanical effects of the gravid uterus on the stomach by displacing the pylorus and altering the anatomy of the gastro-oesophageal junction.

  All these factors predispose to increased risks of aspiration.

— **Hepatorenal system**
  - Decrease in level of pseudocholinesterase even though this is clinically not significant; the use of suxamethonium is not contraindicated in pregnancy.
  - Decrease in total plasma protein concentration.
  - Increase in renal blood flow, glomerular filtration rate and renal clearance.

  Altered drug pharmacokinetics in pregnancy.

— **Nervous system**
  - A 25–40% decrease in minimal alveolar concentration (MAC) for inhalational anaesthetics.
  - A 30% decrease dosage requirement for local anaesthetics in spinal and epidural anaesthesia.

  Anaesthetic requirements are generally reduced.

EFFECTS ON THE FOETUS

1. **Direct effects**

   — Teratogenicity.

   — Maternal drug administration such as β-blockers leading to foetal bradycardia.

   Factors which affect the potential teratogenicity of a drug or anaesthetic agent include individual susceptibility to the agent, timing of administration of the agent and threshold or amount of exposure. One should also consider the spontaneous occurrence of congenital abnormalities unrelated to the use of drugs or anaesthetic agents. The period of organogenesis, corresponding to day 15 to day 90 of gestation, is the period of highest susceptibility to teratogens. Therefore, it is prudent to defer surgery until the period of organogenesis is over.

Most data are derived from animal studies and no clear-cut cause-effect relationships in humans have been established. After organogenesis is complete at 13 weeks, effects on the foetus are primarily growth retardation or functional effects rather than gross structural defects. There are higher risks for abortions, growth restriction, and frequency of low and very low birth weight babies. These are attributed to the patient's primary disease and the surgical procedure rather than the anaesthetic administered.

2. **Indirect effects**

   This relates to the adequacy of utero-placental circulation and oxygen delivery, which may be compromised by:

   — Maternal hypotension due to sympathetic blockade, aorto-caval compression, haemorrhage.
   — Vasoconstriction of utero-placental vessels due to hypocarbia, α-adrenergic drugs such as adrenaline, dopamine and other catecholamines.
   — Maternal hypoxaemia due to any cause.

   Foetal cardiovascular and central nervous systems can also be depressed from transplacental passage of anaesthetic agents.

RECOMMENDATIONS

— Postpone purely elective surgery until after delivery.
— Defer urgent surgery, if possible, until after the first trimester of pregnancy.
— Carry on emergency surgery, inform the patient about possible risks to the foetus and take precautions to safeguard well-being of mother and foetus.

The risks of teratogenicity and abortion are greatest in the first trimester, while those of preterm labour are greatest in the third trimester of pregnancy. Relatively speaking, the second trimester is regarded as the "safest period" for urgent, non-elective surgery.

An obstetrician, whose expertise will be invaluable to diagnose and manage possible preterm labour, and take steps to avert preterm delivery, should be involved in the perioperative management of the pregnant patient.

ANAESTHETIC MANAGEMENT

- Allay anxiety and apprehension by adequate reassurance and premedication. The possibility of abortion or spontaneous preterm labour should be discussed but the patient should also be reassured of the low risk of direct harm to the foetus by anaesthetic drugs or techniques used. Relieve pain, whenever present, with a narcotic analgesic.
- Take precautions against gastric aspiration.
  - Oral H_2 receptor antagonist of either ranitidine 150 mg or cimetidine 200 mg on the night before and on morning of elective surgery.
  - Intravenous stat dose of H_2 receptor antagonist such as ranitidine 50 mg for emergency surgery.
  - Non-particulate antacid with 30 ml of 0.3M sodium citrate before sending the patient to OT.
- Prophylactic tocolysis may be prescribed by some obstetricians in the form of β_2-agonist drugs or magnesium sulphate. Their haemodynamic effects (e.g., tachycardia induced by β_2-agonists) and interactions with anaesthetic agents (e.g., potentiation of action of non-depolarizing neuromuscular blocking drug by magnesium) must be considered.
- The patient should be placed in the lateral decubitus position to minimize the risk of aorto-caval compression, which increases from the second trimester of pregnancy onwards. Uterine displacement should be maintained at all times during transport and in the perioperative period.
- Intraoperative foetal monitoring should be carried out wherever possible. An external Doppler device to monitor foetal heart rate and tocodynamometer to monitor uterine contractility should be used after 16–20 week gestation if these do not interfere with the surgical field. Such monitoring provides additional assurance that the intrauterine environment has been optimized for the foetus.
- The choice of anaesthetic agent is not as critical as the site and nature of surgery in determining the foetal outcome. Pelvic surgery, for example, is associated with greater risks of abortion and preterm labour than peripheral surgery.
- Whenever possible, regional anaesthesia is preferred in order to avoid the hazards of general anaesthesia. Spinal anaesthesia is particularly useful since the amount of local anaesthetic administered is small and unlikely to cause direct adverse foetal effects. However, hypotension should be prevented by fluid preloading, and aggressively treated with intravenous fluids and/or vasopressor. Ephedrine has long

been regarded as the vasopressor of choice during pregnancy because the utero-placental blood flow was shown to be preserved in animal studies. These earlier findings have now been challenged and other vasopressors, phenylephrine in particular, have been advocated either in place of or in combination with ephedrine. Phenylephrine may be preferred when ephedrine is ineffective, when the baseline heart rate is high or in patients with cardiac disease where tachycardia may be deleterious.

— General anaesthesia should be preceded by preoxygenation for 3–5 minutes to avoid maternal and foetal hypoxaemia during induction and intubation. All patients should be regarded as having "full stomach". The airway should be protected by rapid sequence induction, cricoid pressure and intubation with a cuffed endotracheal tube.

— Choose anaesthetic drugs with a history of safe usage over many years. The anaesthetic agents commonly in use are regarded to be safe for both mother and foetus. There is no evidence that any specific drug is more superior to another if maternal tissue perfusion and oxygenation are maintained within normal limits.

— Volatile anaesthetic agents may inhibit uterine irritability by uterine relaxation and improve uterine blood flow by vasodilatation. This is especially desirable in pelvic and intraabdominal procedures although the incidence of postoperative preterm labour has not been shown to decrease with their use.

— Nitrous oxide may be used despite theoretical objections based on its action in inhibiting methionine synthetase, an enzyme involved in DNA synthesis. It is a weak teratogen in rodents when administered for long periods. This effect is not clinically significant since the period of exposure is short. Even when used for oocyte retrieval during *in vitro* fertilization (IVF) procedures, nitrous oxide has not been shown to affect success rate or the incidence of chromosomal abnormalities.

— Maintain adequate oxygenation. Avoid hyperventilating the patient since the resultant hypocarbia may compromise utero-placental blood flow by vasoconstriction.

— Reverse neuromuscular blockade at the end of the procedure. Remove the endotracheal tube only when the patient is awake and with full return of protective airway reflexes.

POSTOPERATIVE MANAGEMENT

— The patient should be reviewed by the obstetrician in the postoperative period. Monitoring of foetal heart rate and uterine activity should be carried out for foetus of viable gestational age and size. Whenever possible, the foetus should be shielded from radiographic exposure. Since residual anaesthetic agents and medications used for postoperative analgesia may blunt the pain of uterine contractions, uterine monitoring should be continued for at least 24 hours to enable early detection and management of preterm labour.

— Appropriate postoperative analgesia should be provided for the site and extent of the surgical procedure. Options include regional blockade with either opioid or local anaesthetic-fentanyl mixture, or intravenous patient-controlled analgesia with opioids. The use of regional anaesthetic technique is preferred since it is not associated with excessive maternal sedation or altered foetal heart rate variability. The use of NSAIDs is inadvisable after 32 weeks of gestation because of concern about premature closure of ductus arteriosus in the foetus.

FURTHER READING

1. Rosen MA. Management of anesthesia for the pregnant surgical patient. Anesthesiology 1999;91:1159–63.
2. Cox PBW, Marcus MAE, Bos H. Pharmacological considerations during pregnancy. Curr Opin Anaesthesiol 2001;14:311–6.
3. Koren G, Pastuszak A, Ito S. Drugs in pregnancy. N Engl J Med 1998;338:1128–37.

Chapter 30

Anaesthetic Management of Preeclampsia

INTRODUCTION

Hypertensive disorders of pregnancy encompass a spectrum of clinical conditions that differ in aetiology, pathophysiology and symptomatology. Lack of universal agreement regarding terminology and even the measurement of blood pressure during pregnancy has resulted in much confusion. Table 30–1 shows one of the more widely adopted classifications of hypertensive disorders of pregnancy based on clinical manifestations.

Table 30–1. Classification of hypertensive disorders of pregnancy

Disorder	Definition	Subtype	Features
Pregnancy-induced hypertension (PIH)	*De novo* hypertension after 20 weeks of gestation and settles within 6 weeks of delivery, characterized by a rise in blood pressure to > 140/90 mmHg	Gestational hypertension	6–7% of pregnancies. Hypertension without proteinuria and associated features
		Preeclampsia	5–6% of pregnancies. Hypertension with proteinuria (> 0.3 g/day)
Preexisting hypertension	Chronic hypertension diagnosed before pregnancy or earlier than 20 weeks of gestation, and persisting after delivery, characterized by a rise in blood pressure to > 140/90 mmHg		3–5% of pregnancies
Preexisting hypertension superimposed with preeclampsia	As above		15–25% of hypertensive pregnancies
Eclampsia	Generalized convulsions during hypertensive pregnancy, labour or within 7 days of delivery		0.05% of pregnancies

These hypertensive disorders contribute significantly to maternal as well as foetal morbidity and mortality. Maternal mortality attributable to preeclampsia is largely secondary to cerebral haemorrhage, heart failure and haematological disorders. The physiologic basis of the disease is still incompletely understood. Treatment is often only symptomatic or supportive, the only curative intervention being delivery of the foetus.

CLASSIFICATION

— **Mild preeclampsia**

- Systolic BP between 140–160 mmHg, diastolic BP between 90–100 mmHg.
- There may or may not be proteinuria > 0.3 g/day.
- There may or may not be oedema.
- No other complications.

— **Severe preeclampsia**

This is diagnosed when one or more of these conditions are present.

- Systolic BP > 160 mmHg or diastolic BP > 110 mmHg, on two readings taken at least 6 hours apart in a pregnant woman who is on bed rest.
- Proteinuria > 5 g/day, or > 3+ on 2 random urine samples collected at least 4 hours apart.
- Oliguria < 500 ml/day.
- Cerebral or visual disturbances: altered consciousness, headache, scotomas, blurred vision.
- Epigastric or right upper quadrant pain.
- Pulmonary oedema or cyanosis.
- Impaired liver function of unclear aetiology.
- Thrombocytopaenia.
- HELLP syndrome: **H**aemolysis, **E**levated **L**iver enzymes, **L**ow **P**latelets.

— **Eclampsia**

- Occurrence of one or more grand mal seizures, not attributable to other cerebral conditions in a patient with preeclampsia.
- May be preceded by warning signs such as headache, hyperreflexia, epigastric pain.
- The presence of fits may not correlate with the degree of hypertension.

PATHOPHYSIOLOGY

The exact aetiology of preeclampsia is still open to debate. Recent hypotheses are focused on the genetic make-up of mother and baby, and on immunological responses triggered by foetal cells and DNA in the maternal circulation. Such factors are thought to interfere with normal trophoblast invasion and placentation resulting in endothelial dysfunction and placental insufficiency.

It has been proposed that one of the consequences of utero-placental ischaemia is a decrease in the production of prostacyclin (a vasodilator prostaglandin). The production of thromboxane A_2 (a vasoconstrictor prostaglandin) is, however, increased. The relative predominance of thromboxane A_2 results in platelet aggregation and uterine vasoconstriction. The former may give rise to coagulation disorder, while the latter causes more utero-placental ischaemia and thus completes the vicious circle.

A meta-analysis of randomized, placebo-controlled trials of low-dose aspirin therapy showed that such therapy reduced the incidence of preeclampsia among women with poor obstetric history and among high-risk nulliparous women, but was ineffective among women with underlying medical illness. Such low-dose aspirin therapy is not expected to cause clinically significant impairment in platelet function and does not contraindicate the use of regional anaesthesia during labour or operative delivery.

PROBLEMS OF ANAESTHESIA

Clinical manifestations of preeclampsia are multi-systemic as a result of widespread maternal vasospasm, volume contraction and organ hypoperfusion. The problems of particular concern to the anaesthesiologist include these.

— Cardiovascular instability
  - Wide BP fluctuations during anaesthesia.
  - Contracted blood volume with poor tolerance of blood loss.
  - Increased risk of left ventricular failure and acute pulmonary oedema.

— Airway concerns
  - Risk of aspiration of gastric contents especially in an obtunded, eclamptic patient.
  - Possibility of difficult intubation secondary to laryngeal oedema.
  - Haemodynamic changes during laryngoscopy and intubation, if not obtunded, can result in hypertensive crisis.

— Peripheral oedema
  - Difficult intravenous access.
  - Indistinct landmarks for central neuraxial block.

— End-organ dysfunction
  - Kidneys: proteinuria with hypoproteinaemia, acute renal failure.
  - Cardiovascular system: cardiac failure.
  - Central nervous system: visual disturbances, increased CNS irritability, hypertensive encephalopathy, convulsions, cerebral haemorrhage.
  - Liver: hepatic failure.
  - Haematological system: thrombocytopaenia, haemolysis, disseminated intravascular coagulation (DIC), HELLP syndrome.

- Placental insufficiency: intrauterine growth retardation, abruptio placentae, foetal distress.

— Poor recovery from general anaesthesia due to a combination of factors.
- Benzodiazepine (diazepam or midazolam) bolus or infusion to abort eclamptic fits.
- Possible presence of metabolic acidosis.
- Poor renal function with prolonged action of renally excreted anaesthetic agents.
- Potentiation of action of non-depolarizing neuromuscular blocking drugs by magnesium administered in the form of magnesium sulphate.

MANAGEMENT OF ECLAMPSIA

Eclampsia is an important risk factor in maternal morbidity and mortality. There is no direct correlation between severity of hypertension and occurrence of eclampsia, as the condition is thought to result from cerebral vasospasm leading to cerebral ischaemia, disruption of blood-brain barrier and cerebral oedema. Complications include transtentorial herniation and intracerebral haemorrhage.

Management of eclampsia is based on the following measures.

— Acute management
- Immediate resuscitation in terms of airway, breathing and circulation; ensure adequate oxygenation and ventilation, protect the airway from aspiration, and prevent trauma to the mother and foetus during seizure.
- Treatment of seizures with IV benzodiazepine or IV magnesium sulphate 4 g over 10–20 minutes.

— Prevention of further seizures with magnesium sulphate infusion at 1 g/hr.

— Control of blood pressure.

— Definitive treatment: plan for delivery once seizures are controlled, severe hypertension treated and hypoxia corrected.

MANAGEMENT PRINCIPLES OF PREECLAMPSIA

Optimal management of patients with severe preeclampsia involves the obstetrician, the anaesthesiologist and the neonatologist. The patient should be admitted to a high dependency area for close monitoring and appropriate management.

— **Consultation**

The anaesthesiologist should be consulted early to assist in resuscitation, fluid management, central venous cannulation, analgesia for labour and delivery, and possibly anaesthesia for caesarean section.

— **Eclampsia prophylaxis**

The patient should be monitored for signs of impending eclampsia. There is clear evidence that magnesium sulphate is the anticonvulsant of choice for women with eclampsia, while its role in eclampsia prophylaxis is less clear. The drug can be administered intravenously or intramuscularly depending on the preference and facilities of the hospital. Watch out for clinical manifestations of magnesium toxicity: loss of patellar reflex, muscle weakness, flushing, somnolence, slurred speech, diplopia. Other anticonvulsants such as diazepam, phenobarbitone and phenytoin have also been used.

— **Control of blood pressure**

Oral therapy, if tolerated, is preferred to intravenous route of administration. The antihypertensives commonly used are labetalol, nifedipine and methyldopa. In severe cases BP control by vasodilatation is achieved by continuous intravenous infusion of hydralazine. The rate of infusion should be titrated to achieve BP < 160/100 mmHg, and concomitant plasma expansion with intravenous fluid may be necessary. Avoid overzealous control as the mother and the foetus may not tolerate large and rapid reductions in BP and perfusion pressure.

— **Fluid management**

Maternal plasma volume expansion that accompanies normal pregnancy is attenuated in preeclampsia. Even though total body water is increased, the patient is chronically vasoconstricted with a contracted blood volume. Intravenous fluids should be administered to restore central venous pressure (CVP) and maintain adequate urine output. However, the potential hazard of this is the development of pulmonary oedema particularly in the presence of impaired renal function. Strict intake/output chart should be maintained and fluid therapy is best guided by serial CVP readings. In selected cases, pulmonary artery pressure monitoring may be necessary.

— **Baseline investigations**

- Check FBC to monitor platelet count.
- Conduct full coagulation studies if coagulopathy is suspected or if platelet count < 100,000/μl and falling.
- Check blood urea, serum creatinine, uric acid and electrolyte concentrations (including magnesium if magnesium sulphate is used).
- Check urine sample for proteins, culture and sensitivity.
- Do liver function test, including total plasma protein and albumin concentrations.

— **Foetal monitoring**

If viable, the fetal heart rate should be continuously monitored by means of cardiotocography (CTG). If the period of gestation is less than 34 weeks, dexamethasone is given to hasten fetal lung maturity prior to delivery.

— **Delivery**

Delivery should be planned for as soon as the above parameters have been met, as there is no advantage in delaying delivery when preeclampsia develops at term. Mode of delivery – vaginal or by caesarean section – should be discussed with the obstetrician. Epidural analgesia/anaesthesia is the method of choice provided contraindications to regional blocks have been excluded. If preeclampsia develops before term, a compromise must be made between maternal and foetal well-being. Maternal BP is controlled for as long as possible to allow for foetal growth, but delivery must be expedited if the maternal condition deteriorates.

MANAGEMENT OF PREECLAMPSIA FOR CAESAREAN SECTION

The choice of regional anaesthesia or general anaesthesia depends on the status of the patient (severity of hypertension, coagulation status, potential airway problems), the state of the foetus and urgency of the surgery.

Regional Anaesthesia

Epidural anaesthesia should be considered if time permits and in the absence of contraindications to performing regional anaesthesia. This is the anaesthetic technique of choice in mild preeclampsia without bleeding disorder or foetal distress.

These factors should be considered.

— Check coagulation status. Regional anaesthesia is contraindicated if:
  - Platelet count < 80,000/μl
  - Prothrombin time > 1½ times normal
  - Fibrinogen concentration < 200 mg/dl
— Avoid the use of adrenaline in local anaesthetic solution as this may cause further vasoconstriction if injected intravascularly.
— The amount of fluid infused for preloading is best guided by serial CVP readings. Care should be taken to avoid fluid over- and underloading, and consider using colloid instead of crystalloid solutions in severe cases.
— Close BP monitoring is essential since hypotension may occur with sympathetic blockade in addition to an already contracted intravascular volume.
— If hypotension occurs:
  - Correct aorto-caval compression if present.
  - Treat hypotension cautiously with intravenous fluids and/or vasopressor such as ephedrine.
  - Avoid overzealous fluid or vasopressor therapy and watch out for complications such as fluid overload, acute pulmonary oedema.

Although controversial, there is growing evidence to suggest that spinal anaesthesia is a reasonable choice for patients with severe preeclampsia, provided that contraindications for regional anaesthesia have been excluded. In addition to the recognized advantages of spinal anaesthesia (rapid onset, reliable and profound blockade), the degree of hypotension or the usage of vasopressor is no different from those encountered in epidural anaesthesia. Furthermore, use of a small 27G spinal needle is expected to result in less tissue trauma compared to a considerably larger 18G epidural needle. Further studies are needed to define the role of spinal anaesthesia in such patients.

General Anaesthesia

— Plan for general anaesthesia for severe preeclampsia complicated by coagulopathy, eclampsia or severe fetal distress.
— Prior to induction of anaesthesia, BP should be controlled with intravenous incremental doses of hydralazine 2.5–5 mg (maximum 20 mg) or labetalol 5–10 mg until systolic BP is below 160 mmHg. Use of esmolol has been questioned by some

anaesthesiologists as prolonged foetal bradycardia has been reported with its use, even though its pharmacologic profile is ideally suited for the purpose. Lignocaine 1–1.5 mg/kg can be used to obtund sympathetic reflexes during laryngoscopy and intubation. Alfentanil 5 μg/kg has also been used for the same purpose but the paediatrician should be forewarned about possible neonatal respiratory depression if this is used.

— Preoxygenate the patient for 3–5 minutes and prepare for difficult intubation. Plan for an awake fibreoptic intubation if difficult airway is anticipated and if the surgery is not emergent. In the absence of a difficult airway, rapid sequence induction and intubation with cricoid pressure is achieved using thiopentone 4 mg/kg and suxamethonium 1–1.5 mg/kg. An ETT one size smaller is advocated in view of the possibility of laryngeal oedema causing airway narrowing.

— Blood pressure and intraoperative blood loss should be closely monitored. Suspect DIC if there is generalized oozing from the surgical field and venepuncture sites. This should be corrected with cryoprecipitate, platelet concentrate, fresh frozen plasma and blood.

— After the baby is delivered, administer oxytocin 5 U diluted to 5 ml by slow intravenous bolus. Infusion of oxytocin 40–80 U in 500 ml solution may be required in the presence of uterine atony. Do not use ergometrine as this causes acute increases in blood pressure. Give an intravenous opioid for intraoperative analgesia. Discontinue hydralazine infusion if diastolic BP < 100 mmHg.

— At the end of the surgery, reverse the neuromuscular blockade and remove the ETT when the patient is fully awake and able to protect her airway. Watch out for problems of poor reversal of neuromuscular blockade or delayed awakening from the effects of general anaesthesia.

— The patient should be admitted to ICU or HDU in the presence of one or more of these conditions.
  - The patient has fitted.
  - The patient is drowsy and the ability to protect the airway is in doubt.
  - There is inadequate reversal of neuromuscular blockade.
  - Presence of clinical features of aspiration pneumonia.
  - Presence of DIC with haemodynamic instability.
  - Unstable CVS: severe hyper- or hypotension, cardiac failure, pulmonary oedema.
  - Marked acidosis or low PaO_2 on ABG.

POSTPARTUM MANAGEMENT

Besides postoperative analgesia, optimal fluid management and blood pressure control are equally important considerations.

— Maintain fluid restriction and control fluid balance.
— Encourage diuresis using low-dose frusemide or dopamine infusion (the latter is controversial) if necessary, especially if CVP continues to rise.
— Gradual reduction of hydralazine and/or magnesium sulphate.
— Conversion to oral antihypertensives such as labetalol, nifedipine if necessary.

FURTHER READING

1. Haddad T. Update on pre-eclampsia. Int Anesthesiol Clin 2002;40:115–35.
2. Schneider MC, Landau R, Mortl MG. New insights in hypertensive disorders of pregnancy. Curr Opin Anaesth 2001;14:291–7.
3. Mortl MG, Schneider MC. Key issues in assessing, managing and treating patients presenting with severe preeclampsia. Int J Obstet Anesth 2000;9:39–44.
4. Heyborne KD. Preeclampsia prevention: Lessons from the low-dose aspirin therapy trials. Am J Obstet Gynecol 2000;183:523–8.
5. Engelhardt T, MacLennan FM. Fluid management in pre-eclampsia. Int J Obstet Anesth 1999;8:253–9.
6. Katz VL, Farmer R, Kuller JA. Preeclampsia into eclampsia: Toward a new paradigm. Am J Obstet Gynecol 2000;182:1389–96.
7. Brodie H, Manilow AM. Anesthetic management of preeclampsia/eclampsia. Int J Obstet Anesth 1998;8:110–24.
8. Hood DD, Curry R. Spinal versus epidural anesthesia for cesarean section in severely preeclamptic patients. Anesthesiology 1999;90:1276–83.
9. Santos AC. Spinal anesthesia in severely preeclamptic women: How safe is it? (Editorial) Anesthesiology 1999;90:1252–4.
10. Howell P. Spinal anaesthesia in severe preeclampsia: Time for reappraisal, or time for caution? (Editorial) Int J Obstet Anesth 1998;7:217–9.
11. Ramanathan J, Vaddadi AK, Arheart KL. Combined spinal and epidural anesthesia with low dose of intrathecal bupivacaine in women with severe preeclampsia: A preliminary survey. Reg Anesth Pain Med 2001;26:46–51.

Chapter 31

Anaesthesia and the Elderly

INTRODUCTION

The process of aging refers to the normal physiological process of degeneration beginning at 30 years and proceeding at variable rates. *Chronological age* refers to the age according to birth date while *biological (or physiological) age* is the estimated age based on the state of body organs. These two may not be well correlated.

There is no universal numerical agreement to "the aged" or "the elderly" because there is no specific clinical marker for the geriatric patient, as aging does not occur abruptly but represents a continuum. A patient aged 65 years and above is empirically regarded as belonging to the geriatric age group.

As a result of increased life expectancy with advances in surgical and anaesthetic techniques, life-supporting systems and infection control, more surgical procedures are now carried out for those patients previously thought to be unfit for anaesthesia and surgery. The incidence of severe complications during the perioperative course increases with age. Mortality rate related to surgery is approximately 3 times higher for patients > 70 years compared with younger patients, and the difference is even more marked in emergency procedures. This is attributed to a combination of factors: a higher prevalence of age-related diseases as well as reduction in basic organ function due to aging *per se.*

ORGAN SYSTEM CHANGES WITH AGING

Age-related physiological changes are characterized by reduction in functional reserve of these organ systems.

1. **Cardiovascular system (CVS)**
   - Changes are observed in cardiac morphology, cardiac function and peripheral vasculature.
   - Cardiac output decreases by approximately 1% per year after the age of 30.
   - Heart valves are thickened and calcified due to ectopic calcification resulting from degeneration of the collagen content.
   - There is increased collagen deposition in the myocardium and conducting system, resulting in:
     - Increased left ventricular (LV) wall thickness with reduced diastolic compliance.
     - Abnormalities in conduction of cardiac impulses, with increased incidence of intraventricular conduction defects and cardiac arrhythmias such as atrial fibrillation.
     - Reduced tachycardic response to atropine and catecholamines.
   - Histologic changes in the vasculature include increased intimal thickness, elastin fragmentation and increased collagen content of arterial wall, resulting in:
     - Decreased compliance and distensibility of the vasculature.
     - Increased systolic blood pressure or "systolic hypertension".
     - Increased LV afterload and further increase in LV wall thickness.
   - Cardiac reserve is reduced and compensatory response to CVS stresses is blunted, resulting in wide BP fluctuations during anaesthetic induction and emergence, and poor tolerance to hypovolaemia or rapid fluid loading.

- Organ perfusion is reduced, resulting in:
  - Slow arm-brain circulation time, with delayed induction of anaesthesia by intravenous induction agents.
  - Preferential delivery of anaesthetic drugs to the brain, with increased sensitivity to centrally depressant drugs.
  - Reduced organ function with poor tolerance to hypoxia.

2. **Respiratory system**
   - Ventilatory reserve is reduced.
   - Airway reflexes and cough effort are suppressed, with increased risks of regurgitation and pulmonary aspiration under anaesthesia.
   - There is a gradual reduction in alveolar surface area with a corresponding increase in interstitial tissue, resulting in decreased efficiency in pulmonary gas exchange and gradual reduction in PaO_2 ($PaCO_2$ remains constant).
   - Reduction in the number of pulmonary capillaries results in raised pulmonary artery pressure and pulmonary vascular resistance.
   - Closing volume encroaches or exceeds functional residual capacity, leading to ventilation/perfusion mismatch with resultant hypoxaemia.
   - There is blunted responsiveness to hypoxia and hypercarbia.

3. **Central nervous system**
   - Brain atrophy correlates well with the extent of cognitive decline.
   - Basal metabolic rate (BMR) and heat production are both reduced, and together with impaired temperature regulation can result in increased tendency to hypothermia during anaesthesia.
   - Local anaesthetic requirement is reduced; central neuraxial blockade in the elderly tends to be more extensive, more intense and lasts longer compared to younger patients.
   - There may be altered response to certain drugs, e.g., scopolamine may cause restlessness rather than sedation.
   - There is increased sensitivity to sedative and centrally depressant drugs; the effects tend to be intense and long-lasting.

4. **Renal system**
   - The renal blood flow, glomerular filtration rate and renal clearance are all reduced, giving rise to accumulation and prolonged effect of renally excreted drugs.

— Fluid shifts, acid-base and electrolyte disturbances are poorly tolerated.
— There is increased susceptibility to nephrotoxic drugs such as aminoglycosides.

5. **Liver and gastrointestinal system**
   — Hepatic blood flow and hepatobiliary function are reduced, resulting in decreased metabolism and excretion of drugs.
   — Plasma albumin concentration is reduced, resulting in decreased protein binding and greater quantities of unbound, pharmacologically active drug.
   — Decreased glycogen storage increases the risk of hypoglycaemia on prolonged starvation.
   — Reduced synthesis of clotting factors may give rise to impaired clotting mechanism.
   — There is an increased susceptibility to hepatic injury from drugs, hypoxia and blood transfusions.
   — There is a higher risk of aspiration because of decreased peristalsis and gastric emptying.

6. **Haematological system**
   — Anaemia is fairly common due to poor nutrition, low iron stores, reduced vitamin B_{12} absorption or reduced haemopoiesis.
   — Poor leukocyte function gives rise to poor wound healing and increased susceptibility to intercurrent infection.

7. **Musculoskeletal system/skin**
   — There is an age-related reduction in bone density resulting in osteoporosis which predisposes to joint damage or fractures.
   — Calcified ligaments may pose difficulty for regional anaesthetic blocks.
   — Senile atrophy of the skin results in easy bruising and increased risk of thermal injury from diathermy or warming mattress.
   — Decreased skin perfusion increases the risk of developing pressure sores if the patient is bedridden.

8. **Common pathological conditions**
   — CVS: hypertension, coronary artery disease, congestive heart failure, valvular heart disease especially aortic stenosis, cardiac conduction defects, peripheral vascular disease.

- Respiratory system: chronic obstructive pulmonary disease (COPD), lung fibrosis.
- CNS: transient ischaemic attacks, stroke, sensorineural deafness, cataracts, senile dementia.
- Endocrine system: diabetes mellitus, hypothyroidism.
- Renal and/or liver disease.

In view of the multiple physiological changes and common pathological conditions associated with the elderly, this group of patients should receive thorough preoperative preparation, optimal intraoperative anaesthetic care as well as careful postoperative management.

PREOPERATIVE ASSESSMENT

- Other than the usual assessment according to ASA status, pay special attention to the patient's mental status, airway (state of dentition, neck mobility, mouth opening), cardiovascular and respiratory systems.
- Find out whether the patient still participates in vigorous physical and mental activities on a regular basis. A patient who is active can be expected to have ample reserves of CVS, respiratory and CNS functions, which may be predictive of a better surgical outcome.
- Identify and evaluate associated medical conditions in terms of end-organ involvement, type of medication and adequacy of treatment. Give clear instruction to the patient and the nursing staff on whether the medication(s) should be continued or withheld on the day of surgery.
- Examine the spine and assess the patient's ability to be optimally positioned if central neuraxial blockade is planned. Explain the proposed anaesthetic technique to the patient.
- An informed consent should be obtained from the patient and/or immediate family member if significant anaesthetic risks are involved. Postoperative ICU admission should be arranged for such patients.
- Premedicant drugs should be omitted or their doses reduced to avoid oversedation and depression of the cardiovascular and respiratory systems. If premedication is deemed necessary and safe, an oral benzodiazepine is preferred over an opioid which may induce respiratory depression. Scopolamine should be avoided in the elderly. Consider H_2 receptor antagonist and antacid to reduce the risk of aspiration.

CHOICE OF ANAESTHETIC TECHNIQUES

Always remember that there is little margin for error in anaesthetizing the elderly patient. No single anaesthetic technique is ideal and individualization is essential.

Regional Anaesthesia

Advantages

- The patient remains conscious or lightly sedated throughout the procedure. Hazards of general anaesthesia – difficult airway, gastric aspiration, delayed recovery, postoperative confusion – are avoided.
- Appropriate regional anaesthetic technique may reduce surgical stress by blocking the input from noxious surgical stimuli and reducing sympathetic efferent activity.
- Certain anaesthetic techniques have provision for effective postoperative analgesia, resulting in less postoperative cardiovascular, respiratory and neurological complications and enabling early ambulation. The latter may result in reduced incidence of deep venous thrombosis, pulmonary embolism and respiratory complications.

Disadvantages

- Patient cooperation is needed; hence, it is not suitable for confused or demented individuals.
- Local anaesthetic requirement is reduced and overdose may occur if its dose is not adjusted.
- Hypotension from central neuraxial blockade is poorly tolerated.
- The block may be technically difficult to perform because of calcified ligaments, or inability of the patient to be optimally positioned for the block.

General Anaesthesia

Anatomical problems

- The patient may be edentulous, or have loose teeth which may be dislodged during airway manipulation.

— Poor supportive tissues at the cheek often results in poor mask fit and difficulty in mask ventilation.
— The possible presence of cervical spondylosis or vertebro-basilar arterial insufficiency should be considered, and hyperextension of the neck during airway manipulation should be avoided.
— Weakened posterior membranous portion of the trachea poses a risk to tracheal trauma during intubation.
— Atrophic skin, pressure areas, osteoporotic bones and arthritic joints require gentle handling and care in ensuring that pressure points are well-padded.

Anaesthetic management

— All intravenous and inhalational anaesthetic agents interfere with cardiovascular performance either by direct myocardial depression or by peripheral vasodilatation. Drugs should be administered slowly and in reduced doses to minimize possible adverse effects.
— The nature and extent of monitoring depend on the patient's medical condition and the extent of surgical procedure. These should be placed prior to induction of anaesthesia as far as possible. Active measures should be taken to prevent perioperative hypothermia.
— It is mandatory to ensure preoxygenation prior to induction of anaesthesia. Intravenous induction agent should be injected slowly and carefully titrated to avoid overdosage, being mindful of the longer circulation time and delayed onset of action in the elderly.
— Instruct the anaesthetic assistant to apply cricoid pressure when consciousness is lost. If not contraindicated, suxamethonium is preferred for intubation because of difficulty in maintaining effective mask ventilation coupled with the risk of aspiration. Direct laryngoscopy should be gentle and undue hyperextension of the neck should be avoided.
— Doses of all anaesthetic drugs should be reduced. Atracurium is suitable for neuromuscular blockade since it is not dependent on liver and kidney for metabolism and excretion. Glycopyrrolate is preferred over atropine since it does not cross the blood-brain barrier to cause confusion.
— The patient's haemodynamic status should be monitored closely. Replace blood loss early and treat hypotension aggressively.

— At the end of surgery, reverse the neuromuscular blockade and remove the endotracheal tube only when the patient is fully awake and with good respiratory effort.

POSTOPERATIVE MANAGEMENT

— Observe the patient closely at the PACU. Use overhead heater, forced-air warming device and blankets to prevent hypothermia. Discharge to the ward when the patient is conscious, comfortable, breathing adequately, and is haemodynamically stable.

— Consider admission to ICU if the patient's general condition is poor, surgery is major or protracted, there is intraoperative instability, or problem occurs with reversal of neuromuscular blockade.

— These patients should be carefully monitored since most surgical morbidity and mortality occur in the postoperative period. Continue supplemental oxygen for 24 hours unless the surgical procedure has been minor and peripheral.

— Postoperative mental confusion, if present, is frequently and sometimes erroneously attributed to senile dementia in the elderly patient. Other causes – uraemia, infection, bladder distension, sedative drugs, electrolyte imbalance, hypo- or hyperglycaemia – should be excluded (see Chapter 74).

— The benefits of effective postoperative analgesia should be weighed against the possible risks of respiratory depression, urinary retention, ileus, constipation and relative overdosage. Options for pain management include:
  - Epidural or other regional blocks.
  - Patient-controlled analgesia if the patient is able to follow instructions.
  - Subcutaneous morphine in reduced doses.
  - Intravenous infusion of morphine if the patient is managed in ICU.

  Although NSAIDs are often used as analgesic adjuncts with opioid-sparing potential, these drugs are often unsuitable in the elderly patients due to frequent occurrence of significant renal dysfunction or peptic ulcer disease.

— Regular chest physiotherapy and breathing exercises are useful especially for patients with COPD and those who have undergone thoracic or upper abdominal surgery.

— Early ambulation should be advocated to reduce the risk of developing deep vein thrombosis. An appropriate form of thromboprophylaxis should be instituted in the perioperative period.

FURTHER READING

1. Cook DJ, Rooke GA. Priorities in perioperative geriatrics. Anesth Analg 2003;96:1823–36.
2. Sielenkamper AW, Booke M. Anaesthesia and the elderly. Curr Opin Anaesthesiol 2001;14:679–84.
3. Priebe HJ. The aged cardiovascular risk patient. Br J Anaesth 2000;85:763–78.
4. Jin F, Chung F. Minimizing perioperative adverse events in the elderly. Br J Anaesth 2001;87:608–24.
5. Rooke GA. Autonomic and cardiovascular function in the geriatric patient. Anesthesiol Clin N Am 2000;18:31–46.
6. Zaugg M, Lucchinetti E. Respiratory function in the elderly. Anesthesiol Clin N Am 2000;18:47–57.
7. Sear JW. Implication of aging on anesthetic drugs. Curr Opin Anaesthesiol 2003;16:373–8.
8. Chelluri L. Critical illness in the elderly: Review of pathophysiology of aging and outcome of intensive care. J Intensive Care Med 2001;16:114–27.
9. Muravchick S. The elderly outpatient: Current anesthetic implications. Curr Opin Anaesthesiol 2002;15:621–5.

C

Anaesthesia for Specific Surgery

Chapter 32

Regional Anaesthetic Techniques I: Central Neuraxial Blockade

INTRODUCTION

This chapter deals with regional anaesthetic techniques practised in the OT and elsewhere, for example, the ICU and delivery suite. The reader is advised to refer to specific textbooks on regional anaesthesia for more detailed descriptions of such techniques.

It is sometimes erroneously assumed that regional anaesthesia carries less anaesthetic risk compared with general anaesthesia, and that less vigilance is required in monitoring the patient. It cannot be emphasized enough that *regional anaesthesia should not be taken lightly*. Morbidity and even mortality can occur as a result of faulty technique, lack of monitoring and failure to institute early management of complications. This is particularly so in central neuraxial blockade. Such patients should receive equivalent standard of care and monitoring accorded to patients under general anaesthesia.

GENERAL CONSIDERATIONS FOR CENTRAL NEURAXIAL BLOCKADE

1. **Explanation and consent**
   - Ideally, suitable patients for the regional anaesthetic technique should be identified during the premedication round. Any contraindications to regional anaesthesia should be ruled out.
   - The option of regional anaesthesia should be discussed with the patient, who should consent to the anaesthetic procedure. In most cases of emergency surgery, this would have to be carried out in the OT itself.

2. **Preparation before procedure**
   - Be familiar with the relevant anatomy, technique and possible complications associated with the regional block.
   - Anaesthetic drugs (thiopentone, ephedrine, atropine, suxamethonium) should be prepared prior to the procedure in case complications to the block develop or if induction of general anaesthesia becomes necessary. Anaesthetic and airway equipment should be checked and ready for use.
   - The patient should be monitored with ECG, BP and pulse oximetry during the procedure.
   - Preload with 10–15 ml/kg intravenous crystalloid (non-dextrose solution) prior to the block.

3. **Performing the block**
   - The block should be performed under strict asepsis. The anaesthesiologist should wear mask, sterile gloves and surgical gown. The block area should be cleaned with antiseptic solution and draped with sterile towels.
   - Determine the appropriate end-point, for example:
     - Backflow of cerebrospinal fluid (CSF) for subarachnoid block.
     - Loss of resistance to air or saline for epidural block.
   - Careful aspiration before injecting the local anaesthetic (LA) lessens the chance of inadvertent intravascular and intrathecal injection in epidural block.
   - Use a test dose in epidural block to detect inadvertent intrathecal or intravas-

cular injection. A commonly used test dose consists of 3 ml of 1.5% lignocaine with 1:200,000 adrenaline (a dose of 45 mg lignocaine and 15 μg adrenaline). Watch for early motor block (for intrathecal injection) and tachycardia or increase in BP (for intravascular injection).

— Fractionate the total dose into aliquots of 3–5 ml, injecting slowly each time.
— Maintain close communication with the patient at all times to detect early signs of LA toxicity or overdose.

4. **After the block**
— Closely monitor the patient's BP, heart rate, oxygen saturation and the intravenous fluids infused.
— Administer oxygen via mask or nasal cannula to selected patients: patients for caesarean section, elderly or ill patients with significant cardiorespiratory disease, or patients who are given supplemental sedation.
— Test the level of sensory block using spirit swab (temperature), pinprick (pain) or touch. Test the degree of motor block using modified Bromage score (see Table 32–1).
— Give adequate time for the block to take effect before allowing the surgeon to commence surgery. Test the incision site for anaesthesia before proceeding with skin incision.
— Consider converting to general anaesthesia if the degree of block is not satisfactory (e.g., patchy block, inadequate level of block) after sufficient time has elapsed and sufficient dose has been administered. Do not supplement inadequate regional anaesthesia with heavy sedation.
— Watch for complications of high block or local anaesthetic toxicity, such as hypotension, bradycardia, nausea or vomiting, circumoral tingling or respiratory distress. Institute treatment early.

Table 32–1. Modified Bromage score

Score	Characteristic
1	Complete block (unable to move feet or knees)
2	Almost complete block (able to move feet only)
3	Partial block (just able to move knees)
4	Detectable weakness of hip flexion (between scores 3 and 5)
5	No detectable weakness of hip flexion while supine (full flexion of knees)
6	Able to perform partial knee bend while standing

5. **Postoperative orders and follow-up**
   - Placement of catheters in certain regional blocks allows continuation of analgesia into the postoperative period. Continued management of such patients can be carried out by the Acute Pain Service (APS) team.
   - Specific orders after spinal anaesthesia (e.g., rest in bed for 6 hours, hourly BP and pulse for 4 hours and 2-hourly thereafter) should be documented in the patient's anaesthesia record and case notes.
   - Follow up patients in the ward, particularly those who developed complications of block, e.g., inadvertent dural puncture in epidural block.

SPINAL ANAESTHESIA

Of the major regional anaesthetic techniques, spinal or subarachnoid block is probably the easiest to perform and master. Its advantages – simplicity with a definite end-point, minimal drug usage, rapid onset, reliability, dense motor and sensory block with provision of good operating conditions – are unsurpassed. Unfortunately it has generated a cavalier attitude among some surgeons and even anaesthesiologists. It needs to be emphasized that things are not as simple as *just give a spinal*. Incidents of sudden, unexpected circulatory collapse have been reported, and the hypotension associated with sympathetic blockade may be poorly tolerated by medically compromised patients.

Indications

Surgery to lower abdomen (e.g., caesarean section, inguinal hernia repair), perineum (e.g., haemorrhoidectomy), lower limbs (e.g., reduction of lower limb fractures).

Problems and Complications

- Hypotension.
- Postdural puncture headache, especially if large-bore bevelled needles are used.
- Transient neurologic syndrome (TNS): incidence 0.01–0.7%; pain or dysaesthesia in the buttocks and lower limbs in the absence of sensory or motor dysfunction. Symptoms usually start within 24 hours after spinal anaesthesia and spontaneously resolve within 2–7 days.

— Cauda equina syndrome: bladder/bowel dysfunction, pain or sensory changes in lower back or buttocks, implicated by high concentration of local anaesthetic associated with the use of microcatheters in continuous spinal anaesthesia.

Technique

1. Position
   - Sitting or lateral, with the neck flexed and hips and knees flexed.
   - The lateral position is more comfortable for patients with painful lower limbs, whereas landmarks are more easily identifiable in the sitting position.

2. Needle
   - 25–27G 9-cm pencil-point spinal needle (or the longer 12-cm spinal needle in obese patients).
   - 22G introducer to guide the spinal needle through the superficial layers.

3. Conduct of block
   - Identify the intervertebral space and the midline. The line joining the iliac crests corresponds to the level of the L4 vertebra in most individuals. Do not go higher than L2–L3 interspace to reduce risks of damage to the conus medullaris.
   - Infiltrate the skin and subcutaneous layer with 1–2% lignocaine. Insert the introducer, then the spinal needle in a slight 15° cephalad direction. The needle passes through the skin, subcutaneous tissue, supraspinous ligament, interspinous ligament and then the ligamentum flavum before entering the epidural space. The ligaments may be calcified and feel "gritty" in elderly patients. Advance the needle until a click is felt as the dura is punctured.
   - An alternative method is the paramedian approach. The needle entry point is 2 cm lateral to the midline and level with the upper border of the spinous process. Insert the needle perpendicular to the skin until the lamina of the vertebra is contacted, then withdraw slightly and redirect 15° medially and 30° cephalad to pass over the lamina. Advance the needle until a click is felt. This approach bypasses the supraspinous and interspinous ligaments which may be calcified in elderly patients.
   - The use of blunt, pencil-point spinal needle enables the operator to appreciate the click as the dura is punctured upon entering the subarachnoid space.

Remove the stylet from the spinal needle and look for CSF to appear at the hub of the needle.

- Inject LA through the spinal needle. Aspirate slightly at midpoint and towards the end of injection to confirm that the spinal needle has not been displaced. Barbotage is not necessary.
- Withdraw the spinal needle. Spray with an antiseptic spray and place a sterile dressing over the puncture site.
- Return the patient to the supine position. If a saddle block is intended, let the patient remain seated for 3–5 minutes. Similarly, if a unilateral block is intended, maintain the patient in the lateral position for 3–5 minutes with the side to be blocked dependent (for hyperbaric LA solution) or non-dependent (for iso- or hypobaric LA solution).

4. Dose of LA
   - 2–3 ml of 0.5% hyperbaric or isobaric bupivacaine is usually adequate.
   - An opioid is often added to the LA solution. Addition of intrathecal fentanyl 15–25 μg improves the quality of block intraoperatively while preservative-free morphine 0.1–0.2 mg provides excellent postoperative analgesia for 12–24 hours.
   - The use of lignocaine for spinal anaesthesia has declined following case reports of TNS.

EPIDURAL ANAESTHESIA

It is technically more difficult to perform epidural than spinal block, but epidural anaesthesia has the advantages of flexibility and ability to extend the period of anaesthesia or analgesia intra- and postoperatively. A more gradual onset of sympathetic and sensori-motor blockade means that hypotension tends to be less frequent and less severe compared with spinal anaesthesia.

Indications

- Same as spinal anaesthesia for lumbar epidural block (see page 398).
- Upper abdominal and thoracic surgery for thoracic epidural block.
- Pain relief for fracture ribs and/or flail chest.

Problems and Complications

- Hypotension.
- Inadvertent intravascular injection resulting in systemic local anaesthetic toxicity.
- Inadvertent intrathecal injection resulting in total spinal.
- Accidental dural puncture with risk of postdural puncture headache.
- Inadequate anaesthesia from unilateral block, missed segments or incorrectly positioned epidural catheter.
- Epidural catheter problems such as kinking, knotting, dislodgement, migration, disconnection, blockage.

Technique for Lumbar Epidural Block

1. Position: sitting or lateral position, as in spinal block (See page 399).
2. Needle: 8- or 9-cm long, 16G epidural needle with 18G epidural catheter, or 18G needle with 20G catheter.
3. Conduct of block
   - Identify the midline and the intervertebral space to be used.
   - Infiltrate the skin and subcutaneous layer with 1–2% lignocaine. Insert the epidural needle with the bevel pointing cephalad. Remove the stylet and attach the loss of resistance (LOR) syringe when the needle reaches the subcutaneous layer. Either saline or air can be used for identifying the epidural space.
   - Exert a steady pressure on the plunger of the LOR syringe as the needle is slowly advanced through the layers until the ligamentum flavum is reached. This is felt as a tough membrane and when this is breached there is a sudden loss of resistance as the epidural space is entered. Avoid injecting more air than is required to elicit LOR since air bubbles in the epidural space have been implicated in causing patchy block or missed segments.
   - Detach LOR syringe from the epidural needle and pass in the epidural catheter. If difficulty is encountered, it may help to inject a few millilitres of saline to "open up" the space.
   - Remove the epidural needle. Leave 3–5 cm of catheter within the epidural space. Aspirate to make sure that no blood or fluid appears in the catheter, and inject 1–2 ml of saline to ensure the whole catheter-connector-filter system is patent.

— Apply an antiseptic spray and secure the catheter with a sterile transparent dressing.

4. Dose of LA
   — Test dose: 3 ml of 1.5% lignocaine with adrenaline 1:200,000.
   — If test dose is negative after 5 minutes, that is, no signs of motor block or increased heart rate, give a total of 10–15 ml of LA – 0.5% bupivacaine, 0.75% ropivacaine or 2% lignocaine – in aliquots of 3–5 ml each time. Rule of thumb: 1–2 ml of LA per dermatome to be blocked.
   — Fentanyl 50–100 μg may be added to improve the quality of block.
   — Test the sensory level and ensure that the block is adequate for the surgical procedure before allowing the surgeon to proceed.

Technique for Thoracic Epidural Block

One should be familiar with lumbar epidural block before attempting a thoracic epidural since this is technically more demanding.

— Anatomical landmarks
- C7: protuberant cervical process
- T3: origin of the spine of scapula
- T7: tip of scapula
- L1: tip of the 12th rib

— The patient's position, epidural equipment and conduct of anaesthesia are similar to those of lumbar epidural anaesthesia with these exceptions.
- The thoracic spines at the mid-thoracic level (T3–T7) are steeply angulated; hence the needle direction should be acutely angled at 45–60° cephalad to get into the interspace. A paramedian approach may be used.
- The ligamentum flavum is thinner in the thoracic spine; hence loss of resistance is more difficult to perceive.
- An alternative way of identifying the epidural space is the "hanging drop" technique. Upon inserting the epidural needle subcutaneously, a drop of saline is placed at the hub of the needle, which is then advanced slowly inwards. As the ligamentum flavum is breached, the drop is sucked into the needle by the negative pressure in the epidural space.
- The dose of LA used is comparatively lower – usually 1 ml or less of LA per thoracic dermatome to be blocked. A total dose of 8 ml is usually adequate.

COMBINED SPINAL-EPIDURAL (CSE) ANAESTHESIA

This is a relatively new technique of regional anaesthesia. It is attractive since it combines the best features of spinal block (fast onset, small LA dose, profound blockade, reliable anaesthesia) and epidural block (titratable levels, ability to prolong block indefinitely) and avoids their respective disadvantages (spinal: inability to extend the block in single-shot technique; epidural: missed segments, incomplete motor block, need for large doses of LA). However, CSE is more than a spinal block followed by an epidural block; spinal blockade can be modified by subsequent epidural drug administration, and prior dural puncture can influence the characteristics of epidurally administered drugs.

There are numerous techniques described in the literature: single pass, needle-through-needle, separate needles (single or separate interspaces) and double-barrel parallel needles. The needle-through-needle technique is the most popular and packaged combination sets are commercially available (e.g., BD Durasafe™, B Braun Espocan™, Portex CSEcure™). This consists of an epidural needle with or without an additional aperture ("back eye") at the end of the longitudinal axis that permits passage of a spinal needle as it is introduced. The back eye is designed to ensure that the dural puncture site is displaced from the epidural catheter and lessen the remote possibility of passing the epidural catheter through the hole made by dural puncture. The spinal needle provided is a 27G pencil-point needle (e.g., BD Whitacre™) that protrudes 10–12 mm beyond the epidural needle when maximally introduced. Various mechanisms for spinal needle stabilization may be incorporated in the CSE set (e.g., ratchet device, "docking" device).

Indications

— Same as that for spinal and epidural anaesthesia. See page 398 and page 400.

Problems and Complications

— Same as that for spinal and epidural anaesthesia. See page 398 and page 401.

— Failure of spinal component of needle-through-needle CSE: 5–10% of cases, this tends to decrease as one becomes more familiar with the technique.

— Failure of the epidural in CSE.

— Problems with epidural after spinal blockade.

- Accidental subarachnoid placement or migration of epidural catheter through the hole created by spinal needle (extremely rare).

- Problem with epidural test dose in the presence of a spinal block.
- Inability to detect paraesthesia during epidural catheter placement.
- Delay in placement of epidural catheter may alter final characteristics of spinal block.

— Intentional dural puncture increases the risk of meningitis from poor aseptic technique.

Note that the incidence of postdural puncture headache is not increased with the use of fine pencil-point spinal needles.

Technique

1. Position
   - — Same as for spinal or epidural. See page 399.
   - — The sitting position is preferred because hydrostatic pressure in the spinal column is greater and CSF backflow can be more readily appreciated in this position.

2. Needle
   - — 9 cm long, 18G epidural needle with or without "back eye".
   - — 27G pencil-point spinal needle.
   - — 20G epidural catheter.

3. Conduct of block
   - — It is important that the midline is accurately identified to increase the success rate of the CSE procedure. It is also important not to go higher than L2–L3 interspace.
   - — The epidural space is located by means of loss of resistance to air. This offers the theoretical advantage over saline in that dural puncture with the backflow of CSF would not be confused with saline. However, anaesthesiologists who are familiar with the saline technique do not find this a problem.
   - — The spinal needle is passed through the epidural needle. For epidural needle with a back eye, the bevel of the spinal needle must face the same way as the Huber opening of the epidural needle to ensure proper passage of the spinal needle through the back eye. Successful dural puncture is often felt as a click.

— The stylet of the spinal needle is removed and CSF should appear in the hub of the needle within a few seconds.
— Local anaesthetic is injected slowly and the spinal needle is withdrawn. The epidural catheter is inserted 3–5cm into the epidural space and anchored at the skin.

4. Dose of LA
— There are various regimes used. In the low-dose ("sequential CSE") technique, a smaller than usual spinal dose (e.g., < 2 ml of 0.5% hyperbaric bupivacaine) is given followed by epidural top-up 15–20 minutes later to achieve the desired block height. Even though this technique is time-consuming, it allows neuraxial blockade to be restricted to the lowest level needed and minimizes sympathetic blockade, making it a useful technique for high-risk patients.
— Most anaesthesiologists use the full dose CSE technique in which the usual dose of spinal anaesthetic is administered initially, and additional doses via the epidural catheter are administered only when necessary.
— A technique of epidural volume expansion to increase the height of spinal blockade has been described. In this technique, 5–10 ml of saline is injected through the epidural needle immediately after placing the spinal block and before inserting the epidural catheter. In doing so, the spinal dose can be reduced by 20% to achieve the same level of blockade.
— If surgery is still in progress when the spinal anaesthetic is wearing off, an aliquot of 3–5 ml of 0.5% bupivacaine is injected slowly through the epidural catheter after aspiration is made to exclude the presence of blood or CSF.
— If surgery has ended, a continuous infusion of 0.1% bupivacaine or ropivacaine with 2 μg/ml fentanyl is started at a rate of 6–8 ml/hr.

CAUDAL ANAESTHESIA

This is an epidural blockade performed through the sacrococcygeal membrane at the sacral hiatus. Caudal anaesthesia is particularly useful in the paediatric age group. In children less than 8 years old, the block is easier to perform, spread of LA in the caudal space is more predictable, and postoperative analgesia can be provided by leaving an epidural catheter *in situ*.

Indications

- Single-shot caudal block can be performed for surgery involving the perineum and lower abdomen, such as circumcision, herniotomy, dilatation and currettage, anal dilatation, haemorrhoidectomy.
- By means of epidural catheter in younger children, the level of anaesthesia can be extended to cover operations in the upper abdomen such as hepatobiliary surgery.
- It has been used in obstetric analgesia during the second stage of labour, either as a sole technique or to supplement epidural block in the event of inadequate perineal analgesia. Its use has declined due to concerns about its complications, in particular accidental puncture of the fetal head.

Complications

- Accidental dural puncture with intrathecal injection of large volumes of LA, leading to total spinal and cardiovascular collapse.
- Intraosseus injection of LA with rapid systemic absorption and toxicity.
- Penetration of pelvic viscera and blood vessels, resulting in bleeding into the caudal space, and injury to fetal head in obstetric analgesia.
- Infection.
- Urinary retention leading to inability to void for 6–8 hours.
- Misplacement of needle into subcutaneous tissue resulting in failed block.

Technique

1. Position
   - Lateral decubitus position with shoulders and knees flexed.
   - Sometimes prone, knee-chest position in an awake patient.

2. Needle
   - 23G for children; 21G for adults.
   - 18G cannula if a 20G epidural catheter is to be inserted.

3. Landmarks
   - Posterior superior iliac spines (PSIS), tip of coccyx.
   - Guteal crease: the sacral hiatus is usually found at the top of the gluteal crease.

4. Point of entry
   - The sacral hiatus, identified by palpating the tip of coccyx and advancing cephalad until defect in the sacral vertebra is felt, or located at the tip of an imaginary equilateral triangle formed by PSIS on both sides.

5. Conduct of block
   - The needle is angled 45° and advanced until a loss of resistance is felt on piercing the sacrococcygeal membrane.
   - Do not advance the needle further than 1–2 mm to avoid puncturing the dura or epidural veins.
   - Inject LA slowly through the needle after aspirating carefully for blood or CSF. There should be minimal resistance to injection and with no evidence of swelling in the subcutaneous tissue of the sacral hiatus.
   - In the catheter technique, a 20G epidural catheter is introduced through the 18G cannula. The length of catheter left in the space corresponds to the level at which the catheter tip is to be sited. This catheter technique should only be performed in children as it is prone to failure in adults.
   - In the adult, the needle is angled 70–80° and inserted to pierce the sacrococcygeal membrane. It is then readjusted and advanced further into the epidural space. This advancement is not recommended in children.

6. Dose of LA
   - Children: 0.25% bupivacaine at 0.5 ml/kg for low lumbar and sacral block.
   - Adult: 20–30 ml of 0.25% bupivacaine is usually required for surgical anesthesia; 10–15 ml of 1% lignocaine with adrenaline is used for perineal analgesia during labour.
   - Countercheck to ensure that the maximum safe dose of 2 mg/kg is not exceeded for bupivacaine.

FURTHER READING

1. Rodgers A, Walker N, Schug S, et al. Reduction of postoperative mortality and morbidity in anaesthesia: Results from overview of randomized trials. Br Med J 2000;321:1493–1510.
2. Rawal N. Combined regional and general anesthesia. Curr Opin Anaesthesiol 2000;13:531–7.
3. Loo SS, MacDonald SB. Current issues in spinal anesthesia. Anesthesiology 2001;94:888–906.
4. Horlocker TT, Wedel DJ. Neurologic complications of spinal and epidural anesthesia. Reg Anesth Pain Med 2000;25:83–98.
5. Reynolds F. Damage to the conus medullaris after spinal anaesthesia. Anaesthesia 2001;56:238–47.
6. Stienstra R. Mechanisms behind and treatment of sudden, unexpected circulatory collapse during central neuraxis blockade. Acta Anaesthesiol Scand 2000;44:965–71.
7. Pollard JB. Cardiac arrest during spinal anesthesia: Common mechanisms and strategies for prevention. Anesth Analg 2001;92:252–6.
8. Freedman JM, Li DK, Drasner K, et al. Transient neurologic symptoms after spinal anesthesia: An epidemiologic study of 1863 patients. Anesthesiology 1998;89:633–41.
9. Cook TM. Combined spinal-epidural techniques. Anaesthesia 2000;55:42–64.
10. Rawal N, Holmstrom B, Crowhurst JA, van Zundert A. The combined spinal-epidural technique. Anesthesiol Clin North Am 2000;18:267–95.
11. Tobias JD. Caudal epidural block: A review of test dosing and recognition of systemic injection in children. Anesth Analg 2001;93:1156–61.

Chapter 33

Regional Anaesthetic Techniques II: Neural Plexus and Nerve Blocks

INTRODUCTION

Regional anaesthetic techniques in the form of neural plexus and nerve blocks are described in this chapter. The reader is again advised to refer to specific textbooks on regional anaesthesia for more detailed descriptions of such techniques.

Peripheral nerve blocks are versatile anaesthetic techniques which do not incur significant haemodynamic changes provided that precaution is taken to avoid complications such as inadvertent intravascular (for most blocks) or intrathecal (for certain blocks such as interscalene block) injections and pneumothorax (for supraclavicular block). As such, they are excellent anaesthetic options for patients who are at high risk for general anaesthesia and central neuraxial blockade. Most of these blocks are not difficult to perform and they require nothing more than practice, experience, as well as a good working knowledge of the relevant anatomy. The anaesthesiologist would then have a whole armament of useful regional blocks at his/her disposal, which can be used as sole anaesthetic techniques, in combination with general anaesthesia, and as a means of providing effective postoperative analgesia.

GENERAL CONSIDERATIONS FOR NEURAL PLEXUS/NERVE BLOCKS

1. **Explanation and consent**
   - As in central neuraxial blockade, patients suitable for peripheral nerve blocks should be identified and any contraindications excluded.
   - Explanation and consent are steps that are equally pertinent in peripheral nerve blocks as in central neuraxial blocks. Patients should be forewarned about the end-points elicited, either in the form of paraesthesia or muscle twitches on stimulation by peripheral nerve stimulator.
   - In adult patients, the nerve blocks should be performed before induction of general anaesthesia if a combined RA–GA technique is planned. Such blocks are usually inserted under general anaesthesia in paediatric patients.

2. **Preparation before procedure**
   - The anaesthesiologist should be familiar with the relevant anatomy, technique and possible complications associated with the regional block. The reader is encouraged to visit www.nysora.com, an excellent website maintained by the New York School of Regional Anesthesia, which contains a wealth of knowledge and practical tips on regional anaesthetic techniques.
   - Drugs such as thiopentone, ephedrine, atropine and suxamethonium should be prepared prior to the procedure in case complications to the block arise, or if conversion to general anaesthesia becomes necessary. Anaesthetic and airway equipment should be checked and ready for use.
   - An intravenous access should be established and the patient should be monitored with ECG, BP and pulse oximetry during the procedure.

3. **Performing the block**
   - All blocks should be performed under aseptic technique.
   - Local anaesthetic (LA) is infiltrated subcutaneously at the designated needle insertion site. The nerves may be shallow in certain blocks, and care should

be taken only to infiltrate LA in the subcutaneous tissue plane. Deeper needle insertion may risk injection into the nerve sheath and a consequent difficulty in obtaining the twitch response.

— Progression of the needle through tissue planes can be better appreciated by using a short-bevelled needle rather than a hypodermic needle. As the needle tip is blunt, the point of entry at the skin should be pierced with an ordinary needle first before introducing the block needle.
— Determine the appropriate end-point, for example:
  - Paraesthesia or muscle twitch on current stimulation with peripheral nerve stimulator for peripheral nerve blocks.
  - Loss of resistance to air or saline for interpleural block.
— Careful aspiration before injecting the LA lessens the chance of inadvertent intravascular injection. This also lessens the chance of inadvertent intrathecal injection in interscalene block.
— Do not persist when resistance is met on injection of LA solution, because it often means that the correct tissue plane has not been entered or that the block needle has been misplaced. Reposition the needle with guidance from the nerve stimulator and attempt to inject once more. If the same problem persists, remove and flush the needle to make sure that it is patent, and repeat the whole procedure.
— Similarly, do not persist when the patient complains of severe pain on injection. The block needle may be located intraneurally and further injection may cause nerve damage.
— Maintain close communication with the patient at all times to detect early signs of LA toxicity or overdose.

4. **Use of peripheral nerve stimulator**
— This is an excellent tool to facilitate the performance of many nerve blocks as it provides an objective end-point without having to elicit paraesthesia from the patient.
— The nerve stimulator should be specifically designed for nerve blocks and should not incorporate features for monitoring neuromuscular blockade.
— The use of plastic coated insulated, short-bevelled block needles specific for the purpose (e.g., Stimuplex® needle) may lessen the likelihood of nerve penetration and intraneural injection, reducing the potential of nerve damage. An insulated needle concentrates current density at the tip of the needle and improves accuracy by allowing a more precise localization of the nerve(s).

- The polarity should be clearly displayed and the block needle should always be connected to the negative lead. Higher currents are required if the polarity is reversed. An ECG electrode is connected to the positive lead and placed on the patient at least 20 cm from the site of the block.
- Usual initial settings of the nerve stimulator when the block is performed are current strength 1.0 mA, pulse duration 0.1 ms and pulse frequency 2 Hz.
- Current strength is reduced stepwise when nerve stimulation and contraction of the relevant muscle group is elicited, usually down to 0.3–0.5 mA when muscle contraction is just visible. The needle should be withdrawn slightly if contraction is still seen at 0.1 mA as this may suggest intraneural placement of needle.
- If visible contractions of the target muscle continue to occur at the threshold current, check that no blood is aspirated then inject the LA solution slowly, 5 ml at a time. There should be no resistance or pain to injection.
- Muscle twitch is seen to be abolished on injection of LA, further confirming the correct placement of the block needle.

5. **After the block**
   - Closely monitor the patient's blood pressure, heart rate and oxygen saturation.
   - Test the level of sensory block using spirit swab (temperature), pinprick (pain) or touch. An effective block should be accompanied by sympathetic blockade in the form of vasodilation with warm extremities, and motor blockade in the form of limb paresis or paralysis.
   - Give adequate time for the block to take effect before allowing surgery to commence. Test the surgical site for anaesthesia before proceeding with skin incision.
   - Consider converting to general anaesthesia if the degree of block is not satisfactory after sufficient time has elapsed and sufficient dose has been given. Do not supplement inadequate regional anaesthesia with heavy sedation.
   - Watch for complications of local anaesthetic toxicity, such as hypotension, bradycardia, nausea or vomiting, circumoral tingling or respiratory distress. Institute treatment early.

6. **Postoperative orders and follow-up**
   - Placement of catheters in certain regional blocks allows continuation of analgesia into the postoperative period. Continued management of such patients can be carried out by the Acute Pain Service (APS) team.

— Follow up patients in the ward particularly those who developed complications of block, e.g., pneumothorax following supraclavicular brachial plexus block.

NEURAL PLEXUS/NERVE BLOCKS OF THE UPPER LIMB

A. Brachial Plexus Block

The brachial plexus is formed by anterior rami of C5–8 and T1. Various techniques have been described to block the branches of the brachial plexus at different levels, namely the interscalene, supraclavicular, infraclavicular and axillary approaches. These are the indications for using this block.

— Surgery of the upper limb.

— Sympathetic blockade in an attempt to promote vasodilation and improve perfusion: microvascular surgery (e.g., reimplantation of digits), management following inadvertent intraarterial injection of thiopentone.

a. Interscalene approach

In the interscalene approach, the nerve roots within the fascial sheath between scalenus anterior and scalenus medius are anaesthetized. This is the regional anaesthetic technique of choice for shoulder surgery and can be performed without having to position the arm – an advantage in painful conditions of the upper limb. However, it is likely that the lower trunk of the brachial plexus which supplies the ulnar nerve sensory distribution may not be well blocked. Since ipsilateral diaphragmatic paralysis secondary to phrenic nerve block almost inevitably occurs, it should be used with caution (if at all) in patients who have severe respiratory disease.

Technique (Figure 33–1)

1. Position
   — The patient is placed supine with the head turned to the opposite side.
   — The arm can be in any position, but preferably on the chest to allow for detection of muscle twitch responses to nerve stimulation.
2. Needle: A 3–5 cm long, 22G or 23G short-bevelled insulated needle is used.

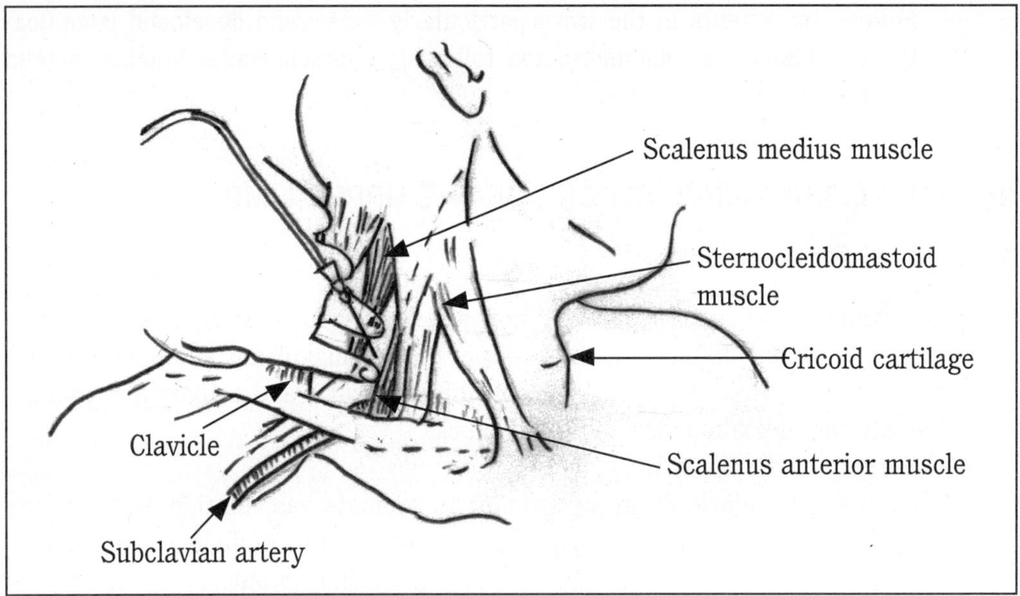

Figure 33–1. Brachial plexus block: Interscalene approach

3. Landmarks
   — The sternocleidomastoid muscle is accentuated by making the patient raise the head slightly off the table. Identify the sternal and clavicular heads of the muscle.
   — The scalene muscles are accentuated by maximal inspiration.
   — The cricoid cartilage denotes the level of transverse process of C6.
4. Conduct of block
   — Feel for the lateral border of clavicular head of sternocleidomastoid at C6 level.
   — Roll the index finger laterally across the belly of scalenus anterior (immediately lateral and deep to the border of the sternocleidomastoid) until the interscalene groove is felt.
   — The needle is inserted into the interscalene groove perpendicular to the skin and aimed caudad and medially.
   — End-points to look out for:
     - A click from the short-bevelled needle is not always obvious because the brachial plexus sheath is thinnest at the interscalene area.

- Twitch at biceps and/or deltoid muscle in response to electrical stimulation may be observed.
- Paraesthesia below the level of the shoulder may be elicited.

  Note that paraesthesia at the shoulder is not acceptable as it may be due to direct stimulation of the supraclavicular nerve.

— If bone is contacted without eliciting the end-point, the needle is "walked" antero-posteriorly along the transverse process of C6 until a positive end-point is elicited.

— Carefully aspirate for blood or CSF before slowly injecting LA. Apply digital pressure above the injection site to aid caudal spread.

— If a catheter technique is planned, the catheter is inserted through the Tuohy-style insulated needle after injection of LA and advanced into the space. The needle needs to be properly stabilized for catheter advancement to ensure that the needle is not displaced. A slight caudal orientation of the needle may facilitate catheter insertion.

— The onset time for this block is short. The first sign of the blockade is the loss of coordination of the shoulder and arm muscles that occurs sooner than the onset of sensory blockade or temperature change.

5. Dose of LA

   — Large volumes are needed to ensure that the lower trunk is anaesthetized. Usual amount: 30–40 ml of 0.25–0.375% bupivacaine in adult, injected at 5 ml aliquots.

   — It is advisable to inject 2 ml first and wait for 30 seconds before injecting the rest of the LA solution. This allows detection of an inadvertent injection into the vertebral artery.

6. Possible complications

   — Inadvertent spinal or epidural anaesthesia.

   — Inadvertent intravascular injection with vessel puncture of internal or external jugular vein, common carotid artery or vertebral artery.

   — Phrenic nerve block.

   — Stellate ganglion block resulting in Horner's syndrome.

   — Recurrent laryngeal nerve palsy.

7. Alternative approach

   — Instead of the C6 level, the needle insertion site may be located wherever the interscalene groove is felt most prominently, usually at the lateral border of the sternocleidomastoid muscle just above the clavicle. The interscalene groove at this level is shallower and easier to identify, and the risk of vascular puncture is less because the needle insertion is more lateral. It is especially useful when the external jugular vein crosses the interscalene groove at the level of the cricoid cartilage.

— Landmarks include the clavicle, lateral border of the clavicular head of the sternocleidomastoid muscle and the external jugular vein.
— Palpate for the interscalene groove as described, at a level just above the clavicle.
— Insert the block needle and advance it at an angle almost perpendicular to the skin plane in a slight caudal direction. Advance the needle slowly until stimulation of the brachial plexus is obtained, typically at a depth of 1–2 cm in almost all patients. The needle should not be advanced beyond 2.5 cm to avoid the risk of complications (cervical cord injury, pneumothorax, carotid artery puncture).
— Once appropriate twitches of the brachial plexus are elicited, slowly inject 35–40 ml of LA with intermittent aspiration to rule out intravascular injection.

b. Supraclavicular approach

In the supraclavicular approach, the trunks emerging from the interscalene groove are blocked in the posterior triangle of the neck. At this point the nerve trunks are most compactly arranged; the required volume is lower and the onset of block is more rapid. The block can be performed with the arm in virtually any position. The drawbacks are risks of pneumothorax and phrenic nerve palsy. Bilateral supraclavicular blocks should not be performed, and this block is contraindicated in patients with significant respiratory disease.

Two methods have been described: the classical method (Patrick) and the subclavian perivascular technique (Winnie). The classical method is not described here; it has become less popular because it is associated with the highest incidence of inadvertent pneumothorax.

Winnie's Subclavian Perivascular Technique (Figure 33–2)

1. Position and needle: these are the same as the interscalene approach. See page 413.
2. Landmarks: these include the interscalene groove, the clavicle and pulsation of subclavian artery identified at the lower end of interscalene groove.

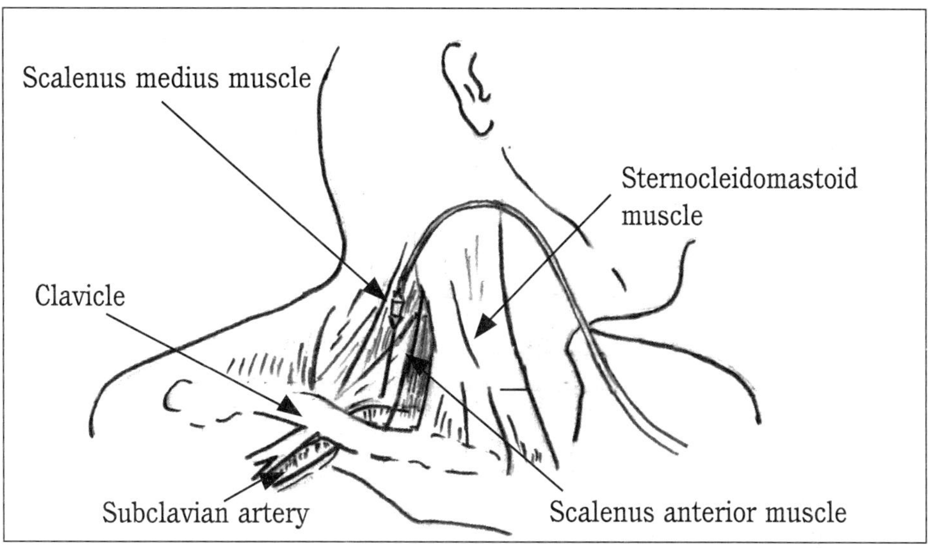

Figure 33–2. Brachial plexus block: Supraclavicular approach

3. Conduct of block
   — The needle insertion site is the base of the interscalene groove directly above the pulsation of the subclavian artery.
   — If the artery is not well palpated, insert the needle as low in the interscalene groove and as close to the scalenus medius as possible. This corresponds to a line between the mastoid process and midpoint of clavicle.
   — Direct the needle caudally until response to electrical stimulation or paraesthesia is elicited. A click may be perceived when the needle pierces the sheath. The optimal response is middle trunk stimulation, shown by hand contraction or paraesthesia, as this response has been associated with higher rates of success for surgery of the hand.
   — If the first rib is contacted without eliciting nerve stimulation or paraesthesia, "walk" the needle antero-posteriorly along the rib until a response is obtained. If the appropriate response is not encountered with either approach, the needle may be further walked more laterally, and lastly more medially seeking stimulation or paraesthesia.

4. Dose of LA
   — Volume of LA solution is comparatively smaller: 20 ml of 0.25–0.375% bupivacaine in adult is usually sufficient for the block.

5. Possible complications include:
   — Pneumothorax.
   — Haemothorax (puncture of subclavian artery).
   — Phrenic nerve palsy.
   — Recurrent laryngeal nerve palsy.
   — Stellate ganglion block.

c. Infraclavicular approach

The infraclavicular approach can be considered an alternative to the axillary approach in cases where arm abduction is painful or difficult, or when infection is present at the axilla. It is devoid of complications associated with the interscalene or supraclavicular approaches, and its popularity has exceeded the supraclavicular approach. If postoperative analgesia is provided via an indwelling catheter, there is less risk of catheter dislodgement or infection since the infraclavicular region is relatively clean and not subjected to excessive movement.

This approach is considered to be the regional anaesthetic technique of choice for surgery of the hand, wrist, elbow and distal arm. It also provides excellent analgesia for application of arm tourniquet. However, this block is technically more difficult to perform and requires the use of peripheral nerve stimulator. Many techniques have been described for infraclavicular block, such as modified lateral technique and the vertical infraclavicular block (VIB) technique. The coracoid approach is described here.

Technique: Coracoid approach (Figure 33–3)

1. Position
   — The patient is placed supine with the head maintained in the neutral position.
   — The arm can be in any position as long as it enables a clear unobstructed detection of the twitches of the hand, either with the elbow flexed and hand on the abdomen, or the arm abducted and flexed at the elbow.
2. Needle: A 10 cm 22G insulated short-bevelled needle is used in conjunction with a nerve stimulator.
3. Landmarks: The coracoid process is identified by palpation of the bony prominence just medial to the shoulder, while the arm is elevated and lowered. As the arm is lowered, the coracoid process meets the fingers of the palpating hand.

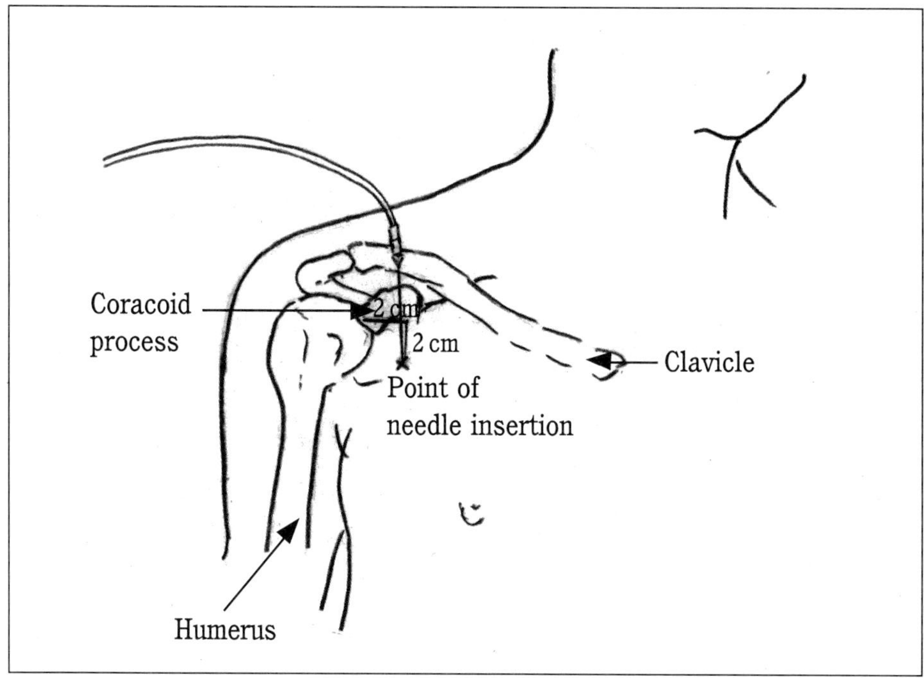

Figure 33–3. Brachial plexus block: Infraclavicular approach

4. Conduct of block
   — The needle insertion point is 2 cm medial and 2 cm caudad from the most lateral aspect of the coracoid process. The needle is passed directly posteriorly.
   — The nerve stimulator is initially set to deliver 1.5 mA. A local twitch of the pectoralis muscle is typically elicited as the needle is advanced beyond the subcutaneous tissue at a depth of 1–3 cm.
   — Once the pectoralis twitches disappear, lower the current to 1.0 mA and advance the needle slowly, looking for stimulation of the brachial plexus at the hand muscles. This is usually encountered at a depth 5–8 cm.
   — Often the axillary or musculocutaneous nerve is first stimulated (biceps or deltoid muscle twitches) but these responses seem to yield lower rates of successful blockade and should be disregarded. Ideal twitch response is that of the median nerve stimulation evident by hand/finger flexion, as this indicates a relatively central position of the needle in the plexus.

— The stimulating current is slowly decreased to 0.3 mA or less. Inject LA after negative aspiration for blood.
— If a catheter technique is planned, the catheter is inserted through the Tuohy-style insulated needle after injection of LA and advanced 5 cm into the space.
— A typical onset time for this block is 5–15 minutes depending on the LA chosen. Waiting beyond 20 minutes will not result in further enhancement of the blockade. The first sign of the impending successful blockade is loss of muscle coordination, which usually precedes onset of sensory blockade.

5. Dose of LA
— Bolus injection: 30–40 ml of 0.25–0.375% bupivacaine; or a mixture of equivolumes of 2% lignocaine and 0.5% bupivacaine.
— Continuous infusion: 0.25% bupivacaine at 20–30 mg/hr (8–12 ml/hr), started approximately 1 hour after the bolus injection.

6. Possible complications
— This is a relatively safe technique with no specific complications other than haematoma, systemic toxicity and nerve injury.
— Pneumothorax is exceedingly rare, as the needle is directed away from the chest cavity.

d. Axillary approach

In the axillary approach, LA is deposited around the origins of the lateral, medial and posterior cords as they form a neurovascular bundle surrounding the axillary artery. This block is indicated for forearm and hand surgery. It is relatively simple to perform with or without the use of a nerve stimulator, and is devoid of serious complications other than haematoma around the axillary artery. However, the arm needs to be abducted for the block to be performed; the radial, axillary and musculocutaneous nerves may be missed resulting in inadequate anaesthesia and poor tolerance to application of upper limb tourniquet.

Technique (Figure 33–4)

1. Position
— The patient is placed supine. The arm is abducted to 80°, externally rotated and with the elbow flexed.
— Overabduction of the arm beyond 90° should be avoided as it makes palpation of the axillary artery pulse difficult, impedes circumferential

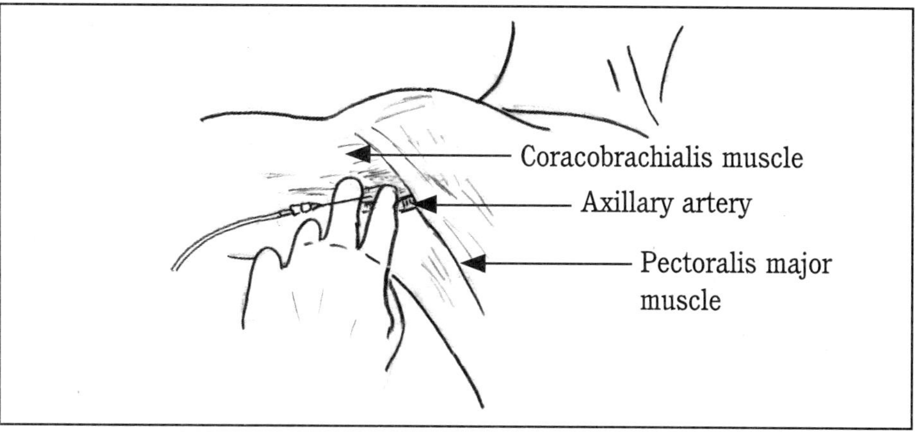

Figure 33–4. Brachial plexus block: Axillary approach

spread of LA, and may stretch the brachial plexus components increasing the risk of nerve injury during needle advancement.
- The anaesthesiologist sits by the patient's side to avoid strain and hand movement during the procedure.

2. Needle: A 3–5 cm long 22G short-bevelled insulated needle is used.
3. Landmarks: These consist of the axillary artery, coracobrachialis and pectoralis major muscles.
4. Conduct of block
   - Palpate for the axillary artery just below the coracobrachialis muscle and lateral to the pectoralis major. The point of entry is at the most proximal pulsation of axillary artery where it disappears under the pectoralis major.
   - Straddle the artery between the index and the middle finger and firmly press against the humerus at the midaxillary fossa level. This manoeuvre compresses the soft tissues of the axilla, provides distal traction and stabilizes the axillary artery during block performance. This hand should not be moved during the entire procedure.
   - Set the nerve stimulator to deliver 1 mA current initially. Insert the needle just in front of the palpating fingers and advance slowly towards the apex of the axilla at an angle 45° cephalad.
   - A definite click is felt as the needle penetrates the axillary sheath. Contractions are sought in the area of the median nerve or the radial nerve.

The needle, if properly positioned within the neurovascular bundle, can be seen to move with arterial pulsation. This occurs at a depth of 1–2 cm in most patients.

- Once the response is elicited, slowly inject LA through the needle after careful aspiration. Aspirate repeatedly to rule out intravascular injection. Firm digital pressure is applied to the artery distal to the injection site to promote proximal spread of LA.
- Multiple stimulation techniques (stimulating and injecting each major nerve of the brachial plexus separately) have been advocated to increase the success rate of the axillary block. However, there is also a corresponding increase in complexity and time required to complete the block.
- If the axillary artery is punctured during the block, insert the needle through the artery to reach the posterior wall, deposit half the amount of LA after aspirating to make sure that the needle is not in the artery. Withdraw the needle until the needle is just out of the artery (no more blood aspirated), deposit the rest of the LA anterior to the artery.
- To block the musculocutaneous nerve, insert the needle above the artery and towards the coracobrachialis muscle. Inject 5 ml of LA when twitches at the biceps are observed on nerve stimulation. Alternatively, the extension of the nerve to the forearm can be located at the elbow 1 cm proximal to the lateral elbow flexion crease in the groove formed by the biceps and brachioradialis muscle. The nerve is blocked by injecting 3 ml of LA.
- Infiltrate subcutaneously around the medial part of the upper arm to block the intercostobrachial nerve.
- The first sign of the blockade is the loss of the coordination of the arm and forearm muscles. This sign can be seen usually sooner than the onset of sensory or temperature change. When this sign is present within 1–2 minutes after injection, it has a very high positive predictive value for a pending successful brachial plexus blockade.

5. Dose of LA
   - Bolus injection: 30–40 ml of 0.25–0.5% ropivacaine; or a mixture of equivolumes of 2% lignocaine and 0.5% ropivacaine.
   - Continuous infusion: 0.2% ropivacaine at 20–30 mg/hr (10–15 ml/hr) started approximately 1 hour after the bolus injection.
   - Some authors advise caution against the use of bupivacaine because of its high cardiotoxicity profile and potential for inadvertent intravascular injection with the axillary block technique.

6. Possible complications
   - This is a relatively safe technique with no specific complications other than haematoma, systemic toxicity and nerve injury.
   - If the axillary artery is inadvertently punctured, firm digital pressure should be applied to the artery to prevent haematoma formation.

B. Wrist Block

The nerves to be blocked are the terminal branches of the ulnar, median and radial nerves. The technique is simple to perform, essentially devoid of systemic complications, and highly effective for a variety of procedures on the hand and fingers. The LA solution used for wrist block should not contain adrenaline.

Technique

The patient lies supine with the arm abducted and a slight dorsiflexion at the wrist.

1. Ulnar nerve block
   - The nerve passes between the ulnar artery and tendon of the flexor carpi ulnaris which is superficial to the ulnar nerve. Identify the flexor carpi ulnaris tendon by asking the patient to flex the wrist against resistance.
   - The ulnar nerve is anaesthetized by inserting the needle under the tendon of the flexor carpi ulnaris just above the styloid process of the ulna. Advance the needle by 5–10 mm to just past the tendon of the flexor carpi ulnaris. Paraesthesia may be elicited. Inject 3–5 ml of LA.
   - Infiltrate 3–5 ml of LA subcutaneously around the ulnar aspect of the wrist to block the cutaneous branches that often extend to the hypothenar area.

2. Median nerve block
   - The nerve is located between the tendons of the palmaris longus and the flexor carpi radialis. Note that the palmaris longus may be absent in some patients.
   - The median nerve is blocked by inserting the needle between the tendons of the palmaris longus and flexor carpi radialis. Advance the needle until it pierces the deep fascia or until it contacts the bone. If bone is contacted, the needle is withdrawn 2–3 mm and 3–5 ml of LA is injected.

- A "fan" technique is recommended to increase the success rate of the block. After the initial injection, the needle is withdrawn back to the skin level, redirected 30° laterally, and advanced again to contact the bone. After pulling back 1–2 mm off the bone, an additional 2 ml of LA is injected. This is repeated with a 30° medial redirection of the needle.
- Paraesthesia may or may not be elicited.

3. Radial nerve block
   - The radial nerve passes along the front of the radial side of the forearm. About 3 inches above the wrist, it pierces the deep fascia and divides into the external and internal branches. On the back of the hand, it forms an arch with the dorsal cutaneous branch of the ulnar nerve.
   - The radial nerve block is essentially a "field block" because of its less predictable anatomic location and division into multiple, smaller, cutaneous branches.
   - Inject 3–5 ml of LA subcutaneously just above the radial styloid, aiming medially. Extend the infiltration around the radial border of the wrist to just past the midline dorsally using an additional 3–5 ml of LA.
   - The ring of infiltration should not extend around the whole circumference of the wrist. Care should be taken not to injure the subcutaneous veins.

A typical onset time for a wrist block is 10–15 min depending primarily on the concentration of LA used. Sensory anaesthesia of the skin develops faster than the motor block. Complications after wrist block are typically limited to residual paraesthesia due to an inadvertent intraneural injection. Systemic toxicity is rare because of the distal location of the block.

C. Intravenous Regional Anaesthesia (IVRA)

This block was first described by a German surgeon August Bier in 1908. The technique is remarkably simple and reliable. Anaesthesia provided is adequate for minor surgery on the forearm and hand that lasts up to 1 hour, such as carpal tunnel release, excision of ganglion, tendon contracture release and foreign body extraction. Its use for longer surgical procedures is precluded by the appearance of the discomfort from the tourniquet. Its drawback is the lack of postoperative analgesia. The duration of block is limited by the duration of tourniquet; this quickly dissipates after release of the tourniquet.

Technique

- Insert an intravenous cannula into a peripheral vein at the dorsum of the hand to be blocked, and another cannula at the contralateral hand for intravenous access if required.
- Place a tourniquet on the arm of the extremity to be blocked. A "double cuff" tourniquet is preferred in order to increase the reliability of the technique and help reduce the tourniquet pressure pain. The tourniquet cuffs should be tested prior to use to ensure that there are no leaks in the system. If the surgeon requires a bloodless field, this can be obtained by using an Esmarch bandage. Otherwise elevate the patient's limb for 1–2 minutes to passively exsanguinate the arm.
- Inflate the proximal cuff of the tourniquet to a pressure 100 mmHg above the systolic BP (cuff pressure is usually set at 200–250 mmHg). Check that the radial pulse is absent.
- Inject LA slowly into the intravenous cannula. Rapid injection can lead to pressures high enough to cause passage of drug into the general circulation.
- When anaesthesia is established, inflate the distal tourniquet then deflate the proximal one.
- The onset of anaesthesia is within 5 minutes, typically starting with "pins and needles" sensation in the extremity. Most patients will report pressure at the site of the tourniquet after 30–45 minutes, sometimes even earlier.
- Allow at least 30 minutes to elapse before deflating the cuff. Maintain cuff inflation even if surgery ends earlier than this time.
- A 2-stage deflation is suggested whereby the cuff is deflated for 10 seconds and re-inflated for 1 minute before the final release. This practice prevents a massive "washout" of LA into the systemic circulation. Monitor the cardiovascular system closely and watch for signs of LA toxicity.
- Since the release of the tourniquet will result in a rapid resolution of anaesthesia and analgesia, the surgeon should be instructed to infiltrate the incision site with LA before skin closure. Alternatively, judicious doses of analgesic may be administered preemptively in anticipation of postoperative pain.

Local anaesthetic in IVRA

- Because of its low toxicity, prilocaine is almost always used in IVRA. The dose is 2–3 mg/kg, equivalent to 30–40 ml of 0.5% solution for an adult of 70 kg. The maximum dose is 8 mg/kg; hence there is a large margin of safety. However, this drug is no longer available in many countries and its use has been superseded by lignocaine.

- 0.5% lignocaine may be used in place of prilocaine. The dose is 3 mg/kg (up to 40 ml).
- Limited study of 0.2% ropivacaine suggests that this local anaesthetic produces longer postoperative analgesia with less central nervous system disturbance after tourniquet deflation.
- Bupivacaine is *not* used in IVRA because of its cardiotoxicity.

Problems and contraindications

- Complications of IVRA are few and are mainly limited to systemic toxicity from LA arising from an inadequate tourniquet application or equipment failure.
- Problems may also arise from venous stasis and formation of methaemoglobin from prilocaine. Hence this technique is not suitable for patients with these conditions.
    - Peripheral vascular or neurological disease.
    - Sickle cell disease.
    - Methaemoglobinaemia.
    - Congestive heart failure.

NEURAL PLEXUS/NERVE BLOCKS OF THE LOWER LIMB

A. Femoral Nerve Block and Three-in-One Block

The femoral nerve, arising from L2–L4 of the lumbar plexus, supplies the anterior aspect of the thigh, most of the femur and knee joint and the medial aspects of the leg (via the saphenous nerve) up to the big toe. A femoral nerve block is easy to perform, has a high success rate and carries a low risk of complications. It is suitable for surgical anaesthesia, analgesia for femoral fractures, as well as postoperative pain management following femur and knee surgery. When this is combined with sciatic nerve block, anaesthesia of almost the entire lower extremity from the mid-thigh level can be achieved.

Since the femoral nerve supplies the antero-medial aspect of the lower limb, blockade of this nerve alone would not be sufficient to provide adequate anaesthesia if surgery involves lateral aspects of the limb. The nerves involved in the three-in-one block are the femoral nerve, obturator nerve and lateral cutaneous nerve of the thigh. The approach is essentially that for femoral nerve block except that larger volumes are used to block the nerves. The obturator nerve is not consistently blocked via this approach.

Technique (Figure 33–5)

1. Position
   — The patient lies supine with the lower limbs fully extended, legs slightly apart and feet turned loosely to the outside.
   — In obese patients, a pillow may be placed under the hips to facilitate palpation of the femoral artery.
2. Needle: A 5 cm 22G short-bevelled needle is used.
3. Landmarks
   — These include the femoral crease and pulsation of the femoral artery.
   — It is useful to think of the mnemonic "VAN" (vein, artery, nerve) going from medial to lateral, when recalling the relationship of the femoral nerve to the vessels in the femoral triangle.

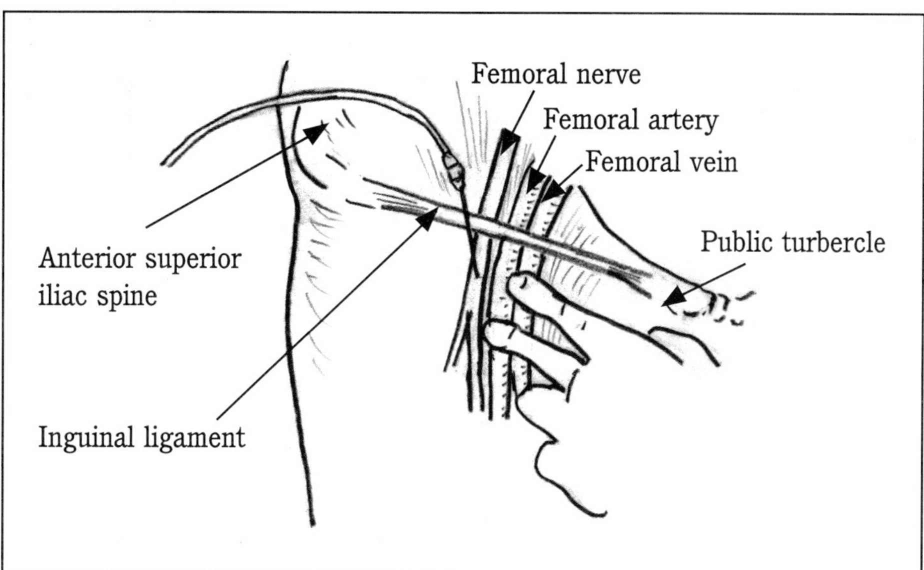

Figure 33–5. Femoral nerve block

4. Conduct of block
   - The needle insertion site is at the femoral crease (approximately 2 cm below the inguinal ligament) immediately lateral to the femoral artery pulse.
   - Insert the needle at an angle 30° to the skin and advance in a sagittal and slightly cephalad plane. As the femoral nerve is covered by the fascia lata and fascia iliaca, two clicks will be felt before the nerve is reached. Distinct paraesthesia is almost never elicited with femoral nerve block and should not be sought.
   - Look for stimulation of the quadriceps muscle – the "patellar twitch" – occurring typically at a depth of 2–3 cm. This is the optimal response and signifies stimulation of the main trunk of the femoral nerve.
   - Often the sartorius muscle is stimulated and results in a band-like contraction across the thigh without movement of the patella. This is not reliable because branches of femoral nerve supplying the sartorius muscle may be outside the femoral sheath. When this occurs, redirect the needle laterally and advance the needle by 1–3 mm.
   - After negative aspiration for blood, inject 15–20 ml of LA (femoral nerve block) or 30–40 ml of LA (three-in-one block). Apply pressure distal to the injection site to promote the spread of LA towards the lumbar plexus.
   - A typical onset time for this block is 10–15 minutes depending on the type, concentration and volume of LA used. The first sign of onset of blockade is the loss of sensation of the skin over the saphenous nerve distribution.

5. Possible complications and precautions
   - This is a relatively safe technique with no specific complications other than haematoma, systemic toxicity and nerve injury.
   - Femoral artery puncture may occur if the needle is directed too medially. The block needle is first inserted just lateral to the femoral artery; subsequent redirections should all be progressively more lateral rather than medial. When vascular puncture occurs, apply a firm and constant pressure over the femoral artery for 2–3 minutes before proceeding with the block.
   - The patient should be instructed regarding precautions for the anaesthetized lower extremity. There should be no weight-bearing until the block has completely resolved.

B. Sciatic Nerve Block

Sciatic nerve, root segments L4–S3, is the largest nerve in the lower limb. It innervates the posterior and lateral aspects of the lower limb including the knee and ankle. Sciatic nerve block results in anaesthesia of the skin of the posterior aspect of the thigh, hamstrings and biceps muscles, part of hip and knee joint, and entire leg below the knee, with the exception of the skin of the medial aspect of the lower leg (innervated by the saphenous nerve).

Various approaches have been described. The two most common ones are the posterior (transgluteal) approach according to Labat and the anterior approach according to Meier.

Posterior approach (Figure 33–6)

1. Position
   - The patient is placed in the lateral decubitus position with the side to be blocked uppermost and tilted slightly forward.
   - The lower leg is extended and the upper knee is flexed with the foot resting on the dependent leg. This enables observation of the twitches at the foot or toes during nerve stimulation.
   - This precise position should be maintained throughout the block, because even slight movements may result in significant shift of the landmarks.

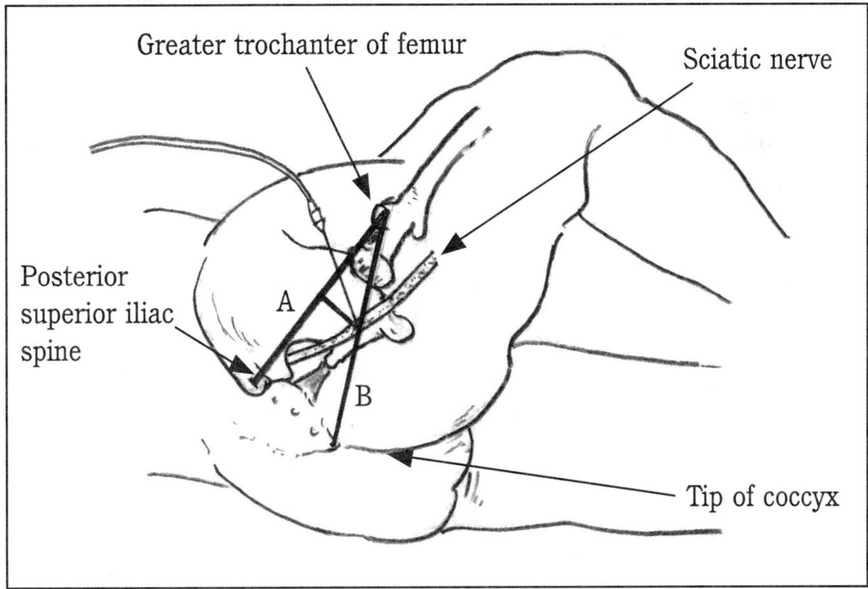

Figure 33–6. Sciatic nerve block: Posterior approach

2. Needle and landmarks: A 10 cm 22G short-bevelled needle is used. Landmarks include the greater trochanter, posterior superior iliac spine and tip of coccyx.
3. Conduct of block
   - Draw a line between the inner aspects of greater trochanter and PSIS (Line A), and another line from greater trochanter to tip of coccyx (Line B). Draw a perpendicular line from midpoint of Line A to Line B: the point of intersection is the needle insertion point.
   - Press firmly on the gluteus muscle with the fingers of the palpating hand to decrease the skin-nerve distance, and stabilize the skin between the index and middle fingers. Set the nerve stimulator to deliver 1.5 mA current and insert the needle perpendicular to the skin. Direct stimulation and contractions of the gluteal musculature will be observed first.
   - Once the gluteal twitches disappear, twitches at the hamstrings, calf musculature with plantar- or dorsiflexion of the foot are elicited. Reduce the stimulating current until twitches are still present at 0.2–0.5 mA. This typically occurs at a depth of 5–8 cm in an average-sized adult.
   - After negative aspiration for blood, slowly inject 20–30 ml of LA. Adrenaline should not be used in view of possibility of nerve ischaemia due to stretching or sitting on the anaesthetized nerve.
   - If no twitches are elicited or if bone is contacted, withdraw the needle to the skin and re-direct at 15° medially. If this fails, repeat this at 15° laterally. Reassess the landmarks and patient position, ensuring that the pelvis is slightly tilted forward, before proceeding further.
   - Onset of the block is approximately 10–25 minutes depending on the type, concentration and volume of LA used. The first signs of blockade are usually a feeling that the foot feels “different” or an inability to wiggle the toes.
4. Possible complications
   - No specific complications are observed.
   - Proper care for the lower extremity which is anaesthetized: frequent body re-positioning is needed to avoid stretching and prolonged ischaemia on the anaesthetized sciatic nerve.

Anterior approach (Figure 33–7)

This approach is technically more difficult than the posterior approach. The only part of the sciatic nerve that is accessible to blockade through an anterior approach is a short segment slightly above and below the lesser trochanter. Compared to

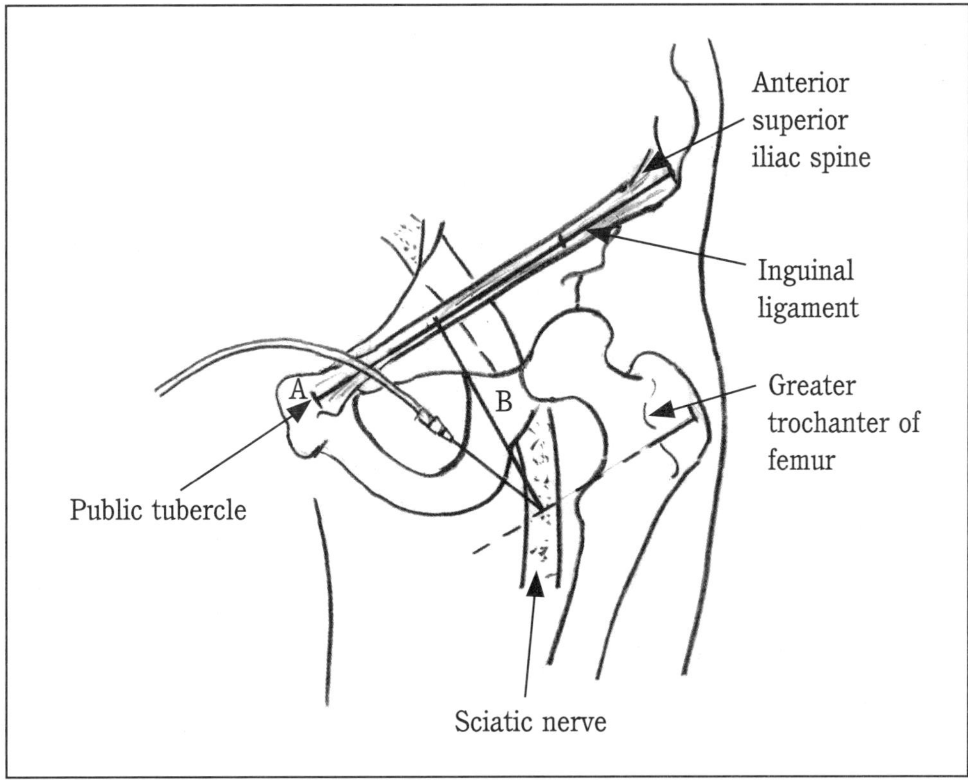

Figure 33–7. Sciatic nerve block: Anterior approach

the posterior approach, the sciatic nerve is blocked more distally and a higher level of skill is required to achieve reliable anaesthesia. This approach is usually reserved for patients who cannot be placed in the lateral position.

1. Position: The patient lies supine with legs fully extended in neutral position (lower extremity not externally rotated as in femoral nerve block).

2. Needle and landmarks: A 15 cm 22G short-bevelled needle is used. Landmarks include the anterior superior iliac spine (ASIS), pubic tubercle and greater trochanter.

3. Conduct of block
   — Trisect a line between ASIS and pubic tubercle (Line A) and draw a perpendicular line (Line B) from the junction of medial and middle third.

Draw another line from the tuberosity of the greater trochanter parallel to Line A. The needle insertion site is the point of intersection of Line B with the parallel line.

- Set the nerve stimulator to deliver 1.5 mA current and insert the needle perpendicular to the skin. Direct stimulation and twitches of the quadriceps muscle are often elicited during needle advancement and should be disregarded. Observe for visible or palpable twitches of the calf muscles, foot or toes at 0.2–0.5 mA current, which typically occurs at a depth of 10–12 cm.
- Unlike the posterior approach, twitches of the hamstrings should not be accepted as a reliable sign of sciatic nerve localization because branches to the hamstrings muscle may depart the main trunk of the sciatic nerve at the level of needle insertion.
- The femur may be contacted (usually at the lesser trochanter) during needle advancement. When this occurs, withdraw the needle by 2–3 cm and get an assistant to internally rotate the foot. This often allows passage of the needle beyond the lesser trochanter towards the sciatic nerve. If this fails, withdraw the needle back to the skin and re-insert at a slightly medial direction.
- Aspirate and inject a small dose of LA to determine ease of injection. There should be minimal resistance to injection. Inject 20–30 ml of LA. Again avoid the use of adrenaline in LA.

4. Possible complications
   - No specific complications are observed.
   - This approach should not be used in anticoagulated patients to lessen the risks of haematoma formation in deep tissue planes.

C. Ankle Block

An ankle block is a basic, peripheral nerve block technique. It is simple to perform, essentially devoid of systemic complications, and highly effective for a wide variety of procedures on the foot and toes.

Five nerves are blocked during the procedure.

- 3 superficial nerves: sural nerve, superficial peroneal nerve, saphenous nerve blocked by subcutaneous LA infiltration.
- 2 deep nerves: anterior tibial (deep peroneal) nerve, posterior tibial nerve blocked by injecting LA underneath the superficial fascia.

All except the saphenous nerve are terminal branches of the sciatic nerve. All 5 nerve blocks at the ankle, undertaken simultaneously, would produce a ring of infiltration around the ankle at the level of malleoli.

Technique

1. The patient lies supine with the foot resting on a foot stand for easy access to all nerves to be blocked. A 3 cm 23–25G needle is used for the block.

2. Conduct of block
   - The 2 deep nerves should be blocked first because subcutaneous injections for the superficial blocks will inevitably deform the surface anatomy.
   - Anterior tibial (deep peroneal) nerve
     - At the ankle level, the nerve lies anterior to the tibia and the interosseous membrane and close to the anterior tibial artery. It is usually sandwiched between the tendons of the extensor hallucis longus and extensor digitorum longus muscles.
     - Palpate for the extensor hallucis longus tendon (ask the patient to dorsiflex the big toe against resistance) and anterior tibial artery at the level of the medial and lateral malleoli.
     - Raise a skin wheal just lateral to the tendon at the area of arterial pulsation.
     - Insert the needle perpendicularly until it hits the bone (tibia). The patient may experience paraesthesia down to the toes.
     - Withdraw the needle by 1–2 mm and inject 3–5 ml of LA in a fanwise manner.
   - Posterior tibial nerve
     - At the level of the medial malleolus, the posterior tibial nerve is lateral and posterior to the posterior tibial artery, and midway between the posterior aspect of the medial malleolus and the Achilles tendon. Just beneath the malleolus, the nerve divides into lateral and medial plantar nerves.
     - Raise a skin wheal midway between medial malleolus and calcaneous adjacent to the Achilles tendon.
     - Palpate for the posterior tibial artery and inject 3–5 ml of LA slightly posterior to the artery in a fanwise manner.
     - Point of injection should be behind the upper border of the medial malleolus to include the calcaneal branch.

- Superficial peroneal nerve
  - The nerve divides into terminal cutaneous branches 5–10 cm above the lateral malleolus.
  - Insert the needle at the tibial ridge and extend laterally towards the lateral malleolus.
  - Infiltrate with 5 ml of LA subcutaneously in a medial and lateral direction.
- Saphenous nerve
  - The saphenous nerve is a terminal cutaneous branch of the femoral nerve. It runs in the subcutaneous tissue of the skin on medial aspect of the ankle and foot.
  - Insert the needle at the level of the medial malleolus and infiltrate 5 ml of LA subcutaneously to the Achilles tendon and anteriorly to the tibial ridge.
- Sural nerve
  - The sural nerve emerges on the lateral aspect of the Achilles tendon, 10–15 cm above the lateral malleolus. After giving lateral calcaneal branches to the heel, the sural nerve descends 1–1.5 cm behind the lateral malleolus, anterolateral to the short saphenous vein and on the surface of the fascia covering the muscles and tendons.
  - Insert the needle midway between lateral malleolus and calcaneous and infiltrate 3–5 ml of LA in an antero-posterior direction.
- A typical onset time for this block is 10–25 minutes depending mainly on the concentration of the LA used. Sensory anaesthesia of the skin develops faster than the motor block.

3. LA used: 0.25–0.5% bupivacaine or 1–2% lignocaine. There is a hazard of vascular occlusion; hence no adrenaline should be added to the LA solution.
4. Possible complications: systemic toxicity is rare because of the distal location of the block.

NEURAL PLEXUS/NERVE BLOCKS AT THE TRUNK

There are many nerve blocks at the trunk but only 4 of these blocks will be outlined here. Other neural plexus/nerve blocks include the coeliac plexus block and the lumbar sympathetic block. These are mainly encountered in chronic pain management where sympatholysis by injection of neurolytic may alleviate the chronic pain condition.

A. Intercostal Nerve Block

Multiple intercostal nerves are often blocked in this technique. These can be unilateral or bilateral depending on site and nature of injury. A single catheter intercostal block technique has been suggested but its effectiveness is controversial.

Systemic absorption of local anaesthetic from intercostal nerve block is found to be the highest among all the nerve blocks both in time course and peak plasma concentration produced. This should be taken into consideration when multiple nerve blocks on both sides of the chest are required, in which the thoracic epidural technique would often be more suitable.

Indications

— Pain relief for chest injury (e.g., fractured ribs).
— Postoperative analgesia for thoracotomy and upper abdominal surgery.
— Pain relief for herpes zoster.
— Minor surgery on the abdominal or chest wall.

Complications

— Pneumothorax
— Systemic toxicity due to rapid absorption of LA (rare)

Technique

1. Position
   — Unilateral block: The patient lies semi-prone with the side to be blocked uppermost and the upper arm raised above the head to elevate the scapula.
   — Bilateral block:
      - The patient is in the prone position with both arms raised above the head.
      - If the patient is conscious and able to sit up, lean the patient slightly forward with arms resting on support provided by a table or multiple pillows.

2. Needle and landmarks:
   — A 3 cm 22G needle attached to a syringe containing LA is used. A longer needle may be required if the patient is muscular or obese. Landmarks include the thoracic vertebrae, paraspinal muscles and ribs.

3. Conduct of block
   — Identify the specific ribs involved in intercostal nerve block.
   — Mark the junction of paraspinal muscles and lower border of the rib. This is about 6–8 cm from the midline and corresponds to the angle of the rib.

— The thumb and index finger of the non-dominant hand bracket the rib.
— Direct the needle between the fingers at the lower portion of the rib at an angle of approximately 20° cephalad.
— Note the depth at which the rib is contacted. Retract the needle slightly, walk it off the lower border of the rib. Advance the needle 2–3 mm further to lie in the subcostal groove.
— Aspirate for blood, inject 3–5 ml of LA if this is negative.
— Repeat for the other intercostal nerves.

B. Interpleural Block

In interpleural block, LA is injected between the parietal and visceral pleura. Analgesia is thought to be produced by retrograde diffusion of LA to reach the intercostal nerves.

Indications

— Postoperative analgesia for cholecystectomy, thoracotomy, renal surgery, breast surgery, cardiac surgery, abdominal surgery.
— Analgesia for multiple fractured ribs.
— Chronic pain management for conditions such as malignancy, chronic pancreatitis, postherpetic neuralgia, reflex sympathetic dystrophy.

Interpleural analgesia has been consistently proven to be effective in patients following cholecystectomy. Studies on its use after thoracic surgery have yielded inconclusive results. For pain relief of multiple fractured ribs, interpleural analgesia has been shown to be effective in unilateral fractures.

Complications

— Pneumothorax
— Unilateral sympathetic block leading to Horner's syndrome
— Pleural effusion

Technique

1. The patient is placed in the lateral position with the upper arm raised above the head. An 18G Tuohy needle from the standard epidural set is used in conjunction with 20G epidural catheter.

2. Conduct of block
   — The technique is similar to an epidural block. The Tuohy needle is inserted at the 5th intercostal space at mid-axillary line. An air- or saline-filled syringe is attached to the needle and advanced slowly using the loss of resistance technique until the pleural cavity is entered.
   — The catheter is inserted 5–6 cm into the pleural space.

3. Dose of LA
   — Bolus dose: 15–20 ml of 0.5% bupivacaine.
   — Continuous infusion: 0.125–0.25% bupivacaine at 8–12 ml/hr.

C. Inguinal Field Block

The inguinal region receives most of its sensory innervation via the ilioinguinal and iliohypogastric nerves. Minor contributions may also be made from T12, L2 and the genitofemoral nerve. Even though a subarachnoid block is usually performed for surgery at the inguinal region, some patients may not be able to withstand the hypotension which commonly occurs following the block. Inguinal field block is a suitable alternative for such patients.

Technique

1. The patient lies supine, and a 7–10 cm 22G needle is used for the block. Landmarks include the anterior superior iliac spine (ASIS), umbilicus and pubic tubercle.

2. Conduct of block
   — A skin wheal is made 1–2 cm medial and inferior to the ASIS. The needle is inserted at right angle to the skin until it pierces the external oblique aponeurosis, and 10–15 ml of LA is infiltrated between ASIS and umbilicus. This blocks the terminal branches of T12 fibres.
   — The needle is readjusted in a caudal and medio-caudal direction and another 10–15 ml of LA is infiltrated between ASIS and pubic spine. This blocks the ilioinguinal and iliohypogastric nerves.
   — A second skin wheal is raised over the pubic tubercle. The needle is inserted in the direction of the umbilicus and 5 ml of LA is infiltrated subcutaneously. This blocks the nerve twigs from the opposite side.
   — A third skin wheal is raised 1.5 cm above the midpoint of the inguinal ligament. The needle is inserted perpendicularly to pierce the aponeurosis

of the external oblique and 10 ml of LA is deposited. This blocks the genitofemoral nerve and autonomic fibres.

— If the spermatic cord is to be manipulated, direct infiltration of 2–3 ml of LA around the cord in the internal ring will complete the anaesthesia.

3. Dose of LA
   — Due to the large volumes of LA needed for the block, the concentration of bupivacaine should be reduced to 0.25% to prevent toxicity. One percent lignocaine may also be used.

4. Ilioinguinal and iliohypogastric nerve block in children
   — Various techniques have been described, including multiple injections to block all the nerves involved. A simplified, singe-injection technique can be used with high success rate.
   — The point of entry for the single-injection technique is at the junction of the lateral ¼ with medial ¾ of the line joining umbilicus to ASIS.
   — The needle is inserted at 45–60° to the skin pointing towards the midpoint of the inguinal ligament until it pierces the external oblique aponeurosis.
   — Inject 0.3–0.4 ml/kg of 0.25% bupivacaine (up to 10 ml) in a fanwise manner.

D. Penile Block

The dorsal nerves of the penis, one on each side, are terminal branches of the pudendal nerve and the major innervation of the penis. Each nerve runs together with the ipsilateral dorsal artery and vein. It passes under the pubic bone, crosses the subpubic space (where it can be easily blocked), enters the suspensory ligament, then runs along the inner surface of the Buck's fascia and enters the corpora cavernosa to supply the skin and glans penis. The genitofemoral nerve via its genital branch innervates the base of the penis and scrotum.

Penile block is often performed for circumcision, either as a sole anaesthetic or for postoperative analgesia.

Technique

1. The patient lies supine. A 23G to 25G needle is used for the block. The sole landmark is the symphysis pubis.

2. Conduct of block
   — Pull down the penis and insert the needle just below the symphysis pubis

about 0.5–1 cm from the midline. The needle is directed almost at 90° to the skin, with a slight inclination caudally and medially.

— A pop is felt as the Scarpa's fascia is pierced. The needle should not move when it is let free.
— Inject half the dose of plain LA solution and repeat the procedure on the other side of midline. *Avoid intravascular injection and do NOT add adrenaline.*
— Inject 1 ml of LA subcutaneously around the ventral side of the shaft of the penis.
— The volume of LA varies depending on the age and body weight.
  - Children: 1 ml + 0.1 ml/kg of 0.25% bupivacaine (maximum 5 ml).
  - Adult: 10 ml.
— Alternative technique: midline, single injection. This may be problematic since the subpubic space is occasionally completely divided into two separate compartments by the suspensory ligament, preventing spread of LA from one side to the other.

FURTHER READING

1. Neal JM, Hebl JR, Gerancher JC, Hogan QH. Brachial plexus anesthesia: Essentials of our current understanding. Reg Anesth Pain Med 2002;27:402–28.
2. De Andres J, Sala–Blanch X. Peripheral nerve stimulation in the practice of brachial plexus anesthesia: A review. Reg Anesth Pain Med 2001;26:478–83.
3. Long TR, Wass T, Burkle CM. Perioperative interscalene blockade: An overview of its history and current clinical use. J Clin Anesth 2002;14:546–56.
4. Murphy D, McCartney C, Chan V. Novel analgesic adjuncts for brachial plexus block: A systematic review. Anesth Analg 2000;90:1122–8.
5. Enneking K, Wedel D. The art and science of peripheral nerve blocks. Anesth Analg 2000;90:1–2.
6. Brill S, Middleton W, Fisher A. Bier's block: 100 years old and still going strong! Acta Anaesthesiol Scand 2004;48:117–22.
7. Ross AK, Eck JB, Tobias JD. Pediatric regional anesthesia: Beyond the caudal. Anesth Analg 2000;91:16–26.

Chapter 34

Anaesthesia for Caesarean Section

INTRODUCTION

Caesarean section is one of the most commonly performed surgical procedures in women of childbearing age. The rate of caesarean delivery varies from institution to institution, depending on the patient demographics, obstetric management protocols and whether the institution is a tertiary referral centre for complicated deliveries.

Obstetric anaesthesia is a unique and specialized field of anaesthesia because the anaesthesiologist is providing care for two lives – that of the mother and the foetus. It must be remembered that the primary responsibility of the anaesthesiologist is towards the mother. If the lives of both are in jeopardy, the anaesthesiologist's priority lies in resuscitating the mother. Hopefully, with improved haemodynamic parameters in the mother, the foetal condition will correspondingly improve.

Audit studies on anaesthesia-related maternal mortality worldwide have repeatedly emphasized that GA is associated with a higher risk of mortality compared to RA. An earlier survey in the United States found a 17-fold increase in relative risk under GA compared to RA for caesarean delivery. The most recent triennial report of the Confidential Enquiry into Maternal and Child Health (CEMACH) in the United Kingdom – "Why Mothers Die 2000–2002" – listed six anaesthetic deaths all of which were related to GA. Causes of death were undiagnosed oesophageal intubation leading to hypoxia and cardiac arrest, inadequately managed hypoventilation, and a case of unsuccessful resuscitation from anaphylaxis.

In view of these grim statistics, it is strongly recommended that caesarean section should be performed under regional anaesthesia (spinal, epidural or combined spinal-epidural) unless specifically contraindicated. While this may raise concern that anaesthetic trainees have limited opportunity to manage an obstetric patient under general anaesthesia, it is the safety and well-being of the mother that is of paramount importance.

PREOPERATIVE ASSESSMENT AND PREPARATION

All patients scheduled for elective caesarean section should be assessed by the anaesthesiologist at least a day before the surgery. This is often not possible for patients scheduled for emergency caesarean section because of time constraints; hence they are usually assessed in the OT just before surgery.

Clinical features to be noted include:

— Patient's age, parity, period of gestation, any complications during pregnancy.

— Relevant medical, surgical and anaesthetic history; history of allergies and drug therapy.

— Indication and consent for caesarean section.

— Physical examination with emphasis on cardiovascular and respiratory systems, careful airway assessment and examination of the lumbar spine if RA is planned.

— Laboratory investigations of FBC, coagulation screen in preeclamptic patients and other relevant tests if indicated.

The anaesthesiologist should spend some time with the patient to answer her queries and help allay her fears about the impending surgery. In the absence of contraindications to RA, this option should be strongly recommended to the patient.

No sedative premedication should be prescribed to avoid foetal depression. All patients should be given acid aspiration prophylaxis as follows irrespective of whether they are planned for caesarean section under GA or RA.

— **Elective caesarean section**
  - Fast from 12 midnight; clear fluids may be allowed until 2 hours before the surgery.
  - Oral ranitidine 150 mg the night before and on morning of surgery.
  - 0.3M sodium citrate 30 ml before transfer to OT.

— **Emergency caesarean section**
  - Stat dose of IV ranitidine 50 mg as soon as decision for caesarean section is made.
  - 0.3M sodium citrate 30 ml before transfer to OT.
  - IV metoclopramide 10 mg may be given at induction of anaesthesia.

GENERAL ANAESTHESIA

The advantages and disadvantages of both GA and RA are listed in Table 34–1. In a well-conducted anaesthesia with no adverse events (e.g., hypotension, hypocarbia, hypoxaemia), the baby's neurobehavioural scores do not show any statistically significant difference between GA and RA. Factors such as the foetal condition *in utero*, and the incision-delivery interval, are more important in determining neonatal outcome than the choice of anaesthetic technique *per se*.

Despite the well-documented advantages of RA for caesarean section, there is always a role for GA under these circumstances.

— When RA is contraindicated: local or systemic infection, coagulopathies.

— When RA may be potentially hazardous: severe aortic stenosis, active bleeding with hypovolaemia.

— When RA takes too long to be established: severe foetal bradycardia or cord prolapse.

— When RA does not produce adequate surgical anaesthesia: failed, inadequate, unilateral or patchy block.

Table 34–1. Advantages and disadvantages of general and regional anaesthesia for caesarean section

Anaesthetic Technique	Advantages	Disadvantages
General anaesthesia	▪ Shorter induction time compared to epidural anaesthesia ▪ Lower failure rate compared to epidural amaesthesia ▪ Better CVS control – avoids hypotension due to sympathetic blockade ▪ Full control of respiratory functions to achieve desired PaO_2 and $PaCO_2$ ▪ Rapid control of convulsion in eclamptic patients ▪ Patient cooperation not required	▪ Difficult airway management – Difficult or failed intubation – Trauma ▪ Risk of regurgitation and pulmonary aspiration of gastric contents ▪ Awareness under anaesthesia ▪ GA problems – PONV – Hangover from GA effect – Lack of effective postoperative analgesia ▪ Stress response during induction and emergence
Regional anaesthesia	▪ Awake patient – Improved maternal-child bonding and early establishment of breastfeeding – Spouse can be present at delivery ▪ Avoid problems of GA – Airway concerns and aspiration risks – Hangover effect – Multiple drug administration ▪ Ability to provide effective postoperative analgesia	▪ Sympathetic blockade with hypotension ▪ Incomplete or patchy block inadequate for surgery ▪ Limited duration of anaesthesia in spinal and single-shot epidural injections ▪ Complications of RA: – Inadvertent intravascular or intrathecal injection of LA – Accidental dural puncture

Table 34–1. *(continued)*

Anaesthetic Technique	Advantages	Disadvantages
Regional anaesthesia *(continued)*	▪ Reduce the incidence of thromboembolic phenomena – Early mobilization – Rheological and micro-vascular effects of RA	

Anaesthetic Management

— Prepare for difficult intubation and check that airway equipment and airway adjuncts are available and in good working order.

— Mandatory monitors include ECG, non-invasive blood pressure monitor, pulse oximeter and capnography. Others such as invasive pressure monitoring devices, peripheral nerve stimulator and temperature probes should be available if needed.

— Place the patient supine with left uterine displacement to prevent aorto-caval compression. This can be achieved by tilting the OT table 15–20° to the left or placing a wedge under the right buttock.

— Reliable intravenous access is necessary especially in potentially difficult cases such as bleeding placenta praevia, previous caesarean section, possible placenta accreta. The intravenous cannula(e) should be 18G or larger.

— The patient should be preoxygenated with 100% oxygen for 3–5 minutes to prevent desaturation during airway instrumentation. In extremely emergent situations this can be achieved by instructing the patient to take 4 vital capacity breaths via a tight-fitting face mask. Both methods produce a similar rise in arterial PO_2, provided a tight mask fit is ensured in the latter method to prevent entrainment of room air.

— General anaesthesia is induced by rapid sequence induction using IV thiopentone 4 mg/kg (or IV ketamine 2 mg/kg) and IV suxamethonium 1.5 mg/kg. Instruct a trained anaesthetic assistant to apply cricoid pressure as the patient begins to lose consciousness. Avoid manual ventilation to prevent gastric insufflation which may provoke regurgitation. Maintain cricoid pressure until the endotracheal tube is inserted, its cuff inflated, its correct position checked and confirmed. Continue application of cricoid pressure if difficulty in intubation is encountered.

- Anaesthetic gas mixture used before delivery is 50% oxygen and 50% nitrous oxide with isoflurane or sevoflurane. The higher than usual FiO_2 serves to ensure adequate oxygenation in the baby, while the volatile anaesthetic agent is used to provide adequate depth of anaesthesia and reduce the incidence of awareness. Problems with uterine relaxation and excessive surgical bleeding are minimal at clinical concentrations of volatile anaesthetic agents used. No opioid analgesic is administered until after the baby is delivered to avoid possible neonatal respiratory depression.
- Ensure adequate oxygenation and normocarbia during IPPV. Avoid hyperventilation as the resultant hypocarbia causes vasoconstriction which decreases utero-placental blood flow. Maintain normal haemodynamic parameters and treat any hypo- or hypertension aggressively.
- When the baby is delivered, change the gas flow of oxygen: nitrous oxide to the usual 1:2 ratio, administer IV syntocinon 5 U slowly followed by an intravenous opioid. Any of the opioids – fentanyl, pethidine, morphine, nalbuphine – can be used although one with a longer duration of action would be helpful in alleviating postoperative pain. This can be supplemented with rectal diclofenac and local anaesthetic infiltration of the wound at skin closure.
- If there is uterine atony, the surgeon may request a dose of intravenous ergometrine or intravenous infusion of syntocinon 40 U in a 500 ml solution. Ergometrine should be avoided in patients with hypertension because it causes a sudden increase in blood pressure.
- Blood loss may be difficult to estimate because blood in the suction bottle is mixed with amniotic fluid. Decision on blood transfusion lies in clinical assessment as well as the degree and speed of blood loss.
- At the end of the surgery, reverse the neuromuscular blockade and awaken the patient in the usual manner. Remove the endotracheal tube only when the patient is fully awake, having good breathing effort and gag reflex, and is able to protect her airway.
- Observe the patient at PACU for at least 30 minutes. Discharge to the ward when she is comfortable, breathing well and haemodynamically stable.

Failed Intubation Protocol (Figure 34–1)

Successful attempt at intubation should be aided by:

- Optimal positioning of the head and neck to ensure proper intubating position.

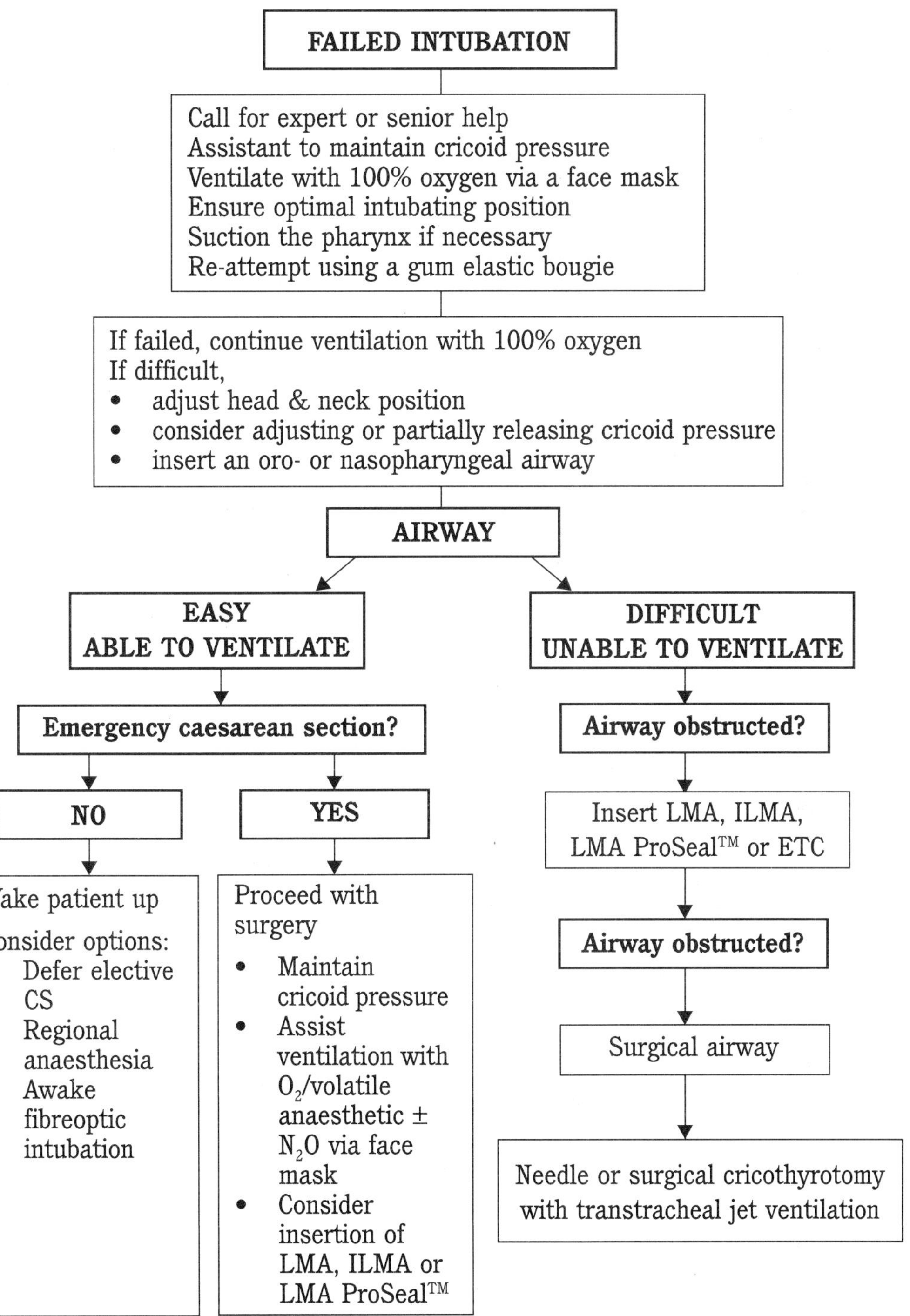

Figure 34–1. Failed intubation protocol

— Smaller sized endotracheal tube with stylet.
— Profound relaxation with adequate dose of suxamethonium.
— Tug on breasts or use laryngoscopes with short handles for easy manoeuvrability.
— Use of McCoy blade in which the tip of the laryngoscope can be manipulated to lift up the epiglottis.
— Correct application of cricoid pressure, sometimes a slight release of cricoid pressure may be needed to ease intubation.

Multiple intubation attempts should not be made without ensuring adequate oxygenation.

The failed intubation protocol for obstetric anaesthesia, originally proposed by Tunstall in 1976, has stood the test of time even though some aspects have been modified over the years. The ultimate goals are to maintain oxygenation and prevent aspiration during a failed intubation scenario. The drill is activated after three failed attempts in Cormack and Lehane Grade III laryngoscopic view, and immediately in Cormack and Lehane Grade IV.

Use of Laryngeal Mask Airway in Failed Intubation

The introduction of laryngeal mask airway (LMA) in 1983 by Dr. AJ Brain represents a major advance in airway management. Its role in obstetric anaesthesia has generated considerable debate as anaesthesiologists attempt to define its place in the failed intubation protocol. Newer variants of the LMA, such as the intubating LMA (ILMA, or Fastrach™) and in particular LMA ProSeal™, represent further advances. The latter holds promise in the context of obstetric anaesthesia with its ability to achieve patent airway while affording some protection against regurgitation of gastric contents. However, these devices are as yet not widely available and require experience to ensure proper and successful insertion.

These points are pertinent.

— The LMA has a definite place in the failed intubation protocol and hence should be readily available on the difficult intubation trolley. The basic principles and guidelines of the failed intubation protocol remain unchanged despite introduction of LMA.
— Anaesthesiologists managing obstetric patients should be skilled and adequately trained in airway management, including the use of LMA and/or other airway

adjuncts such as ILMA, LMA ProSeal™, Trachlight™, oesophageal-tracheal Combitube (ETC). They should also be trained in awake fibreoptic laryngoscopy.

— In the failed intubation scenario, the decision of whether and when to use the LMA is important.
  - If satisfactory ventilation can be achieved with a face mask, it seems prudent not to attempt further manipulation and risk losing the airway altogether. Attempts to insert LMA may provoke laryngospasm and may require release of cricoid pressure with possible regurgitation.
  - If ventilation cannot be achieved with a face mask and oropharyngeal airway, insertion of LMA is indicated and may be life-saving.

  The success rate at first insertion of LMA increases as clinical experience with LMA grows. Some anaesthesiologists argue that the benefit of having LMA *in situ* far outweighs the potential risks of inducing laryngospasm and/or regurgitation during insertion. This is particularly so if emergency surgery is allowed to proceed after having attained satisfactory mask ventilation. The hands holding the face mask are likely to be fatigued over time, resulting in progressively ineffective ventilation and possible airway obstruction.

— There is doubt as to whether cricoid pressure can be applied effectively in the presence of LMA. Furthermore, the presence of cricoid pressure can reduce the success rate of LMA insertion. Cricoid pressure is also shown to significantly impair the success rate of intubation through the ILMA. The recommendation is that cricoid pressure should be maintained when LMA is inserted. It should only be released if this is essential for correct positioning of the LMA to establish a patent airway, and reapplied once the LMA is in place.

— Persistent attempts at inserting the LMA should not be condoned if insertion is found to be difficult. The Difficult Airway Society in the UK recommended not more than two attempts at insertion in their difficult intubation guidelines. Other options, such as establishment of transtracheal ventilation via cricothyrotomy, should not be delayed.

REGIONAL ANAESTHESIA

Regional anaesthesia offers definite advantages over general anaesthesia. These advantages, together with its potential problems, are listed in Table 34–1.

As patient education improves and more patients are aware of the advantages of regional anaesthesia, the rate of spinal and epidural anaesthesia for caesarean section can be expected to increase. There is also a subset of patients with preexisting epidural block, having received epidural analgesia while in the labour room. Surgical anaesthesia in such patients can be achieved by increasing the level and intensity of blockade using local anaesthetic with opioid.

Contraindications to Regional Anaesthesia

These are discussed under absolute and relative contraindications.

a) **Absolute contraindications**

- Patient who is unwilling or unable to cooperate.
- Unskilled, unsupervised operator.
- Local or systemic infection.
- Bleeding tendency or coagulopathy: anticoagulant therapy, severe preeclampsia.
- Hypovolaemia or inadequate volume resuscitation: antepartum haemorrhage.
- Cardiac disease with fixed cardiac output states: severe mitral stenosis, aortic stenosis.
- Known allergy to local anaesthetics (rare).

b) **Relative contraindications**

- Inadequate time to perform regional block: cord prolapse, severe foetal bradycardia, abruptio placentae.
- Anticipated complicated or prolonged surgery with significant blood loss: ruptured uterus, placenta accreta or placenta percreta with possible caesarean hysterectomy.
- Spinal deformity: technically more difficult to perform; higher risk of inadequate surgical anaesthesia.
- Neuromuscular disease.
- Known foetal abnormality such as hydrocephalus (the patient may prefer not to be awake during surgery).

With the advent of combined spinal-epidural (CSE) anaesthesia, some of the "contraindications" have been successfully managed by means of a sequential CSE. In this technique, a small intrathecal dose is initially given and the required level of block is slowly established by small incremental doses via the epidural route. Another proposed technique is the use of epidural volume expansion to increase the height of spinal block established with a small intrathecal dose. This requires skill and experience and should be managed by specialists or obstetric anaesthetists.

Procedure

- The spinal, epidural and CSE techniques are described in Chapter 32.
- Level of insertion is usually at L2–L3 or L3–L4 intervertebral space.

A. Spinal

- The LA most commonly used is 0.5% bupivacaine, at volumes ranging from 1.5 ml (7.5 mg) to 2.5 ml (12.5 mg) depending on the height and build of the patient. An opioid may be added to improve the quality of block, a useful dose being 20 μg fentanyl (0.4 ml) added to 0.5% bupivacaine 1.8 ml for an average build patient.
- Intrathecal dose of preservative-free morphine 0.1–0.2 mg is effective for post-operative analgesia up to 12–24 hours, but has side-effects such as pruritus, nausea, vomiting. Diamorphine has been widely used (intrathecally but more often epidurally) in the UK but is not available elsewhere.

B. Epidural

- Use a test dose of 2% lignocaine with 1:200,000 adrenaline. Watch for signs and symptoms of intravascular or intrathecal injection, such as early but transient increases in heart rate and blood pressure, early onset of profound sensory and/or motor block, circumoral numbness or tingling, dizziness, nausea.
- Any of these LA – 0.5% bupivacaine, 0.75% ropivacaine or 2% lignocaine – may be used alone or together with fentanyl. The usual dose is 10–15 ml in aliquots of 3–5 ml each time. Fentanyl 50–100 μg may be added to improve the quality of block. It does not cause neonatal respiratory depression at this dose. Addition of 2 ml of 8.4% sodium bicarbonate solution and 0.1 ml of adrenaline to 20 ml of 2% lignocaine (resultant strength of adrenaline 1:200,000) may hasten the onset of anaesthesia and improve the quality of block.
- If subarachnoid tap occurs, convert to spinal anaesthesia and follow up the patient for postdural puncture headache.

C. Combined Spinal-Epidural

— Use the same spinal dose as stated above.

— Alternatively, it has been shown that the spinal dose may be decreased by a technique called epidural volume expansion. The spinal dose is 0.5% heavy bupivacaine 5–7.5 mg (1–1.5 ml) with fentanyl 25 μg. After injecting the intrathecal dose, 5–7ml of saline is injected into the epidural space before the epidural catheter is inserted.

After performing the central neuraxial block:

— Place the patient supine with left uterine displacement by tilting OT table or putting a wedge under the right buttock. Avoid supine position as it may cause aorto-caval compression.

— Provide oxygen 4 L/min via a clear face mask.

— Monitor blood pressure every minute for 10 minutes then at 3–5 minute intervals if stable.

  - If systolic BP decreases below 90 mmHg or by more than 20% from preoperative level, administer intravenous fluids and 5–10 mg bolus doses of ephedrine.
  - For spinal anaesthesia, some anaesthesiologists advocate the use of prophylactic ephedrine 30 mg in 500 ml of Ringer's lactate.
  - The role of ephedrine as the vasopressor of choice has now been questioned because neonatal acid-base status does not seem to benefit despite restoration of haemodynamic parameters. Pure α-agonists (e.g., phenylephrine 50–100 μg) have been advocated instead, but the occurrence of bradycardia sometimes necessitates the use of atropine.

— Check the level of block. A block to light touch up to T4 is required for surgery. Consider conversion to GA if the level remains below T10 after adequate time has elapsed.

— The rest of the anaesthetic management for caesarean section is the same as that done under GA. Avoid using IV ergometrine as this may cause severe nausea and/or vomiting in conscious patients.

— For epidural, top up with bupivacaine 0.25% or pethidine 25–50 mg before removing the catheter at the end of surgery. Alternatively the epidural catheter can be left *in situ* and epidural infusion (pethidine or bupivacaine/fentanyl mixture) commenced in PACU. Subsequent management can be carried out by the Acute Pain Service (APS) team. This should be supplemented with oral or rectal analgesics.

Spinal Anaesthesia Following Failed Epidural Block

Occasionally epidural injection of local anaesthetic fails to produce adequate anaesthesia for surgery, and one is left with the options of converting to general anaesthesia, re-siting the epidural block or performing a spinal block instead. The last option may, however, be hazardous as there have been case reports of extensive sensory block with respiratory compromise, which have prompted some anaesthesiologists to declare that spinal anaesthesia is contraindicated following a failed epidural block. Many others, however, believe that it can still be a viable option with appropriate precautions and modifications in technique, provided one is aware of the increased risk of high block and be prepared to intervene quickly if necessary.

This technique is suggested.

— Unless concerned about technical difficulty, reduce the risk of postural hypotension by performing the block in the lateral position.

— Base the dose of local anaesthetic on the extent of the existing epidural block.

— After the spinal block, position the patient supine with left lateral tilt and place an extra pillow under her head.

— Closely monitor the patient's respiration and sensory level. Be prepared to intervene early if excessively high block develops.

PROPHYLAXIS AGAINST THROMBOEMBOLISM

The CEMACH report in the 2000–2002 triennium cited venous thrombosis and thromboembolism as the leading cause of direct maternal death in the United Kingdom. Various measures of thromboprophylaxis are available, and patients are stratified into three categories according to risk factors. Patients undergoing elective caesarean sections, with no other predisposing factors, fall under the low-risk category while those undergoing emergency caesarean deliveries are considered to have moderate thromboembolic risks.

It is recommended that all patients should receive adequate hydration and be encouraged to have early mobilization after delivery, while those who belong to the moderate and high-risk categories should receive additional thromboprophylaxis during the peripartum period. There should also be vigilance to detect and treat early clinical manifestations of deep vein thrombosis or pulmonary thromboembolism.

Enoxaparin, a low molecular weight heparin (LMWH), can be used in the peripartum period at a daily dose of 40 mg subcutaneously, preferably given in the evenings. Alternatively, SC heparin 5000 U may be given in the OT just prior to caesarean section after insertion of the central neuraxial block.

After the surgery the removal of the epidural catheter should be timed at least 2 hours after the dose of standard heparin, or 12 hours after LMWH. Although heparin at this dose is not expected to increase the risk of excessive bleeding during surgery or bleeding into the epidural or intrathecal space, vigilance is required to detect numbness, weakness or bladder/bowel dysfunction suggestive of epidural haematoma.

The exact protocol for thromboprophylaxis should be adapted for individual hospitals. There should also be close communication among the obstetricians and anaesthesiologists so that confusion and misunderstanding do not arise. Wider use of thromboprophylaxis and better investigation of classic symptoms, particularly in high-risk women, are urgently recommended.

NEONATAL RESUSCITATION

Knowledge of neonatal resuscitation is essential because the anaesthesiologist may be called upon to help in resuscitating the baby in the OT in the absence of a paediatrician. Since the primary responsibility of the anaesthesiologist lies with the mother, the anaesthesiologist should help in neonatal resuscitation only if the mother's condition is stable and does not require any immediate active management.

Assessment

The Apgar score (Table 34–2) is the most widely used scoring system for newborn. A rapid evaluation of the newborn's condition is performed at 1 minute and 5 minutes after delivery. If the 5-minute Apgar score is less than 7, additional scores are obtained every 5 minutes for a total of 20 minutes.

The Apgar score at 1 minute reflects the condition of the baby at birth and is said to correspond to its survival; while that of 5 minutes reflects the resuscitative efforts and may be related to the neurological outcome.

Note that the Apgar score cannot be used to determine the need for resuscitation. If resuscitative efforts are required, they should be promptly instituted and should not be delayed while the Apgar score is being obtained.

Table 34–2. Apgar score chart

Sign	0	1	2
Heart rate (beats/min)	Absent	< 100	> 100
Respiration	Absent	Slow, irregular gasps	Good, crying
Tone	Flaccid	Some flexion	Active motion
Reflex irritability	No response	Grimace	Cough or sneeze
Colour	Pale and cyanosed	Pink body, peripheral cyanosis	Completely pink

Equipment for Resuscitation

These should be checked and ready for use.

— Sterile gloves.

— Towels, warmed blankets.

— Heat source: radiant warmer or heating lamps.

— Oxygen source.

— Face masks of different sizes.

— Self-inflating bag.

— Laryngoscopes with straight blades.

— Endotracheal tubes of different sizes: 2.0, 2.5, 3.0, 3.5 with stylets.

— Suction catheters.

— Resuscitation drugs: adrenaline 1:10,000, naloxone 0.4 mg/ml (dose 0.1 mg/kg), sodium bicarbonate 4.2% solution, dextrose 50%.

— Intravenous fluids, 24G cannulae, needles, syringes.

— Umbilical catheters.

— Stop clock, stethoscope.

Resuscitation Procedure

1. **Drying and warming**
   - Dry the amniotic fluid covering the baby.
   - Place the baby under radiant heater and remove wet linens from contact with the baby.

2. **Airway positioning**
   - The baby should be placed supine with the neck in neutral position and a slight head down tilt.
   - Place the baby on the side with neck slightly extended if copious secretions are present.

3. **Airway suctioning**
   - In the presence of thick meconium:
     - Immediate laryngoscopy with suctioning of the hypopharynx, followed by intubation and direct tracheal suctioning using meconium aspirator; this is done before drying, stimulation and assisted ventilation.
     - After the baby has been stabilized, insert an orogastric tube to minimize the amount of meconium in the stomach, which could later be regurgitated and aspirated.
   - Suction the mouth before the nose if meconium is absent.
   - Suctioning should be gentle and should be limited to 3–5 seconds per attempt.
   - Deep suctioning of the oropharynx may produce a vagal response with bradycardia and/or apnoea.

4. **Stimulation**
   - Mild stimulation by drying, warming and suctioning is usually adequate. This can be combined with tactile stimulation by flicking the soles of the feet and rubbing the back of the baby.
   - Avoid more vigorous methods of stimulation.

5. **Oxygen**
   - Oxygen can be given via a self-inflating bag, face mask or by a head hood.
   - If oxygen is needed during resuscitation, it should not be withheld because of its potential hazards.

6. **Ventilation**
   - Positive pressure ventilation is indicated in babies with:
     - Apnoea or gasping respirations.
     - Bradycardia, heart rate < 100/min.
     - Persistent central cyanosis despite administration of 100% oxygen.
   - Ventilation can be instituted initially via bag-valve-mask device, at a ventilatory rate of 40–60/min.
   - Endotracheal intubation is indicated in:
     - Ineffective bag-valve-mask ventilation.
     - Tracheal suctioning for aspiration of thick meconium.
     - Prolonged intermittent positive pressure ventilation.

7. **Chest compressions**
   - Bradycardia and cardiac arrest can usually be avoided by prompt initiation of effective ventilation and oxygenation.
   - Chest compressions should be started if the heart rate is less than 60–80/min and not rapidly increasing despite effective IPPV with 100% oxygen for 30 seconds.
   - The middle third of the sternum is compressed by approximately ½–¾ inch at a rate of 120/min.

8. **Medications and drugs**
   - Drugs are rarely indicated in newborn resuscitation.
   - Profound hypoxaemia is the most common cause of bradycardia and shock in neonates.
   - Adrenaline (0.01–0.03 mg/kg or 0.1–0.3 ml/kg of a 1:10,000 solution) should be administered in asystole or if heart rate remains less than 60/min after a minimum of 30 seconds of adequate ventilation with 100% oxygen and chest compressions.
   - Consider volume expansion with crystalloid (Ringer's lactate or normal saline) or colloid (blood or albumin) at 10 ml/kg when there has been suspected blood loss, or if the baby appears to be in shock and has not responded to other resuscitative measures.
   - Naloxone (0.1 mg/kg of a 0.4 mg/ml solution) is indicated for the reversal of neonatal respiratory depression induced by opioids administered to the mother within 4 hours of delivery.

- — There is no evidence that atropine, calcium or sodium bicarbonate is beneficial in the acute phase of neonatal resuscitation.
- — Sodium bicarbonate should only be administered in the presence of adequate ventilation, when resuscitation is prolonged and other therapies are ineffective; further doses should be guided by arterial blood gas results.
- — The umbilical vein is the most rapidly accessible route for volume expanders and administration of adrenaline, naloxone or sodium bicarbonate.
- — Adrenaline and naloxone may be given via the endotracheal route, which is generally the most rapidly accessible site of administration.
- — Alternative routes include the peripheral vein or the intraosseous route. These are not commonly used in newborn resuscitation because of accessibility of the umbilical vein.

Hand over the care of the baby to your paediatric colleague with full details of the resuscitation procedure. The resuscitation details should also be documented fully in the patient's case notes.

FURTHER READING

1. Confidential Enquiry into Maternal and Child Health. Why Mothers Die 2000–2002: The Sixth Report of the Confidential Enquiries into Maternal Death in the United Kingdom. London: RCOG Press, 2004.
2. Chestnut DH. Anesthesia and maternal mortality. Anesthesiology 1997;86:273–6.
3. Hawkins JL, Koonin LM, Palmer SK, Gibbs CP. Anesthesia-related deaths during obstetric delivery in the United States, 1979–1990. Anesthesiology 1997;86:277.
4. Stamer UM, Stuber F. Anaesthesia for non-scheduled caesarean delivery. Curr Opin Anaesthesiol 2002;15:293–8.
5. Schneck H, Scheller M. Acid aspiration prophylaxis and caesarean section. Curr Opin Anaesthesiol 2000;13:261–5.
6. Lee A, Ngan Kee WD, Gin T. A quantitative, systematic review of randomized controlled trials of ephedrine versus phenylephrine for the management of hypotension during spinal anesthesia for cesarean delivery. Anesth Analg 2002;94:920–6.
7. Ngan Kee WD, Lee A. Multivariate analysis of factors associated with umbilical arterial pH and standard base excess after caesarean section under spinal anaesthesia. Anaesthesia 2003;58:125–30.

8. Stoneham M, Souter A. Spinal anaesthesia for caesarean section in women with incomplete extradural analgesia. Br J Anaesth 1996;77:301–2.
9. Gupta A, Enlund G, Bengtsson M, Sjoberg F. Spinal anaesthesia for caesarean section following epidural analgesia in labour: A relative contraindication. Int J Obstet Anaesth 1994;3:153–6.
10. Tiberu E, Szmuk P, Evron S, Geva D, Hagay Z, Katz J. Difficult airway in obstetric anesthesia: A review. Obstet Gynecol Survey 2001;56:631–41.
11. Harry RM, Nolan JP. The use of cricoid pressure with the intubating laryngeal mask. Anaesthesia 1999;54:656–9.
12. American Heart Association. Newborn resuscitation. Textbook of Pediatric Advanced Life Support. 1994; Chapter 9.
13. Kattwinkel J, et al. Resuscitation of the newly born infant: An advisory statement from the Pediatric Working Group of the International Liaison Committee on Resuscitation. Circulation 1999;99:1927–38.
14. Casey BM, McIntire DD, Leveno KJ. The continuing value of the Apgar score for the assessment of newborn infants. N Engl J Med 2001;344:467–71.

Chapter 35

Epidural Analgesia for Labour

INTRODUCTION

> ...In the absence of a medical contraindication, maternal request is a sufficient justification for pain relief in labour.
>
> *American College of Obstetricians & Gynaecologists,* 2002 ACOG practice bulletin

Pain relief during labour can be achieved by various means. Traditionally the two commonest methods of pain relief are intramuscular injections of pethidine and inhalation of entonox (50% nitrous oxide in oxygen). In the majority of cases these methods do not effectively abolish the pain during labour, and they are associated with many side-effects such as nausea, vomiting, sedation, neonatal depression.

Lumbar epidural analgesia is undoubtedly a highly effective means of pain relief during labour, enabling the parturient to have a pleasant and relatively pain-free delivery.

While the benefits of epidural analgesia are desirable for every parturient, this is particularly useful in parturients with associated medical conditions, such as preeclampsia and heart disease, where hypertension and tachycardia, stimulated by pain and straining, can be deleterious.

MANAGEMENT OF OBSTETRIC EPIDURAL ANALGESIA

1. **Assessment before the procedure**
   - Do a quick assessment of the parturient before the procedure, noting these in particular.
     - Any co-existing medical condition.
     - Past history of anaesthesia and surgery.
     - History of allergies.
     - Obstetric history.
     - Progress of the labour including the strength and frequency of uterine contractions, latest finding on vaginal examination, use of oxytocin for induction or augmentation of labour.
   - Rule out contraindications to central neuraxial blockade, such as:
     - Coagulation abnormalities.
     - Local or systemic sepsis.
     - Severe haemorrhage and hypovolaemia.
     - Refusal by the parturient despite adequate explanation.
   - Explain the procedure and possible side-effects of central neuraxial blockade.
     - The amount of information offered is often individualized and dependent on the stage of labour, intensity of pain experienced, receptiveness and educational level of the parturient.
     - Obtain a written consent for the procedure.

2. **Preparation before the procedure**
   - These items should be checked and prepared.
     - Resuscitation trolley including resuscitation drugs and airway equipment.
     - Monitoring equipment: non-invasive BP monitor is mandatory, while pulse oximetry and ECG are required in selected cases such as maternal heart disease.
   - A trained assistant should be available to assist during the procedure and monitor the parturient thereafter.

— Insert an 18G or 16G intravenous cannula and infuse 500 ml of Ringer's lactate solution. Do not use dextrose-containing solutions. Preload is not routinely required when using low doses of local anaesthetic, but the parturient should not be hypovolaemic before instituting epidural analgesia.
— Place the parturient in the preferred position (sitting or lateral decubitus); re-check the maternal blood pressure and foetal heart rate after positioning.
— If the parturient is on oxytocin infusion, this may be turned off momentarily during the procedure so as to minimize uterine contractions.

3. **The epidural procedure**
   — The conduct of the epidural block is similar to the technique described in Chapter 32, with these notable differences.
   - The parturient is often in varying degrees of pain; hence the procedure should be expedited and completed in the shortest possible time.
   - Communicate with the parturient at all times during the procedure especially concerning uterine contractions. Wait until each contraction has eased off before proceeding as the risk of inadvertent dural puncture is high during contractions.

4. **Test dose in obstetric epidural analgesia**
   — While the test dose aims to detect intravascular or intrathecal placement of the epidural catheter, it is not fool-proof since false positives and false negatives can still occur.
   — The standard recommended test dose is 3 ml of 1.5% lignocaine with 5 μg/ml of adrenaline.
   — Sign of intravascular injection:
   - Heart rate increase > 20 bpm within 1 minute.
   - Increase in systolic BP > 15 mmHg within 2 minutes.

   — Sign of intrathecal injection: rapid onset (within 5 minutes) of
   - sympathetic blockade – warm extremities.
   - numbness of lower limbs.
   - motor blockade to lower limbs.

   — The value of test dose in modern-day obstetric epidural analgesia has been questioned, due to these reasons.
   - Altered sensitivity to chronotropes and vasopressor during pregnancy – attenuated and/or varied response in normal parturients, exaggerated

response in parturients with preeclampsia – precludes the use of set criteria for diagnosis of intravascular injection.

- Requirement for continuous ECG or pulse oximetry monitoring to detect transient heart rate changes may not be practical in all cases.
- There are confounding heart rate changes during labour, with significant tachycardia during each painful uterine contraction.
- Hypertensive and tachycardic effect of adrenaline to the maternal circulation may not be well tolerated in the presence of hypertensive disorder or cardiac disease.
- Issue of foetal safety remains unresolved. Adrenaline-induced vasoconstriction and reduction in the utero-placental circulation may adversely affect the foetus, particularly in the presence of placental insufficiency, intrauterine growth retardation or foetal compromise.
- Effect of the traditional test dose on lower limb sensation, proprioception and motor function may impair the parturient's ability to walk in the context of ambulatory ("walking") epidural.

— The use of very dilute local anaesthetic solutions seems inherently safe, as intravascular injections usually manifest as loss of analgesic efficacy and are unlikely to be large enough to cause systemic toxicity, while intrathecal injections produce increasingly dense motor blockade without severe haemodynamic changes.

5. **Subsequent management**

— Once the test dose is negative, a further dose of local anaesthetic is injected slowly after careful aspiration. Fentanyl 50 μg may be added to improve the quality of block.

— Remember "*every dose is a test dose*". Injection of local anaesthetic should be done slowly after negative aspiration for blood or CSF, and given in small aliquots of 3–5 ml each time.

— Monitor maternal BP and heart rate every 5 minutes for the first 15 minutes after each top-up dose, then every 15 minutes for the first hour, then half-hourly after that.

— Foetal heart rate should be monitored either intermittently or by continuous cardiotocography (CTG). In 3–15% of parturients there may be foetal bradycardia secondary to uterine hypertonus. This is a transient phenomenon with no neonatal sequelae and in most cases respond to these conservative measures.

- Left lateral position to avoid aorto-caval compression.
- Supplemental oxygen via nasal prongs or face mask.
- Intravenous fluids and/or vasopressor if hypotension is present.
- Vaginal examination to check progress of labour and rule out emergencies such as cord prolapse.
- Temporary cessation of oxytocin infusion.
- Bolus dose of IV nitroglycerin 50 μg or SC terbutaline 0.25 mg to treat uterine hypertonus. Nitroglycerin causes a rapid and short-lived uterine relaxation with a quick return to a normal labour pattern, whereas terbutaline can slow the labour by 30–60 minutes.

There is usually no need for operative intervention.

— Test the sensory level of the block with pin or spirit swab. During the first stage of labour a block of up to T10 is usually adequate. This should be checked every 1–2 hours. Assess motor block according to the modified Bromage score (see Table 32–1, Chapter 32). An increasingly dense motor block may indicate intrathecal or subdural placement of the epidural catheter.

— Stay with the parturient until her condition is stable. Any complications arising from the epidural should be treated early and aggressively.

— Avoid supine position which may result in aorto-caval compression. As labour progresses, the parturient should be propped up progressively to allow diffusion of local anaesthetic to the vicinity of the sacral nerve fibres.

— The parturient should not eat any solid food during labour but may have sips of water or clear fluids if desired.

6. **Alternative technique: Combined spinal-epidural analgesia**

— The CSE technique is gaining popularity because of its rapid onset and minimal amount of drug to achieve excellent pain relief. The conduct of this block is described in Chapter 32.

— The sensory level is tested in the usual manner and the epidural infusion is commenced immediately. In parturients who receive only intrathecal fentanyl, no sensory level is elicited until approximately 30 minutes after starting the infusion, although some parturients may have subjective sensation of "numbness" initially.

— Breakthrough pain may occasionally occur 1½–2 hours after the procedure, as the effect of intrathecal medication wears off while the epidural infusion has not achieved sufficient drug concentration. Reassess the sensory level and administer 3–5 ml bolus of 0.25% bupivacaine or 0.2% ropivacaine epidurally.

— There is a high incidence of pruritus associated with the use of intrathecal opioid. This should be explained to the parturient before the procedure. In most cases this is transient and most do well with simple reassurance. Drugs used for treatment of pruritus include small amounts of propofol, nalbuphine and naloxone, all of them with various degrees of success.

7. **Dose recommendations**
   - — The trend in labour analgesia is towards the use of more dilute solutions in an attempt to minimize motor blockade. This also facilitates the practice of mobile or "walking" epidural. This has to be balanced against the obvious drawback of inadequate pain relief achieved with solutions that are too dilute.
   - — Maintenance of epidural analgesia may be achieved in one of three ways:
     - Continuous infusion (see Table 35–1 for dose recommendations).
     - Intermittent bolus doses: 10–15 ml of 0.1% bupivacaine or ropivacaine and 2 μg/ml fentanyl.
     - Patient-controlled epidural analgesia (PCEA): Background infusion: 6–8 ml/hr; bolus dose: 5 ml; lockout interval: 15 minutes.
   - — The level of block should be checked 1- to 2-hourly. If the block extends up to T8, reduce the infusion rate or withhold top-up doses.

8. **Protocol for ambulation**
   - — Even though the popularity of mobile, "walking" or ambulatory epidural has been spurred on by the widespread use of the CSE technique, ambulation is also possible by means of dilute, low-dose local anaesthetic/opioid solution in conventional epidural analgesia.
   - — There must be no obstetric contraindication to the parturient ambulating or to intermittent CTG monitoring.
   - — Allow ambulation after a 30-minute period of observation following insertion of the central neuraxial block. Both the mother and the foetus should be stable before ambulation.
   - — Assess motor strength before ambulation in this sequence.
     - Straight leg raising on the bed.
     - Sit at the edge of the bed.
     - Stand by the side of the bed.
     - Slight knee bend to be sure that motor function is fully intact.
   - — Allow the parturient to sit on a chair, walk to the bathroom and walk in the room but always with someone in attendance.

Table 35–1. Dose recommendations for epidural and CSE

Stage of Labour	Initial Bolus		Infusion Regime	Additional Bolus
	Epidural	CSE		
Very early labour Mild pain or no pain (cervical os ≤ 2cm)	50 μg fentanyl in 5 ml saline	fentanyl 25 μg or sufentanil 5 μg	0.0625% bupivacaine or ropivacaine with 2 μg/ml fentanyl at 12–15 ml/hr	0.125% bupivacaine or 0.1% ropivacaine 5–10 ml
Active labour Mild to moderate pain (cervical os ≥ 3 cm)	10–15 ml of 0.125% bupivacaine or 0.1% ropivacaine with 50 μg fentanyl	intrathecal 1 ml of 0.25% bupivacaine (2.5 mg) or 0.2% ropivacaine (2 mg) with fentanyl 20–25 μg*	0.0625–0.1% bupivacaine or ropivacaine with with 2 μg/ml fentanyl at 12–15 ml/hr	0.25% bupivacaine or 0.2% ropivacaine 5–10 ml with 50 μg fentanyl
Established labour Severe pain	10–15 ml of 0.25% bupivacaine or 0.2% ropivacaine with 50–100 μg fentanyl	intrathecal 1 ml of 0.25% bupivacaine (2.5 mg) or 0.2% ropivacaine (2 mg) with fentanyl 20–25 μg*	0.0625–0.1% bupivacaine or ropivacaine with 2 μg/ml fentanyl at 12–15 ml/hr	2% lignocaine 5–10 ml with 50 μg fentanyl

* Note that half the local anaesthetic dose – bupivacaine 1.25 mg or ropivacaine 1 mg – is found to be sufficient for smaller Asian women.

— Instruct the parturient to inform the midwife or anaesthesiologist as soon as she feels a return of contraction pain, so that an additional epidural dose may be administered before the pain becomes too intense.

9. **Management of epidural at late first stage and second stage of labour**
   — The parturient should be advised not to strain and bear down prematurely before the second stage of labour is reached. When the cervical os is fully dilated, she may experience an urge to bear down during uterine contraction and the attending staff should be informed.
   — Towards late first stage and second stage of labour, the parturient may complain of inadequate pain relief as afferent fibres from S2–4 may not be well blocked. Administer a bolus dose with the parturient in the semi-sitting position in order to block the sacral nerve fibres.
   — The epidural infusion should not be discontinued during the second stage of labour unless it is evident that the parturient is unable to bear down because of significant motor blockade.

10. **Emergency caesarean section**
   — If emergency caesarean section becomes necessary, the parturient should be prepared in the usual manner: consent, GXM blood, acid aspiration prophylaxis using IV ranitidine 50 mg, sodium citrate and/or metoclopramide.
   — Check the level of the block. If epidural is functioning and the sensory block is at T10, add 3–5 ml aliquots of 0.5% bupivacaine or 0.75% ropivacaine to increase the level of block to T4–T6. Administer fentanyl 50 μg in addition to the local anaesthetic to improve the quality of the block.
   — If there is an urgent need for caesarean section to be performed immediately, administer 2% lignocaine with fentanyl 50 μg instead of bupivacaine or ropivacaine.
   — This mixture may be administered (in aliquots of 3–5 ml) to further hasten the onset of epidural anaesthesia.
   - 20 ml of 2% lignocaine
   - 2 ml of 8.4% sodium bicarbonate
   - 0.1 mg adrenaline, constituting a dilution of 1:200,000 in the resultant solution

   Omit the use of adrenaline if the foetus is compromised.
   — If the epidural is not functioning, alternative methods – re-establishment of epidural block or general anaesthesia – should be considered depending on

the suitability and urgency of the situation. Spinal anaesthesia following an epidural block should be used with caution because of the possibility of causing an inadvertently high block.

— If the problem of inadequate anaesthesia arises intraoperatively, available options include:
  - Additional doses of local anaesthetic (use 2% lignocaine or lignocaine-sodium bicarbonate-adrenaline mixture with fentanyl).
  - Verbal reassurance if anxiety-induced.
  - Entonox delivered via a face mask and anaesthetic circuit.
  - Small doses of IV ketamine 10 mg (0.2–0.4 mg/kg).
  - IV pethidine after the baby has been delivered.
  - Conversion to general anaesthesia.

— Continue postoperative analgesia using epidural infusion of 0.1% bupivacaine or ropivacaine with 2 μg/ml fentanyl or pethidine 2 mg/ml at 5–10 ml/hr.

— Alternatively, administer pethidine 50 mg or morphine 3–5 mg diluted to 5 ml via the epidural catheter and observe the patient in the PACU. Remove the epidural catheter before discharge from PACU.

— In patients with no contraindications to the use of NSAIDs, these drugs (orally or rectally administered) are useful as adjuncts to improve the quality of postoperative analgesia.

11. **Removal of epidural catheter**

— After delivery, remove the epidural catheter, spray the site of needle puncture with antiseptic spray and cover with gauze. Inspect the epidural catheter for integrity.

— Each parturient should be followed up in the obstetric ward postdelivery. Besides getting feedback about her epidural experience, the visit is part of total patient care and serves to enhance the image of the anaesthesiologist in the eyes of the general public.

PROBLEMS ENCOUNTERED

Epidural analgesia is a remarkably safe technique with an excellent track record worldwide. Various factors are contributory; among them are proper selection of patients who are generally healthy, good anaesthetic practice, the use of smaller local anaesthetic doses compared to surgical and obstetric anaesthesia, as well as monitoring and vigilance by trained medical and nursing staff. In spite of this, it is a major neuraxial block which should not be taken lightly. Training and supervision, monitoring, awareness of potential problems, early diagnosis and management of such problems are key issues which should not be compromised.

Problems encountered range from the common and "trivial" (pruritus, shivering, nausea, vomiting), to those which require intervention by the anaesthesiologist (inadequate analgesia, hypotension, postdural puncture headache), and rare but catastrophic events (total spinal, epidural haematoma or abscess). Some of the problems are discussed next.

1. **Hypotension**
   - Avoid aorto-caval compression by making sure that the parturient is in the lateral position.
   - Measure BP on the dependent arm, and monitor every minute until stable.
   - Infuse an intravenous fluid bolus of a crystalloid solution.
   - Administer IV ephedrine 6 mg or phenylephrine 50 μg and repeat as necessary.
   - Check the level of the sensory block and test for motor block. Withhold epidural infusion if block extends above T8 or if the parturient has a significant motor block.
   - Administer supplemental oxygen if hypotension is prolonged.
   - Check the foetal heart rate and inform the obstetrician if necessary.
   - See also "Total Spinal" below.

2. **Inadequate analgesia** (see Table 35–2)
   - Assess the site and severity of pain, and its relation with uterine contractions.
   - Check level of block.
   - Identify possible cause and treat accordingly.

3. **Total spinal**
   - Clinical features of total spinal
     - Rapidly rising block, with dense motor and sensory block to lower limbs, trunk, upper limbs and lower cranial nerves.
     - Reduced cough effort, difficulty with breathing and swallowing, respiratory paralysis.
     - Hypotension and bradycardia leading to cardiovascular collapse.
     - Loss of consciousness.

Table 35–2. Causes and management of inadequate analgesia

Possible Causes	Management
Mechanical causes ▪ Infusion pump malfunction ▪ Epidural catheter problem: kinking, leaking, disconnection, dislodgement	Replace infusion pump Reconnect epidural catheter Re-site epidural
Failed epidural: no detectable block	Re-site epidural
Inadequate dose	Administer 3–5 ml of local anaesthetic Increase infusion rate if there is positive response to the bolus dose
Unilateral block	Administer 3–5 ml of local anaesthetic and 50–100 μg fentanyl with painful side in a dependent position Withdraw epidural catheter by 1 cm or until a minimum of 2 cm length lies in the epidural space and give a further top-up Re-site epidural if this does not work
"Patchy" analgesia or segments	Administer 3–5 ml of local anaesthetic with fentanyl Re-site epidural if this does not work
Back pain: common in occipitoposterior position of the foetus	Administer 3–5 ml of local anaesthetic with fentanyl Consider increasing the concentration of local anaesthetic infusion to 0.1% or 0.125%
Perineal pain: usually during late first stage or second stage of labour	Administer a bolus dose with the parturient in the sitting position Get the obstetric staff to check progress of labour and catheterize a full bladder

Table 35–2. *(continued)*

Possible Causes	Management
Intravascular migration of epidural catheter: this should be considered if no pain relief occurs with repeated bolus doses	Re-site epidural
Uterine rupture: breakthrough pain unrelieved by epidural analgesia	Look for other signs of uterine rupture: foetal distress, scar tenderness, vaginal bleeding, shock, recession of presenting part, readily palpable foetal parts per abdomen, peritoneal irritation Prepare for immediate caesarean delivery

— Management of total spinal
- Maintain airway and ventilation, early intubation for respiratory support and airway protection may be necessary.
- Avoid aorto-caval compression, provide cardiovascular support with intravenous fluids and vasopressor.
- Discuss with obstetrician regarding further obstetric management; caesarean section is not an immediate requirement in the absence of foetal distress.

4. **Subdural block**

— This occurs when the epidural catheter is misplaced between the dura mater and arachnoid mater.

— Characteristics of subdural block
- Slow onset (15–20 minutes) block which is unexpectedly extensive for the amount of local anaesthetic administered: may reach cervical dermatomes and affect cervical sympathetic chain, resulting in Horner's syndrome.
- Sensory block may be patchy and asymmetrical.
- Motor block is usually not dense.
- Blood pressure is remarkably well preserved given the extent of sensory block.

— Management of subdural block
  - Mainly supportive and symptomatic.
  - Monitor BP and pulse oximetry, administer supplemental oxygen if indicated.
  - Check for regression of block and re-site the epidural.

5. **Effects of intrathecal opioids**
   — Intrathecal opioids, in the form of sufentanil 5–10 μg or fentanyl 15–25 μg, are commonly used alone or in conjunction with local anaesthetic in the CSE technique.
   — Reported side-effects include pruritus, hypotension, nausea and vomiting, urinary retention, foetal bradycardia. Uncommon side-effects include respiratory depression, respiratory arrest, high sensory blockade associated with facial tingling, dysphagia and dyspnoea, altered level of consciousness and aphasia.
   — Management of side-effects
     - Pruritus: often self-limiting and most parturients require nothing other than reassurance. Drugs which have been tried include small IV doses of propofol (10–20 mg), naloxone (40 μg increments or an infusion) and nalbuphine (2.5–10 mg). Since pruritus is unrelated to histamine release, diphenhydramine is unlikely to be helpful except in providing sedation.
     - Respiratory and CNS side-effects: supportive management including supplemental oxygen, assisted ventilation and/or endotracheal intubation, cessation of epidural infusion and close monitoring until symptoms resolve; consider administering a small dose of IV naloxone to reverse the opioid effect.

6. **Inadvertent dural puncture** – See **Appendix**.

CONTROVERSIES REGARDING OBSTETRIC EPIDURAL ANALGESIA

Despite its efficacy and overall safety, epidural analgesia is still being regarded with suspicion by some obstetricians and nursing staff, the public, and even among some non-obstetric anaesthetists themselves. Controversies abound regarding the effect of epidural analgesia on the progress and outcome of labour, as well as uncertainties about its possible side-effects and complications, both immediate and long term. Meta-analyses and systematic reviews may not represent the true picture because of heterogeneity in both obstetric and anaesthetic management protocols in different hospitals and over the years. It cannot be ruled out that modifications in obstetric anaesthetic practice – the use of more dilute solutions of newer local anaesthetic agents (ropivacaine, levobupivacaine), supplementation with opioids (fentanyl, sufentanil), means of maintenance of epidural analgesia (intermittent bolus, continuous infusion or patient-controlled epidural analgesia), the CSE technique and practice of ambulatory ("walking") epidural – may influence labour progress and outcome.

Effects of epidural analgesia on labour are summarized here.

1. There is a correlation between painful labour (hence increased likelihood for epidural analgesia) and abnormal labour progress.
2. Prospective studies show that epidural analgesia does not affect the duration of first stage of labour, amount of oxytocin usage, incidence of dystocia and caesarean delivery rate. Effects on the duration of second stage of labour and instrumental delivery rate are less consistent.
3. Retrospective population-based (or "before and after") studies demonstrate that changes in availability of obstetric epidural service do not have impact on the caesarean delivery rate.
4. The COMET (Comparative Obstetric Mobile Epidural Trial) Study Group in the UK demonstrated that both CSE and low-dose infusion epidural techniques (0.1% bupivacaine with 2 μg/ml fentanyl) resulted in significantly more normal vaginal deliveries and lower instrumentation rate compared to the traditional epidural technique (0.25% bupivacaine) in an unselected population of nulliparous women. No differences were observed in both caesarean delivery rates and quality of pain relief between the low-dose and traditional epidural groups.
5. There are no demonstrable differences between low-dose epidural analgesia and CSE analgesia in terms of labour characteristics, obstetric and neonatal outcome.

APPENDIX: MANAGEMENT OF ACCIDENTAL DURAL PUNCTURE

1. **Preventive measures**
   — During the epidural procedure, always keep in mind the structures and tissue planes traversed by the epidural needle. Do not blindly advance the epidural needle without appreciating the structures involved. Withdraw the needle and re-attempt at a slightly different angle if there is doubt as to the precise location of the needle.

— Do not continue to advance the needle if the parturient is having a contraction. She may find it difficult to keep still and this might result in a dural puncture. Wait for the contraction to ease off.

2. **Management during labour**
   - All dural taps must be documented clearly and managed in an appropriate manner.
   - At the time of dural puncture, consider giving the intrathecal dose of local anaesthetic-fentanyl mixture through the epidural needle. This should offer partial pain relief to the parturient while attempt is being made to insert the epidural catheter in another level, preferably one intervertebral space higher than the site of dural puncture.
   - If it has been a difficult epidural block, consider inserting the epidural catheter in the subarachnoid space and use it as a spinal catheter. If this is done, it is vital that this should be clearly documented in the anaesthesia record and the catheter prominently labelled as "Spinal Catheter". All personnel involved in managing the parturient should be made aware of this, and subsequent top-ups should only be administered by the anaesthesiologist.
   - The parturient should be informed about the complication. Subsequent follow-up and management should be outlined to the parturient.
   - Prophylactic epidural blood patch has been advocated after delivery but its success rate has been queried.

3. **Postdelivery**
   - The patient should be followed up daily and more often if necessary. Explanation and encouragement should be given as needed.
   - Conservative measures include bed rest; oral fluids including coffee, simple analgesics such as paracetamol, mefenemic acid or other NSAIDs may be prescribed.
   - If the patient is pain-free after 24 hours, she should be gradually mobilized but discouraged from lifting or straining. The progress should be checked daily.
   - If she has a postdural puncture headache, or if one should start when she ambulates, she should be returned to complete bed rest and appropriate analgesic given. At this stage the possibility of an epidural blood patch should be discussed.

4. **Epidural blood patch**
   - The procedure should be done in the OT under aseptic conditions, after having explained the procedure and obtained a written consent from the patient.
   - Intravenous access and monitors (NIBP, SpO_2) are established.
   - The patient is placed in the upright or lateral position for the procedure. If the patient is having a severe headache, she would prefer to be in the lateral position.
   - Two operators are required: one to withdraw blood and the other to locate the epidural space and perform the blood patch.
   - The epidural space should be located at the same interspace as the one where dural puncture has occurred.
   - Once the epidural space has been located, the assistant withdraws 15–20 ml of blood under aseptic condition.
   - The blood is injected slowly into the epidural space; usually a total volume of 15 ml is sufficient. Injection is stopped when the patient experiences fullness at the back, complains of backache or if the headache disappears.
   - The remainder of the blood is injected into the culture medium and sent to the laboratory for blood culture.
   - The patient is returned to the ward in the supine or lateral position. She should remain in bed for the first 4 hours and then gradually allowed to ambulate. A second blood patch may be necessary in some patients if headache recurs.

FURTHER READING

1. Mulroy MF, Norris MC, Liu SS. Safety steps for epidural injection of local anesthetics: Review of the literature and recommendations. Anesth Analg 1997;85:1346–56.
2. Practice guidelines for obstetrical anesthesia: A report by the American Society of Anesthesiologists Task Force on Obstetrical Anesthesia. Anesthesiology 1999;90: 600–11.
3. Segal S. Epidural analgesia and the progress and outcome of labor and delivery. Int Anesthesiol Clin 2002;40:13–26.
4. Howell CJ. Epidural versus non-epidural analgesia for pain relief in labour [Cochrane review]. Cochrane Database Syst Rev 2000;2:CD000331.
5. Segal S, Su M. The effect of a rapid change in availability of epidural analgesia on the cesarean delivery rate: A meta-analysis. Am J Obstet Gynecol 2000;183:974–8.

6. COMET Study Group UK. Effect of low-dose mobile versus traditional epidural techniques on mode of delivery: A randomised controlled trial. Lancet 2001;358:19–23.
7. Eisenach JC. Combined spinal-epidural analgesia in obstetrics. Anesthesiology 1999;91:299–302.
8. Birnbach DJ, Ojea LS. Combined spinal-epidural (CSE) for labor and delivery. Int Anesthesiol Clin 2002;40:27–48.
9. Norris MC, Fogel ST, Conway-Long C. Combined spinal-epidural versus epidural labor analgesia. Anesthesiology 2001;95:913–20.
10. Brown J, Cyna AM, Simmons SW. Combined spinal epidural versus epidural analgesia in labour. Cochrane Database Syst Rev 2002; Vol 1.
11. Van de Velde M, Vercauteren M, Vandermeersch E. Foetal heart rate abnormalities after regional analgesia for labor pain: The effect of intrathecal opioids. Reg Anesth Pain Med 2001;26:257–62.
12. Nielsen PE, Erickson JR, Abouleish EI, Perriatt S, Sheppard C. Foetal heart rate changes after intrathecal sufentanil or epidural bupivacaine for labor analgesia: Incidence and clinical significance. Anesth Analg 1996;83:742–6.
13. Porter J, Bonello E, Reynolds F. Effect of epidural fentanyl on neonatal respiration. Anesthesiology 1998;89:79–85.
14. Davignon KR, Dennehy KC. Update on postdural puncture headache. Int Anesthesiol Clin 2002;40:89–102.
15. Turnbull DK, Shepherd DB. Post-dural puncture headache: Pathogenesis, prevention and treatment. Br J Anaesth 2003;91:718–29.
16. Butler R, Fuller J. Back pain following epidural anaesthesia. Can J Anaesth 1998;45:724–8.
17. Loo CC, Dahlgreen G, Irestedt L. Neurological complications in obstetric regional anesthesia. Int J Obstet Anesth 2000;9:99–124.
18. Scavone BM. Altered level of consciousness after combined spinal-epidural labor analgesia with intrathecal fentanyl and bupivacaine. Anesthesiology 2002;96:1021–2.

Chapter 36

Anaesthesia for Cardiac Surgery

INTRODUCTION

Patients presenting for cardiac surgery belong to various age groups – infants and children for correction of congenital cardiac lesions, adults with valvular heart lesions for valve replacement or valvuloplasty, and older patients for coronary artery bypass grafting (CABG). Many of them have multi-organ diseases affecting the cardiovascular, pulmonary, cerebrovascular, endocrine and hepato-renal systems. These co-morbid conditions need to be carefully identified, assessed and optimized preoperatively.

The development of interventional cardiology has made an enormous impact on the treatment of coronary artery disease (CAD). Its impact on the use of CABG as intervention for CAD are 2-fold: the use of percutaneous transluminal coronary angioplasty (PTCA) with intraluminal coronary stenting obviates the need for CABG in a proportion of patients with CAD; there is also the occasional patient with failed angioplasty and in near-arrest state who requires emergency CABG to correct life-threatening ischaemia.

Newer surgical, monitoring and anaesthetic techniques are constantly being developed in an attempt to improve efficiency and to reduce perioperative morbidity and mortality. These are supported by advances in cardiovascular pharmacology and perfusion technology. An example is the drive towards fast-track cardiac anaesthesia, (FTCA), with the objectives of achieving early tracheal extubation and decreased length of Cardiothoracic ICU (CICU) and hospital stay. FTCA techniques entail the use of short-acting hypnotic drugs, lower opioid dose regimens or use of ultrashort-acting opioids. A recent systematic review found no evidence of increased mortality and major morbidity rates in FTCA compared to traditional high-dose opioid techniques.

Surgical procedures in the form of minimally invasive direct-access coronary artery bypass (MIDCAB) and off-pump coronary artery bypass (OPCAB) have been developed and performed in selected patients. While OPCAB is gaining popularity worldwide, MIDCAB has largely been abandoned because it allows only a single-vessel surgery, is technically demanding and may yield suboptimal results. Whatever the techniques and new innovations, good teamwork and close communication among the cardiologists, surgeons, anaesthesiologists, perfusionists and CICU staff are essential in ensuring good outcome in cardiac surgery.

CARDIOPULMONARY BYPASS (CPB)

— Cardiopulmonary bypass (CPB), a common procedure in cardiac surgery, facilitates surgery by providing a bloodless and motionless surgical field.

— Components of the CPB machine are the venous reservoir, auxiliary filter, oxygenator, heat exchanger, roller pump and arterial inflow filter. These replace the work of the heart and lungs during cardiac arrest by providing gas exchange, temperature regulation and delivery of a non-pulsatile flow. The filters trap bubbles and remove particulate matter such as fat globules, tissue particles and microthrombi that may arise during the surgery.

— Blood is siphoned from the inferior vena cava (IVC) and superior vena cava (SVC) into the reservoir, where it is filtered and pumped through the oxygenator, then the heat exchanger, and returned to the patient via an arterial cannula in the aortic root.

— CPB causes major physiological aberrations such as alterations of pulsatility and blood flow patterns, exposure to non-physiological surfaces and shear forces, and exaggerated stress and systemic inflammatory responses. Complications of CPB include these.
  - Haematological stresses: haemodilution, haemolysis, thrombocytopaenia, platelet dysfunction, consumption of coagulation factors, accelerated fibrinolysis.
  - Mechanical effects: poor venous drainage, aortic dissection, gas and particulate embolization.
  - Organ dysfunction: cerebrovascular events, subtle neuropsychiatric dysfunction, renal failure, full-blown acute respiratory distress syndrome (ARDS) or "pump lung".

Commencement of CPB

— When the pericardium is opened and the surgeon asks for heparin, inject heparin 3 mg/kg (or 300 U/kg) into the central vein. Check ACT after 3 minutes.

— The surgeon proceeds with cannulation of the aorta and vena cavae if ACT is more than 1½ times the baseline value. Maintain mean arterial pressure 60–70 mmHg or systolic BP 80–100 mmHg to reduce the risk of aortic dissection during cannulation.

— Atrial arrhythmias, usually premature atrial contractions but occasionally atrial fibrillation, are common during cannulation. If this is associated with deteriorating haemodynamic status, treat by either cardioversion or going on bypass after expeditious cannulation.

— CPB may be instituted when ACT exceeds 400 seconds, after ensuring that:
  - There are no air bubbles in the arterial line.
  - All clamps are removed from arterial and venous lines.
  - Anaesthesia is maintained by bolus doses of fentanyl and midazolam, infusion of propofol or inhalational anaesthetic agent via vaporizer mounted on the CPB machine.

- The patient is adequately paralyzed.
- Pupil size is checked and recorded (as a baseline for subsequent assessment of neurologic state or anaesthetic depth).
- Intravenous infusions are turned off.

— Observation during commencement of CPB:
- Flow of venous blood into cannula with no air locks.
- Fluid flow through arterial cannula: first clear prime then red oxygenated blood.
- Patient's head and face: plethora indicates obstruction to SVC return, right-sided blanching indicates innominate artery cannulation.
- Evidence of distension of the heart, due to inadequate venous drainage or over-zealous transfusion from the pump.

— Discontinue ventilation after the heart ceases to eject. One can either administer oxygen at low flow rates, or discontinue all gas flows and leave the lungs flaccid.

— After the aorta is cross-clamped, the cardioplegia solution is administered either into the aortic root (anterograde cardioplegia) or directly into the coronary sinus (retrograde cardioplegia). Initial dose of cardioplegia is 10 ml/kg. Observe the flow, pressure and amount given, and note the volume at which asystole occurs. Repeat ⅓ – ½ of the initial volume every 30 minutes or earlier if cardiac electrical activity appears.

Maintenance of CPB

— These are monitored by the perfusionist during CPB.
- Venous reservoir level, indicating adequacy of venous return.
- Pump flow rate.
- Arterial inflow line pressure.
- Perfusate temperature.
- Vent and pump suction: check that they are not occluded or exert too much suction pressure, which traumatizes blood.

— The perfusionist maintains the perfusion pressure at 50–70 mmHg by modifying flow and filling and by means of vasoactive drugs.

— The patient's temperature is lowered to between 28–34°C depending on the type of surgical procedure and the surgeon's preference.

— Check ABG, electrolytes, haematocrit half-hourly and make necessary corrections. Alpha-stat regime of ABG interpretation is used (pH and $PaCO_2$ values are not corrected for temperature and are kept in the normal range when measured at 37°C).

Weaning from CPB

— This is an important period when the heart and lungs are allowed to re-establish normal physiological functions. There should be close communication among the surgeon, the anaesthesiologist and the perfusionist to ensure that the patient is successfully weaned from the CPB machine.

— The surgeon asks for rewarming on completion of the cardiac procedure. It is important to avoid warming the blood too fast with subsequent formation of small air bubbles as gas solubility decreases.

— Air is evacuated if the heart has been opened during surgery. This is done by venting the ascending aorta. Inflating the lungs during this time removes the air from the pulmonary veins and helps to fill the heart with blood.

— The venous cannula is progressively occluded and the heart gradually allowed to eject. The patient should be relatively underfilled to avoid overdistension of the ventricles as additional volumes are infused. Closely observe the heart performance and filling; commence infusion of inotrope(s) if necessary. Intraaortic balloon pump counterpulsation may be required in problematic cases.

— Optimum heart rate should be 80–100/min and in sinus rhythm if possible. If the heart fibrillates on releasing the aortic cross clamp, prepare to defibrillate starting with low energy settings (10 J). Cardiac pacing may be required using a programmable pacemaker with the ventricular demand pacing mode (VVI) being most commonly used (see Chapter 14).

— Commence ventilation when the heart begins to eject. Inflate the lungs manually to assess lung compliance. Reduced tidal volumes are preferred prior to separation from CPB so that the lungs do not interfere with surgical exposure. The patient is ventilated with 100% oxygen; no nitrous oxide is used due to risk of small air emboli from CPB. Anaesthesia is maintained with volatile anaesthetic and opioid.

— Checks prior to coming off bypass
  - Heart performance is satisfactory in terms of size, contractility and rhythm, with no major bleeding in the surgical field.
  - Ventilation is satisfactory.
  - Investigation results are normal or corrected: serum potassium concentration 4–5 mmol/L; haematocrit 22–25%, ABG within the normal range.
  - The patient is warm and well perfused, with nasopharyngeal temperature at 37°C.
  - Inotropes are available and being infused via the central venous cannula if inotropic support is required.

- Pacemaker is ready or working.
- Blood and/or blood products are available and checked.

— With increasing cardiac ejection, the arterial pump flows are gradually reduced. The venous line is completely occluded first while blood is gradually returned in aliquots of 50–100 ml via the aortic cannula. When filling is optimized, the pump is turned off and bypass ceases.

— When it is certain that the heart can sustain an adequate cardiac output, slowly commence administration of protamine 3 mg/kg via a peripheral line. The systemic arterial pressure is likely to decrease as a result of vasodilatation, and pulmonary hypertension can occasionally occur. *Do not prepare protamine until the patient is off bypass* in case this is accidentally administered while on bypass. The venous cannula is clamped and removed first; the arterial cannula is removed near the end of protamine infusion when the patient is haemodynamically stable.

— Check ACT to ensure that it returns to the baseline value, signifying adequate reversal of heparin.

— Transfuse blood and/or blood products if necessary. Additional protamine may be needed when pump blood is transfused.

— Treatment options if problems are encountered on coming off bypass:
- Volume status: volume replacement if hypovolaemic; return blood to pump if overdistended.
- Calcium chloride to improve myocardial contractility.
- Vasoactive drugs: inotropes (dobutamine, dopamine, adrenaline), inodilators (milrinone), vasodilators (GTN), vasoconstrictors (noradrenaline) as appropriate.
- Antiarrhythmic treatment, pacing, isoprenaline.
- Intraaortic balloon pump or other ventricular assist device.

BLOOD CONSERVATION STRATEGIES IN CARDIAC SURGERY

The use of allogeneic blood transfusion may be reduced by various blood conservation techniques. These measures are applicable for cardiac surgery.

— Acute normovolaemic haemodilution technique: this is feasible in selected patients.

— Limit prime volume, smaller calibre tubing, limited haemodilution in CPB.

— Use of heparin-bonded circuits for CPB.

— Consider "primeless pump" to maintain higher intraoperative haematocrit, achieved by arterial and then venous side evacuation of crystalloid prior to CPB.
— After CPB, concentrate residual oxygenator contents and reinfuse to patient.
— Individualize and optimize heparinization and protamine reversal; avoid standard weight-based dosing to prevent over- or underdosage with haemostatic consequences.
— Postoperative cell salvage technique (see Chapter 55).

ANAESTHETIC MANAGEMENT FOR CABG

Preoperative Assessment

— There should be careful and detailed assessment of the cardiovascular system and left ventricular function in particular. This includes pertinent history, physical findings, cardiac catheterization and other laboratory data, and the patient's usual vital signs recorded in the ward.
— Patients undergoing CABG are generally older with concomitant medical conditions such as hypertension, diabetes mellitus, chronic obstructive pulmonary disease, cerebrovascular disease and renal dysfunction. These should be carefully identified, assessed and optimized preoperatively.
— The patient's medication should generally be continued except these.
  - Antiplatelet drugs such as aspirin, clopidogrel: stop for 7–10 days.
  - Angiotensin converting enzyme (ACE) inhibitors: withheld by some anaesthesiologists due to problems of reduced systemic vascular resistance and hypotension post-CPB.
  - Hypoglycaemic agents.
— Reserve and confirm blood and blood products. Usually 4 units of blood are requested, while complicated procedures such as re-do CABG require 6 units of blood together with blood products in the form of fresh frozen plasma, cryoprecipitate and platelets.
— Premedication can be in the form of oral benzodiazepine or intramuscular opioid with anticholinergic.
  - Oral benzodiazepine (diazepam, midazolam, lorazepam) as night sedation and/or as premedication 2 hours before surgery.
  - IM morphine 0.3–0.4 mg/kg (maximum 10 mg) or pethidine 1–1.5 mg/kg and hyoscine 0.01 mg/kg.

— Note that intramuscular injections are not recommended in patients who are on anticoagulants with prolonged International Normalized Ratio (INR).
— Reduce the dose of premedicant drugs in patients with severe left main stem disease.
— Ensure that the patient receives a nitroglycerin (GTN) patch and supplemental oxygen on transport to the OT. Some GTN tablets should accompany the patients in case anginal symptoms arise during transport.

Induction of Anaesthesia

— Check the anaesthetic machine; prepare anaesthetic drugs and vasoactive agents as required (GTN, adrenaline, dopamine).
— Establish monitors before induction of anaesthesia. These include:
  - 5-lead ECG for simultaneous monitoring of Lead II and V_5 with automated ST-segment analysis.
  - Non-invasive blood pressure measurement.
  - Pulse oximetry.
  - Capnography.
  - Temperature via nasopharyngeal temperature probe.
  - Urine output via indwelling urinary catheter.
  - Invasive haemodynamic monitors: intraarterial blood pressure and central venous pressure monitoring; cannulation is done under local anaesthesia.
  - Pulmonary artery pressure monitoring in patients with very poor left ventricular function (ejection fraction < 30%) and/or pulmonary hypertension.
  - Transoesophageal echocardiography (TEE) to monitor intraoperative regional wall motion abnormalities and cardiac valve functions.
— Consider insertion of intraaortic balloon pump (IABP) in patients with unstable angina and poor ventricular function.
— Send arterial blood samples for baseline ABG analysis, haematocrit, electrolyte concentration and activated clotting time (ACT). Check blood glucose concentration for diabetic patients.
— The use of thoracic epidural anaesthesia is controversial. While it may provide attenuation of stress response, cardiac sympathetic blockade and postoperative analgesia, concerns persist regarding risk of epidural haematoma formation in the face of full intraoperative heparinization.

- The choice of anaesthetic agents is less important than the manner of its use. Traditionally, induction of anaesthesia is achieved with high-dose fentanyl (up to 50 μg/kg) supplemented with midazolam. High-dose opioids result in less myocardial depression compared to hypnotic agents but may delay extubation due to prolonged respiratory depression. The trend is towards use of short-acting intravenous induction agents (e.g., etomidate or propofol) supplemented with remifentanil and/or inhalational anaesthetic agents (e.g., isoflurane or sevoflurane).
- A non-depolarizing neuromuscular blocking drug is administered to facilitate tracheal intubation. Laryngoscopy and intubation should be done atraumatically in view of intraoperative anticoagulation.
- Beware of hypotension postinduction, usually caused by absence of stimulation while the patient is being prepped and draped. This is usually transient but treatment is indicated if hypotension is severe (reduction in BP > 20% preinduction value) particularly in a patient with poor left ventricular function. Treatment options include reduction of concentration of volatile anaesthetic, infusion of intravenous fluid if CVP is low, small doses of vasopressor (e.g., phenylephrine) to maintain adequate myocardial perfusion pressure.

Intraoperative Management

- Anaesthesia is maintained by using oxygen, oxygen-air or oxygen-nitrous oxide mixture with isoflurane. Maintain haemodynamic stability by aiming for blood pressure and heart rate within 20% of baseline value; this is achieved by judicious use of intravenous fluids, vasopressor and GTN infusion where appropriate.
- The period from skin incision to commencement of CPB may be associated with haemodynamic changes due to intense surgical stimulation and cardiac manipulation. Sympathetic responses are often seen following skin incision, sternotomy, spreading the sternal retractor, reflecting and suturing the pericardium, and manipulation of the aorta in preparation for cannulation. These should be anticipated and attenuated by increasing the anaesthetic depth prior to these events. Options include bolus doses of fentanyl, increasing concentration of volatile anaesthetic and use of vasodilators such as GTN or sodium nitroprusside.
- Grafts may be harvested from the saphenous veins, the internal mammary or radial artery. Arterial grafts are prone to vasospasm and this is overcome by local application of papaverine by the surgeon.

— If myocardial ischaemia is evident or worsens before CPB:
  - Ensure adequacy of anaesthesia, oxygenation, ventilation and volume status.
  - Check surgical status such as profuse bleeding, mechanical disturbance to the heart.
  - Institute treatment pending clinical situation: vasodilator such as GTN if BP is high, intravenous fluids and vasopressors such as phenylephrine if BP is low, β-blockers for tachycardia (in the absence of hypovolaemia), antiarrhythmic treatment if ischaemia develops secondary to arrhythmias.
  - Administer heparin and institute early CPB if ischaemia is severe and refractory to treatment.

— Management of the patient on CPB is as described on pages 480–484.

Postoperative Management

— Send the patient to CICU with full monitoring during transport. Pass over relevant information to the CICU staff, including intraoperative events and further management plans.

— Aim for early extubation (within 1–6 hours) if the intraoperative course has been uneventful. Otherwise continue overnight ventilation or until further assessment. Adjust ventilator settings to maintain $PaCO_2$ 30–35 mmHg and PaO_2 90–100 mmHg.

— Commence infusion of sedative and analgesic drugs: midazolam, propofol, morphine or fentanyl, alone or in combination. The use of dexmedetomidine infusion, at a range of 0.2–0.7 μg/kg/hr, is especially advantageous for short-term sedation prior to extubation.

— Check CXR, ABG, FBC and electrolyte concentration.

— Continue close haemodynamic monitoring and treat cardiovascular derangements accordingly. Watch out for complications such as cardiac failure, cardiac tamponade, arrhythmias or excessive bleeding due to surgical causes or coagulation problems.

— Transfuse additional blood and/or blood products if necessary. Shed mediastinal blood can be collected through the cardiotomy reservoir and reinfused into the patient.

— The patient is ready for extubation when these criteria are met.
  - Intact central nervous system with no gross neurological deficit.
  - Stable cardiovascular parameters with MAP > 70 mmHg, LA pressure < 20 mmHg, stable heart rate and rhythm with minimal inotropic support.

- Adequate respiratory excursions with normal ABG.
- Adequate neuromuscular function with full return of airway reflexes.
- Absence of excessive bleeding from the drains or elsewhere.
- Adequate urine output > 0.5 ml/kg/hr.
- Temperature > 36°C.

Re-do CABG

— Patients who require re-do CABG are often ill and have poor left ventricular function. Surgery is technically more difficult and there is often a risk of torrential bleeding and risk of ventricular fibrillation during sternotomy and dissection of adhesions.

— Additional management includes these measures.
- A lateral CXR is useful to assess the distance between the heart shadow and the sternum. Dense adhesions are likely to be present if these structures are closely apposed to each other on CXR.
- Group and cross match 6 units of blood in reserve, with additional blood products in the form of fresh frozen plasma, cryoprecipitate and platelets.
- Place external defibrillator pads *in situ* in case defibrillation becomes necessary.
- Consider insertion of PA catheter and intraaortic balloon pump.
- Prepare automated cell saver for intraoperative cell salvage as bleeding is often substantial during chest opening and dissection prior to instituting CPB.
- Consider prophylactic use of antifibrinolytic agent such as aprotinin or tranxenamic acid during the procedure. Other useful adjuvants include desmopressin (deamino D-arginine vasopressin, DDAVP) and activated recombinant factor VII.

OFF-PUMP CORONARY ARTERY BYPASS (OPCAB)

— This is a surgical technique in which no CPB is utilized and was developed with the intention of avoiding pump-associated deleterious effects. This is particularly beneficial for patients at high risk of neurological injury, renal insufficiency, respiratory dysfunction and coagulopathy.

— OPCAB is technically more demanding compared to the conventional on-pump CABG. The surgeon needs to obtain optimal cardiac positioning to access target coronary vessels, stabilize and dampen local cardiac wall motion around the distal anastomotic site, and minimize myocardial injury from temporary occlusion of the target coronary vessel during anastomosis.

— The anaesthesiologist often encounters significant cardiovascular instability produced by cardiac manipulation and acute intraoperative myocardial ischaemia during coronary artery flow interruption.

— Close communication among the cardiac team members, already a prerequisite in cardiac surgery, is even more essential in OPCAB surgery. The team must be prepared to rapidly institute CPB in the event of sustained ventricular fibrillation or cardiovascular collapse.

— The use of volatile anaesthetic agents in OPCAB is particularly beneficial, as they have been shown to induce significant pharmacological preconditioning to confer protection against ischaemia. In contrast, intravenous anaesthetics do not seem to have significant cardioprotective effects.

— The ambient OT temperature is increased to 23–24°C during surgery and intraoperative normothermia is maintained.

— Partial heparinization (heparin 1–1.5 mg/kg) with ACT 250–300 seconds is considered adequate. Heparin reversal with protamine is optional.

— OPCAB appears to produce better results than conventional surgery in high-risk patient populations, elderly patients and those with compromised renal function or cerebrovascular disease. Other benefits include shorter time requiring ventilatory support, less blood loss or transfusion requirement, decreased systemic inflammatory response and a shorter hospital stay. Early and mid-term (1–3 years) outcomes after OPCAB are favourable but long-term outcome has not been evaluated. The potential for decreased graft patency due to the technical difficulty of grafting onto a beating heart is always a possibility. This awaits longer follow-up and further evaluation.

CARDIAC VALVE REPLACEMENT

— Patients presenting for cardiac valve replacement are generally younger than those for CABG and may have mixed valvular heart disease requiring double valve replacement.

— Clinical features are varied and include dyspnoea, angina, syncope, heart failure and palpitations. These are elaborated in Chapter 13. It is important for the anaesthesiologist to be familiar with the pathophysiology of the cardiac lesion in order to better appreciate the physiological and anaesthetic requirements in each category of patients.

— Prosthetic valves can be mechanical valves or bioprosthesis depending on the patient's age. Mechanical valves tend to be used in younger patients and lifelong anticoagulation is required to prevent clot formation around the prosthetic valves. Porcine tissue valves, with an expected lifespan of 15 years, may be used in older patients, and long-term aspirin therapy alone would suffice in such cases.

— The following are special considerations for the specific valve lesions. In cases where both the stenotic and regurgitant components are present, the dominant lesion will be more pertinent.

a. **Aortic stenosis**
   - An opioid-based technique may be more appropriate as it is associated with less myocardial depression.
   - A decrease in systemic vascular resistance (SVR) may be detrimental to coronary perfusion.
   - Haemodynamically significant atrial arrhythmias may occur during atrial manipulation, which may necessitate expeditious commencement of CPB.
   - Adrenaline may be required to improve LV performance, while alpha-agonists may be used to maintain SVR.

b. **Mitral stenosis**
   - The patient has a fixed cardiac output, may be in atrial fibrillation and may have elevated pulmonary pressures.
   - Maintain heart rate < 100/min and in sinus rhythm if possible in order to provide a more favourable oxygen supply: demand ratio and maximize coronary perfusion during diastole.
   - Pulmonary artery pressure should be monitored to assess intravascular volume and guide inotrope therapy. Nitric oxide may be considered to reduce pulmonary arterial pressure.
   - Both CVP and left atrial pressure (LAP) should be monitored after termination of CPB, especially in patients with severe pulmonary hypertension, to detect postbypass right heart failure manifested as a rise in CVP and a fall in LAP.

c. **Aortic regurgitation**
   - Preload is essential in the face of a stiff and dilated LV. Afterload should be kept low to augment forward flow.

- Cardiac output is rate-dependent; increasing the rate shortens time for regurgitation and encourages forward flow.
- Refractory bradycardia may occasionally occur, causing severe left ventricular distension. Treat with isoprenaline infusion or direct atrial pacing once the pericardium is opened.
- Abnormal myocardial contractility may be present as shown by elevated pulmonary capillary wedge pressure. An inodilator such as milrinone will improve LV function and reduce SVR at the same time.
- Meticulous blood pressure control is important in patients with aortic root dilatation or dissection. Maintain systolic BP < 120 mmHg with GTN if required.

d. **Mitral regurgitation**
- The condition may be acute (secondary to papillary muscle rupture due to myocardial infarction or trauma) or chronic (usually rheumatic in origin).
- Chronic MR may be asymptomatic or present with features of LV failure, while acute MR results in acute increases in LA pressure, pulmonary venous pressure, acute pulmonary oedema and congestive heart failure.
- Maintain preload and a relatively high heart rate to encourage forward flow.
- Inotropes are rarely needed prebypass for chronic MR, while intraaortic balloon pump may be necessary in acute MR. Adrenaline may be indicated postbypass as the LV may fail against a competent valve.

CONGENITAL HEART DISEASE FOR CARDIAC SURGERY

— The patients are often children (ranging from neonates to school-going children), adolescents or young adults.

— There may be congenital anomalies in other systems such as the gastrointestinal system, kidneys.

— Anaesthetic management requires an understanding of the pathophysiology of the cardiac defect and the nature of the surgical procedure, which may be curative (e.g., ligation of patent ductus arteriosus, closure of atrial or ventricular septal defect), corrective (e.g., Tetralogy of Fallot repair) or palliative (e.g., Fontan procedure to separate the pulmonary and systemic circulations in a patient with a single ventricle).

— The child with cyanosis suffers from chronic systemic hypoxaemia from a right-to-left shunting of blood, as a result of obstruction to pulmonary blood flow, presence of a common mixing chamber or transposition of the great vessels. Care must be taken during the perioperative period not to aggravate factors that may result in worsening hypoxaemia.

FURTHER READING

1. Lampa M, Ramsay J. Anaesthetic implications of new surgical approaches to myocardial revascularisation. Curr Opin Anaesthesiol 1999;12:3–8.
2. Chaney MA. Intrathecal and epidural anesthesia and analgesia for cardiac surgery. Anesth Analg 1997;84:1211–21.
3. Ahonen J, Salmenpera M. Brain injury after adult cardiac surgery. Acta Anaesthesiol Scand 2004;48:1–19.
4. Chassot PG, van der Linden P, Zaugg M, Mueller XM, Spahn DR. Off-pump coronary artery bypass surgery: Physiology and anaesthetic management. Br J Anaesth 2004;92:400–13.
5. Heames RM, Gill RS, Ohri SK, Hett DA. Off-pump coronary artery surgery. Anaesthesia 2002;57:676–85.
6. Angelini GD, Taylor FC, Reeves BC, Ascione R. Early and midterm outcome after off-pump and on-pump surgery in beating heart against cardioplegic arrest studies (BHACAS 1 and 2): A pooled analysis of two randomized controlled trials. Lancet 2002;359:1194–9.
7. Greenspun HG, Adourian UA, Fonger JD, Fan JS. Minimally invasive direct coronary artery bypass (MIDAB): Surgical techniques and anesthetic considerations. J Cardiothorac Vasc Anesth 1996;10:507–9.
8. Wake PJ, Cheng DCH. Postoperative intensive care in cardiac surgery. Curr Opin Anaesthesiol 2001;14:41–5.
9. Myles PS, Daly DJ, Djalani G, Lee A, Cheng DCH. A systematic review of the safety and effectiveness of fast-track cardiac anesthesia. Anesthesiology 2003;99:982–7.

Chapter 37

Anaesthesia for Thoracic Surgery

INTRODUCTION

Thoracic surgery involves surgical procedures on any thoracic structures (airways, lungs, heart, oesophagus, mediastinum, great vessels) via sternotomy, thoracotomy or performed endoscopically. These include:

— Lung-related surgery: lobectomy, pneumonectomy, drainage of empyema, closure of bronchopleural fistula, lung volume reduction surgery (LVRS), video-assisted thoracoscopic surgery (VATS).

— Surgery to the heart or great vessels.

— Mediastinal surgery: resection of thymus, retrosternal thyroid or other mediastinal tumours, mediastinoscopy.
— Oesophagectomy via the thoraco-abdominal approach.
— Trauma surgery: repair of ruptured airways, aorta or pulmonary vessels, lung resection.

Risks of postoperative pulmonary complications in the form of pneumonia, atelectasis, hypoxaemia or respiratory failure are high in patients undergoing thoracic surgery. This is especially so in the elderly, those with preexisting chronic pulmonary diseases and chronic smokers. As many of the patients have co-existing cardiac impairment, postoperative cardiac complications are not uncommon in such patients.

Thoracic anaesthesia is often challenging because of these aspects:

— **Patients** often pose significant anaesthetic risks due to severe cardiovascular and respiratory impairment.
— **Surgery** often involves significant physiological changes and massive blood loss.
— **Anaesthesia** requires skill and experience in the management of one lung ventilation (OLV), including correction of hypoxaemia during OLV.

PREOPERATIVE ASSESSMENT

— The patient's cardiorespiratory reserve should be carefully assessed; consultation with the respiratory physician and/or cardiologist is often necessary.
— Endocrinopathies, though rare, may be seen in patients with carcinoma of bronchus. Examples include myasthenic syndrome (Eaton-Lambert syndrome) and secretion of ectopic hormone such as adrenocorticotropic hormone (ACTH), parathyroid hormone (PTH).
— Patients with myasthenia gravis may present for thymectomy.
— Investigations
  - Blood tests: FBC, urea, electrolytes, creatinine, blood glucose concentration.
  - 12-lead ECG, with more detailed tests to the cardiovascular system if indicated.
  - CXR and CT scan/MRI of chest: assess abnormalities related to the heart and lungs; delineate nature and extent of the lesion. It is important to check for evidence of compression, tumour infiltration or distortion of the tracheobronchial anatomy as this may complicate endobronchial intubation.

- Baseline arterial blood gases (ABG).
- Baseline lung function test.

— Preoperative tests (spirometry, ABG analysis) have been used to assess suitability of patient for lung resection. Traditionally, limits have been defined for values of forced expiratory volume in 1 second (FEV_1), forced vital capacity (FVC) or $PaCO_2$ beyond which pulmonary resection is considered inadvisable.
  - Generally accepted minimum preoperative FEV_1: > 55% (pneumonectomy); > 40% (lobectomy); > 35% (wedge resection) of predicted value.
  - Predictors of increased operative morbidity and/or mortality: $PaCO_2$ > 45 mmHg; FEV_1 < 2 L (pneumonectomy); < 1 L (lobectomy); < 0.6 L (wedge resection); FEV_1 < 50% FVC.

  Note that these limits have recently been challenged particularly in cases of VATS and LVRS.

Preoperative Preparation

The following measures have been taken to prepare the patient for surgery, with the objective of reducing perioperative morbidity and mortality.

— Cessation of smoking.

— Optimization of concomitant medical conditions.

— Improvement of nutritional status especially for carcinoma of oesophagus: total parenteral nutrition (TPN) may be indicated if enteral feeding is not adequate.

— Treatment of any lung infection with relevant antibiotics.

— Use of bronchodilators in the perioperative period for prevention and/or treatment of bronchospasm.

— Chest physiotherapy and breathing exercises in the form of postural drainage, physiotherapy and suction, deep breathing and coughing exercises, incentive spirometry.

— Prophylactic digitalization (controversial): digitalis has long been used to reduce the incidence of supraventricular arrhythmias and postpneumonectomy pulmonary oedema. Its use is now limited since there are doubts as to its effectiveness, coupled with concerns about digitalis toxicity during the perioperative period.

The nature of premedication depends on the general status of the patient. It should be omitted in cachexic, malnourished patients. Intramuscular opioid premedication is preferable to oral sedation in carcinoma of oesophagus because of uncertain drug absorption from the gastrointestinal tract. Consider using an antisialogogue to facilitate insertion of bronchoscope and tracheal intubation.

INTRAOPERATIVE MANAGEMENT

In addition to routine monitoring of ECG, non-invasive BP, pulse oximetry and capnography, invasive monitoring such as intraarterial BP and CVP are indicated for most thoracic surgical procedures. Other parameters to be monitored are urine output, temperature and neuromuscular blockade.

If a thoracic epidural block is planned for intra- and postoperative analgesia, this is established before induction of general anaesthesia. This enables early detection of complications, such as spinal cord injury or paraesthesia, in a conscious patient.

Methods of Lung Isolation

These devices are commonly used for lung isolation.

1. **Double-lumen endobronchial tube (DLT)**
   - This is the most versatile and most commonly used method of lung separation.
   - Examples of DLT:
     - Robertshaw (red rubber tube).
     - Single-use polyvinyl chloride tube, e.g., Broncho-Cath™.
     - Carlens (left-sided DLT with a carinal hook).
   - Various sizes are available: 3 sizes (small, medium, large) for Robertshaw; sizes 28–41 Ch for Broncho-Cath™. The Charriere (Ch) gauge corresponds to the external circumference in millimetres.
   - DLT is described as "right" or "left" according to the main bronchus it is designed to intubate. The right-sided DLT has a slit in the wall of the endobronchial section to facilitate ventilation of the right upper lobe.

Choice of DLT

- The use of DLT is contraindicated in the presence of an extremely distorted tracheobronchial anatomy or an intraluminal lesion. These should be ruled out by prior assessment of CXR, CT scan and any previous bronchoscopy reports.

- The left-sided DLT is almost always used because of the ease in placement, versatility and greater margin of safety. It also gives a better tolerance to shifts in tube position that frequently occurs when the patient's position is altered.
- If clamping of the left main bronchus is necessary (e.g., in left pneumonectomy), the left-sided DLT cuffs are deflated, the tube withdrawn into the trachea and the tracheal cuff re-inflated. It then functions as a single-lumen tube with both lumens ventilating the right lung.
- The left-sided DLT is contraindicated if the left main bronchus is stenosed, disrupted, distorted or infiltrated with tumour.
- The right-sided DLT has a lower margin of safety in ensuring that the right upper lobe is well ventilated. However, by using fibreoptic bronchoscope to confirm placement, right-sided DLTs can be used with a higher rate of reliability than previously appreciated.

Size of DLT

- The DLT lumen is small compared to a standard single-lumen endotracheal tube, hence the largest DLT that will pass easily through the glottis should be chosen. This corresponds to 41 or 39 Ch gauge PVC tube (large or medium Robertshaw) for males; 37 Ch gauge PVC tube (medium Robertshaw) for females; and 35 Ch gauge PVC tube (small Robertshaw) for small individuals.
- It is important to use DLT of the correct size: an inappropriately small tube will be prone to displacement, may fail to provide adequate lung isolation or require large bronchial cuff volumes or pressures that could damage the bronchus; while too large a DLT can rupture the trachea or bronchus.
- It is important to test for leaks around the bronchus. The bronchial cuff should only be inflated to the minimal volume that provides lung isolation: recommended volume of air for cuff inflation: 1–3 ml (bronchial); 5–7 ml (tracheal).

2. **Bronchial blocker**
   - This consists of a balloon-tipped catheter either within or external to a single-lumen tracheal tube; it is advanced into the bronchus to be occluded under bronchoscopic guidance.
   - It is occasionally useful in patients who are difficult to intubate, have distorted tracheobronchial anatomy or have a tracheostomy *in situ*.

— Disadvantages of the bronchial blocker
  - Reliability with complete isolation is not as good compared to DLT.
  - It tends to become dislodged during manipulation.
  - There is no easy access for suctioning the non-ventilated lung.

— The Univent® tube is a single-lumen tube with a moveable bronchial blocker enclosed in a separate channel within the tube. It has the advantage of being stabilized by the cuff of the tracheal tube.

3. **Single-lumen endobronchial tube**
   — This is a standard ETT inserted into the trachea and later advanced under bronchoscopic guidance into the bronchus to act as an endobronchial tube when OLV is needed.

Insertion and Checking of Correct Placement of DLT

Many anaesthetic trainees are confused about the steps taken to check the correct placement of DLT. It is actually not difficult if one has a clear picture of what one is checking for in each step of the checking sequence.

1. **Preliminary steps**
   — Check the DLT especially the cuffs; have various sizes of DLT available.
   — Make sure the Y-connector, the clamps and the 15-mm connectors for the DLT lumens are available.
   — Establish venous access and monitoring.
   — Preoxygenate the patient for 3–5 minutes.
   — Commence induction of anaesthesia with IV fentanyl, thiopentone, suxamethonium.

2. **Intubation**
   — Perform laryngoscopy when the patient is adequately anaesthetized.
   — Insert DLT with the tip facing anteriorly.
   — Rotate DLT 90° anticlockwise (for left-sided DLT) or 90° clockwise (for right-sided DLT) once the tip is past the glottis.
   — Gently advance DLT until resistance is felt.
   — Connect to the breathing system.

3. **Checking by auscultation**
   - Inflate the tracheal cuff and ventilate.
     - Both lungs should expand and breath sounds should be equal bilaterally.
     - This indicates the DLT is in the trachea and not in the oesophagus.
   - Inflate the bronchial cuff and ventilate.
     - Again both lungs should expand and breath sounds should be equal bilaterally.
     - This indicates the bronchial tube is in place and the bronchial cuff does not occlude the bronchial lumen by over-inflation.
   - Clamp off the gas flow to the tracheal lumen at the Y-connector and open sealing cap on the tracheal lumen to air.
     - Only the lung ventilated through the bronchial lumen (left lung in left-sided DLT, or right lung in right-sided DLT) should expand.
     - Listen at the open lumen to detect air leak around the bronchial cuff. If a reasonable seal cannot be obtained, the DLT is either incorrectly positioned or too small for the patient.
     - Assess compliance by manual ventilation. Very poor compliance (peak pressure > 35 cmH_2O) not explained by the patient's pathology suggests malposition of the DLT.
   - Re-connect the tracheal tube and repeat the manoeuvre on the other lumen.
     - The opposite lung to the above manoeuvre should expand, i.e., right lung for left-sided DLT or left lung for right-sided DLT.
     - Listen at the disconnected bronchial lumen to detect air leak.

4. **Bronchoscopic confirmation**
   - Proper positioning of the DLT should be confirmed with the fibreoptic bronchoscope, because a significant number of critically malpositioned tubes will be missed by reliance on clinical signs alone.
   - The bronchoscope is passed down the tracheal lumen first. There should be a clear straight-ahead view of the carina indicating the tracheal tube is positioned above the carina. For left-sided DLT the left tube is seen going into the left main bronchus with the upper surface of the left bronchial cuff visible just below the carina. The opposite applies for the right-sided DLT.
   - The bronchoscope is then passed down the bronchial lumen to determine whether there is any cuff herniation that may partially occlude the bronchial lumen. For right-sided DLT, the slit in the wall of the bronchial lumen should be aligned with the upper lobe bronchus.

- DLT is re-positioned under bronchoscopic guidance if necessary. The bronchoscope is inserted via the bronchial lumen, DLT is partially withdrawn to lie in the trachea and the carina is located with the scope. The scope is then advanced into the appropriate bronchus and the DLT railroaded into its correct position.

5. Anchor the DLT securely. After the patient has been placed in the lateral decubitus position, check that the DLT has not been displaced by means of auscultation and/or fibreoptic bronchoscope.

6. *Note:* If lung isolation should be achieved urgently to prevent soiling of the unaffected lung (e.g., empyema or active pulmonary haemorrhage), the bronchial cuff should be inflated first before the above steps are taken.

Maintenance of Anaesthesia

1. **Two-lung ventilation**
   - This should be maintained for as long as possible during surgery, with typical ventilatory settings at FiO_2 0.33, tidal volume 10 ml/kg, respiratory rate 10–12/min, airway pressure < 25 cmH_2O.
   - Closely monitor the patient's haemodynamic and ventilatory status.
   - Continuous display of the airway pressure/volume loop is useful in monitoring and managing OLV. Check baseline ABG while on two-lung ventilation.

2. **During one-lung ventilation (OLV)**
   - Increase FiO_2 to 0.5 and supplement anaesthesia with fentanyl or morphine and a volatile anaesthetic (avoid halothane because of its arrhythmogenicity in the presence of possible hypercarbia).
   - Check ABG while on OLV, maintain tidal volume at 8–10 ml/kg and adjust respiratory rate to maintain $PaCO_2$ between 30–40 mmHg.
   - Closely observe the airway pressure: it often increases by 30–40% but if excessive (peak pressure > 35 cmH_2O) may be due to other causes such as obstruction or DLT malposition.
   - Check with the surgeon that the lung is collapsed and the mediastinum is not displaced.

3. **If severe hypoxaemia occurs**
   - Exclude other causes – *these are still possible!* – oxygen supply failure, breathing system problems such as disconnection, obstruction, malfunctioning of unidirectional valves.
   - Increase FiO_2 to 1.0.
   - Check haemodynamic status, correct hypovolaemia and hypotension if present.
   - Check DLT position and patency.
     - Auscultate the dependent lung to check for breath sounds and adventitious sounds.
     - Suction DLT to clear secretions.
     - Rule out DLT cuff problem by deflating then re-inflating the cuffs.
     - Re-check the DLT position with fibreoptic bronchoscope.
   - Apply continuous positive airway pressure (CPAP) of 5–10 cmH_2O to the non-dependent lung. This requires a separate oxygen source and a pressure gauge to determine the amount of CPAP applied.
   - Apply positive end-expiratory pressure (PEEP) to the dependent lung, starting with 5 cmH_2O. This can be increased to 10 cmH_2O if the patient's cardiovascular status is not compromised.
   - Re-check patient's oxygenation and haemodynamic parameters.
     - Send blood sample for ABG analysis.
     - Inform the surgeon if the patient's oxygenation is not satisfactory.
     - Resume two-lung ventilation until SpO_2 improves.
   - For pneumonectomy, get the surgeon to clamp the pulmonary artery as soon as possible. This eliminates the problem of shunting blood to the non-ventilated lung resulting in hypoxaemia.

Other Considerations

- Good intravenous access is essential since blood loss may be substantial. CVP monitoring may be unreliable in the lateral position with an open chest but the central venous catheter may be a useful source of venous access and for postoperative monitoring.
- Radial artery on the dependent arm should be cannulated since this arm is extended on lateral decubitus position during surgery.

— Titrate intravenous fluid replacement to intraoperative losses. Avoid overzealous fluid administration especially in pneumonectomy as this may contribute to post-pneumonectomy pulmonary oedema.
— Watch out for cardiac arrhythmias and/or hypotension as a result of surgical manipulation that causes compression to the heart and great vessels. Inform the surgeon if this occurs.
— The airway to the collapsed lung should be suctioned prior to re-inflation. Following lung resection, the bronchial suture line is "leak tested" by manual inflation to 40 cmH_2O.
— Following an uneventful surgery in an otherwise healthy patient, aim to extubate the patient awake at the end of the surgery. Ensure adequate postoperative analgesia to facilitate postoperative recovery.

POSTOPERATIVE MANAGEMENT

Postoperative management is just as important as intraoperative management, with particular attention to these aspects.

1. Postoperative ICU/HDU management
   — Early extubation should be the aim since postoperative IPPV stresses suture lines, increases air leaks and risk of chest infection.
   — For the patient who has undergone pneumonectomy, check the position of the trachea before extubation.
   — Continue oxygen therapy to compensate for increased V/Q mismatch.

2. Postoperative analgesia
   — Effective analgesia is important to prevent hypoventilation and atelectasis leading to hypoxaemia.
   — Options for postoperative analgesia include:
   - Thoracic epidural analgesia by means of continuous infusion, intermittent bolus doses or patient-controlled epidural analgesia.
   - Intercostal nerve block under direct vision at the time of chest closure.
   - Paravertebral block with catheter inserted by the surgeon at the time of chest closure.
   - Interpleural block inserted at the end of the surgery.
   - Wound infiltration during skin closure.

- Intravenous infusion of opioid such as morphine while in ICU or HDU.
- Intravenous patient-controlled analgesia with morphine or pethidine.

— In the absence of contraindications, NSAIDs are useful as adjuncts to local anaesthetics and opioids.

3. Close monitoring
   — Cardiovascular system: BP, heart rate, CVP, SpO_2; watch out for cardiac arrhythmias such as atrial fibrillation particularly following pneumonectomy.
   — Respiratory system: adequacy of ventilation, serial ABGs.
   — Fluid balance and urine output.
   — Haematology and biochemistry: urea, creatinine, electrolyte concentrations, FBC (consider blood transfusion if Hct < 30%).
   — Repeat CXR, 12-lead ECG.

4. Care of intercostal drains
   — Make sure that the intercostal drain is patent and functioning.
   — Check with CXR to confirm positions of intercostal drain and mediastinum.
   — Note the amount and nature of fluid drained out: the surgeon should be alerted if the drain consists of fresh blood exceeding 150–200 ml/hr.

5. Postpneumonectomy intercostal drains
   — This is a contentious issue.
   — Some surgeons do not insert any intercostal drain after pneumonectomy since there is no remaining lung tissue on the operated side for re-expansion. The cavity fills up gradually with a sero-sanguinous exudate that is allowed to accumulate provided there are no postoperative complications (e.g., active bleeding) and the mediastinum is not displaced.
   — Some surgeons feel that closing the chest without intercostal drain is dangerous since there may be concealed bleeding into the chest cavity. A single basal drain with underwater seal is inserted. The intercostal drain is clamped and released intermittently every 2–4 hours. Suction is absolutely contraindicated since it predisposes to a mediastinal shift that may cause cardiovascular embarrassment.

6. Postpneumonectomy pulmonary oedema
   — This occurs in 2–4% of cases and is more frequently seen following right pneumonectomy.

- Symptoms usually begin 48–72 hours after surgery although the radiologic changes may occur before the onset of symptoms.
- Histologically it is compatible with acute respiratory distress syndrome (ARDS), and mortality rate is high (> 50%).
- Causes may be multi-factorial. Fluid overload, abnormal lung lymphatic drainage, increased capillary permeability, right ventricular dysfunction are some of the mechanisms proposed.
- The patient should be fluid restricted. Total positive fluid balance in the first 24 hours should not be more than 20 ml/kg. In an average adult this translates to < 2 L intraoperatively and < 50 ml/hr postoperatively. Diuretics may be administered to increase urine output.
- If increased tissue perfusion is required postoperatively, consider use of inotropes under invasive haemodynamic monitoring rather than excessive fluid administration.

7. Chest physiotherapy and breathing exercises, which began preoperatively, should be re-instituted as early as the patient's condition permits. Early ambulation is also necessary to reduce the incidence of deep vein thrombosis and pulmonary thromboembolism.

8. Watch out for these complications
   - Respiratory insufficiency: sputum retention with atelectasis, respiratory distress, respiratory failure.
   - Cardiovascular instability: hypotension, cardiac arrhythmias, pericarditis, acute right heart failure, myocardial infarction, pulmonary oedema, heart herniation in radical pneumonectomy which involves resection of part of the pericardium.
   - Acute haemorrhage into the chest cavity.
   - Empyema in the pleural cavity.
   - Bronchopleural fistula due to dehiscence of the bronchial stump.
   - Acute renal failure, pulmonary infarction, spinal cord ischaemia, paraplegia.

ANAESTHESIA FOR MEDIASTINAL TUMOURS: GENERAL PRINCIPLES

- Patients with anterior mediastinal masses may present for diagnostic or definitive surgical procedures and pose serious challenges to the anaesthesiologist.
- Main problems encountered include:
  - Compression of the heart leading to haemodynamic instability.

  - Compression of the large vessels, specifically superior vena cava (SVC) obstruction.
  - Compression of the trachea and main bronchi, with potential for total airway obstruction under general anaesthesia and muscle paralysis leading to hypoxaemia and death.
- The presence and degree of airway obstruction should be assessed.
  - Dyspnoea or noisy breathing at rest, on exertion and in different positions.
  - Stridor, wheezing, rhonchi, reduced breath sounds on examination.
  - Radiological examinations (plain X-rays, CT scan or MRI) to determine the level and extent of compression of tracheobronchial tree.
  - Lung function tests with flow-volume loop studies in supine and upright positions to quantify the degree of impairment, and differentiate between extra- and intrathoracic obstruction.
- Note that airway compression may be insidious when it is intrathoracic and occurs at the bronchial level. The patient may be asymptomatic and airway obstruction only manifests itself at induction of anaesthesia when voluntary control of the airway is lost.
- These considerations are pertinent in the choice of anaesthetic technique.
  - General anaesthesia should be avoided wherever possible given the extreme anaesthetic risks involved. If possible the tissue biopsy should be obtained under local anaesthesia.
  - If general anaesthesia is unavoidable, intubate the trachea by means of awake fibreoptic bronchoscopy under topical anaesthesia.
  - If awake fibreoptic intubation is not suitable or possible, induction of anaesthesia is by means of inhalation of sevoflurane. No intravenous induction agent or neuromuscular blocking drug should be administered.
- The patient should adopt the position of greatest comfort on the operating table prior to induction of anaesthesia.
- Venous access should be established on the lower limb in view of SVC obstruction.
- The ENT surgeon and cardiothoracic team should be available with rigid bronchoscope and cardiopulmonary bypass equipment for immediate use if necessary.
- If ventilation is difficult and desaturation occurs, an attempt should be made to pass the endotracheal tube down the least obstructed bronchus, failing which the ENT surgeon should try to pass the rigid bronchoscope. Cardiopulmonary bypass may be instituted as a life-saving measure if this fails.

— The patient should be managed in ICU postoperatively because airway obstruction can occur on emergence or after extubation.

VIDEO-ASSISTED THORACOSCOPIC SURGERY

— Thoracoscopy is a minimally invasive procedure that involves intentionally creating a pneumothorax and introducing a telescope through an intercostal incision to visualize intrathoracic structures.

— Video-assisted thoracoscopic surgery (VATS) was initially used for simple diagnostic procedures involving the pleura, lungs and mediastinum. New innovative applications of the technique have now been developed, and surgical procedures done under thoracoscopy now include lobectomy, oesophageal surgery and transthoracic sympathectomy for treatment of hyperhidrosis.

— Compared to thoracotomy, thoracoscopic surgery is much less invasive, gives rise to less postoperative pain, fewer respiratory complications and shorter hospital stay.

— Preoperative assessment similar to that for thoracotomy should be carried out even though the procedure is less invasive.

— The procedure is done under general anaesthesia with DLT insertion and OLV. Commence OLV before insertion of the trocar to minimize the risk of lung injury. CO_2 insufflation may be used during VATS to improve surgical exposure.

— The use of short-acting anaesthetic agents is important to allow rapid emergence and recovery of airway reflexes. Total intravenous anaesthesia (TIVA) with infusions of propofol and remifentanil (or bolus doses of fentanyl) is an attractive option.

— Management of hypoxaemia during OLV is similar to that during thoracotomy.

— Options of postoperative analgesia include intercostal nerve or paravertebral blocks and intravenous PCA with morphine. Epidural analgesia is seldom necessary unless the procedure is extensive or conversion to open thoracotomy is a distinct possibility.

— The patient is extubated and nursed propped up with supplemental oxygen after the procedure.

— A CXR is required postoperatively to confirm full re-expansion of the collapsed lung.

LUNG VOLUME REDUCTION SURGERY

- Lung volume reduction surgery (LVRS) involves resection of 20–30% of diseased lung tissue in selected patients with severe emphysema. It has been shown to improve dyspnoea and pulmonary function in such patients. However, consensus regarding issues such as patient selection criteria, best surgical approach (median sternotomy versus thoracotomy versus bilateral VATS), and cost-effectiveness has yet to be established.
- LVRS should only be performed in specialist centres as part of a multi-disciplinary programme with close coordination among the surgeon, anaesthesiologist, respiratory physician, intensivist, physiotherapist and dietician. Careful preoperative assessment and optimization is required.
- Premedication should be light or omitted altogether.
- Invasive monitoring of BP and CVP should be established under local anaesthesia before induction.
- Thoracic epidural block, inserted prior to induction of anaesthesia, is indicated for intraoperative and postoperative analgesia.
- Anaesthetic technique consists of general anaesthesia with propofol or etomidate, muscle relaxation, intubaton with DLT and maintenance with TIVA. Short-acting anaesthetic agents should be used to enable rapid postoperative recovery.
- The patient may be volume depleted, and hydration before induction should be guided by CVP. The induction to incision interval should be shortened as much as possible.
- Mechanical ventilation with IPPV should be instituted cautiously taking into account the problem of hyperinflation and air trapping in emphysema. Recommended ventilator settings are tidal volume 6–8 ml/kg, respiratory rate 10–12 breaths/min, I:E ratio 1:4, peak airway pressure < 30 cmH_2O. Allow permissive hypercapnia.
- Nitrous oxide is contraindicated since there is a serious risk of rupturing the emphysematous bullae with IPPV causing leaks and tension pneumothorax.
- Aim for smooth emergence and early tracheal extubation at the end of surgery as postoperative mechanical ventilation is undesirable.
- The patient should be managed in HDU or ICU.
- Look out for postoperative air leaks: this may occur for more than 7 days in 50% of patients.
- Ensure adequate postoperative analgesia, chest physiotherapy and early mobilization.
- Other postoperative therapy includes bronchodilators, corticosteroids, diuretics.

FURTHER READING

1. Beckles MA, Spiro SG, Colice GI, Rudd RM. The physiologic evaluation of patients with lung cancer being considered for resectional surgery. Chest 2003;123:105S–114S.
2. Campos JH. Current techniques for perioperative lung isolation in adults. Anesthesiology 2002;97:1295–301.
3. Pennefather SH, Russell GN. Placement of double lumen tubes – time to shed light on an old problem (Editorial). Br J Anaesth 2000;84:308–10.
4. Slinger P. Lung isolation in thoracic anesthesia: State of the art. Can J Anaesth 2001;48:R1–R10.
5. Brodsky JB. Approaches to hypoxemia during single-lung ventilation. Curr Opin Anaesthesiol 2001;14:71–6.
6. Azad SC. Perioperative pain management in patients undergoing thoracic surgery. Curr Opin Anaesthesiol 2001;14:87–91.
7. Plummer S, Hartley M, Vaughan RS. Anaesthesia for telescopic procedures in the thorax. Br J Anaesth 1998;80:223–34.
8. Conacher ID. Anaesthesia for thoracoscopic surgery. Best Prac Res Clin Anaesthesiol 2002;16:53–62.
9. Mets B. Current status of lung volume reduction. Curr Opin Anaesthesiol 2000;13:61–4.
10. Hillier J, Gillbe C. Anaesthesia for lung volume reduction surgery. Anaesthesia 2003;58:1210–9.
11. Slinger PD. Post-pneumonectomy pulmonary edema: Is anesthesia to blame? Curr Opin Anaesthesiol 1999;12:49–54.
12. Goh MH, Liu, XY, Goh YS. Anterior mediastinal masses: An anaesthetic challenge. Anaesthesia 1999;54:670–82.

Chapter 38

Anaesthesia for Vascular Surgery

INTRODUCTION

Aneurysms and occlusive diseases involving the vascular tree are due to atherosclerosis in over 90% of the patients. Atherosclerosis results in occlusion and ischaemia when perfusion becomes critical, while the atheromatous plaque may break off and result in embolic phenomena. The generalized atherosclerotic process may involve the coronary vasculature as well. Such patients presenting for vascular surgery are high-risk candidates for perioperative ischaemic events, be it coronary, cerebrovascular or peripheral vascular. They need close monitoring and early aggressive therapeutic intervention if required.

Vascular surgery involves repair or reconstruction of blood vessel for aneurysmal disease, vascular insufficiency or trauma. It also removes atheromatous plaque from within the artery, and creates shunts to bypass areas of occlusion. Common procedures performed in vascular surgery include:

- Aneurysm surgery: repair of abdominal aortic aneurysm (AAA), thoracic aortic aneurysm (TAA) or thoracoabdominal aortic aneurysm (TAAA).
- Aortic surgery on the ascending aorta, aortic arch.
- Peripheral revascularization surgery: femoropopliteal bypass, femorodistal bypass, femorofemoral crossover graft, axillobifemoral bypass.
- Carotid artery surgery: carotid endarterectomy (CEA).
- Embolectomy, amputation, varicose vein surgery (often done by the orthopaedic and general surgeon).

The perioperative mortality in vascular surgery is largely determined by the patient's co-morbid condition as well as the type and extent of surgery. Certain procedures such as repair of ruptured aortic aneurysm carry a high mortality because of the severity of the surgical condition and the urgency of the procedure necessitating resuscitation and anaesthesia on an often-moribund patient. On the other end of the spectrum, perioperative mortality is much lower in procedures such as peripheral vascular bypass surgery. This does not involve extreme haemodynamic derangements during surgery, and most patients have an uneventful intraoperative course and postoperative recovery.

PREOPERATIVE ASSESSMENT

Patients suffering from vascular disease are considered to be high-risk candidates for surgery and anaesthesia because of their numerous co-morbid conditions. They are often elderly and arteriopathic, and there is a high prevalence of cardiovascular disease and other age-related diseases.

Thorough assessment and optimization of the cardiovascular system is extremely important. This is reflected by the fact that in AAA surgery 40–60% of perioperative deaths are due to acute myocardial infarction. Preoperative assessment involves consultation with a cardiologist for a thorough cardiac work-up to determine the severity of underlying cardiac disease and the cardiorespiratory reserve of the patient. This is elaborated in Chapter 12.

Other concomitant diseases such as hypertension (Chapter 11), chronic respiratory disease (Chapter 15), diabetes mellitus (Chapter 19), renal and hepatic diseases (Chapters 16 and 17) should be assessed and the treatment optimized before surgery.

Approximately 30–40% of vascular procedures are semi-urgent or emergent, and it may not be feasible to carry out a complete preoperative evaluation including investigative procedures. This entails discussion among the surgeon, anaesthesiologist and the physician; the risks of delaying urgent surgery should be balanced against those of undue haste at the expense of preoperative assessment and optimization.

INTRAOPERATIVE MANAGEMENT

Regional Anaesthesia in Vascular Surgery

Several studies have investigated whether regional anaesthesia is beneficial in terms of outcome following vascular surgery compared with general anaesthesia alone. The Multicentre Australian Study of Epidural Anaesthesia (the MASTER Anaesthesia Trial), for example, found no evidence that perioperative epidural analgesia significantly influences major morbidity or mortality after major abdominal surgery.

The advantages of regional anaesthesia, commonly epidural and sometimes spinal anaesthesia, include improvement in blood flow to the lower limbs, effective postoperative analgesia, reduced risk of deep vein thrombosis and early recovery. Regional anaesthesia also acts as a form of preemptive analgesia for amputations and possibly reduces the problem of phantom limb pain.

As an alternative, peripheral nerve blocks (cervical or lumbar plexus, sciatic, femoral) may be utilized to provide anaesthesia for peripheral vascular surgery in selected patients. This would avoid the haemodynamic disturbances associated with central neuraxial blockade. A combination of femoral and sciatic nerve blocks can be used for virtually all lower limb procedures, but care must be taken with the dose of local anaesthetic used for both blocks to avoid overdosage. Carotid artery surgery can also be performed under cervical plexus blocks to facilitate intraoperative monitoring of the patient's neurological status.

The most common side-effects of regional anaesthesia involve insufficient blockade and hypotension due to sympathetic blockade and vasodilatation. The use of intraoperative anticoagulation is also a cause for concern, as there is a small (but reported) risk of epidural haematoma, even though the amount of heparin used for vascular surgery is lower than that used in cardiac surgery. The choice of anaesthetic technique should again be individualized, weighing the risks versus benefits of regional anaesthesia for each patient.

In many instances a combined regional and general anaesthesia technique is adopted. This provides patient comfort as well as effective intra- and postoperative analgesia. The regional block should be established before induction of anaesthesia to enable detection of problems during insertion of block in a conscious patient.

Intraoperative Monitoring in Vascular Surgery

The extent and invasiveness of monitoring depends on the status of the patient, the nature of surgery and the intraoperative haemodynamic stresses anticipated. In certain procedures such as AAA repair, the cardiovascular system should be closely monitored while in CEA, the emphasis should be on cerebral perfusion.

Intraoperative monitors include these.

- Cardiovascular parameters
  - ECG (lead II, CM_5), pulse oximetry for all patients.
  - Intraarterial BP, CVP for major vascular surgery.
  - Pulmonary artery catheterization, transoesophageal echocardiography (TEE) for patients at increased risk of myocardial ischaemia or with severe ventricular dysfunction.
- Respiratory parameters: capnography, spirometry for patients under general anaesthesia.
- Renal parameters: urine output via indwelling urinary catheter.
- Neurophysiologic parameters
  - Monitoring for spinal cord ischaemia: somatosensory evoked potential (SSEP) or motor evoked potential (MEP).
  - Monitoring for cerebral ischaemia: electroencephalography (EEG), SSEP, transcranial Doppler, internal carotid artery stump pressure, jugular venous oxygen saturation, *and the awake patient!*
- Biochemistry: ABG, electrolytes, haemoglobin and haematocrit, glucose, coagulation screen.

POSTOPERATIVE MANAGEMENT: GENERAL GUIDELINES

Postoperative management is no less important because the risk of postoperative myocardial event is ever present. Postoperative metabolic stresses produce undesired cardiovascular responses, which may precipitate cardiac failure and acute coronary insufficiency. The stresses may also induce a coagulation response, which results in hypercoagulability.

Following a major vascular surgery, postoperative management should be carried out in ICU or HDU especially if the patient belongs to the high-risk category. A reasonably healthy patient who underwent an uneventful peripheral vascular surgery may be managed in the ward.

These aspects of management should be considered.

— **Ventilatory support**
  - Most patients do not require prolonged mechanical ventilation in the postoperative period. Early extubation is imperative in CEA to enable early assessment of neurological status.
  - If in doubt, continue sedation and ventilation in ICU until the haemodynamic status is stable, hypothermia is corrected, respiratory effort is adequate, the patient is sedated but alert and ABG is satisfactory.
  - Usual criteria for extubation apply.

— **Analgesia**
  - Adequate postoperative analgesia is important to reduce pulmonary complications and allow early ambulation.
  - Options include epidural analgesia, intravenous morphine or pethidine infusion (in ICU/HDU) and patient-controlled analgesia when the patient is conscious.

— **Cardiovascular system**
  - Continue invasive monitoring of haemodynamic parameters.
  - Check 12-lead ECG and compare with preoperative ECG for any changes suggestive of further ischaemic events.
  - Send blood samples for plasma creatinine kinase-MB fraction (CK-MB) or cardiac Troponin I if acute myocardial infarction is suspected.
  - Treat hypo- or hypertension aggressively. Inotropic support may be indicated if BP is low and hypovolaemia is excluded.
  - Development of hypotension in the later postoperative period is usually associated with sepsis syndrome, likely causes being pneumonia, intravascular device-related infection, and urinary tract and intraabdominal infection. Management with low-dose noradrenaline infusion 0.02–0.08 μg/kg/min may be indicated.

— **Renal function**
  - Maintain urine output > 0.5–1 ml/kg/hr.
  - Send blood samples for urea, creatinine, electrolyte concentrations. Correct abnormalities if present.

- Consider renal replacement therapy. Refer to nephrologist if patient shows signs of acute renal failure.

— **Fluids**
- Sequestration of fluid in the third space is common immediately following surgery, but greater-than-expected volume requirements would demand exclusion of on-going haemorrhage.
- Volume requirement may also be increased when the effective blood volume decreases with vasodilation as warming of the patient occurs.
- Subsequent diuresis usually occurs as the body excretes the excess extracellular fluid.
- Check FBC and maintain Hct > 30% by transfusing packed cells if indicated.

— **Areas of concern**
- There are certain "at risk" areas associated with specific vascular surgery. In CEA the cerebral perfusion is obviously an area of concern, and a full neurologic examination is indicated when the patient has recovered from the effects of general anaesthesia.
- Areas of concern following AAA surgery include the kidneys, spinal cord and intestines, with risks of acute tubular necrosis, paraplegia and ischaemic colitis respectively.
- Perforation of gangrenous necrotic segments with peritonitis may be associated with 40–75% mortality.
- Stress ulceration may be associated with AAA surgery: consider routine prophylactic measures against stress ulcers.

ABDOMINAL AORTIC ANEURYSM

Abdominal aortic aneurysm is a pathologic dilatation of the abdominal aortic wall, commonest at or near the aortic bifurcation at L4 level. The normal size of abdominal aorta is approximately 3 cm. An AAA greater than 5 cm occurs in 1.5% of patients more than 50 years old. The risk of rupture is approximately 10% per year if AAA is 5 cm, increasing to 40% per year if AAA is 7 cm or more.

Based on the patient's clinical presentations, surgery can be divided into 3 categories:

— Asymptomatic (painless pulsatile mass): "*elective*" surgery.

— Acute expansion with impending rupture (abdominal pain/discomfort with mass): "*urgent*" surgery.

— Ruptured AAA (pain, in shock): "*emergency*" surgery.

The operative mortality rate for elective AAA repair (1–8%) is significantly higher than 0.2–0.4% in other surgery. This is attributed to older patient age group with co-existing medical problems, and major surgery involving haemodynamic changes which may be poorly tolerated in compromised patients. Ruptured AAA carries an even higher operative mortality of 40–80%.

Conventional surgical approach to AAA repair involves replacement of the aneurysmal segment with a prosthetic graft. It requires cross-clamping and declamping of the aorta, which produce a complex array of pathophysiological changes that may not be tolerated by patients with significant cardiovascular disorders. Such patients may require less invasive surgery in the form of axillobifemoral bypass, where shunts are placed extraperitoneally from axillary artery to both femoral arteries.

The endovascular stent-graft is another alternative. In this technique, the endograft is placed under fluoroscopic guidance within the aorta, extending above and below the aneurysm. The site of arterial access is usually through a femoral artery cutdown, thus avoiding large surgical incisions in standard open techniques. This procedure can be performed under local or regional anaesthesia for most patients, thus obviating problems of general anaesthesia. This is a relatively new technique and a degree of learning curve is involved, while perigraft leaks and reports of endoprosthesis rupture are causes of concern. Its role in AAA management awaits further evaluation.

Premedication

— It is important to explain the anaesthetic procedure to the patient during premedication round, including postoperative management and possible ventilation in ICU.

— Discuss anaesthetic risks and obtain informed consent from the patient and/or next-of-kin if significant anaesthetic risks are involved.

— Anxiety and excitement can be potentially dangerous because the resultant hypertension may lead to aneurysm rupture, while tachycardia increases myocardial oxygen consumption and may precipitate an acute coronary event.

— Premedication is provided by oral benzodiazepine or intramuscular injection of opioid analgesic if the patient is reasonably fit. The dose should be reduced or omitted in patients with significant cardiorespiratory disease.

Anaesthetic Technique

The surgery is usually done under combined epidural and general anaesthesia. This combination provides good intraoperative surgical condition and effective postoperative analgesia.

Induction

— Prepare anaesthetic drugs and vasoactive drugs likely to be used during surgery, such as nitroglycerin (GTN) or sodium nitroprusside (SNP), and dobutamine in high-risk patients with poor ventricular function.

— Perform epidural block and establish monitoring before induction of anaesthesia.

— Take steps to prevent perioperative hypothermia. Normothermia is important to prevent coagulopathy, allow early extubation and maintain normal metabolic function.

— Large bore intravenous cannulae are necessary as blood loss may be substantial. Rapid infusion devices should be utilized if available.

— This is a good candidate for intraoperative cell salvage as part of the autologous blood transfusion technique. However, this technique requires the estimated blood loss to exceed 1 L to be cost-effective.

— Use incremental doses of opioid such as fentanyl and small dose of thiopentone for induction of anaesthesia in patients with poor cardiovascular status.

— Aim for smooth induction of anaesthesia with minimal haemodynamic disturbances. Use IV esmolol or lignocaine to obtund sympathetic responses during laryngoscopy and intubation.

Maintenance

— A balanced anaesthetic technique is commonly employed, with opioid, neuromuscular blocking drug, volatile anaesthetic, oxygen and nitrous oxide. Some anaesthesiologists omit nitrous oxide because of its myocardial depressant effect and its effect on bowel distension, which compromises surgical exposure.

— Maintain urine output > 0.5–1 ml/kg/hr. Check baseline ABG, electrolytes, haematocrit.

— Administer IV heparin 1 mg/kg prior to aortic cross-clamping.

Aortic cross-clamping

- This causes an immediate increase in systemic vascular resistance (SVR) and left ventricular afterload by 40%. This may be poorly tolerated by patients with poor left ventricular function and may lead to increases in CVP, pulmonary artery pressure (PAP), pulmonary capillary wedge pressure (PCWP), left ventricular failure or myocardial infarction.
- SNP or GTN is usually required to control the precipitous increase in BP.
- Gradual clamp application, carefully coordinated with anaesthetic and vasoactive drug administration, is required to avoid this problem.
- Aortic cross clamping results in ischaemic vasodilatation and vasomotor paralysis to the blood vessels distal to the clamp. Hepatic and renal blood flows are severely compromised. There is a build up of lactate and other anaerobic metabolites in the ischaemic areas giving rise to metabolic acidosis.

Aortic declamping

- Release of the aortic cross-clamp causes an acute decrease in SVR and results in central hypovolaemia or "declamping hypotension". As the lower extremities are re-perfused, the washout of anaerobic metabolites and vasoactive mediators cause vasodilation and myocardial depression.
- SNP or GTN should be discontinued. The patient should be kept relatively hypervolaemic with fluid therapy guided by CVP and/or PCWP.
- Close communication with the surgeon is essential. The surgeon should release the aortic clamps slowly while keeping a close watch on the BP. The anaesthesiologist should be prepared for rapid fluid infusion. If systolic BP falls below 100 mmHg, administer fluids and ask the surgeon to re-apply the aortic clamp. If BP cannot be elevated with fluid administration alone, vasopressors (e.g., phenylephrine) should be administered. Attempt declamping again when BP stabilizes.

Renal protection

- The risks of renal insufficiency are increased in patients with preexisting renal disease, high level of AAA (juxta- and suprarenal aneurysms worse than infrarenal AAA) as well as prolonged aortic cross-clamp time.
- Preventive measures suggested include IV mannitol before aortic clamping, maintenance of urine volume with frusemide and renal cooling when long clamp times are anticipated.

— Endovascular insertion of stents or grafts appear to cause less systemic inflammatory response than open repairs. There is some evidence that endovascular aortic aneurysm repair causes less renal injury compared to open repair.

Emergency AAA Surgery

This is a critical emergency with high morbidity and mortality rates despite advances in anaesthesia, surgery and intensive care. The patient typically presents with hypotension, shock, abdominal pain and a pulsatile mass. This poses a difficult challenge for the anaesthesiologist who must resuscitate and anaesthetize a shocked, hypotensive patient who has not been assessed preoperatively.

Anaesthetic management

— Once the clinical diagnosis is made, the patient should be taken promptly to the OT while resuscitation is on-going. The surgical team should be scrubbed and ready to begin, and usually the patient is prepped and draped before induction of anaesthesia.

— Large bore 14–16G intravenous cannulae are inserted and sufficient intravenous fluid infused to achieve a systolic BP between 80–100 mmHg. Further elevation of BP or Valsalva manoeuvre should be avoided as this may overcome the tamponade effect and increase risk of further rupture.

— Blood should be sent for laboratory tests and emergency GXM for blood and plasma. Unmatched Group O negative blood may be transfused in dire circumstances although most times it is possible to resuscitate with a combination of crystalloid and colloid solutions until emergency cross-matched blood is available. Facilities for intraoperative cell salvage should be utilized if available.

— Rapid sequence induction is performed with administration of fentanyl, ketamine or etomidate and suxamethonium followed by intubation using a cuffed endotracheal tube.

— Monitoring is only minimal to begin with: ECG, non-invasive BP, pulse oximetry, capnography. *Priority is on intravascular replacement rather than monitors*, i.e., more intravenous cannulae for rapid infusion of fluid and blood, *then* intraarterial cannula, *then* CVP or PA catheter (if indicated).

— More complications in terms of coagulopathy, renal dysfunction and hypothermia are to be expected in this category of patients.

— Postoperative ICU management is as outlined above. Postoperative complications include cardiac events, respiratory failure, ischaemic colitis, stroke, paraplegia and limb ischaemia.

THORACOABDOMINAL AORTIC ANEURYSM

Thoracoabdominal aneurysms (TAAA) are aneurysms that extend from the descending thoracic aorta into the abdomen and also those that involve the visceral segments of the upper abdominal aorta.

Open surgical repair of TAAA carries elevated mortality and complication rates. This is due to difficulties with surgical exposure, as well as potential complications arising from the temporary interruption of renal, splanchnic and spinal cord perfusion. Haemorrhagic shock, cardiac arrest and multi-system organ failures are the most frequent causes of death, and paraplegia and renal failure are the major complications. The aetiology of ischaemic and reperfusion injury to the spinal cord is multi-factorial and its prevention remains a formidable and as yet unresolved task. To select patients for surgical repair, the risk of TAAA rupture should be balanced against risks of perioperative mortality, paraplegia and renal failure.

As in AAA, endovascular stent-graft technique is being developed for TAAA. This method will be an attractive option for patients too ill to undergo extensive thoracic and abdominal surgery with cross-clamping and declamping of aorta.

Anaesthetic Management

— As this is a high-risk major vascular surgery, the patient should be extensively monitored for both cardiovascular and spinal cord functions. Arterial cannula should be placed in the upper limb after confirming equal BP reading on both arms. If aortic clamping is to be proximal to the left subclavian artery then the right radial artery should be cannulated. A PA catheter and TEE are also indicated. Spinal cord monitoring is by means of MEP or SSEP, the former being more useful than the latter.

— Anaesthesia is induced with titrating doses of an intravenous induction agent and an opioid, followed by a neuromuscular blocking drug to facilitate intubation. Care must be taken not to increase the BP during airway manipulation for fear of rupturing the aneurysm.

— Double-lumen tube (DLT), usually a left-sided DLT, is inserted after the patient is fully paralyzed. If the aneurysm compresses the left main bronchus, either a right-sided DLT or a bronchial blocker is used instead. Optimal placement of the DLT is confirmed with fibreoptic bronchoscope. Subsequent management of one-lung ventilation (OLV) is described in Chapter 37.

— Cerebrospinal fluid (CSF) drainage is commonly done to improve spinal cord perfusion pressure and hence reduce the risk of ischaemia. The patient is turned on the side and a CSF drain is placed in the lumbar region. A thoracic epidural catheter may be placed at the T10 level if epidural cooling of the spinal cord is used as another technique to reduce the risk of spinal cord ischaemia.

— Position for surgery is a modified lateral position: the patient's abdomen and pelvis are placed supine with a slight rotation, and the thorax is rotated to a right lateral decubitus position. This enables exposure to both thoracic and abdominal areas.

— Before aortic cross-clamping, mannitol or frusemide is administered to promote diuresis in an attempt to reduce renal complications as a result of aortic cross-clamping.

— Surgical techniques are employed depending on the extent of the aneurysm and the preference of the surgeon. Some surgeons use a "clamp-and-sew" technique with rapid surgical repair to limit the length of cross-clamp time. Many others make use of extracorporeal support in the form of partial left heart bypass and distal aortic perfusion, usually left atrium to left iliac artery. For the latter technique, the patient is heparinized before cannulation to go on bypass. The proximal thoracic aorta and abdominal aorta are clamped and the aortic pressure proximal to the clamp is adjusted by varying venous drainage into the bypass circuit.

— Transfusion of blood and blood products should be started early as blood loss is expected to be substantial, and coagulopathy is frequently encountered. Intraoperative cell salvage is useful in minimizing allogeneic blood transfusion.

— Significant haemodynamic changes occur during aortic declamping. Intravenous fluids and judicious use of vasopressors are necessary to treat the ensuing hypotension.

— The patients are managed in ICU postoperatively. Early assessment of lower limb neurologic function is necessary, hence epidural analgesia should be provided by opioid alone to avoid confusion of local anaesthetic-induced motor block with neurological complication. CSF pressure is maintained at < 10 mmHg for 24–48 hours after the surgery. The neurologic assessment should be carried out regularly as spinal cord dysfunction can develop over 24 hours after surgery.

— Use of partial left heart bypass and visceral organ ischaemia contribute to occurrence of coagulopathy which often persists into the postoperative period. This requires frequent evaluation of the coagulation status and correction of abnormalities with blood component therapy.

LOWER EXTREMITY ARTERIAL OCCLUSIVE DISEASE

Thromboembolic obliteration of the artery is most commonly atherosclerotic in origin. The patient typically presents with symptoms of intermittent claudication or rest pain signifying limb-threatening ischaemia. Symptoms suggestive of insufficiency of the coronary and cerebral vasculature may also be present; as many as 86% of patients have CAD, 52% have carotid artery disease and 10% have AAAs.

The type of procedure to be performed is based on the patient's symptoms, location of disease and overall condition. Options are:

— Aorto-iliac occlusive disease: aortobifemoral bypass graft or extraanatomic bypasses (axillofemoral or femorofemoral crossover graft).

— Infrainguinal occlusive disease: femoropopliteal ("fem-pop") or femorodistal bypass grafting.

— Endovascular procedures: percutaneous transluminal angioplasty with intraluminal stenting.

Surgery may be elective or urgent for attempted limb salvage. The principles of perioperative anaesthetic management are similar to those pertinent in AAA surgery. Unlike AAA surgery, these procedures do not often involve large fluid shifts or extreme haemodynamic changes, but the duration of surgery may be long. There is a finite risk of cardiac complications even with these procedures, and the long-term patency and limb salvage following extraanatomical bypass may be inferior compared with aorto-iliac reconstruction.

Studies thus far have failed to demonstrate differences in cardiac outcome between regional anaesthesia and general anaesthesia. Nonetheless, epidural anaesthesia should be encouraged as it provides increased graft flow, good postoperative analgesia and conditions for early ambulation. The use of central neuraxial blockade is contraindicated if the patient has been on anticoagulant therapy – likely in patients undergoing urgent surgery for threatened limb loss. In such cases, peripheral nerve blocks (lumbar plexus, sciatic, femoral) may be viable alternatives to central neuraxial blockade.

OCCLUSIVE CAROTID ARTERY DISEASE

Carotid artery disease, like occlusive diseases in the aorto-iliac vessels, is often a manifestation of generalized atherosclerosis. Severity of the carotid artery disease often parallels that in the coronary and cerebral vasculature. Atheromatous plaques occur most commonly at the carotid bifurcation and undergo cellular proliferation, lipid accumulation, calcification, ulceration, haemorrhage and thrombosis with resultant stenosis to the vessel.

Occlusive carotid artery disease may manifest in this manner.

— Transient ischaemic attack (TIA).
— Reversible ischaemic neurological deficit.
— Stroke: majority are preceded by one or more episodes of TIAs.
— Asymptomatic carotid bruits.
— Flow reduction as demonstrated by Doppler ultrasound or angiographic evidence of stenosis.

Treatment involves the use of antiplatelet drugs (aspirin, clopidogrel), anticoagulant (warfarin) or carotid endarterectomy (CEA), a surgical procedure where atheromatous plaque is removed from the lumen of the affected carotid artery. The surgical procedure necessitates systemic heparinization and occlusion of the artery proximal and distal to the lesion. A bypass shunt may or may not be used depending on patient's condition and surgeon's preference.

Not all cases of carotid artery disease are suitable for CEA. Its place in asymptomatic patients is controversial as CEA itself carries significant risks of perioperative morbidity and mortality. The risk of perioperative stroke and myocardial infarction may approach 5%.

Currently the accepted indications are:

— Transient ischaemic attack.
— Selected cases of stable stroke with good functional recovery.
— Angiographic evidence of > 70% of internal carotid artery (ICA) stenosis in a symptomatic patient.
— Angiographic evidence of ulcerated plaque with or without stenosis.

As in the case for AAA, minimally invasive techniques in the form of angioplasty and percutaneous stenting of carotid stenosis have been successfully performed. However, most studies have shown a perioperative stroke rate significantly higher than that achieved with CEA.

These problems are present in CEA.

— Elderly patient with co-morbid conditions.
— Presence of other occlusive vascular diseases, coronary artery disease in particular.
— Intraoperative monitoring of cerebral perfusion.
— Perioperative stroke and other neurological deficits.
— Carotid sinus and carotid body dysfunction.

Anaesthetic Management for Carotid Endarterectomy

Preoperative assessment

— Emphasis is on preoperative neurological status, cardiovascular and respiratory functions.
— Close attention should be paid to preoperative control of hypertension. Poorly controlled hypertensive patients are at risk for large BP fluctuations postoperatively due to malfunctioning of the carotid sinus and loss of baroreceptor activity in the carotid bulb.
— Light premedication using an oral benzodiazepine is useful to allay anxiety. Over-sedation should be avoided as this may result in respiratory depression.
— All patients with carotid artery disease should be receiving antiplatelet therapy, unless contraindicated, and it should not be stopped before CEA. There have been no reports showing an increased risk of postoperative bleeding.

Monitors

— Standard monitors include ECG, pulse oximetry and capnography.
— Intraarterial cannulation should be performed under local anaesthesia; CVP or pulmonary artery catheterization is unnecessary unless the patient's cardiac status warrants it.
— Monitoring for adequacy of cerebral perfusion is best done in an awake patient; failing which the parameters mentioned below are proposed. However, not all monitors are practical or freely available. Many are non-specific and require expertise for interpretation, and are influenced by anaesthetic agents and other drugs.
  - Internal carotid artery stump pressure is the mean arterial pressure in the carotid artery cephalad to the common carotid artery cross-clamp. It represents

the back pressure generated by collateral flow through the Circle of Willis and the vertebrobasilar system. Although simple and inexpensive, its accuracy in determining adequacy of collateral circulation has never been validated.

- Other monitors include electroencephalography (EEG), transcranial Doppler at the middle cerebral artery, somatosensory evoked potential (SSEP), measurements of regional cerebral blood flow (rCBF) and jugular venous bulb oxygen saturation ($SjvO_2$).

Anaesthetic technique

CEA can be done under regional or general anaesthesia, each with its own merits and problems. These are summarized in Table 38–1.

— Patients managed under regional anaesthesia may be given a small dose of IV benzodiazepine for anxiolysis during block insertion. Further sedation is best avoided if possible to allow meaningful neurological assessment during surgery. Frequent verbal contact should be made with the patient, and motor power is assessed by grip strength on the contralateral arm.

— Both hypotension and excessive hypertension should be avoided. Systolic BP should be maintained at or slightly above normal (within 20% of the preoperative level). This may require the use of vasoactive drugs such as phenylephrine to treat hypotension; or vasodilators and β-blockers to treat hypertension. Blood sample should be sent for ABG analysis to check that PaO_2 is adequate and $PaCO_2$ is maintained between 30–35 mmHg.

— Blood loss is usually not sufficient to warrant blood transfusion. Fluid administration should only replace estimated losses, and care must be taken to avoid fluid overload. Glucose-containing solutions should not be used unless specifically indicated in view of the deleterious effects that hyperglycaemia may have on potentially ischaemic areas of the brain.

— Hypotension and bradycardia may develop when the carotid sinus is stimulated during surgery. This may be overcome by local infiltration of 1% lignocaine or a small dose of IV atropine.

— Administer IV heparin 1 mg/kg immediately before surgical occlusion of the carotid artery. Reversal with protamine is not necessary at the end of the procedure.

— Vascular clamps are applied to the external and common carotid arteries. Carotid stump pressure is measured and decision made on the need for a bypass shunt. A stump pressure of less than 50 mmHg is generally regarded as indicative of inadequate collateral circulation. In an awake patient, cerebral ischaemia

Table 38–1. Comparisons between regional and general anaesthesia for CEA

Anaesthetic Technique	Advantages	Disadvantages
Regional anaesthesia: ▪ Deep and superficial cervical plexus block or ▪ cervical epidural anaesthesia supplemented with ▪ local anaesthetic infiltration of surgical site	▪ Awake patient, repeated neurological evaluation possible. ▪ Problems of GA avoided in high-risk patients. ▪ Lower requirement for bypass shunting. ▪ Lower CVS and respiratory morbidity. ▪ Shorter ICU and hospital stay.	▪ High degree of patient cooperation and contact required throughout procedure. ▪ Unfamiliarity with regional technique. High failure rate (20%) even in experienced hands. ▪ Potential for RA complications – Total spinal – Seizures – Cardiovascular collapse ▪ Inability to manipulate PaO_2, $PaCO_2$ intraoperatively. ▪ Problems with emergency airway control under physically awkward conditions.
General anaesthesia: ▪ Balanced anaesthesia with IPPV (short-acting anaesthetic agents preferred; nitrous oxide best avoided)	▪ Patient cooperation not required. ▪ Motionless operative field facilitates surgery; surgery less hurried and technically easier. ▪ Easy control of airway, oxygenation and ventilation. ▪ Anaesthetic agents (e.g., barbiturates) may be cerebral protective.	▪ No reliable signs to correlate with adequacy of cerebral perfusion. ▪ Haemodynamic changes during anaesthetic induction and emergence. ▪ Problems of GA in elderly, high-risk patients. ▪ Prolonged hangover effects of GA preclude early neurological assessment.

may manifest as slurring of speech, altered grip strength or decreased conscious level.

— If bypass shunt is not required, internal carotid clamp is then applied and endarterectomy performed. The internal carotid artery cross-clamp time should be noted.

— Bypass shunting allows flow to be maintained and reduces hypoperfusion during occlusion of the artery, but opinions differ on the usefulness of the shunt. Surgical practice ranges from shunting all patients, shunting selected patients if evidence of ischaemia occurs during cross-clamping, to not shunting any patient at all. Regardless of the surgical practice, the overall stroke rate is approximately 5%. Hazards of bypass shunts include air or particulate embolism, and elevation of distal intimal flap resulting in further thrombosis. The surgical exposure is restricted with the bypass shunt *in situ.* This adds to technical difficulty of the procedure and prolongs operative time.

— Aim for reversal of neuromuscular blockade and extubation at the end of the procedure to enable early assessment of neurological function. Give oxygen supplementation in the postoperative period and monitor the patient closely for complications.

Postoperative problems

The major complications following CEA are stroke, myocardial infarction and respiratory dysfunction.

1. **Cardiovascular instability**
   - This may be due to carotid sinus dysfunction or myocardial ischaemia.
   - Both hypo- and hypertension should be treated early and aggressively.

2. **Respiratory insufficiency**
   - Rule out and treat possible causes.
     - Laryngeal dysfunction from superior or recurrent nerve palsy.
     - Haematoma at the operative site compressing the airway.
     - Venous and lymphatic congestion resulting in tissue oedema, laryngeal oedema and upper airway obstruction.
     - Tension pneumothorax, pneumomediastinum.
     - Loss of chemoreceptor-mediated ventilatory response to hypoxia.
   - Mask ventilation and intubation may be difficult in the presence of significant. supraglottic oedema, and awake intubation or tracheostomy may be required.

3. **Neurological dysfunction**
   — Stroke is commonly due to embolization of atheromatous plaques.
   — Cranial nerve dysfunction (commonly vagus, hypoglossal, glossopharyngeal and facial nerves) may occur as a result of nerve injury during surgical dissection. Symptoms include vocal cord paresis, hoarseness of voice and dysphagia.
   — "Central hyperperfusion syndrome" is uncontrolled hypertension secondary to disturbance in cerebral autoregulation. Patients may present with migrainous-type headache, seizures, cerebral oedema and intracerebral haemorrhage.

FURTHER READING

1. Foex P. Preoperative evaluation and risk assessment of patients undergoing vascular surgery. Best Prac Res Clin Anaesthesiol 2000;14:1–16.
2. Thomson DA. Anaesthesia for patients with an abdominal aortic aneurysm. Best Prac Res Clin Anaesthesiol 2000;14:187–97.
3. Peyton PJ, et al. Perioperative epidural analgesia and outcome after major abdominal surgery in high-risk patients. Anesth Analg 2003;96:548–54.
4. Posner M, Gelman S. Pathophysiology of aortic cross-clamping and unclamping. Best Prac Res Clin Anaesthesiol 2000;14:143–60.
5. Papworth D. Intraoperative monitoring during vascular surgery. Anesthesiol Clin N Am 2004;22:223–50.
6. De Bels D, Coriat P. Post-operative management following major vascular surgery. Best Prac Res Clin Anaesthesiol 2000;14:209–23.
7. Colombo JA, Truman KJ. Peripheral vascular surgery: Does anaesthetic management affect outcome? Curr Opin Anaesthesiol 1998;11:23–7.
8. Stoneham MD, Knighton MD. Regional anaesthesia for carotid enarterectomy. Br J Anaesth 1999;82:910–9.
9. Bower MW, Zierold D, Loftus JP, Inglis KJ. Carotid endarterectomy: A comparison of regional versus general anesthesia in 500 operations. Ann Vasc Surg 2000;14:145–51.
10. Carling A, Simmons M. Complications from regional anaesthesia for carotid endarterectomy. Br J Anaesth 2000;84:794–9.

Chapter 39

Anaesthesia for Ear, Nose and Throat Surgery

INTRODUCTION

Airway management issues dominate all other anaesthetic considerations in ear, nose and throat (ENT) surgery. There are many potential problems in airway management of the ENT patient, such as:

— Sharing the patient's airway with the surgeon with reduced accessibility to the airway during surgery.

— Possibility of difficult intubation in patients with laryngeal tumours or upper airway obstruction.

— Compromised airway, as a result of:
  - Preoperative causes: oedema, infection, abnormal anatomy, tumours, haematoma or trauma.
  - Intraoperative causes: bleeding, oedema, surgical manipulation, alteration in the patient's head position, kinking of endotracheal tube or accidental extubation.
  - Postoperative causes: laryngospasm due to irritation by blood, secretions or vomitus in the airway, foreign body inhalation, laryngeal or upper airway oedema, inadequate surgical haemostasis with postoperative bleeding or inadequate reversal of neuromuscular blockade.

As in all other surgical disciplines, there are many advances and innovations in ENT surgery, in particular upper airway endoscopic procedures and surgery for tracheal reconstruction. The anaesthesiologist should keep abreast with these new developments and be familiar with the anaesthetic requirements in such surgical procedures.

EAR SURGERY

These are examples of procedures.

— Myringotomy with gromet insertion.

— Myringoplasty: reconstruction of perforated tympanic membrane with autograft, usually temporalis fascia.

— Stapedectomy, tympanoplasty: excision and reconstruction of damaged middle ear structures.

— Mastoid exploration, mastoidectomy: clearance of cholesteatoma from mastoid cavity.

— Ossiculoplasty, cochlear implant.

— Excision of tumours: acoustic neuroma, glomus tumour.

— Parotidectomy with facial nerve exploration.

Some of these are relatively long procedures performed under the microscope and the patient should be kept immobile throughout the surgery. Some degree of hypotension is usually requested in order to decrease intraoperative blood loss.

These are some pertinent considerations for ear surgery.

— **Adrenaline**
  - Adrenaline is commonly used as a vasoconstrictor, either alone or in combination with a local anaesthetic, to reduce intraoperative blood loss.
  - The concentration of adrenaline used for local infiltration should be no greater than 1:100,000 to 1:200,000. Total adult dose should be no greater than 10 ml of 1:100,000 dilution in 10 minutes, or no greater than 30 ml of 1:100,000 dilution in 1 hour.
  - Close monitoring of ECG and BP for tachyarrhythmias and hypertension is essential, as precipitous increases may be deleterious for patients with hypertension and coronary artery disease.
  - Ensure ventilation is adequate as certain volatile anaesthetics (especially halothane) may sensitize the myocardium and cause arrhythmias in the presence of hypercarbia. Such problems are rarely seen with newer, non-arrhythmogenic volatile anaesthetics such as sevoflurane, desflurane and isoflurane.

— **Controlled hypotension**
  - This is often requested by the surgeon for microsurgery of the ear in order to decrease intraoperative bleeding, improve visibility and facilitate surgery.
  - Formal hypotensive techniques using potent antihypertensive drugs such as sodium nitroprusside are usually not required.
  - These are further measures to decrease intraoperative blood loss.
    — Adequate premedication and smooth induction of anaesthesia.
    — Positioning with slight head up tilt to avoid venous congestion of the head and neck.
    — Adequate depth of anaesthesia using balanced anaesthetic technique, avoiding hypoxia and hypercarbia.
    — Local infiltration with adrenaline, or use of adrenaline packs.
    — Intravenous bolus doses of β-blocker (esmolol, labetalol) or vasodilator (hydralazine), keeping a close watch on the blood pressure.

— **Use of nitrous oxide**
  - Due to its high solubility, nitrous oxide may diffuse into the middle ear cavity and increase its pressure during surgery. The reverse occurs when diffusion occurs out of the cavity at the end of the surgery. This may cause displacement of the graft used in myringoplasty.
  - In order to overcome this problem, one may:
    — Turn off nitrous oxide 15 minutes before closure of middle ear, use an air-oxygen mixture while ensuring adequate depth of anaesthesia with additional doses of opioid and volatile anaesthetic.

  - — Use total intravenous anaesthesia (TIVA) technique with infusion of propofol, bolus doses or infusion of opioid (fentanyl, alfentanil, remifentanil), neuromuscular blocking drug and oxygen-air mixture.
- Advances in surgical technique have made this a less important issue. It is best to discuss with the surgeon to discover his/her preference.

— **Facial nerve stimulation**
- For surgical procedures which require facial nerve exploration, the surgeon may wish to check for the integrity of facial nerve intraoperatively. Use of neuromuscular blocking drug may interfere with results of facial nerve stimulation.
- This should be discussed with the surgeon and the anaesthetic technique modified accordingly, either by using a non-relaxant technique or monitoring the extent of neuromuscular blockade such that the train-of-four (TOF) count returns to 4 before the surgeon performs facial nerve stimulation.
- The latter technique usually entails a single dose of neuromuscular blocking drug to facilitate intubation, monitoring of neuromuscular blockade with peripheral nerve stimulator and maintaining adequate anaesthetic depth by means of opioid and volatile anaesthetic without further doses of neuromuscular blocking drugs.

— **Postoperative nausea and vomiting**
- This is a common postoperative complication following middle ear surgery.
- Consider prophylactic PONV therapy especially for patients with other risk factors, such as female gender, paediatric age group and history of motion sickness or PONV from previous anaesthetic.
- Choice of antiemetic includes serotonin (5-HT_3) receptor antagonist such as ondansetron or granisetron, dexamethasone and droperidol (see Chapter 61).

NOSE AND SINUS SURGERY

These are examples of procedures.

— Nasal surgery:
- Septoplasty, turbinectomy, nasal polypectomy, removal of foreign body from nose.
- Correction of nasal fracture, rhinoplasty (reconstruction of nose using bone or cartilage graft).

— Sinus surgery
- Functional endoscopic sinus surgery (FESS).

- Maxillary sinus: antral washout, intranasal antrostomy, Caldwell Luc procedure.
- Fronto-ethmoidal sinus, intranasal/transnasal ethmoidectomy, external fronto-ethmoidectomy.

These are considerations for nasal/sinus surgery.

— **Airway protection**
  - The airway should be protected from aspiration of blood and foreign body by means of endotracheal intubation.
  - A moist pharyngeal pack should be inserted to absorb blood and secretion.
  - At the end of the surgery, perform a direct laryngoscopy to check these.
    — The pharynx is clear of blood and secretions.
    — The pharyngeal pack has been removed.
    — There is no active bleeding.
    — Protective airway reflexes have returned.
  - The endotracheal tube should be removed with the patient on his/her side.

— **Cocaine**
  - This ester local anaesthetic with vasoconstrictor action is used to provide a relatively dry, bloodless surgical field.
  - Cocaine 4–10% is supplied in the form of nasal spray, paste/gel or solution to be applied in the form of nasal pack. The drug is well absorbed from the nasal mucosa and its maximum safe dose is 3 mg/kg.
  - The maximum safe dose is also dependent on the type of preparation (solution, paste), the site of administration (nasal, tracheal) and the rate of metabolism of cocaine by the patient. Greater toxicity occurs with intratracheal injection, concentrated (10%) solution or use of cocaine flakes instead of solutions.
  - Synergistic effect exists with adrenaline and it is unnecessary to use both drugs simultaneously.
  - Signs of sympathetic overactivity such as hypertension, tachyarrhythmias should be monitored and treatment instituted if necessary.

UPPER AIRWAY SURGERY

These are examples of procedures.

— Tonsillectomy, adenoidectomy or adenotonsillectomy.

— Uvulopalatopharyngoplasty (UPPP).

— Incision and drainage of peritonsillar abscess or retropharyngeal abscess.
— Endoscopic procedures and/or laser surgery
  - Endoscopic laryngeal microsurgery (ELMS): diagnosis, biopsy, tumour excision.
  - Rigid bronchoscopy: diagnosis, tissue biopsy or tracheobronchial foreign body removal
  - Panendoscopy – direct laryngoscopy, bronchoscopy, oesophagoscopy for tumour diagnosis and biopsy.
— Laryngectomy, pharyngolaryngooesophagectomy, radical neck dissection and/or muscle flap.
— Tracheostomy.
— Tracheal resection/tracheoplasty for tracheal stenosis.

Airway considerations are always pertinent in upper airway surgery. Airway management should be tailored to the patient's clinical condition, in particular the degree of upper airway obstruction. These anaesthetic options are available.

— Severe airway obstruction with stridor at rest
  - Preoperative supplemental oxygen
  - No premedication.
  - Urgent tracheostomy under local anaesthesia.
— Moderate airway obstruction which may worsen after induction of anaesthesia
  - No premedication.
  - Awake fibreoptic intubation or inhalational induction with volatile anaesthetic agent.
— Small lesions with no evidence of airway obstruction
  - Benzodiazepine premedication.
  - Intravenous induction and intubation under direct laryngoscopy.

Be prepared for difficult intubation with the necessary equipment, including laryngeal mask airway, ready and checked before induction of anaesthesia.

TONSILLECTOMY AND ADENOIDECTOMY

Lymphoid hyperplasia in the tonsils and adenoids can lead to upper airway obstruction, obligate mouth breathing and may, in severe cases, present with pulmonary hypertension and cor pulmonale. Enlarged tonsils have been regarded as one of the causes of obstructive sleep apnoea. The patient may also give a history of quinsy or frequent tonsillitis.

1. **Preoperative assessment**
   - The patient frequently belongs to the paediatric age group.
   - Inquire about history of snoring, obstructive sleep apnoea, frequent tonsillitis or respiratory tract infections, recent aspirin ingestion.
   - Examine the airway, look at the size of tonsils, determine ease of intubation.
   - Investigations are usually confined to full blood count, checking haemoglobin, haematocrit and platelet count. Bleeding time, clotting time and other coagulation studies have little predictive value for surgical bleeding tendencies. They should be reserved only for patients with known or suspected coagulation disorders.
   - It is not necessary for blood to be grouped and cross-matched in routine cases; a group and antibody screen (G&S) should suffice.
   - The surgery should be deferred if there is evidence of active respiratory tract infection with fever, cough, coryza or enlarged hyperaemic tonsils.
   - Sedative premedication should be omitted if there is likelihood of upper airway obstruction; otherwise a oral benzodiazepine premedication is suitable.

2. **Anaesthetic management**
   - The anaesthetic technique for induction depends on whether the airway is likely to be obstructed under anaesthesia. Options of airway management include:
     - Awake fibreoptic intubation: usually not feasible in the paediatric age group.
     - Prior topical anaesthesia to the airway with lignocaine spray; inhalational induction with oxygen, sevoflurane and/or nitrous oxide; gentle laryngoscopy and intubation with or without use of neuromuscular blocking drug.
     - Intravenous induction and intubation following muscle paralysis if airway obstruction is deemed unlikely.
   - The trachea is intubated using preformed endotracheal tube (RAE tube), which is secured in the midline for placement of the self-retaining mouth-gag (Boyle-Davis gag) over it.
   - A moist pharyngeal pack is necessary to prevent blood and secretions from tracking down the trachea and soiling the lungs. This may be inserted by either the anaesthesiologist or the surgeon.
   - Analgesia is provided by intravenous opioids and rectal paracetamol or diclofenac.

- The patient's lungs should be manually ventilated until airway integrity is assured. Make sure that the endotracheal tube is not obstructed during insertion of the Boyle-Davis gag or displaced by hyperextension of the neck.
- Blood transfusion is usually not required but the amount of intraoperative blood loss should be noted.
- At the end of the procedure, do a careful suction under direct laryngoscopy to remove blood or secretion in the pharynx, check for active bleeding, make sure that the pharyngeal pack has been removed and observe for the return of gag reflex to indicate readiness for reversal of neuromuscular blockade.
- The patient is turned to the lateral position with head down and neck extended, and the upper hand placed under the chin – the so-called "tonsil" position – so that secretions or blood can drain out instead of being aspirated.
- The patient is extubated when the respiratory effort is adequate. Deep extubation minimizes coughing or laryngospasm and lessens the risk of bleeding.
- In PACU, the patient should be closely monitored and observed for bleeding from the oral cavity. The surgeon should be informed immediately if bleeding is excessive.

Posttonsillectomy Bleed

- This is a surgical emergency which may manifest in PACU or several hours later. These problems are relevant to the anaesthesiologist.
    - It may be difficult to accurately assess the amount of bleeding since much of this may have been swallowed, which contributes to an emergency "full stomach" scenario.
    - The patient may be in hypovolaemic shock with pallor, hypotension, tachycardia and peripheral vasoconstriction.
    - The shocked patient with decreased cerebral perfusion may be restless and uncooperative, but sedation is not advisable as this may further compromise the cardiovascular and respiratory functions.
    - Residual effects of anaesthetic agents may result in relative overdosage during the second anaesthetic and prolong recovery from anaesthesia.
    - Intubation may be problematic as a result of possible laryngeal oedema, upper airway obstruction and poor visualization due to presence of blood in the oropharynx.

  - Bleeding may be worsened by a preexisting but previously undiagnosed bleeding disorder.

— The surgeon should be immediately informed and preparations for emergency surgery undertaken.

— The G&S blood packs should be collected from the Blood Bank and more blood should be requested if necessary. Blood samples should also be sent for FBC and coagulation tests.

— Resuscitate the patient with intravenous fluids and obtain more intravenous access. This may not be easy in a shocked and restless patient with peripheral vasoconstriction.

— Prepare anaesthetic drugs and equipment in anticipation of difficult intubation, which includes functioning laryngoscopes, smaller-sized endotracheal tubes (both RAE and ordinary polyvinyl chloride tubes), gum elastic bougie.

— Ensure that the suction device is functioning and with rigid Yaunkeur sucker attached. Have another one on standby in case the first one fails to function.

— Bring the patient into the operating room. Attach monitors. Preoxygenate the patient even though this may not be feasible in a restless patient.

— Maintain the patient in the supine position and turn the patient's head to the side for suctioning if there is active bleeding. Some anaesthesiologists prefer to place the patient in the lateral position, but intubation may be technically more difficult for someone unfamiliar to intubating patients this position.

— Use a rapid sequence induction technique with ketamine and suxamethonium.

— Apply cricoid pressure when the patient loses consciousness.

— Suction the oropharynx to improve visibility if necessary. A smaller-sized endotracheal tube may be required for intubation.

— Insert an orogastric tube when the airway is secured. Aspirate as much blood from the stomach as possible.

— Doses of anaesthetic drugs should be reduced and titrated according to patient's haemodynamic status. Be mindful of residual effects of anaesthetic drugs previously administered.

— Resuscitation is continued intraoperatively with intravenous fluids and blood.

— At the end of the procedure the neuromuscular blockade is reversed and endotracheal tube removed when the patient is fully awake and breathing well. The patient should be closely monitored for further bleeding and airway obstruction in the postoperative period.

UPPER AIRWAY ENDOSCOPY

Upper airway endoscopic procedures vary from routine examination to complex microsurgery and laser surgery of the larynx. Endoscopic removal of laryngeal and tracheal lesions is generally performed using laser technology or microlaryngeal instrumentation. A new development, the laryngeal shaver or microdebrider, provides an alternative to conventional endoscopic surgery and laser resection of most airway lesions. The claimed advantages of the microdebrider over conventional endoscopic surgery include improved access to the anterior commissure, subglottic and tracheal lesions. Relative to laser surgery, the laryngeal microdebrider is safer because it eliminates the risks of airway fire, thermal injury and potentially infectious laser plume. There is also decreased postoperative oedema with a shorter duration of postoperative hoarseness.

Whatever the surgical technique, anaesthetic requirements for upper airway endoscopy include:

— Adequate oxygenation and carbon dioxide elimination.
— Adequate surgical access with clear uninterrupted view.
— Relaxation of jaw and vocal cords with immobility of airway structures.
— Ability to observe vocal cord movement in certain conditions such as laryngomalacia.
— Obtundation of autonomic reflexes associated with airway manipulation.
— Quick return of airway reflexes without laryngospasm after surgery.

These are the problems faced by the anaesthesiologist.

— Possibility of perioperative upper airway obstruction due to various causes.
— Inadequate ventilation with hypoxaemia and carbon dioxide retention.
— Sympathetic stimulation with hypertension and tachycardia during the procedure.
— Unprotected airway in non-intubation technique, with risks of uncontrolled bleeding and distal dissemination of tumour tissue or blood along the airway,
— Excessive airway pressure with risk of barotrauma from ventilating via a small-diameter microlaryngeal tube (MLT) or during jet ventilation.
— Increased risk of awareness if anaesthesia is not adequately maintained with intravenous agents, since the lungs are ventilated with 100% oxygen during jet ventilation.
— Postoperative laryngeal oedema with stridor following surgical manipulation.

1. **Preoperative assessment**
   - It is important to do a thorough airway assessment to determine severity of airway obstruction and potential difficulty in intubation. Findings from indirect laryngoscopy provide useful information regarding the site and nature of the lesion. Radiological examinations (CXR, CT scan or MRI), if available, are also helpful to delineate the extent of the lesion and the degree of compression or deviation of the tracheobronchial tree.
   - A baseline ABG should be obtained in patients with evidence of airway obstruction or respiratory distress.
   - If indicated, supplemental oxygen should be given under pulse oximetry monitoring.

2. **Anaesthetic management**
   - There is no single ideal or universally accepted anaesthetic technique to cover the wide range of endoscopic procedures. Anaesthetic management depends on the condition of the patient's airway, the surgical technique and in part the surgeon's preference. It is always advisable to discuss with the surgeon before the procedure.
   - Induction of anaesthesia is by means of inhalational or intravenous induction. Means of airway access includes:
     - Intubation techniques, by means of standard ETT, small microlaryngeal tube or laser tube for laser surgery.
     - Non-intubation techniques, by ventilating via the breathing system attached to the side-arm of a ventilating bronchoscope.
     - Jet ventilation techniques, by using a Venturi device such as Sander's injector and performing supraglottic or subglottic (via Benjamin tube) ventilation.
   - There are two techniques for maintenance of anaesthesia.
     - Conventional balanced anaesthesia technique with volatile anaesthetic, neuromuscular blocking drug and opioid. Short-acting drugs are preferred in order to hasten recovery. This is possible when anaesthetic is delivered via the breathing system.
     - Total intravenous anaesthesia (TIVA) technique using propofol, opioid, neuromuscular blocking drug, 100% oxygen or oxygen-air mixture. This is often used in conjunction with jet ventilation.

   In the TIVA-jet ventilation technique, target-controlled infusion (TCI) of propofol is often utilized with the target blood concentration in the range of

4–7 μg/ml. This is used together with a short-acting opioid (remifentanil infusion, fentanyl or alfentanil) and neuromuscular blocking drug (atracurium or mivacurium). The inflation pressure is adjustable in some jet ventilators and ranges of inflation pressures recommended for adult and child are indicated on the dial of the pressure gauge. Jet ventilation is performed at a rate of 8–10 breaths/min with inspiratory duration of 1 second. Expiration should be allowed to occur passively between inflations to prevent barotrauma.

- Close communication with the surgeon is essential. Inform the surgeon if difficulty is encountered during ventilation because of leaks or obstruction, if the patient's oxygen saturation decreases or if frequent cardiac arrhythmias occur.
- A dose of IV dexamethasone should be administered at induction to reduce airway oedema resulting from surgical manipulation.
- At the end of the procedure, maintain mask ventilation or insert a laryngeal mask airway if the patient has not recovered from muscle paralysis. Endotracheal intubation is usually not necessary.
- On return of spontaneous respiration, reversal agent for neuromuscular blockade is administered, the oropharynx is suctioned to remove blood and secretion and the LMA is removed when the patient is awake.
- The patient should be closely observed for airway obstruction in PACU (see Chapter 67).

Laser Airway Surgery

- LASER, an acronym for light amplification by stimulated emission of radiation, is a form of monochromatic, coherent radiation energy. It is defined by the medium used to produce their radiation, such as carbon dioxide, KTP (potassium-titanyl-phosphate), or Nd-YAG (neodymium-yttrium aluminium garnet). Carbon dioxide laser is widely used in airway surgery. As it is invisible (wavelength at far infra-red range), a visible red light is used as an aiming beam to direct the laser to its target.
- Laser surgery enables precise surgical cutting and coagulation with little surface bleeding or damage to surrounding tissue. It results in minimal postoperative oedema or scarring and permits rapid pain-free healing. As such it is considered to be advantageous over conventional surgical techniques.
- A laser beam striking a surface can be reflected, transmitted to deeper layers, scattered or absorbed and converted to heat energy. Precautions must be taken to prevent laser-induced ETT ignition resulting in airway burns, and damage to normal

tissue for both the patient and OT personnel. Damage to normal tissue may be due to overshoot or deflection of laser beam, or mal-alignment of aiming and vaporizing beams. It can also occur if the patient coughs or moves unexpectedly, so muscle paralysis is often required to avoid a "moving target" problem. Eye protection is also essential. The patient's eyes should be closed and covered with moist pads, while OT personnel should wear protective goggles. There should be prominent signs on the doors leading to the OT that laser surgery is in progress.

These aspects are pertinent in the anaesthetic management for laser airway surgery.

— Problems associated with airway surgery (airway calibre, intraoperative sharing of airway and haemodynamic changes) are just as relevant in anaesthesia for laser airway surgery.
— Choice of anaesthetic agents
  - FiO_2 used should be kept as low as possible to maintain $SpO_2 > 96\%$.
  - Nitrous oxide should not be used as it supports combustion at high temperatures; it is recommended to use oxygen in air, nitrogen or helium.
  - Volatile anaesthetics may be used.
— Modifications in anaesthetic technique and ETT
  - Use of tubeless anaesthesia with intermittent apnoea or insufflation, or jet ventilation techniques with supraglottic, subglottic or transtracheal ventilation.
  - Use of special laser-proof tubes such as flexible metal tube which may be double-cuffed (e.g., Laserflex™) or non-cuffed (e.g., Norton laser tube). Note that the ETT cuff is not protected and may be damaged by the laser beam; it should be inflated with water or saline rather than air.
  - Use of conventional ETT wrapped in aluminium foil. This is often unsatisfactory because of multiple problems: laser reflection damage, exposed areas that may ignite, an unprotected cuff, airway damage from sharp edges of the foil wrapping, possibility with unwrapping of foils interfering with surgery and making tube removal difficult.

Management of airway fires

Summary of the essential steps.

— **Primary emergency care**
  - Immediately discontinue oxygen administration.
  - Remove ETT.
  - Flood the field with saline or water.

— **Secondary emergency care**
  - Insert an oropharyngeal airway and ventilate via face mask.
  - Perform immediate bronchoscopy to evaluate extent of injury to the tracheobronchial tree.
  - Remove fragmented mucosa and debris.
  - Re-intubate, or perform low tracheostomy if airway oedema is severe or injury is extensive.

— **Subsequent management**
  - Overnight observation is necessary even if there is no evidence of damage on bronchoscopy.
  - Patient should be placed on reverse isolation and closely monitored for features of airway compromise.
  - Consider antibiotics and short-term steroids.
  - Provide oxygen supplementation in the form of humidified gases.
  - If mechanical ventilation is indicated, add positive end-expiratory pressure (PEEP) to intermittent positive pressure ventilation (IPPV); aim for early weaning off the ventilator.
  - Send daily tracheal aspirate for culture and sensitivity (C&S).
  - Perform bronchoscopy 3–5 days later to re-assess the extent of injury.

FURTHER READING

1. Patel A. The shared airway. Curr Anaesth Crit Care 2001;12:213–7.
2. Reed AL, Flint P. Emerging role of powered instrumentation in airway surgery. Curr Opin Otolaryngol Head Neck Surg 2001;9:387–92.
3. Jaeger JM, Durbin CG. Specialized endotracheal tubes. Clin Pulm Med 2001;8:166–76.

Anaesthesia for Ophthalmic Surgery

INTRODUCTION

There have been significant changes in ophthalmic anaesthesia over the years. The widespread use of the surgical technique of phacoemulsification has simplified cataract surgery. As a result more can be done under regional or local/topical anaesthesia. Compared to conventional endotracheal intubation, the use of laryngeal mask airway (LMA) is associated with lesser degrees of changes in haemodynamic parameters and intraocular pressures (IOP), which are important considerations in patients who are medically compromised or have elevated IOP.

These are common ophthalmic surgical procedures.

— Cataract extraction with intraocular lens implant.

— Corneal surgery: corneal transplant.

— Vitreoretinal surgery: vitrectomy, cryotherapy, laser surgery, scleral buckling.

— Strabismus (squint) surgery.

— Lacrimal surgery: dacrocystorhinostomy (DCR).

- Orbital surgery: enucleation, evisceration.
- Ocular trauma: penetrating eye injury, toilet and suture of corneal laceration.
- For babies: examination under anaesthesia, syringing of lacrimal ducts.

PROBLEMS ASSOCIATED WITH OPHTHALMIC SURGERY

These aspects of management should be considered while anaesthetizing the patient for ophthalmic surgery.

- The ophthalmic patients comprise those from extremes of age group ranging from the very young (including the "ex-premie") for procedures relating to retinopathy of prematurity, to the elderly patients for cataract surgery. The anaesthesiologist should be well versed in paediatric and geriatric anaesthesia.
- The anaesthetic drugs and technique should not adversely affect the patient's IOP, particularly if the IOP is already elevated.
- Oculocardiac reflex (OCR) may manifest intraoperatively and should be optimally managed.
- One should be aware of systemic effects of ophthalmic drugs prescribed to the patients.
- Use of nitrous oxide in retinal detachment surgery may be inadvisable and alternative anaesthetic technique should be employed.
- In patients with penetrating eye injuries for emergency surgery, attempts should be made to minimize the possibility of extrusion of intraocular contents.

Intraocular Pressure

Normal IOP is approximately 16 ±5 mmHg. The magnitude of IOP depends on the production and drainage of aqueous humour as well as blood volume. While production of aqueous humour is relatively constant, the latter two are subject to changes and can be manipulated by pharmacological and physical means.

Steps to reduce IOP

- The patient should receive adequate premedication and anxiolysis.
- Measures should be taken for smooth anaesthetic induction and intubation
  - Ensure adequate depth of anaesthesia and allow sufficient time for the patient to be fully paralyzed before attempting laryngoscopy and intubation.

  - Obtund sympathetic reflexes with an intravenous bolus of lignocaine or esmolol, or a small dose of intravenous induction agent just prior to intubation.

— Drugs which increase IOP, such as ketamine and suxamethonium, should be avoided unless specifically indicated.

— Avoid external compression of the globe by a tightly fitting face mask.

— The use of LMA or LMA ProSeal™ instead of endotracheal tube results in smoother anaesthetic induction and emergence. This avoids surges in IOP seen during intubation and extubation particularly if the patient coughs or bucks on the tube.

— The patient should be placed at a 15–20° reverse Trendelenburg position.

— Adequate oxygenation and normocarbia should be maintained intraoperatively.

— Prophylaxis against postoperative nausea and vomiting (PONV) should be considered especially in high-risk patients. This aims to avoid postoperative retching and vomiting which would increase IOP (see Chapter 61).

— Aim for smooth emergence from anaesthesia. Deep extubation is advocated in the absence of difficult airway or full stomach.

— If the patient is positioned on his/her side postoperatively, ensure that the side with the operated eye is placed up in order to avoid increase in IOP.

Oculocardiac Reflex

The oculocardiac reflex (OCR) is usually caused by traction on the extraocular muscle, ocular manipulation such as pinching of the conjunctiva or manual pressure on the globe. It occurs most commonly in paediatric patient undergoing surgical correction of strabismus but can be evoked in all age groups and during a variety of procedures. Possible contributing factors include preoperative anxiety, light anaesthesia, hypoxia and hypercarbia. Manifestations include sinus bradycardia, bigeminy, ectopic beats, nodal rhythm, atrioventricular block and even cardiac arrest in susceptible individuals.

Management

— Monitoring of ECG, blood pressure, pulse oximetry and capnography is mandatory for all patients under anaesthesia.

— Check blood pressure, heart rate and rhythm when bradycardia occurs. Check that SpO_2 and $ETCO_2$ readings are within normal range.

— Inform the surgeon if bradycardia is severe or if there is significant hypotension associated with the bradycardia. It may be necessary to stop the surgical stimulation.

— Administer IV atropine 0.01 mg/kg if bradycardia is profound, persists despite cessation of surgical stimulation or is associated with significant hypotension.

— The surgeon may need to infiltrate the rectus muscles with local anaesthetic in recalcitrant cases.

Systemic Effects of Ophthalmic Drugs

Ophthalmic drugs may be absorbed via the conjunctiva or mucosal surfaces through nasolacrimal ducts. The anaesthesiologist should be aware of the nature of medications and watch out for possible side-effects or interaction with anaesthetic agents.

Common ophthalmic drugs

— Timolol
- Long-acting β-adrenergic blocker for treatment of glaucoma.
- Side-effects: bradycardia, congestive heart failure, exacerbation of bronchial asthma.

— Phenylephrine
- Sympathomimetic drug used as a mydriatic.
- Side-effects: reflex bradycardia, hypertension, nervousness in conscious patients.

— Atropine
- Anticholinergic used as mydriatic.
- Side-effects: tachycardia, flushing, agitation in elderly, central anticholinergic syndrome.

— Acetazolamide
- Carbonic anhydrase inhibitor to reduce IOP.
- Side-effects: alkaline diuresis leading to metabolic acidosis, increased excretion of sodium and potassium.

Use of Nitrous Oxide

Sulphur hexafluoride (SF_6) gas may be used in vitreoretinal surgery. It is an inert gas with a high molecular weight, and is odourless and colourless. It is poorly water soluble and poorly diffusible, properties which enable it to remain in the eye for a long period to exert a tamponade effect. When injected intravitreally, it takes 7–10 days for total resorption to occur.

During nitrous oxide anaesthesia, nitrous oxide diffuses rapidly into the intravitreal air bubble. This may result in raised IOP or retinal bleed. When nitrous oxide is discontinued at the end of the surgery, diffusion occurs in the opposite direction and IOP may decrease to lower than control level. This is detrimental to retinal repair since it may cause the retina to re-detach when the tamponade effect is lost.

Management

- Discontinue nitrous oxide at least 15 minutes before intravitreal gas injection.
- Use oxygen-air mixture and supplement with volatile anaesthetic and opioid to ensure adequate depth of anaesthesia.
- Total intravenous anaesthesia (TIVA) technique using propofol, fentanyl, neuromuscular blocking drug and oxygen-air mixture may also be used.
- Nitrous oxide should be avoided up to 10 days after SF_6 injection.

The introduction of silicone oil has somewhat lessened the problems associated with the use of nitrous oxide in vitreoretinal surgery. Silicone oil is used in cases where the tamponade effect is desirable over a longer period of about 3 months, after which it is removed from the vitreous cavity.

Penetrating Eye Injury

Problems

- There may be trauma to other organs, in particular injury to the head and neck; these should be assessed and excluded prior to surgery.
- The patient may have a full stomach, which increases the risk of regurgitation and aspiration.
- IOP control is essential since a raised IOP risks extrusion of the vitreous, lens prolapse and haemorrhage.

Management

- The condition is seldom urgent enough to warrant immediate surgery. Fasting times should be observed – 6 hours in adults and 4 hours in children. Note that fasting does not guarantee empty stomach because of delayed gastric emptying following trauma.

— Metoclopramide may be administered to hasten gastric emptying and increase the lower oesophageal sphincter tone.
— A thorough preoperative assessment should be carried out to exclude injury to the cervical spine and other organs, and to exclude potential airway problems.
— Discuss the prognosis of the affected eye with the surgeon. If the eye is salvageable, one should take active measures to avoid increases in IOP; otherwise the anaesthetic management is along the lines of any other emergency surgery.
— Suxamethonium causes a transient increase in IOP, which may be related to the transient period of muscle fasciculation seen before onset of paralysis. The adverse effect of suxamethonium on IOP should be balanced against the risks associated with a full stomach.
— The anaesthetic technique may be modified in these ways.
    - Use suxamethonium in a rapid sequence induction technique following a large dose of intravenous induction agent. Induction agents reduce IOP; hence the effects of suxamethonium may be moderated to a certain extent. However vasodilation and hypotension postinduction may be a problem.
    - Precurarize using 1/10 the dose of non-depolarizing neuromuscular blocking drug prior to administration of suxamethonium. This may reduce or prevent muscle fasciculation, thereby preventing a rise in IOP.
    - Attenuate the pressor response during intubation, which may increase the IOP, by using IV lignocaine, esmolol or an additional dose of induction agent prior to intubation.
    - If no intubation problem is anticipated, use high dose of vecuronium (0.15–0.2 mg/kg) or rocuronium (1 mg/kg) instead of suxamethonium. It is claimed that intubation may be performed within 60–90 seconds but the intubating condition is often not as good as compared to suxamethonium.

CHOICE OF ANAESTHESIA

An ideal anaesthetic technique for ophthalmic surgery should provide anaesthesia to the globe and lids and ensure immobility of the operated eye. In addition, it should not cause an elevation in IOP or cause bleeding into the eye cavity. It should also provide some form of analgesia in the immediate postoperative period.

As in anaesthesia for other forms of surgery, there are advantages and disadvantages associated with both regional anaesthesia and general anaesthesia. These are summarized in Table 40–1.

Table 40–1. Advantages and disadvantages of regional and general anaesthesia for ophthalmic surgery

Anaesthetic Technique	Advantages	Disadvantages
Regional anaesthesia: ▪ Retrobulbar block ▪ Peribulbar block ▪ Sub-Tenon's block ▪ Facial nerve blocks	▪ Awake patient ▪ Complications of GA avoided – especially suitable for elderly and medically compromised patients ▪ Residual analgesia in the immediate postoperative period ▪ Early ambulation and recovery ▪ Reduced incidence of postoperative nausea and vomiting (PONV)	▪ Patient's cooperation is required; not suitable for children and patients who are unable or unwilling to cooperate ▪ Patients with cardiovascular or respiratory diseases may not be able to lie flat ▪ Sudden coughing may disrupt surgery ▪ Risk of inadequate anaesthesia necessitating conversion to GA ▪ Not suitable for long, complicated surgical procedures ▪ Serious life-threatening and sight-threatening complications of block (*see text*)
General anaesthesia: ▪ Balanced anaesthesia with IPPV ▪ Spontaneous ventilation	▪ Patient's cooperation is not required ▪ Patient is anaesthetized and immobile ▪ Surgeon is free to concentrate on his work especially for long, complex surgery ▪ Full control of the airway ▪ Ability to manipulate PaO_2 and $PaCO_2$	▪ Risks of anaesthesia especially for patients ASA III and above ▪ Problems with IOP control during anaesthetic induction and emergence ▪ No provision of postoperative analgesia ▪ Increased incidence of PONV ▪ Hangover effects from GA; longer recovery period compared to RA

Regional Anaesthesia

There are two major regional ophthalmologic blocks: retrobulbar and peribulbar block. This is supplemented by blocking the facial nerve or its terminal branches in order to prevent blepharospasm. Another technique, the sub-Tenon's block, has also been described.

Retrobulbar block

In retrobulbar block, the local anaesthetic is deposited within the muscle cone of the orbit, providing akinesia to the extraocular muscles and anaesthesia to the conjunctiva, cornea and uvea. The block requires a single injection of a small volume of local anaesthetic. The onset of the block is rapid (within 5 minutes) and the success rate is high. However, it has fallen out of favour in some centres because of the risk of these serious complications.

- Life-threatening complications: intravascular or intrathecal injection of local anaesthetic leading to seizures, brainstem anaesthesia or cranial nerve block.
- Sight-threatening complications: retrobulbar haemorrhage, scleral perforation, retinal vascular occlusion, optic nerve damage.

Procedure

- The patient lies supine with eyes in primary gaze position.
- Apply local anaesthetic eyedrops to anaesthetize the conjunctiva.
- Use needle size 25G, length 25 mm.
- Local anaesthetic used: 2% lignocaine or 0.5% bupivacaine. Hyaluronidase (10 units/ml of local anaesthetic), if available, may be added to facilitate the spread of local anaesthetic.
- Percutaneous site: above the inferior orbital rim, at the junction of lateral and middle thirds of the margin. Pull the lower lid down and out to expose the globe.
- Insert the needle tangentially towards the floor of the orbit. After the tip has passed the equator of the globe, direct the needle cephalad towards the middle of the eye to enter the muscle cone.
- Aspirate for blood or CSF, and then slowly inject 2–3 ml of local anaesthetic solution, feeling the tension of the globe at the same time.

— Apply gentle massage to the globe with gauze, then apply Honan's balloon at 30 mmHg for 15–20 minutes to reduce orbital pressure and promote the spread of local anaesthetic.
— Signs of orbital akinesia will be seen within 5 minutes of a successful retrobulbar block.

Peribulbar block

In this technique, two injections are required to deposit a larger volume of local anaesthetic outside the muscle cone. The onset of action is longer (15–30 minutes) because the local anaesthetic has to diffuse into the muscle cone. Complications similar to those associated with retrobulbar block are comparatively less frequent, but scleral perforation is still a possibility with this technique.

Procedure

— The patient's position and the type of needle used are the same.
— Landmark for inferior injection is the same as for retrobulbar block. The needle is directed posteriorly along the inferior orbit to the equator of the globe. It is then angled supero-medially and 4 ml of local anaesthetic is injected, after aspiration, at a depth of 2.5 cm. A further 1 ml is injected on withdrawing the needle.
— Landmark for superior injection is just medial and inferior to the supraorbital notch. The needle is directed posteriorly over the globe to a depth of 2.5 cm; 2–3 ml of local anaesthetic is injected after aspiration, a further 1 ml is injected on withdrawing the needle.
— Orbital compression using Honan's balloon is applied as in retrobulbar block.

Facial nerve block

Various techniques of facial nerve blocks have been described for blocking different branches of the facial nerve. Examples are the Van Lindt, O'Brien, Atkinson and Nadbath techniques. Of these, the Van Lindt technique is most commonly employed.

Van Lindt technique

— Only the zygomatic branches of the facial nerve are blocked.
— Local anaesthetic is deposited along the upper and lower temporal orbital rim, forming a V-shaped wheal.

Sub-Tenon's block

The Tenon's capsule is a dense fascial layer of elastic connective tissue surrounding the globe and extraocular muscles in the anterior orbit. The sub-Tenon's or episcleral space is a potential cavity bound by Tenon's capsule and the sclera.

The sub-Tenon's block is usually performed by the ophthalmologist after anaesthetizing the conjunctiva with a topical anaesthetic. It consists of blunt dissection through the Tenon's capsule and insertion of a curved, blunt irrigating cannula to instil local anaesthetic into the posterior sub-Tenon's space. The local anaesthetic commonly used is 3–4 ml of equivolume of 2% lignocaine and 0.5% bupivacaine. Hyaluronidase 75–150 units may be added to promote the rate and extent of diffusion to the peri- and retro-orbital tissues.

The block is relatively easy to perform and offers excellent quality of anaesthesia. Compared with the peribulbar block, it provides a more rapid onset of anaesthesia, better akinesia and a lower rate of incomplete blockade requiring re-injection. It is safer compared to the retrobulbar block, in which a sharp needle is passed blindly into the orbit and retrobulbar space.

Both retro- and peribulbar blocks are contraindicated in high myopic with axial length ≥ 25 mm because of the increased risk of globe perforation. A sub-Tenon's block may be used but extra care should be taken with these patients. The technique is relatively contraindicated where there is a history of previous retinal detachment surgery with scleral buckles, or scleral disease with possibility of scarring and friability of the sclera.

General Anaesthesia

The standard technique used to be GA with endotracheal intubation and balanced anaesthesia with intravenous induction agent, neuromuscular blocking drug, volatile anaesthetic and opioid analgesic. This is no longer so with the increasing popularity of laryngeal mask airway, either the flexible LMA or LMA ProSeal™. Unless contraindicated, the LMA is ideal in ophthalmic anaesthesia because it obviates laryngoscopy with the undesirable haemodynamic changes and IOP surges; it is better tolerated while *in situ* and permits a lighter plane of anaesthesia with better emergence and recovery characteristics. For short and medium-length procedures the patient can be managed on spontaneous ventilation, thus avoiding the need for neuromuscular blockade and its subsequent reversal. For long procedures it is advisable to use controlled ventilation with neuromuscular blockade. This allows a more precise control of CO_2 and permits benefits of a balanced anaesthetic technique. The LMA ProSeal™, with an oesophageal drain tube incorporated into the device, prevents inadvertent gastric insufflation and is ideally suited for GA with IPPV.

Points to remember

- Take active measures to prevent surges of IOP at all times.
- Closely monitor the ECG to detect and treat oculocardiac reflex.
- Ensure adequate neuromuscular blockade to avoid sudden cough or movement, which may be disastrous in eye surgery.
- Consider the use of antiemetics to prevent PONV especially in high-risk patients.
- Consider extubation in a deep plane of anaesthesia to avoid coughing and bucking on the endotracheal tube in suitable patients.

It has been suggested that a combination of GA and a regional block – analogous to a combination of general and epidural anaesthesia in general surgery – may offer excellent condition for surgery while providing postoperative analgesia. However, one should also consider the potential complications that the patient may be subjected to if both techniques are utilized in combination. Perhaps the only indication for such GA-RA combination is vitreoretinal surgery; and sub-Tenon's block, with minimal complications, should be performed in preference to retro- or peribulbar blocks.

FURTHER READING

1. Venkatesan VG, Smith A. What's new in ophthalmic anaesthesia? Curr Opin Anaesthesiol 2002;15:615–20.
2. Canavan KS, Dark A, Garrioch MA. Sub-Tenon's administration of local anaesthetic: A review of the technique. Br J Anaesth 2003;90:787–93.
3. Ahmad S, Ahmad A. Complications of ophthalmologic nerve blocks: A review. J Clin Anesth 2003;15:564–9.

Chapter 41

Anaesthesia for Urological Surgery

GENERAL CONSIDERATIONS

Surgical procedures in urology include endoscopic procedures and open surgery. Conditions which require surgical intervention include benign prostatic hyperplasia, stones in the renal calyces and anywhere along the urinary tract, strictures, tumours and chronic renal failure for creation of arteriovenous fistula (AVF) or renal transplantation.

These are examples of surgical procedures.

— Endoscopic procedures: cystoscopy, transurethral resection of prostate (TURP), transurethral resection of bladder tumour (TURBT), bladder neck incision, ureteroscopy and/or stone removal, insertion of ureteric stent.

— Open surgery: nephrectomy, pyelolithotomy, open (retropubic) prostatectomy, radical prostatectomy, cystectomy and/or ileal conduit, urethroplasty, renal transplantation.
— Others: percutaneous nephrolithotripsy (PCNL), nephrostomy, insertion of Tenckoff catheter, surgery for AVF.

The majority of patients undergoing urological surgery are elderly patients with multiple co-morbid conditions. There are also a smaller number of patients belonging to the paediatric age group who undergo hypospadias repair or circumcision for phimosis.

These patients may have normal, marginally impaired or grossly deranged renal function. Many patients present with features of obstructive uropathy which in turn results in varying degrees of renal impairment. Drug pharmacokinetics may be altered in such patients. Reduced renal clearance and drug excretion result in prolonged duration of action, and hypoalbuminaemia decreases protein binding and increases free drug concentration. These are elaborated in Chapter 16. Drugs which may be nephrotoxic, such as non-steroidal antiinflammatory drugs (NSAIDs), aminoglycosides, should be used with caution, if at all, in these patients.

Because of their unique anaesthetic requirements, anaesthetic management for these surgical procedures is elaborated further.

— Transurethral prostatectomy.
— Renal transplantation.
— Extracorporeal shock wave lithotripsy (ESWL).
— Percutaneous nephrolithotripsy (PCNL).

TRANSURETHRAL PROSTATECTOMY

Transurethral resection of the prostate is performed by application of a high frequency current to a wire loop in the resectoscope. Prostatic tissue is removed by successive cuts under direct endoscopic vision. Haemostasis is achieved by sealing the blood vessels with the coagulating current. Continuous irrigation of the bladder and prostatic urethra is required to maintain visibility, remove dissected tissue and blood and distend the operative site. The most commonly used irrigation fluid is 1.5% glycine in water, which is hypotonic with an osmolality of 220 mosm/L.

Preoperative Assessment

- The patient is likely to be elderly with concomitant medical illnesses. These should be identified and optimized. There may also be renal impairment secondary to obstructive uropathy.
- Examine the patient's spine to determine ease of performing a regional block and explain the planned anaesthetic procedure to the patient.
- Assess the patient's mental status preoperatively; this will aid in evaluation of intra- or postoperative changes in conscious level or neurological status.
- Premedication is either omitted or with reduced dose of an oral benzodiazepine. Drugs which may give rise to postoperative confusion (e.g., scopolamine) should be avoided.

Problems and Complications of TURP

- **TURP syndrome** – see page 562.
- **Blood loss**
  - Blood loss is usually variable and difficult to quantify.
  - The amount of blood loss depends on the size of the prostate, duration of surgery – estimated to be 7–20 ml/g of resected tissue or 2–5 ml/min of resection time – and expertise of the surgeon.
- **Hypothermia**
  - Elderly patients are especially prone to hypothermia, worsened by the use of cold irrigation fluid and low ambient OT temperature.
  - Every attempt should be made to minimize hypothermia, e.g., by using warming blankets, and warmed intravenous and irrigation fluids.
- **Bladder perforation**
  - This may occur as a result of instrumentation or overdistension of bladder.
  - Clinical features include abdominal pain, distension, rigidity, pallor, nausea, vomiting, sweating, shock. These features are not masked by spinal anaesthesia, but diagnosis may be difficult under general anaesthesia.
- **Bacteraemia and infection**
  - Antibiotic is indicated when there is a proven urinary tract infection.
  - Bacteria from infected urinary tract may enter the bloodstream and spread systemically, resulting in septic shock.

— **Obturator spasm**
  - This results from direct stimulation by diathermy current of the obturator nerve which runs adjacent to the lateral walls of the bladder. It may impair surgical access by causing adduction of the lower limbs and increase the risk of bladder perforation.
  - Reduction of the diathermy current usually helps, but in severe cases it may be necessary to convert to general anaesthesia with muscle relaxation.

— **Problems with lithotomy and Trendelenburg position**
  - The head-down position may cause splinting of the diaphragm, impair ventilation and result in hypoxaemia in obese patients and those with chronic pulmonary diseases.
  - The increase in venous return may precipitate cardiac failure in patients with poor cardiac reserve.
  - Take particular care in positioning patients with degenerative diseases of the hip joints or those with prior joint replacements.
  - Hypotension may occur when the legs are lowered abruptly at the end of the procedure, because of a sudden reduction in the effective blood volume.

Anaesthetic Options

1. **Spinal anaesthesia**

   Spinal anaesthesia works well for TURP and other cystoscopic procedures, and is the anaesthetic technique of choice in patients with no contraindication to regional anaesthesia. Sensory supply to the urethra, prostate and bladder neck is from S2–S4, while that of bladder is from T10–T12. A block height of at least T10 is required for adequate anaesthesia. The subarachnoid block is performed at the L3–L4 or L4–L5 interspace in the sitting position. A dose of 2.5–3 ml hyperbaric 0.5% bupivacaine is usually adequate. Judicious fluid preload is essential since overzealous infusion may lead to volume overload in medically compromised patients.

   — **Advantages**
     - Awake patient, able to provide early warning of complications.
     - Atonic bladder with large capacity aids in reducing the infusion pressure.
     - Postoperative pain relief is available, albeit limited to the duration of spinal anaesthesia.

— **Disadvantages**
  - Usual problems with spinal anaesthesia, such as failed block, limited duration of anaesthesia, postdural puncture headache (lower incidence in geriatric patients).
  - Sympathetic blockade with decreased vascular tone accentuates the effects of hypovolaemia resulting in hypotension which is poorly tolerated in the elderly.

2. **General anaesthesia**

   General anaesthesia may be necessary in patients who are unable to cooperate with a regional technique, or in whom regional anaesthesia is contraindicated. Both spontaneous ventilation technique using a laryngeal mask airway or controlled ventilation technique using an endotracheal tube can be utilized. Consider protecting the airway with endotracheal intubation in patients who are obese or give history of reflux oesophagitis.

   — **Advantages**
   - Controlled ventilation eliminates problems of diaphragmatic splinting and impaired ventilation in the lithotomy position.
   - Better control of vascular tone and relative volume status.
   - Ability to control PaO_2 and $PaCO_2$.
   - Patient cooperation is not required; this may be the only anaesthetic option available in demented, uncooperative patients.

   — **Disadvantages**
   - Unconscious patient with inability to provide early warning of complications such as TURP syndrome, bladder perforation.
   - Longer recovery with disturbance in mental status especially in the very old.
   - No provision for postoperative analgesia.

Postoperative Management

Bladder irrigation with saline via a 3-way catheter is carried out for a few hours postoperatively until the bleeding is reduced. There is usually little pain even though discomfort from the indwelling urinary catheter or bladder spasm may be a problem. Clot retention can cause a painful distended bladder which may necessitate bladder washout, occasionally under anaesthesia.

TURP Syndrome

This is a clinical syndrome which may occur during TURP as a result of absorption of large quantities of hypotonic irrigation fluid into the general circulation through open prostatic veins. This gives rise to volume overload with cardiovascular compromise in susceptible patients, water intoxication, hypo-osmolality and hyponatraemia with associated neurological manifestations.

The TURP syndrome may occur as quickly as 15 minutes after resection starts or up to 24 hours postoperatively. It ranges in severity from mild to life-threatening, with a mortality of 0.2–0.8%.

No consistent correlation has been found between the volume of fluid absorbed, the duration of TURP and the weight of prostatic tissue removed. Contributory factors include the hydrostatic pressure of the irrigation fluid, the number and size of venous sinuses opened, the patient's peripheral venous pressure, duration of surgery as well as experience of the surgeon.

Clinical Manifestations

— **Cardiorespiratory systems**
- Initial rise in systolic blood pressure and widening of pulse pressure.
- Increased central venous pressure and reflex bradycardia.
- Chest pain in conscious patients.
- Acute pulmonary oedema in patients with poor left ventricular function.
- Respiratory distress, cyanosis.
- Finally bradycardia, hypotension, shock and cardiac arrest.
- ECG shows arrhythmias, nodal rhythm and U waves.

— **Central nervous system**
- Mental confusion, restlessness.
- Visual disturbances, nausea, vomiting.
- Headache, malaise, weakness.
- Convulsions, coma.
- Failure to awaken from general anaesthesia.

— **Laboratory investigations**
- Hyponatraemia, hypo-osmolality.
- Low haemoglobin concentration from haemolysis.
- Features of acute renal failure.
- If glycine is used as irrigation fluid:

- High plasma glycine levels (normal 176–332 μmol/L)
- High blood ammonia levels (normal 11–35 μmol/L)
- High urinary oxalate levels

Management

Prevention

- The anaesthesiologist should avoid sodium-free intravenous fluids such as dextrose 5% for preloading and intraoperative fluid replacement unless specifically indicated.
- Hypotension should be treated early and aggressively since the amount of fluid absorption depends on the venous pressure. More fluid is absorbed if the patient is hypovolaemic or hypotensive.
- Reduce the hydrostatic pressure of irrigation fluid to less than 70 cmH_2O (height of infusion bag should not be more than 70 cm above the level of the OT table).
- Haemostasis should be promptly secured to reduce the number of open veins facilitating fluid absorption into the systemic circulation. Limit duration of resection to 1 hour because the fluid absorption rate is about 20 ml/min.

Treatment

- *The mildly symptomatic patient* (nausea, vomiting, confusion and/or visual disturbances; stable cardiovascular system)
  - Alert the surgeon to coagulate bleeding points and terminate surgery as soon as possible.
  - Administer IV frusemide 0.5–1 mg/kg.
  - Give reassurance and continue observation until symptoms resolve.
  - Send blood sample for laboratory investigation: haemoglobin and serum sodium concentration.
- *The unconscious patient* (comatose, fails to awaken from general anaesthesia or shows signs of cardiovascular compromise)
  - **Supportive treatment**
    - Unstable, comatose patients require ICU management with intubation, ventilatory support and/or inotropes.
    - Correct volume overload using diuretics such as frusemide, mannitol.
    - Send blood sample for coagulation screen if there is evidence of coagulopathy.

- Maintain postoperative urine output; consider early renal support if indicated.
- Treat infection with broad-spectrum antibiotics if sepsis develops.
- Consider blood transfusion if indicated.

- **Correction of hyponatraemia**
  - This is based on the formula: sodium deficit = (140 – serum sodium) × 0.6 × body weight
  - Usually 0.9% normal saline is sufficient for correction; 3% hypertonic saline is used only in severe cases.
  - Extreme caution should be taken as rapid correction can lead to dangerous changes in osmotic gradients in the intravascular, interstitial and intracellular spaces. Correction rate should not be more than 2 mmol/L/hr; optimal rate of correction being 0.6–1.0 mmol/L/hr or 100 ml/hr. Monitor serum sodium concentration and osmolality 4-hourly during correction.
  - Treatment end-point is the improvement in clinical signs rather than full biochemical correction. Stop infusion of hypertonic saline once serum sodium concentration exceeds 102 mmol/L. Complete correction is gradually achieved by fluid restriction over the next few days

RENAL TRANSPLANTATION

Renal transplantation is a treatment option that gives the patient with end-stage renal disease a new lease of life. With a very good survival rate at 10 years, renal transplantation provides a good quality of life for such patients. Similar to transplant programmes involving other organs, the success of renal transplantation is closely linked to recent advances in immunosuppressive therapy. The use of azathioprine and prednisone produces an acceptable renal graft survival rate. New organ preservation methods allow for retrieval and shipment of cadaveric organs; and the introduction of cyclosporin, a powerful immunosuppressant, increases survival rates among patients undergoing transplantations.

The donor kidney can be from a living-related donor, a living-unrelated donor or from a cadaver. Living-donor transplants are performed electively with the donor and recipient anaesthetized simultaneously but in separate operating rooms, while cadaveric transplants are done as emergency procedures. Problems of emergency anaesthesia, namely full stomach with risk of regurgitation and aspiration, inadequate time for assessment and preparation, are present in addition to the patient's medical problems that require additional care and expertise in anaesthetic management.

These are descriptions for living-related transplants.

Preoperative Considerations

The donor and recipient are registered in the Transplant Registry and are managed by the nephrologist. Preoperative checklist for the recipient includes:

- Personal data.
- Clinical data
  - Underlying disease causing end-stage renal disease.
  - Co-morbid conditions.
  - Infection risk: serological screening tests.
  - Renal replacement therapy: duration and frequency of haemodialysis, peritoneal dialysis.
- Donor data and relationship with recipient.
- Immunosuppressive therapy.
- Physical examination and investigations.

The donor goes through a thorough evaluation of the renal function, with tests which include ultrasonography, radionuclide scans, glomerular filtration rate and renal clearance studies and renal angiogram. Additional tests include HLA typing and matching with recipient and serological tests for infections.

Anaesthetic Management

1. **The donor**

   Anaesthetic management for the donor is essentially management of a patient presenting for nephrectomy. General anaesthesia supplemented with epidural anaesthesia is the anaesthetic technique frequently employed. Measures are taken to ensure renal perfusion and urine production are adequate. These include:
   - Adequate hydration with intravenous fluids 100 ml/hr during the period of fasting.
   - Intraoperative infusion of mannitol 1 g/kg.
   - Maintenance of stable haemodynamic parameters.
   - Maintenance of urine output > 1 ml/kg/hr.

2. **The recipient**

   The transplant is carried out by placing the donor kidney in the iliac fossa, anastomosing the renal vessels to the iliac vessels and the ureter to the bladder.

Nephrectomy is only performed in the presence of intractable hypertension or chronic infection. Anaesthetic management is essentially one for a patient with end-stage renal disease. General anaesthesia is again the usual anaesthetic technique employed.

These special considerations should be noted.

— Monitors include continuous ECG, non-invasive BP, pulse oximetry and capnography. Central venous pressure monitoring is useful in guiding fluid therapy, and indwelling urinary catheter is necessary to measure urine output. Arterial catheterization for invasive blood pressure monitoring is usually not necessary.
— Maintain adequate fluid status and stable haemodynamic parameters throughout the surgery.
— Prior to graft insertion, maintain CVP at 10–12 mmHg to ensure optimal graft perfusion and urine production.
— Administer IV frusemide 0.5–1 mg/kg after anastomosis of renal vessels to promote diuresis. Some surgeons would also ask for mannitol and hydrocortisone to enhance graft survival.

Reversal of neuromuscular blockade and extubation are carried out for both the donor and recipient at the end of the surgery. They are managed in ICU or HDU during the postoperative period. Postoperative analgesia by means of intravenous patient-controlled analgesia is frequently used for the recipient and donor (if not on epidural).

EXTRACORPOREAL SHOCK WAVE LITHOTRIPSY

This form of therapy is used for selected patients with renal calculi or calculi in the upper two-thirds of the ureter above the iliac crest. The procedure is minimally invasive and in successful cases it obviates the need for open pyelo- or ureterolithotomy.

In extracorporeal shock wave lithotripsy (ESWL), high energy shock waves are generated and focused on the renal calculus, causing tear and shear forces there, and disintegrating the stone into fragments small enough to be passed down the urinary tract. Ureteric stents are often placed cystoscopically prior to the procedure to facilitate passage of the stone particles.

Anaesthesia for ESWL used to be problematic because in the older ESWL units it was necessary to immerse the patient in a heated water bath on a hydraulic chair. Water immersion is not required in the newer ESWL units, and the majority of the patients do not need anaesthesia other than some form of light sedation.

Problems of ESWL

- — Cardiac arrhythmias
  - Arrhythmias can be induced by shock waves: these are usually self-limiting but may be reduced by synchronizing the shock waves to the R wave of the ECG.
  - Relative contraindications to ESWL include history of cardiac arrhythmias and presence of cardiac pacemaker, which may be deprogrammed by the shock waves.
- — Tissue destruction
  - Shock waves cause damage at interfaces with different acoustic densities such as the tissue-stone interface.
  - Body tissue has the same acoustic density as water hence the waves travel through the body without causing damage; however, energy from shock waves is released if the waves are focused on air-tissue interface (e.g., lung, intestine).

Anaesthetic Techniques

Pain during the procedure arises from the dissipation of a small amount of energy as shock waves enter the body through the skin. This is tolerated by most patients and no anaesthesia is required. Light sedation is sometimes requested for the procedure.

If epidural anaesthesia is employed, saline rather than air should be used to locate the epidural space. Very rarely general anaesthesia is provided. Balanced anaesthesia with muscle paralysis is preferred since it allows control of diaphragmatic excursion and keeps the stone in the wave focus.

PERCUTANEOUS NEPHROLITHOTRIPSY

Percutaneous nephrolithotripsy (PCNL) is yet another procedure for fragmentation of stone in the renal calyces. In this procedure, ultrasonic waves are used to fragment the stones. If successful, patient would be spared the need for open surgery.

The procedure requires placement of a ureteric stent by cystoscopy to distend the renal pelvis. The patient is then placed in the semi-prone position, and a tract from the skin to the renal pelvis is established under radiographic control. The stone is disrupted by a percutaneous ultrasound probe. Irrigation fluid is used to flush away stone fragments and blood. A Foley catheter is needed to drain the irrigation fluid which passes down the ureter.

Anaesthetic Management

General anaesthesia with endotracheal intubation and intermittent positive pressure ventilation is the anaesthetic technique which is most commonly employed. Epidural anaesthesia, though less popular, has also been used. The block height needs to be T8 or above.

Reported complications include hypothermia, pneumothorax, Gram-negative septicaemia, retroperitoneal bleeding and accidental rupture of the renal pelvis with extravasation of irrigation fluid into the retroperitoneal space. The amount of irrigation fluids instilled and recovered should be checked. Extravasation is likely if there is a deficit of 2 litres or more. Retroperitoneal haemorrhage is suggested by a drop in haematocrit and may necessitate renal angiography and/or surgical exploration. Nephrostomy is placed posterolaterally below the 12th rib and close to the diaphragm, and the pleura may be breached with development of a pneumothorax or hydrothorax.

FURTHER READING

1. Gravenstein D. Transurethral resection of the prostate (TURP) syndrome: A review of the pathophysiology and management. Anesth Analg 1997;84:438–46.
2. Colson P. Renal disease and transplantation. Curr Opin Anaesthesiol 1998;11:345–8.

Chapter 42

Anaesthesia at the Radiology Department

INTRODUCTION

In keeping with advances in other fields of medicine, imaging techniques have come a long way from the early days of simple plain X-rays. The role of the radiologist is not only confined to interpretation of X-ray films; there is a new exciting range of diagnostic and therapeutic interventions which can be performed under radiologic guidance.

These are common radiological procedures.

— Computed tomography (CT) scanning.

— Magnetic resonance imaging (MRI).

— Angiographic studies.

— Interventional radiology: embolization of feeder blood vessels to tumours, endovascular procedures with stent insertion, ultrasound-guided diagnostic and therapeutic procedures, interventional neuroradiology.
— Cardiac catheterization (carried out in the OT complex in some hospitals).
  - Diagnostic procedures for shunts, valvular heart diseases, ischaemic heart diseases.
  - Invasive procedures such as balloon atrial septostomy, coronary angioplasty.

The role of the anaesthesiologist in the delivery of services outside the OT is ever expanding; one of the areas frequented by the anaesthesiologist is the Radiology Department. The anaesthesiologist may be called upon to anaesthetize paediatric patients, and those unwilling or unable to cooperate with the imaging procedure without some form of anaesthesia.

The anaesthesiologist should be informed about the patient 1–2 days before the planned procedure. The preanaesthetic visit and assessment should be carried out as for any patient undergoing an elective surgical procedure.

PROBLEMS

The many problems encountered in the Radiology Department are highlighted here.

— **The work environment**
  - This unfamiliar work environment is often in a remote location from the OT or ICU.
  - It may not have adequate resuscitation facilities or personnel familiar with resuscitation procedures.
  - Good, experienced anaesthetic assistant is often not available.
  - The work area is often cramped and congested with bulky machines and scanners.
  - Scavenging facilities for inhalational anaesthetic agents are usually inadequate.
  - The modern radiological equipment with its attendant computing technology has a requirement to remain cooled or risk malfunction. The low ambient temperature may result in hypothermia in susceptible patients such as small babies.
  - Space, facilities and personnel are usually not adequate for recovery of patients following anaesthesia.

— **The procedure**
  - Accessibility to the patient is reduced, giving rise to problems with monitoring and the use of long breathing circuits which increase the risk of kinking or disconnection.
  - The room is darkened during the imaging procedure, making clinical observation and assessment of the patient difficult if not impossible.
  - The patient may be placed in many positions with a risk of accidental extubation or kinking of the endotracheal tube.
  - There is a risk of anaphylaxis or allergic reaction to the X-ray contrast agent administered to the patient.
  - There is radiation hazard to the staff. Appropriate radiation protection should be afforded to the anaesthesiologist if it is necessary to remain with the patient during the imaging procedure.

— **The patient**
  - The patient may be an infant or small child, or an adult with psychological, behavioural or movement disorder.
  - The patient's underlying condition which necessitates the imaging procedure (e.g., intracranial lesion, arteriovenous malformation, cardiac lesion) warrants due consideration for anaesthetic management.
  - It is not uncommon to find patients with multiple medical conditions being listed for the procedure under monitored anaesthesia care. Beware of rare syndromes which involve the airway and/or cardiovascular system.

In view of those problems, a junior anaesthetic trainee who is unfamiliar with the Radiology Department setting should not undertake to anaesthetize the patient alone and unsupervised. He/she should be accompanied by a senior colleague or specialist who can provide assistance and guidance.

ANAESTHETIC MANAGEMENT

Preoperative Assessment

— Although paediatric patients constitute the majority of patients requiring anaesthetic care, adults who are uncooperative or critically ill may be encountered.

— Identify patient's problems and check indication for the scan procedure, for example:
  - Very young patients or those who are mentally retarded.
  - Problems with airway management.

- Cardiovascular abnormality.
- Neurological deficits.

— Keep the patient nil orally as per fasting guidelines.

— Avoid premedication in the very young, the very ill and those with airway problems. Others may receive oral benzodiazepine premedication.

Conduct of Anaesthesia

— The same standard of care – preoperative assessment, trained anaesthetic assistant, minimum monitoring standards, resuscitation facilities, recovery care – should be maintained.

— The goal of anaesthesia is to provide immobility, safety and comfort for the patient while achieving the best condition for the diagnostic study.

— It is mandatory to have a proper check of the anaesthetic and resuscitation equipment before the start. These include:

- Anaesthetic machine and breathing system.
- Oxygen/nitrous oxide supply, whether these are piped gases or from cylinders; if it is the latter, ensure that a full spare oxygen cylinder is available.
- Airway equipment: airways, masks, stylets, endotracheal tubes and laryngeal mask airways of appropriate sizes, laryngoscopes with different sized blades
- Working suction device.
- Resuscitation drugs and equipment, including a self-inflating bag and a defibrillator.

— Monitors include ECG, non-invasive BP, pulse oximetry and capnography. The latter is especially useful in cases with potentially difficult airway and for monitoring airway integrity during the procedure.

— A variety of general anaesthetic techniques may be used – inhalational or intravenous induction with spontaneous or controlled ventilation via laryngeal mask airway or endotracheal tube. The actual choice depends on the anaesthetic requirement for each individual, e.g., whether there is a need for airway protection, respiratory support or control of intracranial pressure.

— In some older children or adults, intravenous sedation with monitored anaesthesia care may be all that is required. Various means of drug delivery using various drugs are available.

- Intravenous fentanyl and midazolam in small titrating doses.

  - Patient-controlled sedation (PCS) with propofol.
  - Target-controlled infusion (TCI) of propofol for sedation, target range 0.5–2.0 μg/ml.

— The anaesthetic technique should be individualized for each patient; and the anaesthesiologist should be comfortable and familiar with the selected technique.

— Scans of the thorax or abdomen may be affected by artefacts caused by respiratory movements. They may require brief periods of apnoea to perform certain sections of the scan. A conscious or lightly sedated patient should be able to follow instructions to breath-hold. A patient under general anaesthesia can be manually ventilated and the lungs held in inspiration for a few seconds when required.

— Intravenous contrast media are sometimes used during the procedure to enhance the X-ray images obtained. These may occasionally trigger allergic reactions in susceptible individuals, even to the extent of full-blown anaphylactic reaction. The patient should be adequately hydrated because some of these contrast agents are known to cause renal failure in the presence of dehydration or impaired renal function.

Postoperative Management

— At least one nurse should be available to take care of the patient in the recovery area.

— Supplemental oxygen is administered to the patient, and monitoring should be done according to PACU guidelines in OT (see Chapter 10).

— Firm digital pressure must be maintained on the site of arterial cannulation following angiographic procedures. Make sure that the bleeding has stopped before the patient is discharged to the ward.

— Usual discharge criteria are applicable.

ANAESTHESIA FOR INTERVENTIONAL NEURORADIOLOGY

Neuroradiological treatment of vascular diseases of the central nervous system (CNS) has undergone significant advances in terms of technology as well as expertise. As procedures become more complex and time-consuming, the requirement for anaesthesia correspondingly increases.

Examples of neuroradiological procedures include:

- Embolization of cerebral arteriovenous malformations (AVM), especially for those with several feeding vessels and with a location unsuitable for surgical intervention.
- Management of brain tumours in terms of embolization or delivery of chemotherapeutic agents.
- Endovascular coiling of cerebral aneurysm by means of stainless steel platinum coils placed inside the aneurysm to initiate thrombosis.
- Cerebral angioplasty for vasospasm.
- Carotid artery stenting.

Many of the procedures require general anaesthesia despite its disadvantage of being unable to evaluate the patient's neurologic status during the procedure. This is because the procedure is often lengthy and uncomfortable for the patient who frequently requires some form of sedation and/or anaesthesia. Other advantages of GA include the provision of a motionless patient for the imaging procedure; ability to achieve control of the airway, oxygenation and ventilation, and in doing so provide improved control of elevated intracranial pressure (ICP). The haemodynamic parameters can be better manipulated if controlled hypotension or augmentation of blood pressure is required. In cases of complications arising from the procedure, such as acute subarachnoid haemorrhage, an already anaesthetized patient enables rescue operations to be instituted immediately.

The anaesthetic goal is to maintain haemodynamic stability and to improve intracranial dynamics so that cerebral perfusion is not jeopardized during the procedure. Anaesthetic agents that do not increase cerebral metabolic rate for oxygen ($CMRO_2$) and allow rapid emergence are preferred, with propofol, fentanyl and sevoflurane being frequently used. Airway maintenance is by means of endotracheal tube or laryngeal mask airway. Blood pressure should be monitored invasively as controlled hypotension is often necessary to reduce the risk of rupture of aneurysm or AVM. Emergence from anaesthesia should be smooth to prevent potential cerebral oedema and bleeding.

ANAESTHESIA FOR MAGNETIC RESONANCE IMAGING

Magnetic resonance imaging (MRI) represents a major development in medical diagnostics through its enhanced resolution of anatomical structures. The images produced by MRI may be superior to CT scan especially for neurologic and soft tissue examination. Structures within the cranium, thorax, spinal column and pelvis are well delineated, and easy differentiation can be made between fat, vessels and tumour.

The increasing use of MRI as a diagnostic modality has led to an increased demand for monitoring and sedation/anaesthesia during the procedure. The anaesthesiologist is often called upon to manage an occasional "difficult" patient, or one in whom sedation has failed. The anaesthesiologist should, therefore, be familiar with the problems and principles of anaesthetic management for such procedures.

Principles of MRI

MRI is a non-invasive diagnostic technique based on the fact that atomic nuclei with an unpaired number of protons and/or neutrons (e.g., ^{1}H, ^{31}P, ^{13}C) have intrinsic magnetic properties and behave like miniature bar magnets. When a sample containing such nuclei is placed within a large magnetic field, the nuclei tend to rotate and align themselves parallel to the magnetic field. Nuclei with an even number of protons or neutrons will offset their ability for rotation.

The atoms are subjected to radio-frequency (RF) pulses that deflect the orientation of the atoms. As the RF pulses are removed, the nuclei rotate back into alignment with the static magnetic field. The energy that is released by the movement of the atoms is used to create the MRI image.

The MRI magnet is a liquid nitrogen-cooled superconductor capable of producing a 0.5–2.0 Tesla magnetic field (a Tesla is a unit measuring the strength of a magnetic field). It is cooled to a temperature of 4.2 degrees Kelvin. Once the magnet is turned off, it takes up to 24 hours to produce a stable magnetic field when it is turned on again.

Problems of MRI

— **Hazards to the patient**
- Electronic implants (e.g., pacemakers, cochlear implants) may malfunction and hence patients with these implants are not suitable for MRI.
- Heat may be generated in metallic implants (e.g., hip prostheses), metallic-based substances (e.g., eye make-up, tattoo) and body tissue (e.g., testes, lenses).
- Loose ferromagnetic objects are pulled towards the magnetic centre with dangerous speed.
- Ferromagnetic implants (e.g., aneurysm clips, prosthetic heart valves, joint prostheses, intraocular implants) may be dislodged.

- Damage can occur to analogue watches, credit cards, floppy disc and cassette tapes.
- Uncomfortable conditions in the MRI room such as excessive noise, cold environment and enclosed space can lead to anxiety and claustrophobia in some individuals.
- Note that there is no evidence of increased risk of carcinogenesis or teratogenesis.

— **Anaesthetic machine, airway and monitoring equipment**
  - Inaccessibility to the patient following placement in the MRI scanner poses problems with airway management and visualization of the patient.
  - Signals from the monitoring equipment can distort the magnetic field and interfere with the images produced. Hence only equipment known to be compatible with MRI should be used in the MRI suite.
  - The anaesthetic machine and monitoring equipment can be located either outside the magnetic field, in which case long tubings and extensions are required; or within the magnetic field, where they should be non-ferromagnetic and wall-mounted. Medical gas cylinders should be made of aluminium.

Anaesthetic Management

Preoperative evaluation

— Indication for MRI should be confirmed, and relevant history, physical examination and investigations reviewed.

— Sedative premedication is usually omitted, but an antisialogogue may be useful as it would be difficult to suction secretions during the procedure.

Anaesthetic techniques

— The procedure may be carried out under general anaesthesia, or sedation with monitored anaesthesia care.

— General anaesthesia may be induced in an adjacent induction room and then the patient transferred into the MRI room on a non-ferromagnetic stretcher. Alternatively, anaesthesia may be induced within the MRI room itself if the equipment used is non-ferromagnetic and MRI-compatible.

— Airway control is achieved by means of endotracheal intubation or laryngeal mask airway.

— The breathing system used is either a modified Ayre's T-piece for paediatric patient or a Bain circuit for adult.
— Anaesthesia is maintained by total intravenous anaesthesia (TIVA) or by inhalational anaesthesia.
— The patient may be allowed to breathe spontaneously during the procedure. Ventilation may be assisted or controlled in cases where control of intracranial pressure is required, or if spontaneous respiration interferes with image qualities.
— At the end of the procedure, the patient is removed from the magnetic field prior to emergence from general anaesthesia. Emergence and recovery from anaesthesia are managed as outlined in page 573.

Critical events

— If a critical event were to occur, the patient must be taken out of the magnetic field immediately. It is impossible to conduct cardiopulmonary resuscitation within the magnetic field because of space constraints. Resuscitation equipment may also malfunction or be propelled towards the magnet.
— Resuscitation equipment required include these.
  - Defibrillator, placed outside the magnetic field with extended paddle leads.
  - Laerdal® resuscitation bag.
  - Plastic Penlon® laryngoscope with lithium batteries.
  - Hand-held emergency suction or wall-mounted suction with extended suction tubing.

Ideally the anaesthesiologist should be consulted when the MRI suite is being designed, so that suitable equipment and adequate space can be provided for anaesthesia and recovery. Unfortunately this is not always possible, and the anaesthesiologist is often forced to work within the equipment and space constraints. With sound anaesthetic practice and the use of suitable MRI-compatible monitoring and anaesthetic equipment, anaesthesia for MRI can be safely carried out and the information gained from the procedure can be extremely useful.

FURTHER READING

1. Kotob F, Twersky RS. Anesthesia outside the operating room: General overview and monitoring standards. Int Anesthesiol Clin 2003;41:1–15.

2. Luney SR. Interventional radiology. Curr Opin Anaesthesiol 2002;15:449–54.
3. Conlay LA. Special concerns in the cardiac catheterization lab. Int Anesthesiol Clin 2003;41:63–7.
4. Gooden CK, Dilos B. Anesthesia for magnetic resonance imaging. Int Anesthesiol Clin 2003;41:29–37.
5. Osborn IP. Magnetic resonance imaging anesthesia: New challenges and techniques. Curr Opin Anaesthesiol 2002;15:443–8.
6. Farling PA. Anaesthesia in the magnetic resonance unit: A hazardous environment (Editorial). Anaesthesia 2002;57:421–3.

Chapter 43
Anaesthesia for Electroconvulsive Therapy

INTRODUCTION

Electroconvulsive therapy (ECT) is a well-established mode of treatment in psychiatry. It has assumed an important role in the treatment of severe and medication-resistant depression and mania, as well as in the management of schizophrenic patients with affective disorders, suicidal drive, delusional symptoms, vegetative dysregulation and catatonic symptoms. Compared to drug therapy, it is often quicker to produce benefit, safer, more effective and has fewer side-effects. The mortality rate of ECT is quoted as 0.02–0.04%, while morbidity includes cognitive impairment in the form of memory loss and confusion.

Typically, the acute phase of ECT is performed 3 times a week for 6–12 treatments; initial clinical improvement is usually evident after 3–5 treatments in successful cases. Maintenance therapy can be performed to prevent relapses at progressively increasing intervals from once a week to once a month.

The safety of the procedure has improved with the use of suxamethonium to prevent overvigorous muscle contractions and fractures during seizure. Anaesthesia is indicated for the procedure to prevent recall of the event. Successful ECT requires close collaboration between the psychiatrist and the anaesthesiologist, who should have an in-depth knowledge of the physiologic effects of ECT and the pharmacology of the drugs administered. As the procedure is usually carried out in the psychiatric ward itself, care must be taken to ensure that the anaesthetic, monitoring and resuscitation equipment are in good working order; and that adequate assistance is available during the conduct of anaesthesia.

PHYSIOLOGIC RESPONSES TO ECT

All ECT devices produce electrical stimuli, the frequency and duration of which can be adjusted. A typical setting is pulse frequency of 60 Hz; pulse duration of 0.75 millisecond (ms); and a total stimulus time of 1.25 seconds. Electrically produced seizures are characterized by an initial brief period of muscle contraction from direct stimulation of muscle, followed by a tonic phase lasting up to 20 seconds which is then replaced by a clonic phase.

It has been generally accepted that seizures are an integral part of the treatment, even though there is as yet no general consensus on the features and duration of the therapeutic seizure. Insufficient seizure duration renders ECT ineffective while increasing seizure duration augments unwanted side-effects such as confusion and memory impairment. Seizure duration of 25–60 seconds appears to be adequate for its antidepressive effect.

Activation of the autonomic nervous system is a prominent feature during ECT. These are the physiological effects of ECT.

— *Cardiovascular effects:* immediate (10–15 seconds) parasympathetic stimulation leading to bradycardia, hypotension; followed by sympathetic stimulation leading to tachycardia, hypertension, dysrhythmias, increased myocardial oxygen consumption, lasting ≥ 5 minutes.

— *Cerebral effects:* elevations in cerebral blood flow, oxygen consumption, intracranial pressure.

— *Others:* increases in intraocular and intragastric pressures.

CONTRAINDICATIONS TO ECT

Cardiovascular complications such as myocardial infarction, congestive heart failure, arrhythmias and cardiac arrest are the most frequent causes of peri-ECT mortality. As a result of the physiologic effects of ECT that may be detrimental to the CVS and CNS in particular, these are the contraindications for ECT.

— **Absolute contraindications**
  - Recent myocardial infarction < 3 months.
  - Recent cerebrovascular accident (CVA) < 3 months.
  - Intracranial mass lesion.
  - Unstable cervical spine.
  - Aortic aneurysm.

— **Relative contraindications**
  - Angina pectoris, congestive cardiac failure.
  - Severe pulmonary disease.
  - Severe osteoporosis or major bone fractures.
  - Glaucoma, retinal detachment.
  - Thrombophlebitis, venous thromboembolism.

REQUIREMENTS FOR SAFE CONDUCT OF ANAESTHESIA FOR ECT

As the procedure is usually conducted in the treatment room in the psychiatric ward, the anaesthesiologist may not be familiar with the staff and the anaesthetic, monitoring and resuscitation equipment available. These should be carefully checked before starting the procedure. Requirements for safe conduct of anaesthesia include:

— **Staffing**
  - An anaesthesiologist trained in basic anaesthesia, skilled in maintaining the airway and in treating any complications arising from the procedure.
  - An anaesthetic assistant whose sole duty is to assist the anaesthesiologist during conduct of anaesthesia.
  - Adequate personnel to help restrain and transfer the patient.

— **Facilities and equipment**
  - A tiltable OT table or trolley with a cardiac board support.
  - A fully equipped anaesthetic machine with oxygen/nitrous oxide source and reserve cylinders.
  - Airway equipment consisting of various sizes of face masks, oropharyngeal

airways, laryngoscopes, endotracheal tubes with stylets, gum elastic bougie, laryngeal mask airways.

- A functioning suction device.
- Monitors consisting of ECG, non-invasive BP monitor, pulse oximeter.
- Facilities for resuscitation with emergency drugs used during cardiopulmonary resuscitation (CPR) and a functioning defibrillator.
- A designated area with staff and facilities to monitor patients recovering from the effects of anaesthesia.

CONCURRENT MEDICATIONS

One should be aware of interactions between the psychotropic drugs, ECT and the anaesthetic agents administered. Furthermore, the effects of the anaesthetic agents and other medications on seizure intensity are important determinants influencing outcome of the therapy. Traditionally it has been recommended that psychotropic drugs be tapered and discontinued before starting a course of ECT. This policy is being reconsidered as concomitant use may improve efficacy and prevent relapse. The anaesthesiologist should remain vigilant at all times, as untoward responses during ECT may occur suddenly due to interactions between psychotropic drugs, anaesthetic agents and/or ECT.

These drug interaction may be of relevance during ECT.

— Antidepressants: tricyclic antidepressants and ECT can be combined safely and beneficially. Earlier concerns about anticholinergic effects, cardiac dysrhythmias, and exaggerated effects of direct-acting sympathomimetics have not been reported.

— Monoamine oxidase inhibitor (MAOI): care is required especially for the older irreversible varieties of MAOI and in patients recently placed on such therapy (< 3 months): watch out for exaggerated responses to indirect-acting sympathomimetics, fatal reactions to pethidine, increased duration of block with suxamethonium.

— Lithium: this is associated with significant risk of delirium and/or acute organic syndromes, potentiation of effects of barbiturates and suxamethonium; hence recommendation to discontinue lithium before ECT.

— Benzodiazepines: anticonvulsant properties might interfere with the therapeutic efficacy of ECT.

— CNS stimulants: may prolong seizures, produce dysrhythmias and elevate blood pressure.

— Calcium channel blockers: may cause significant cardiovascular depression.

ANAESTHETIC MANAGEMENT

— Anaesthetic requirements for a successful ECT include rapid induction of anaesthesia, effective attenuation of the haemodynamic responses to ECT, minimal interference with seizure activity, and rapid emergence and recovery from anaesthesia.

— A thorough preanaesthetic assessment should be carried out, which might not be possible if the patient is delusional, paranoid or uncommunicative. These should be noted.
  - General status: ASA classification, co-existing diseases.
  - Concurrent medications.
  - Minimal laboratory investigations unless medically indicated; young, healthy patients may not require any lab investigations.
  - Indication for ECT; rule out possible contraindications.
  - Number of treatments carried out so far, anaesthetic drugs and doses, response during each ECT: further dose adjustments may be made on the basis of earlier responses.

— The patient should be fasted for at least 6 hours while clear fluids may be allowed up to 2 hours before the procedure. Premedication with opioid or benzodiazepine is not warranted. If indicated, acid aspiration prophylaxis should be administered before the procedure.

— Methohexitone 1 mg/kg has been the most widely used intravenous induction agent for ECT because it has no effect on the duration of ECT-induced seizure activity. The use of propofol 1–1.5 mg/kg can significantly shorten the duration of seizure activity, which may be of concern to the psychiatrist. Recovery characteristics are similar; hence there are no clear advantages to the use of propofol for ECT. Etomidate 0.25–0.3 mg/kg may be considered for patients with significant cardiac disease and, unlike propofol, it does not seem to shorten the seizure duration.

— A sub-paralyzing dose of suxamethonium 0.5 mg/kg is used to reduce the intense muscle contractions associated with ECT-induced seizure activity. Low-dose mivacurium 0.08 mg/kg may be used as an alternative for patients in whom suxamethonium is contraindicated.

— Atropine should be drawn up, diluted and ready for use if needed to treat severe bradyarrhythmia. Glycopyrrolate (0.1–0.3 mg IV) is preferable because it produces anticholinergic effects without CNS side-effects. These drugs are also useful for their antisialogogue properties. Esmolol (0.5–1 mg/kg) should be available to attenuate the acute sympathetic responses to ECT.

— A bite-block is inserted after the patient loses consciousness. This protects the oral structures from laceration and provides a patent airway in case mask ventilation is necessary during the tonic phase of the seizure. Allow the psychiatrist to apply the electrical stimulus and note the distribution, intensity and duration of seizure in response to the current delivered. Assistants should be present to restrain the patient during seizure.

— After the procedure, gently ventilate the patient with 100% oxygen until adequate spontaneous respiration has returned. Transfer the patient onto the trolley and to the recovery area. The patient should be observed in the recovery area until he/she is fully awake.

— Side-effects of ECT – confusion, agitation, amnesia, and headache – may be encountered during the recovery period. The patient should be closely observed so that no self-inflicted injury occurs. A small dose of benzodiazepine (e.g., IV midazolam 0.5–1 mg) can be used to treat post-ECT agitation. Rare complications of ECT include acute cardiovascular and neurologic events, splenic rupture and pulmonary oedema.

FURTHER READING

1. Ding Z, White PF. Anesthesia for electroconvulsive therapy. Anesth Analg 2002;94:1351–64.
2. Simpson KH, Lynch L. Anaesthesia and electroconvulsive therapy. (Editorial) Anaesthesia 1998;53:615–7.
3. Naguib M, Koorn R. Interactions between psychotropics, anaesthetics and electroconvulsive therapy: Implications for drug choice and patient management. CNS Drugs 2002;16:229–47.
4. Folk JW, Kellner CH, Beale MD, Conroy JM, Duc TA. Anesthesia for electroconvulsive therapy: A review. J ECT 2000;16:157–70.

Chapter 44

Anaesthesia for Neurosurgery

INTRODUCTION

Anaesthetic management of neurosurgical patients requires an understanding of the basic physiology of the central nervous system (CNS) and the effects of anaesthetic intervention on cerebral function. There are marked advances in the field of neurosurgery as more complex and intricate surgical techniques are being developed. These include minimally invasive neurosurgery, functional neurosurgery for treatment of epilepsy and Parkinson's disease, interventional neuroradiology and the use of image guidance during neurosurgical procedures. For neuroanaesthesia, newer anaesthetic agents (e.g., sevoflurane, desflurane, remifentanil), newer anaesthetic techniques (e.g., management of awake craniotomy), and advances in neuro-monitoring make it an interesting area of subspecialty.

Anaesthetic management for neurosurgery aims to achieve these objectives.

- Provision of optimal operating conditions.
- Maintenance of stable intracranial pressure (ICP), or reduction of elevated ICP by physical or pharmacological means.
- Maintenance of stable haemodynamic, oxygenation and ventilation parameters; use of controlled hypotensive anaesthesia as required in certain procedures.
- Maintenance of an appropriate cerebral perfusion pressure (CPP) and cerebral oxygenation, while minimizing cerebral metabolic rate for oxygen ($CMRO_2$) to protect against ischaemia.
- Early detection and prompt management of intraoperative complications, such as venous air embolism (VAE) in posterior fossa surgery, intracranial bleeding during cerebral aneurysm rupture.
- Controlled but rapid emergence from anaesthesia to enable early assessment and monitoring of neurological status.

Common neurosurgical procedures include:

- Drainage procedures
    - Ventriculo-peritoneal (VP) or ventriculo-atrial (VA) shunt.
    - External ventricular drainage (EVD).
    - Evacuation of extradural or subdural haematoma via Burr hole or craniotomy.
- Craniotomy for excision or debulking of tumour
    - Frontal, temporal or parietal approach for supratentorial tumour.
    - Posterior fossa surgery for cerebellar, cerebellopontine (CP) angle tumour.
    - Frontal or trans-sphenoidal approach for pituitary tumour.
- Cerebrovascular surgery: excision of cerebral aneurysm or arteriovenous malformation (AVM).
- Surgery of the spine or spinal cord
    - Laminectomy: cervical, thoracic, lumbar.
    - Excision of myelomeningocele.

— Surgery on the skull: cranioplasty, elevation of depressed fractures.
— Stereotactic surgery

ANAESTHESIA FOR CRANIOTOMY

Preoperative Assessment

— Confirm diagnosis, indication and consent for surgery. The history and consent may have to be obtained from the patient's next-of-kin if the patient himself/herself is not able to do so.
— Routine preoperative assessment
  - Airway, cardiovascular and respiratory system.
  - Details of concomitant medical illnesses, nature of treatment and compliance to therapy.
  - Investigations appropriate for age, general status of patient and type of surgery.

— Detailed CNS assessment
  - Check the level of consciousness, presence and extent of neurological deficit. This should be clearly documented in the anaesthetic record.
  - Observe the respiratory effort in terms of tachypnoea, laboured breathing or Cheyne-Stokes pattern of breathing.
  - Assess the presence of cough and gag reflex if bulbar involvement is suspected.
  - Look for clinical manifestations of raised ICP such as headache, vomiting, seizures, focal neurological signs and papilloedema. The late signs of increased ICP include deteriorating level of consciousness, Cushing's reflex (hypertension with bradycardia), dilated pupils, decorticate then decerebrate posturing and coma.
  - Review the CT scan or MRI films for the size and location of the space-occupying lesion, size of the ventricles, presence of midline shift and evidence of generalized or peri-tumour cerebral oedema.

— Other considerations
  - Assess the fluid status: possibility of dehydration and electrolyte abnormalities in a patient who has been vomiting, fluid restricted or receiving diuretic therapy.
  - Assess glycaemic status: rule out hyperglycaemia in a patient with preexisting diabetes mellitus or on treatment with dexamethasone.
  - Rule out endocrine dysfunction especially in pituitary tumours: hypo- or hyperthyroidism, acromegaly, hypo- or hyperadrenalism.

- Based on the overall assessment, identify patients who would require postoperative ventilation in ICU, such as Glasgow Coma Scale (GCS) score ≤ 6 (see Appendix), evidence of raised ICP, large or deep-seated tumour, presence of midline shift and/or significant cerebral oedema.

— Premedication
- Opioid premedication is often avoided because of the risk of respiratory depression leading to hypercarbia, increased cerebral blood flow and ICP; and possibility of disrupting early postoperative neurological assessment.
- A small dose of benzodiazepine may be prescribed for patients coming for spinal procedures, or if the patient is conscious, alert and anxious. Alternatively, a small intravenous dose of benzodiazepine can be administered in OT prior to induction of anaesthesia while monitoring is initiated. As long as hypotension is avoided, the cerebral effects of benzodiazepines are not detrimental.

— Other preparations
- GXM appropriate quantity of blood and/or blood products.
- Fasting instruction for the patient: 4 hours for a child, 6 hours for an adult.
- Serve the patient's usual medication on the morning of surgery.

Anaesthetic Management

— Reassess the patient's neurological status before induction of anaesthesia. Confirm availability of ICU or HDU bed for postoperative management.

— Establish venous access with large bore intravenous cannulae. As the anaesthesiologist is situated at the foot end of the patient, intravenous cannulae placed in the long saphenous veins avoids the use of long extension tubing.

— Monitors consist of ECG, non-invasive BP, pulse oximetry and capnography for minor cases (e.g., VP shunt, EVD, Burr hole, cranioplasty). Additional monitors for urine output, temperature, neuromuscular blockade, and invasive BP and CVP measurements are required for major cases.

— Preoxygenate the patient with 100% oxygen for 3–5 minutes before induction of anaesthesia. Common drugs used at induction include fentanyl 2–3 μg/kg, thiopentone 4 mg/kg or propofol 2 mg/kg, atracurium 0.6 mg/kg, vecuronium 0.1–0.15 mg/kg or rocuronium 0.6 mg/kg. Lignocaine 1–1.5 mg/kg or esmolol 0.5–1 mg/kg may be used to obtund sympathetic reflexes during airway manipulation.

- Suxamethonium transiently increases ICP and is best avoided in elective cases, *except* in suspected difficult intubation. Its use should not be withheld in emergency cases where airway protection against aspiration should take precedence over concerns about transient effects on ICP.
- Monitor the degree of neuromuscular blockade with peripheral nerve stimulator. Allow adequate time for the non-depolarizing neuromuscular blocking drug to take effect. Laryngoscopy and intubation should be attempted only when the patient is adequately anaesthetized and fully paralyzed.
- Use an oral RAE tube or a flexometallic tube of appropriate size. Fasten the ETT securely after its correct placement is confirmed. Protect the eyes by using eye pads; this is particularly important if the patient is placed prone with the head on a horseshoe headrest.
- Allow the surgeon or assistant to shave the head and position the patient for surgery. Various positions may be adopted depending on the site of the tumour and the planned surgical approach: supine, prone, semi-prone, lateral or even sitting. Maintain a head-up tilt of 15–20°, and avoid extreme neck flexion or rotation. Re-check the position of the ETT after positioning. The head is often secured in place using a Mayfield 3-point fixator. An additional dose of fentanyl before the pins are inserted helps to prevent a marked hypertensive and tachycardic response.
- In cases of intracranial hypertension, it may be necessary to lower ICP by administering mannitol 0.5–1 g/kg, and/or frusemide 0.5 mg/kg. Mannitol infusion is best started at the time of skin incision so that the peak effect becomes available upon dural opening.
- Send arterial blood sample for ABG. Maintain PaO_2 >100 mmHg and $PaCO_2$ between 30–35 mmHg. Avoid overventilation since hypocarbia may result in cerebral vasoconstriction and reduced cerebral perfusion.
- Maintenance of anaesthesia
  - The choice is between an intravenous or inhalational technique with or without nitrous oxide.
    - A total intravenous anaesthesia (TIVA) technique with propofol infusion, neuromuscular blocking drug, opioid and IPPV with oxygen-air mixture.
    - An inhalational technique with a volatile anaesthetic agent, neuromuscular blocking drug, opioid and either oxygen-nitrous oxide or oxygen-air mixture.
  - Neuromuscular blocking drug is administered by means of intermittent bolus doses or continuous infusion.

- Analgesia is maintained with intermittent bolus doses of fentanyl or infusion of remifentanil.
- Isoflurane and sevoflurane are the preferred volatile anaesthetic agents. The CNS effects of both are similar in terms of maintenance of cerebral autoregulation up to a MAC of 1.5, and maintenance of CO_2 reactivity of cerebral blood vessels. Sevoflurane has a further advantage of smooth induction, rapid onset and offset of action.
- The role of nitrous oxide in neuroanaesthesia is waning. Nitrous oxide should be avoided in patients with cerebral ischaemia or reduced intracranial compliance; and in surgery that carries a significant risk of venous air embolism (e.g., posterior fossa surgery). It causes cerebral vasodilation, increased cerebral blood volume and ICP. It may also contribute to the development of pneumoencephalocele.

— Fluid management
- Intravenous fluids should be used judiciously and be sufficient to maintain intravascular volume and haemodynamic stability.
- Dextrose-containing solutions should be avoided unless specifically indicated because they are hypo-osmolar; furthermore the resultant hyperglycaemia may impair neurological recovery from cerebral ischaemia.
- Ringer's lactate is also hypo-osmolar and may risk increasing plasma glucose concentration through lactate metabolism.
- 0.9% saline is the preferred crystalloid solution but it may cause hyperchloraemic acidosis when large quantities are infused.
- Blood loss is often difficult to estimate but may be torrential. It is important to have adequate venous access as rapid volume replacement may be necessary.

— Temperature control
- There has been a resurgence of interest in controlled hypothermia as a neuroprotective strategy even though improved outcome has not been conclusively demonstrated.
- A moderate, "permissive hypothermia" to 33–35°C decreases $CMRO_2$ and may increase the period of ischaemia tolerated intraoperatively.
- Normothermia should be achieved before the patient awakens in order to avoid shivering, which markedly increases oxygen demand.

— Thromboembolic prophylaxis
- Neurosurgical patients are at risk for development of deep vein thrombosis (DVT) and pulmonary embolism; hence thromboprophylaxis is indicated.

    - Heparin should not be used because of the nature of surgery and risk of bleeding in a confined cavity.
    - Mechanical means of prophylaxis in the form of graduated compression stockings and intermittent pneumatic leg compression are used instead.
- Management of emergence
    - Most patients do not require prolonged intubation and mechanical ventilation after an uneventful craniotomy procedure. In these patients, controlled emergence with an early return to consciousness is desired so that full neurological assessment can be made in the earliest possible time. Anaesthetic agents with short duration of action and little hangover effect are preferred.
    - The patient should not be allowed to cough on the ETT, as this invariably leads to tachycardia, hypertension and increased ICP.
    - A practical approach is to turn off volatile anaesthetic agent at the time of bone flap replacement; maintain anaesthesia with nitrous oxide (if used) and continued infusion of remifentanil or residual concentration of fentanyl.
    - At completion of surgical dressing, reverse the neuromuscular blockade, turn off remifentanil infusion and administer 100% oxygen. Another longer-acting opioid should be administered before discontinuation of remifentanil infusion to provide subsequent analgesia.

Postoperative Management

- Decision for postoperative ventilatory support depends on the patient's preoperative neurological status, intraoperative events (duration and complexity of surgery, haemodynamic stability, complications such as venous air embolism, hypovolaemia, massive transfusion), and evidence of raised ICP, as shown by tense dura or tight brain. Communication with the surgeon is essential to avoid any misunderstanding regarding postoperative management plans.
- Regular neurological observations, including ICP monitoring if available, should be recorded. Any neurological deterioration should raise the suspicion of intracranial bleeding or oedema. An urgent CT scan should be considered.
- Other aspects of postoperative care
    - The patient's haemodynamic status should be closely monitored to maintain adequate cerebral perfusion pressure.
    - Postoperative pain is not often severe and can be managed by intermittent bolus doses or infusion of morphine or other opioids.

- Electrolyte imbalance, especially abnormalities in sodium concentration, may be common in patients with neurological disorders. This should be checked and corrected if present.
- Urine output should be closely monitored as diabetes insipidus may occur.

SPECIAL CONSIDERATIONS

Posterior Fossa Surgery

— Indications for posterior fossa surgery include resection or biopsy of tumours such as glioma, astrocytoma, meningioma, medulloblastoma, acoustic neuroma or haemangioblastoma and resection of vascular lesions such as aneurysm, angioma, AVM. Other lesions include abscess, haematoma or congenital lesion (e.g., Arnold-Chiari malformation).

— Posterior fossa tumours pose special problems for these reasons.
- The confined space does not allow much room for bleeding or oedema, which if uncontrolled may result in coning through the foramen magnum.
- Structures in close proximity to the tumour include the main motor and sensory pathways, the lower cranial nerve nuclei and vital centres controlling the cardiovascular and respiratory functions in the brainstem.
- Obstruction of CSF flow at the aqueduct or fourth ventricle results in obstructive hydrocephalus.
- Patients may have altered level of consciousness with impaired airway reflexes leading to silent aspiration.

— Surgery is often done with the patient in the prone, lateral or semi-prone ("park-bench") position. The sitting position is rarely, if ever, adopted nowadays.
- Extreme care must be taken while turning the patient to the desired position for surgery.
- Avoid extreme flexion of the neck which may cause venous and lymphatic obstruction (resulting in upper airway oedema) and cord hypoperfusion (resulting in quadriparesis) especially in the elderly.

— Insert a nasogastric tube if there is a possibility of lower cranial nerve dysfunction with bulbar paresis. The gag reflex, swallowing and laryngeal function may be impaired.

— Nitrous oxide should be avoided in posterior fossa surgery because of its deleterious effects on $CMRO_2$ and cerebral blood flow, and its propensity to aggravate venous air embolism or pneumocephalus. Anaesthesia using the TIVA technique is preferred.

- Be familiar with early diagnosis and management of venous air embolism (see Chapter 76).
- Closely monitor the cardiovascular system for acute changes such as cardiac arrhythmias or hypertension as a result of surgical interference with the vital centres. A precipitous decrease in heart rate often signifies brainstem ischaemia and should be promptly notified to the surgeon. This often resolves spontaneously when surgical retraction is adjusted but atropine is required in severe bradyarrhythmias. Close communication with the surgeon is essential.
- Postoperative management in ICU is often indicated. Consider mechanical ventilation if the patient's GCS score is low, there is evidence of airway oedema or bulbar paresis, the surgical resection is extensive or complicated, or if there are intraoperative complications.

Pituitary Surgery

- Most of the lesions are benign adenomas of the anterior pituitary which present with different effects.
  - Mass effects: headache, visual disturbance typically bitemporal hemianopia, cranial nerve palsies, hyposecretion of pituitary hormones.
  - Hormone hypersecretion syndromes: hyperprolactinaemia, acromegaly, Cushing's disease, thyrotoxicosis, multiple endocrine neoplasia syndromes.
- Surgical approach can be trans-sphenoidal or transcranial depending on the size of the tumour and the presence of suprasellar extension. Uncomplicated trans-sphenoidal surgery imposes only a minimal physiological disruption and is generally well tolerated.
- During preoperative assessment, it is important to identify significant endocrine abnormalities and modify anaesthetic management accordingly.
  - Acromegaly: potential for difficult intubation which requires a thorough airway assessment and strategy for airway management (e.g., awake fibreoptic intubation via the orotracheal route), increased incidence of obstructive sleep apnoea, possibility of hypertension, cardiomyopathy, glucose intolerance and nerve entrapment syndromes.
  - Cushing's disease: presence of hypertension, cardiac disease, glucose intolerance, electrolyte abnormalities, osteoporosis.
  - ACTH hyposecretion: requirement for perioperative steroid replacement therapy (see Chapter 20).

— Induction and maintenance of anaesthesia are carried out in the usual manner. In the absence of potential airway problem, the commonest anaesthetic technique consists of intravenous induction and balanced anaesthesia with short-acting opioid, non-depolarizing neuromuscular blocking drug, nitrous oxide, volatile anaesthetic and controlled ventilation with IPPV.

— A moist pharyngeal pack is inserted after intubation to absorb blood and secretion at the pharynx. This is removed at the end of surgery and the pharynx cleared of residual secretions under direct vision.

— Consider all patients to be at risk of potential airway difficulties. Instruct the patients to breathe through the mouth because of the presence of nasal packs.

— Postoperative neurological evaluation includes assessment of visual function and conscious level. Monitor fluid balance, changes in plasma and urine concentrations and osmolarity to identify patients developing diabetes insipidus, characterized by large volumes of urine of low osmolarity and sodium concentration despite clinical and biochemical evidence of dehydration.

ANAESTHESIA FOR CEREBROVASCULAR SURGERY

Abnormalities in the cerebral vasculature include intracranial aneurysms, arteriovenous malformations (AVMs) and atheromatous plaques at the branches of extracranial and intracranial vessels. Patients with occlusive disease of the carotid artery often present for carotid endarterectomy, the anaesthetic management of which is described in Chapter 38.

AVMs are dilated arteries and veins with no intervening capillaries; they may present clinically with haemorrhage (subarachnoid or intracerebral), headaches or seizures. High blood flows through such shunts may cause ischaemia and loss of vascular reactivity in the underlying brain tissue. AVMs are treated by excision or devascularization by interventional neuroradiology. Surgery is not urgent unless haemorrhage results in a haematoma causing pressure effects.

The prevalence of unruptured intracranial aneurysms is estimated at 2–5%. The majority of cerebral aneurysms are saccular ("berry") aneurysms. About 90% of aneurysms occur on the anterior part of the circle of Willis, the commonest of which are on the anterior communicating and anterior cerebral arteries.

The patient may present with subarachnoid haemorrhage (SAH) if the aneurysm is ruptured, classically with sudden onset of an unusually severe headache followed by a period of unconsciousness. Alternatively, the aneurysm may cause compression on adjacent neural structures, presenting with headache or cranial nerve palsies. Some patients are completely asymptomatic and diagnosis is only made on an incidental CT scan finding.

The optimal timing of surgery after SAH is controversial:

— Early surgery (< 48 hours after SAH) may be associated with suboptimal surgical conditions but may reduce the incidence of re-bleeding and vasospasm.
— Worst outcome is associated with surgery between 7 and 10 days after SAH, the period that carries the greatest risk for angiographic and clinical vasospasm.
— Delayed surgery provides time for oedema to subside and may be technically easier, but increases the risks of re-bleeding and complications associated with prolonged bed rest.

Anaesthetic concerns in aneurysm surgery include these.

— Problems common to neurosurgical procedures as outlined earlier.
— Problems associated with ruptured intracranial aneurysm.
  - Control of severe intracranial hypertension.
  - Prevention and treatment of cerebral vasospasm.
— Problems during intraoperative management.
  - Stringent control of intraoperative BP within narrow limits.
  - Intraoperative rupture of aneurysm may cause rapid and massive blood loss.

Preoperative Assessment

The asymptomatic patient with unruptured aneurysm is assessed in the manner outlined in page 587. The patient with ruptured aneurysm requires these additional considerations.

— CNS
  - Assess clinical manifestations of SAH (headache, vomiting, neck stiffness or seizures), level of consciousness and presence of neurological deficit.
— CVS
  - The patient's BP is often elevated. Hypertension may be preexisting, secondary to Cushing's reflex in an attempt to maintain cerebral perfusion, or as part of the triple-H therapy with the use of inotropes *(vide infra)*.
  - Various ECG changes are observed following SAH, including peaked P waves, short PR intervals, long QTc intervals, pathological Q waves, ST-T wave abnormalities, prominent U waves; cardiac arrhythmias.

- ECG changes may mimic changes due to myocardial injury. A cardiology consult should be made in doubtful cases.

— Respiratory system
- Examine for basal atelectasis in patients on prolonged bed rest, and evidence of aspiration pneumonia in comatose patients unable to protect the airway.
- Neurogenic pulmonary oedema may occur following SAH.

— Fluid and electrolyte balance
- Assess the hydration status, as the patient may be dehydrated due to vomiting and lack of oral intake.
- Fluid and electrolyte imbalance may result from inappropriate antidiuretic hormone (ADH) secretion or cerebral salt wasting syndrome. These should be diagnosed and corrected before surgery.

— Management of SAH
- The preoperative management is aimed at maintaining a normal CPP, avoidance of extreme hypertension and maintenance of normal fluid balance.
- The patient may be on the triple-H therapy (hypertension, hypervolaemia, haemodilution) in an attempt to improve CPP and prevent ischaemic neurological deficit caused by vasospasm.
- Oral nimodipine, a calcium channel blocker with vasodilating effect on cerebral vessels, is often used for the treatment of cerebral vasospasm. Use of nimodipine in the intravenous route may result in hypotension, and extra vigilance is required in its detection and treatment.

Anaesthetic Management

— It is essential to establish good communication between surgeon and anaesthesiologist concerning surgical conditions and haemodynamic parameters.

— Invasive haemodynamic monitoring in the form of intraarterial BP and CVP should be established before commencement of anaesthesia. A pulmonary artery catheter is indicated in the presence of significant myocardial damage and ventricular dysfunction.

— Close monitoring and stringent control of BP throughout anaesthesia is required to prevent wide fluctuations. This includes smooth induction of anaesthesia with measures to prevent hypertension during intubation and hypotension postinduction. Intraoperative BP should be maintained within 10–20% of the baseline BP:

hypertension risks aneurysm rupture while hypotension risks cerebral ischaemia, both being undesirable occurrences.

— Large bore intravenous cannulae are essential because of the potential for rapid catastrophic haemorrhage especially in AVM surgery. Rapid transfusion devices should be primed and ready for volume resuscitation if necessary.
— Induced hypotension is commonly used for excision of AVM to reduce intra-operative blood loss. A systolic BP of 60–80 mmHg should be adequate for the purpose, achieved by using volatile anaesthetics, β-blockers and/or sodium nitroprusside. When the AVM is excised, a relative hyperperfusion to the previously ischaemic tissue surrounding the AVM may result in cerebral oedema and increased ICP.
— Induced hypotension is used with caution, if at all, in cerebral aneurysm surgery due to the concern that hypotension may increase the risk of cerebral ischaemia in patients with vasospasm and impaired autoregulation. It may be indicated in complex cases or if intraoperative aneurysm rupture occurs.
— Consider other neuroprotective measures in selected cases, such as difficult aneurysm surgery or intraoperative aneurysm rupture. These include induced hypothermia to 32°C and thiopentone infusion to further reduce $CMRO_2$.
— All patients should be admitted to ICU for close monitoring of haemodynamic and neurological status. Even though early assessment of neurological status is ideal, prolonged surgery or intraoperative complications may necessitate sedation and ventilation in the immediate postoperative period.
— Haemodynamic monitoring and fluid management should be receiving close attention in the ICU. Vasoactive drugs and the judicious use of fluids may be required to maintain haemodynamic stability. The patient's neurological status should be assessed as soon as feasible and regular assessments should be made thereafter. A decrease in GCS or development of new neurological deficit may indicate vasospasm, intracranial bleed or hydrocephalus. The patient may need an urgent CT scan to make a definitive diagnosis and further management plan.

ANAESTHESIA FOR HEAD INJURY

Brain damage due to head injury must be considered in terms of primary mechanical effects of force applied to the skull at the time of injury, and secondary effects due to haemorrhage, oedema and infection. It is important to ensure best circumstances are available for recovery from primary insult and to anticipate and, if possible, prevent secondary brain damage.

The anaesthesiologist may be involved in the initial assessment and resuscitation at the Accident and Emergency Department, provision of anaesthetic services in the Radiology Department and/or OT, and management of such patients in the ICU in an attempt to reduce the impact of secondary brain injury.

Anticipated Problems in Head Injury

These are pertinent in the head-injured patient presenting for emergency craniotomy to evacuate intracranial haematoma.

— Problems of emergency surgery
- Presence of full stomach with risks of aspiration.
- Insufficient time for thorough preoperative assessment and preparation.
- Inability to perform proper clinical evaluation in a patient who is intoxicated, uncooperative or unconscious.

— Problems with associated injuries
- Cervical spine fracture-dislocation may result in spinal cord injury with initial period of spinal shock.
- Maxillofacial trauma with potential for acute upper airway obstruction, bleeding into the airway and difficult intubation.
- Thoracic injuries with involvement of the lungs, heart, great vessels or the tracheobronchial tree which may be life-threatening.
- Intraabdominal injury may necessitate emergency laparotomy to repair injured viscus and secure haemostasis.
- Pelvic or bone injuries may present with problems of concealed bleeding and fat embolism syndrome.

— Potentially difficult intubation
- Particularly so in the presence of cervical and/or maxillofacial trauma.
- Urgent intubation may be required in an area where intubating conditions are suboptimal in terms of anaesthetic assistance, airway and resuscitation equipment.

— Presence of raised ICP
- This requires preoperative resuscitation, urgent surgery and postoperative ICU management.
- Measures of cerebral protection need to be instituted.

Anaesthetic Management

— Adequate venous access and monitors are required. The necessity for invasive monitors depends on the status of the patient, extent of head injury and urgency of surgery.

— The anaesthetic technique of choice is rapid sequence induction and intubation with precalculated doses of fentanyl, thiopentone, suxamethonium and with application of cricoid pressure. Suxamethonium causes a transient rise in ICP but the effect is short-lived. Methods suggested to obtund this rise in ICP are not uniformly successful.

— If cervical fracture is suspected or confirmed, intubation should be done with the patient's head and neck in the neutral position. An assistant should apply manual in-line stabilization in order to avoid movement of the cervical spine during airway manipulation.

— Intraoperative management is similar to that for an elective procedure.

— The patient may require elective ventilation postoperatively depending on these factors.
  - Extent and nature of head injury.
  - Initial GCS.
  - Evidence of raised ICP.
  - Intraoperative complications.
  - Associated injuries especially chest injury.

Management in ICU

— Positioning and monitoring
  - The patient should be kept in a slight (15–20°) reverse Trendelenburg position, keeping the head straight to avoid kinking of blood vessels in the neck.
  - Regular neuro-monitoring and haemodynamic monitoring, with early aggressive treatment if deterioration occurs; repeat CT scan if clinically indicated.

— Respiratory care
  - Ensure adequate oxygenation by adjusting FiO_2 to maintain $PaO_2 > 90$ mmHg.
  - Maintain normocarbia with $PaCO_2$ 30–35 mmHg. Avoid hyperventilation and hypocarbia as this may result in cerebral vasoconstriction.
  - Regular chest physiotherapy and tracheal suction. Provide adequate sedation and analgesia to prevent rise in ICP during physiotherapy.

— Blood pressure control
  - Maintain BP within 20% of baseline value to ensure adequate CPP, where CPP = MAP – ICP. CPP should be kept above 70 mmHg.
  - Treat hyper- or hypotension with vasoactive drugs and appropriate fluid management.

— Treatment of increased ICP
  - Maintain the patient on controlled ventilation with IPPV and sedation for 24–48 hours. Muscle paralysis is usually not required when adequate sedation is provided.
  - Administer diuretics in the form of mannitol 0.5–1 g/kg and/or frusemide 0.5–1 mg/kg.
  - Restrict maintenance fluid to maintenance, or approximately 1.5 L/24 hr in an average adult. Do not use dextrose-containing solution unless specifically indicated.
  - Consider the use of hypertonic saline or high-dose barbiturate, e.g., thiopentone in selected cases.
  - Use of corticosteroids such as dexamethasone, even though these are more useful in reducing focal cerebral oedema due to tumours. The effectiveness of steroids in head injury is questionable.
  - Prescribe antiepileptic drugs such as benzodiazepine, barbiturate, phenytoin for both immediate and long-term control of epileptic seizures.

— Others areas of care include:
  - Haematology, biochemical, microbiological investigations.
  - Infection control with appropriate antibiotics.
  - Correction of electrolyte abnormalities.
  - Management of diabetes insipidus if this occurs.
  - Gastric ulceration prophylaxis using ranitidine or cimetidine.
  - Limb physiotherapy, nursing, bladder care, early enteral nutrition.

— Lastly, the possibility of organ donation in a brain dead patient should be borne in mind. Suitable candidates should be identified and the process of organ procurement set into motion as and when appropriate.

STEREOTACTIC SURGERY

Stereotactic surgery uses images of the brain to guide the surgeon to a target within the brain. This technique may utilize an external frame attached to the head (frame-based) or imaging markers attached to the scalp (frameless or image-guided surgery) for orientation.

With frame-based stereotactic surgery, general anaesthesia is induced and a lightweight frame is attached to the patient's head. Imaging is done by means of CT or MR in the Radiology Department to identify the target in relationship to the external frame. Surgical apparatus attached to the head frame can be adjusted to the 3-dimensional coordinates of the target, which can then be accurately approached by the surgeon.

A common example is stereotactic brain biopsy. Deep-seated tumours within the brain may be difficult and dangerous to approach by an open operation. Under image guidance, a biopsy probe is passed through a small hole in the skull to sample tissue for diagnosis. Deep brain stimulator electrodes can also be placed inside specific areas of the brain to treat movement disorders such as Parkinson's disease, Huntington's chorea, and aid location of abnormal tissue in epilepsy.

Further refinement of the technique is the development of frameless stereotactic surgery. This relies on real-time radiologic images obtained by means of CT or MRI, with reference points around the tumour displayed on the monitor. The data acquired are entered into computer software and converted into anatomically distinct structures that show the relationship of surgical instruments to the imaged brain. This 3-dimensional display of the tumour and surrounding tissue enables an accurate approach for removal of the lesion and with reduced injury to normal tissue.

AWAKE CRANIOTOMY

Awake craniotomy is not a new surgical technique as it has been used in epilepsy surgery for removal of epileptic foci since the 1980s. It is now used for the excision of tumours located in the functional ("eloquent") cortex, namely the motor strip, Broca's and Wernicke's speech areas. Intraoperative neurological testing allows optimal tumour resection while preserving functional tissue so that there will be minimal postoperative neurological dysfunction.

Anaesthetic management for awake craniotomy poses an interesting challenge for the anaesthesiologist because optimal analgesia and sedation should be provided during the initial stages of craniotomy, an awake and cooperative patient is expected during the period of brain mapping, and continuous assessment of neurologic status is mandatory during tumour resection to prevent impending damage. Throughout the procedure, the anaesthetic technique should ensure haemodynamic stability without compromising ventilation and oxygenation.

Careful patient selection is necessary. Contraindications include patient refusal, communication difficulties, and patients who are confused, extremely anxious or unable to lie still for many hours. Those with obesity, oesophageal reflux and large vascular tumours may pose problems and are best excluded. A good rapport between the patient and the anaesthesiologist is essential.

Various anaesthetic techniques have been described, including neurolept anaesthesia, dexmedetomidine infusion for sedation, local anaesthesia combined with appropriate sedation and monitored anaesthesia care, or an asleep-awake-asleep technique using general anaesthesia. Whichever technique is employed, it is important to maintain airway and ventilatory control to avoid problems of hypoxaemia and/or hypercarbia.

It is recommended that bispectral index (BIS) is monitored in addition to routine monitors. The asleep-awake-asleep technique makes use of TIVA with a target-controlled infusion of propofol and a remifentanil infusion. Controlled ventilation is maintained via a laryngeal mask airway (LMA) or LMA ProSeal™. The infusion rates of propofol and remifentanil are adjusted in response to changes in haemodynamic variables, response to surgical stimulation, and are guided by the BIS value. Remifentanil has a very short half-life and provides greater haemodynamic stability but more respiratory depression than fentanyl. It is thus safer to control ventilation than to allow spontaneous ventilation and risk hypoventilation.

When the tumour is exposed, infusion of remifentanil is reduced until spontaneous respiration resumes. The propofol infusion is stopped and the LMA is removed as the patient awakens. A background infusion of remifentanil of 0.005–0.01 μg/kg/min is used to provide additional analgesia during the awake period. When tumour resection is completed, the patient is re-anaesthetized and the LMA re-inserted. Ventilation is again controlled until completion of surgery.

The TIVA technique with propofol-remifentanil combination is ideal as this allows titratable levels of anaesthesia as well as fast and reliable awakening when required. The LMA technique is superior to other methods of achieving airway control (e.g., endotracheal tube, nasopharyngeal airway) because it minimizes the risk of coughing or straining and subsequent vomiting during lightening of anaesthesia, complications which are highly undesirable in awake craniotomy. Controlled ventilation via the LMA obviates the problems of apnoea, hypoventilation or airway obstruction. It also enables manipulation of the patient's PaO_2 and $PaCO_2$ by adjusting the FiO_2 and ventilatory parameters.

APPENDIX

GLASGOW COMA SCALE

Criteria	Points
A. Eye opening	
spontaneous	4
to speech	3
to pain	2
nil	1
B. Best motor response	
obeys commands	6
localizes to pain	5
withdraws to pain	4
abnormal flexion	3
extensor response	2
nil	1
C. Best verbal response	
orientated	5
confused	4
inappropriate words	3
incomprehensible sounds	2
nil	1
Maximum possible score = 15	
Minimum possible score = 3	

FURTHER READING

1. Brian JE Jr. Carbon dioxide and the cerebral circulation. Anesthesiology 1998;88:1365–86.
2. Hancock SM, Nathanson MH. Nitrous oxide or remifentanil for the 'at risk' brain (Editorial). Anaesthesia 2004;59:313–7.

3. Fabregas N, Gomar C. Monitoring in neuroanaesthesia: Update of clinical usefulness. Eur J Anaesthesiol 2001;18:423–9.
4. Warner DS. Anesthesia for craniotomy. Can J Anesth 2002;49:R1–8.
5. Girling KJ. New developments in anaesthesia for neurological surgery. Curr Opin Anaesthesiol 2000;13:503–7.
6. Durieux M. Changes in neurosurgery: Implications for neuroanesthesia. Curr Opin Anaesthesiol 2001;14:467–8.
7. Duff CM, Matta BF. Sevoflurane and anesthesia for neurosurgery: A review. J Neurosurg Anesth 2000:12:128–40.
8. Moss E. Anaesthetic management of intracranial aneurysms, arteriovenous malformations and carotid endarterectomy. Best Prac Res Clin Anaesthesiol 1999;13:545–56.
9. Morgan RJ. Anaesthetic management of aneurismal subarachnoid haemorrhage. Curr Anaesth Crit Care 2003;13:277–86.
10. Sarang A, Dinsmore J. Anaesthesia for awake craniotomy – Evolution of a technique that facilitates awake neurological testing. Br J Anaesth 2003;90:161–5.
11. Hans P, Bonhomme V, Born JD, et al. Target-controlled infusion of propofol and remifentanil combined with bispectral index monitoring for awake craniotomy. Anaesthesia 2000;55:255–9.

Chapter 45

Anaesthesia for Minimally Invasive Surgery

INTRODUCTION

Endoscopic surgical procedures are examples of minimally invasive surgery. These procedures are fast gaining popularity, particularly with technological advances in video imaging as well as optics and light transmission. Laparoscopic procedures in gynaecology have been well established while an increasingly greater number of procedures in the general surgical disciplines are being done endoscopically.

Compared with conventional open procedures, minimally invasive surgery produces significantly less trauma in terms of wound size and tissue retraction to gain surgical exposure. Its potential advantages include reduced incidence of postoperative ileus, reduced postoperative pain, improved respiratory function, shorter hospital stay and earlier return to the patient's normal activities.

However, the intraoperative requirements of laparoscopic surgery can cause serious physiological disturbance and risk to patients. Since many surgeons are in the learning process to master this relatively new surgical technique, the duration of surgery is understandably long – an important consideration particularly for the ill or elderly patients. Conversion to an open procedure is always a possibility especially if complications develop or if surgical access is deemed difficult.

Perioperative mortality for gynaecologic laparoscopic procedures is estimated at 4–8 per 100,000. Increased incidence of perioperative mortality is expected for patients presenting for general surgical laparoscopic procedures since they are generally older and may suffer from acute surgical conditions. It is, therefore, important for both the surgeon and the anaesthesiologist to be aware of the potential complications, weigh the risks against the potential benefits of laparoscopic surgery and select the approach in the best interest of the patient.

Examples of such procedures include:

— **Gynaecology:** diagnostic laparoscopy for infertility or pelvic pathology, laparoscopic sterilization, salpingectomy in ectopic pregnancy, ovarian cystectomy, laparoscopic assisted vaginal hysterectomy.

— **General surgery:** laparoscopic cholecystectomy, fundoplication, vagotomy, appendicectomy, oesophagectomy, hernia repair, adhesiolysis, adrenalectomy, nephrectomy, ureterolithotomy.

— **Thoracic surgery:** video-assisted thoracoscopic surgery (VATS), mediastinoscopy.

— **Orthopaedic surgery:** shoulder or knee arthroscopy.

This chapter discusses laparoscopic procedures done in gynaecology and general surgery. Anaesthesia for VATS requires special considerations and is discussed in Chapter 37.

PREOPERATIVE ASSESSMENT

In addition to routine preoperative assessment, these points are pertinent.

— Cardiovascular system: up to 25–30% of adult patients have potentially patent foramen ovale through which paradoxical embolism can occur, and all previously undiagnosed murmurs should be investigated prior to laparoscopy.

— Respiratory system: patients with chronic pulmonary disease may not tolerate CO_2 insufflation and positioning during laparoscopic surgery.

— Acid aspiration risks: patients with significant risk factors should be identified, as pneumoperitoneum and the resultant increase in intraabdominal pressure may promote regurgitation and aspiration of gastric contents.

— The possibility that the procedure may be converted to an open procedure should be explained, and appropriate consent should be obtained from the patient prior to the surgery.

Premedication in the form of oral benzodiazepine is usually adequate. Premedication is not necessary for laparoscopic procedures done as day-case unless the patient is extremely anxious. Acid aspiration prophylaxis should be prescribed for high-risk patients, such as obese patients and those with hiatus hernia or oesophageal reflux.

ANAESTHETIC TECHNIQUE

General anaesthesia with muscle paralysis, tracheal intubation and intermittent positive pressure ventilation is the preferred anaesthetic technique. The laryngeal mask airway, in particular LMA ProSeal™, has been successfully used in place of endotracheal tube especially in short day-case procedures. Use of spontaneous ventilation technique is not advisable in view of intraoperative pneumoperitoneum and positioning of the patient. However, some short procedures (e.g., laparoscopic sterilization) may be performed without neuromuscular blockade in the presence of a skilled surgeon and non-obese patient.

Regional anaesthesia is not advisable as a sole anaesthetic technique because of the level of block required for adequate surgical anaesthesia, positioning requirements, presence of a pneumoperitoneum that may cause embarrassment to respiratory mechanics, and the possibility of shoulder tip pain as a result of diaphragmatic irritation.

Points to Note

— Propofol is the intravenous induction agent of choice as it is non-emetogenic and has good recovery characteristics. Short-acting opioids (e.g., fentanyl, alfentanil, remifentanil) can be used intraoperatively to cover the surgical stimulus that can be intense but usually short-lived.

— Use of nitrous oxide is controversial. There are concerns regarding its ability to cause bowel distension and impair surgical access, even though this is often not clinically significant in short- and medium-length procedures. More significant is the role of nitrous oxide in causing postoperative nausea and vomiting (PONV). It seems prudent to omit nitrous oxide in patients at risk of PONV or when surgical difficulties are anticipated.

— The use of halothane has been superseded by newer inhalational agents such as isoflurane, desflurane and sevoflurane, which are less myocardial depressant and less arrhythmogenic. These are important properties when there is potential hypercarbia associated with carbon dioxide insufflation.

— Other than mandatory monitoring of ECG, BP, pulse oximetry and capnography, one should keep a close watch on the respiratory parameters (airway pressure, tidal volume and minute ventilation) as well as intraabdominal pressure. Modern CO_2 insufflator has an adjustable limit on the intraabdominal pressure (usually set at 15 mmHg), above which an audible alarm is activated and the gas flow is cut off.

— Avoid excessive stomach inflation from overzealous ventilation by mask. Insert a nasogastric tube to decompress the stomach after induction of anaesthesia in laparoscopic cholecystectomy. This reduces the risk of gastric injury during trocar insertion and facilitates surgery around the liver and gall bladder.

— Pay particular attention to pressure areas and avoid nerve injuries during positioning. This is particularly important in steep Trendelenburg and lithotomy positions.

— Adjust the ventilatory pattern according to the patient's respiratory and haemodynamic status. It may be necessary to increase the respiratory rate and fresh gas flow to improve CO_2 removal, or reduce the tidal volume to prevent an excessively high airway pressure.

— The incidence of PONV is high following laparoscopic surgery, and some form of antiemetic prophylaxis is indicated. Combinations of antiemetics are more effective than single agents. A multi-modal approach to prevention of PONV includes use of combinations of droperidol 0.625–1.25 mg, 5-HT_3 antagonists (ondansetron 4 mg), and dexamethasone 8 mg, together with adequate intraoperative hydration and multi-modal pain management with strategies to minimize opioid usage.

— At the end of the procedure, the surgeon should evacuate as much of the CO_2 from the peritoneal cavity as possible. This lessens the incidence of PONV and shoulder-tip pain. The residual CO_2 is absorbed into the bloodstream and excreted via the lungs.

— Postoperative pain may be quite severe in some patients even though it is usually less intense and less prolonged compared to open surgery. There is more visceral pain after laparoscopic procedures compared with parietal (i.e., abdominal wall) pain after open abdominal procedures. This is made worse by shoulder-tip pain secondary to diaphragmatic irritation. In the absence of contraindications, postoperative pain may be controlled with non-steroidal antiinflammatory drugs (NSAIDs) as part of the multi-modal analgesic regimen combining short-acting opioid, NSAID and local anaesthetic infiltration at the wound site (preemptive rather than postoperative). This reduces opioid dose and minimizes side-effects such as PONV. Intraperitoneal instillation of 20 ml of 0.25% bupivacaine at the end of the surgery has also been advocated.

INTRAOPERATIVE PROBLEMS AND COMPLICATIONS

The intraoperative course of laparoscopic procedures is often uneventful even though potential complications exist. Awareness of these complications should allow early detection and treatment, and improve patient care and safety.

1. **Effects of pneumoperitoneum**

   This can lead to these changes.
   - Reduced functional residual capacity due to Trendelenburg positioning (in gynaecological laparoscopy) and diaphragmatic splinting.
   - Decrease in pulmonary compliance, increase in peak airway pressure with risk of barotrauma.
   - Hypoxaemia due to V/Q mismatch.
   - Compression of venous capacitance vessels causing an initial increase followed by a sustained decrease in preload.
   - Compression of arterial vasculature causing increases in afterload and systemic vascular resistance.
   - Increased secretion of catecholamines and vasopressin.
   - Alterations in regional organ perfusion, with increased cerebral perfusion and decreases in renal, hepatic and splanchnic blood flow.
   - Increased risk of regurgitation and/or aspiration.

2. **Carbon dioxide insufflation**

   This may give rise to these problems.
   - Significant hypercapnia and acidosis from peritoneal absorption and/or suboptimal ventilation.
   - Venous carbon dioxide embolism.
   - Paradoxical arterial embolism in patient with patent foramen ovale.

3. **Extra-peritoneal gas insufflation**

This may be due to misplaced Veress needle or trocar, or through anatomic defects in the diaphragm. This can result in pneumothorax, pneumomediastinum, pneumopericardium and/or subcutaneous emphysema. Clinical signs are variable, and one should maintain a high index of suspicion to facilitate early diagnosis and treatment, which can be life-saving.

Pneumothorax can occur from insufflated CO_2 tracking into the thorax through a tear in the visceral peritoneum, breach of the parietal pleura during dissection around the oesophagus or a congenital defect in the diaphragm. These are clinical manifestations of pneumothorax.

— Increase in peak airway pressure.
— Fall in SpO_2.
— Increase in end-tidal CO_2.
— Cardiac arrhythmias.
— Presence of subcutaneous emphysema.
— Reduced breath sounds on the affected side with tracheal deviation to the contralateral side.
— Severe cardiovascular compromise with hypotension in the presence of a tension pneumothorax.

Management of pneumothorax includes these steps.

— Exclude endobronchial intubation and other causes of unequal breath sounds.
— Inform the surgeon, who should stop the surgery and deflate pneumoperitoneum immediately.
— Turn off nitrous oxide and administer 100% oxygen.
— Assess severity of pneumothorax in terms of haemodynamic stability, oxygenation and ventilation
— Order an immediate CXR on OT table, but do not wait for radiological confirmation in the event of haemodynamic instability or clinical evidence of tension pneumothorax.
— Depending on the size of pneumothorax and cardiorespiratory compromise, the management is either conservative or immediate needle aspiration and chest drain insertion in severe cases.
— Further management depends on haemodynamic status. If the patient remains stable the procedure may be continued and terminated as expeditiously as possible. Conversion to an open procedure may be necessary after stabilization to avoid further problems of laparoscopic surgery.

4. **Trauma to intraabdominal structures**

   Any intraabdominal structure may be traumatized, either through blind insertion of the Veress needle or trauma from surgical instrumentation.
   - The Veress needle may be inserted in the subcutaneous space, vascular space, viscus, omentum, mesentery or retroperitoneum.
   - Surgical instrumentation with major vessel injury may lead to massive haemorrhage, CO_2 embolism and cardiovascular collapse.
   - Concealed bleeding from vascular injury can present postoperatively as a fall in hematocrit values.
   - Undiagnosed intestinal injuries may present later with peritonitis and septicaemia.

   These following measures should be taken to minimize trauma.
   - Gastric decompression with nasogastric tube, particularly for general surgical laparoscopies.
   - Urinary bladder catheterization, or ask the patient to void prior to surgery to avoid bladder injury.
   - Placement of the first trocar through a minilaparotomy incision to avoid complications associated with the Veress needle.

5. **Positioning**

   Trendelenburg and lithotomy positions (for most gynaecological procedures)
   - Reduced functional residual capacity with atelectasis and hypoxaemia.
   - Increased intrathoracic, intraocular and intracranial pressures.
   - Increased risk of regurgitation and/or aspiration.
   - Possible endobronchial migration of the tracheal tube.
   - Nerve injuries due to improper positioning, e.g., brachial plexus injury from overabduction of the arm, common peroneal nerve injury from improper application of stirrups.

   Reverse Trendelenburg position (in some general surgical procedures)
   - Hypotension if the patient is volume-depleted.
   - Possible nerve injuries due to improper positioning.

6. **Miscellaneous problems**

   These include:
   - Long duration of surgery (learning phase for surgeons!).
   - Intense vagal stimulation during manipulation of peritoneal structures may cause bradycardia or even asystole.

— Crowding of OT with instruments and personnel.
— Postoperative problems such as shoulder-tip pain, PONV.

The scope of laparoscopic surgery is expected to expand further with improvements in technology and surgical expertise. This will include more extensive and prolonged procedures performed in a wide range of patients. The complex cardiorespiratory changes during laparoscopic procedures should be well understood by all, and vigilance towards early detection and prompt management of complications would contribute to patient safety. Furthermore, a multi-modal approach to the prevention of common postoperative complaints such as pain and PONV would improve patient satisfaction and allow early recovery.

FURTHER READING

1. Coskun F, Salman MA. Anesthesia for operative endoscopy. Curr Opin Obstet Gynecol 2001;13:371–6.
2. Wedgewood J, Doyle E. Anaesthesia and laparoscopic surgery in children. Paed Anaesth 2001;11:391–9.
3. Leonard IE. Anaesthetic considerations for laparoscopic cholecystectomy. Best Prac Res Clin Anaesth 2002;16:1–20.

Chapter 46

Anaesthesia for Orthopaedic Surgery

INTRODUCTION

Orthopaedic surgery, like other surgical disciplines, has seen much progress and refinement of technique over the decades. New procedures in the form of arthroscopic and minimally invasive techniques are less traumatic and allow faster recovery. Such patients can be discharged on the same day of surgery or on the first postoperative day. While hip and knee arthroplasty continue to be common procedures in an orthopaedic surgical OT list, replacements for shoulder, elbow, wrist and ankle are growing in frequency.

The range of orthopaedic procedures includes:

— Arthroplasty for hip, knee, shoulder.

— Arthroscopic surgery for knee, shoulder.

— Spine surgery for scoliosis correction, discectomy, laminectomy, spinal decompression.

— Orthopaedic oncology: biopsy and excision of tumour, amputation.
— Others: congenital talipes equinovarus (CTEV) correction, Achilles tendon release.

Trauma surgery, with reduction and fixation of fractures and dislocations, is another domain of the orthopaedic surgeon. This should be separate from elective orthopaedic workload so that patients under the elective load are not deprived of operating time in preference for trauma surgery.

Patient age group ranges from the very young to the very old, hence anaesthetic management should include considerations for paediatric as well as geriatric anaesthesia. Some of the young patients may suffer from cerebral palsy or some congenital disorders such as osteogenesis imperfecta. The elderly patients, on the other hand, have a high level of co-morbidity. They may suffer from severe arthritis that limits mobility and masks poor exercise tolerance, posing problems for preoperative evaluation of their cardiorespiratory status.

REGIONAL ANAESTHESIA IN ORTHOPAEDIC SURGERY

Many of the orthopaedic procedures are amenable to regional anaesthesia either as a sole anaesthetic technique with or without sedation, or in combination with general anaesthesia. Central neuraxial blockade has had a longstanding history in providing anaesthesia for lower limb surgery. In the past few decades, numerous peripheral nerve block techniques have become increasingly popular in surgery for various parts of the upper and lower extremities.

Advantages of Regional Anaesthesia

— Studies to compare the effects of regional anaesthesia with those of general anaesthesia in orthopaedic surgery are largely centred on elderly patients undergoing hip arthroplasty.
— Perceived advantages of regional anaesthesia include:
  - Reduction in intraoperative blood loss.
  - Provision of postoperative analgesia.
  - Preservation of mental function in the elderly.
  - Reduced incidence of perioperative respiratory complications.
  - Early mobilization with reduced risks of deep vein thrombosis (DVT) and pulmonary thromboembolism.

— There are, however, no significant differences between the two techniques in terms of total blood loss (intraoperative and postoperative), length of hospital stay and long-term outcome.

Disadvantages of Regional Anaesthesia

— Practical problems of regional anaesthesia include difficulty in positioning old patients or patients in pain, and difficulty in performing the block because of calcified ligaments or spinal deformities.

— Regional anaesthesia is unsuitable for demented or uncooperative patients.

— Central neuraxial blockade is contraindicated in patients on anticoagulant therapy; it should be used with caution in patients on thromboprophylaxis, with adjustments to the timing of insertion and removal of epidural catheter.

— Risks associated with central neural blockade include hypotension, inadvertent intravascular or intrathecal injection, high spinal or total spinal, and failed or inadequate block.

— It is difficult to control the patient's oxygenation and ventilation under regional anaesthesia.

The increasing use of peripheral nerve blocks in preference to central neuraxial blockade means that many of these disadvantages of regional anaesthesia are no longer relevant. Success rate is increased with more experience and greater familiarity with the technique. Specific nerve and plexus location is further enhanced by the use of specially designed insulated, short-bevelled block needles and peripheral nerve stimulator. For example, the quality of analgesia in combined femoral-sciatic nerve block is found to be comparable or even better than central neuraxial blockade, with fewer complications. Improved peripheral nerve block equipment, with finer catheters, has allowed catheter placement into the nerve sheath to provide effective postoperative analgesia.

ANAESTHESIA FOR HIP SURGERY

Operative procedures involving the hip include internal fixation for fractures (hemiarthroplasty, plating) and total hip replacement for the diseased joint, usually secondary to osteoarthritis or rheumatoid arthritis. These are major surgery with the potential for significant blood loss. The patients are usually elderly with concomitant medical problems that should be identified and optimized before surgery.

Regional anaesthesia is desirable in this category of patients for the reasons indicated. Central neuraxial blockade with or without sedation is the preferred anaesthetic technique. If the general anaesthetic technique is employed in a patient with rheumatoid arthritis, one should be aware of potential airway difficulty with atlanto-axial subluxation, temporomandibular joint immobility and cricoarytenoid joint inflammation.

Supplemental oxygen is required as there may be marked hypotension and/or desaturation during impaction and insertion of hip prosthesis with or without bone cement (methylmethacrylate). During the reaming process, the intramedullary pressure is increased and cement, fat or surgical debris may be forced into the systemic circulation and give rise to pulmonary microemboli. The use of methylmethacrylate may result in mast cell degranulation with histamine release, causing peripheral vasodilatation, hypotension, bronchospasm and hypoxaemia. The patient should be closely monitored, and supportive treatment (oxygen, intravenous fluids and vasopressors) administered as indicated. The incident is usually transient and readily corrected with the above measures. If hypotension persists, other causes such as hypovolaemia or perioperative myocardial infarction should be considered. If hypoxaemia persists, significant fat embolism may have occurred.

ANAESTHESIA FOR SCOLIOSIS SURGERY

Scoliosis may be idiopathic or secondary to virtually any neuromuscular disease. If left untreated, the patient may present with severe restrictive lung disease with pulmonary hypertension and respiratory failure. The most common disease associated with secondary scoliosis is Duchenne muscular dystrophy. In addition to neuromuscular problems, these patients present with dysrhythmias, cardiomyopathy, respiratory dysfunction and abnormal response to suxamethonium. Its relationship with malignant hyperthermia is less clear-cut.

Fortunately, most of the patients with idiopathic scoliosis presenting for surgery do not have life-threatening respiratory embarrassment. Many are children or adolescents being treated for cosmetic reasons.

The degree of scoliosis is described in terms of its angle. On the anterior-posterior X-ray film of the spine, lines are drawn from the top of the uppermost affected vertebra and the bottom of the lowermost affected vertebra. The angle made by intersection of the perpendicular lines drawn from the two lines is called the Cobb's angle. The greater the angle, the more severe will be the respiratory and subsequent cardiovascular impairment.

Intensive care and respiratory support will be required for most patients with secondary scoliosis and those presenting late with juvenile idiopathic scoliosis. This is especially so if the baseline ABG is abnormal and lung function test shows a vital capacity of less than 40% of predicted value.

The surgical approach can be either posterior or anterior. The most frequently performed surgery for adolescent idiopathic scoliosis involves posterior spinal fusion with instrumentation and bone grafting. In some cases the surgeon uses the anterior approach via a thoracotomy, which requires intraoperative one-lung ventilation. A combined posterior-anterior approach is occasionally used.

Preoperative Assessment

— Besides routine preoperative evaluation, the cardiovascular, respiratory and musculoskeletal systems should be assessed in detail. Look for clinical features of neuromuscular disease. Inquire about past history of anaesthesia and any family history of anaesthetic morbidity or mortality.

— If the surgeon intends to perform an intraoperative wake-up test to check the spinal cord integrity, this should be explained to the patient during the premedication round. Inform the patient that he/she would be awakened during the surgery to test the movement of his/her legs, and that he/she must follow the instruction given by the anaesthesiologist. Emphasize to the patient that there would be no pain during the test and no recall of the incident postoperatively. Most patients are anxious about waking up in pain in the middle of the surgery and they should be fully reassured. This should again be reinforced in OT before induction of anaesthesia.

— Other than routine preoperative tests, CXR, ABG and lung function test are indicated in patients with restrictive respiratory disease. Blood should be cross-matched ahead of the surgery.

— Postoperative management depends on the respiratory status of the patient as well as the extent and complexity of the procedure. Most patients with minimal or no respiratory impairment and following an uneventful surgery can be managed in the general ward.

— If postoperative ICU or HDU management is planned, this can be explained to the patient during the preoperative visit. Postoperative analgesia, usually by means of intravenous patient-controlled analgesia (PCA) technique, should also be explained to the patient. Oral benzodiazepine is usually prescribed for night sedation and premedication.

Anaesthetic Management

General anaesthesia with endotracheal intubation and IPPV, using intravenous induction agent, neuromuscular blocking drug, volatile anaesthetic and oxygen-nitrous oxide is the usual anaesthetic technique. The anaesthetic agents selected should be short-acting and non-cumulative especially if an intraoperative wake-up test is planned.

The use of total intravenous anaesthesia (TIVA) is gaining popularity because of its titratability and good recovery characteristics. This is achieved by administering a target-controlled infusion (TCI) of propofol together with a non-depolarizing neuromuscular blocking drug, a short-acting opioid such as fentanyl, alfentanil and, more recently, remifentanil infusion 0.05–0.5 μg/kg/min, and ventilating the patient with oxygen-air mixture.

One should pay particular attention to these issues.

— Monitoring and venous access
  - Monitors include ECG, non-invasive BP, pulse oximetry, capnography, invasive haemodynamic monitoring in the form of intraarterial BP and/or CVP, peripheral nerve stimulator, temperature and urine output via an indwelling urinary catheter.
  - There should be at least two large bore intravenous cannulae for rapid transfusion of fluid or blood if necessary.
  - Insertion of additional intravenous cannula, arterial cannulation and central venous cannulation should be performed while the patient is anaesthetized and in the supine position; it is impossible to insert a central venous catheter once the patient is turned to the prone position.

— Patient positioning
  - Enough personnel should be at hand to ensure that the patient is turned "in one piece" to the prone position.
  - Pay special attention to ETT, infusion and monitoring lines, pressure areas, limbs and eyes.
  - Use pillows to support the head, neck, chest and pelvis, while the abdomen should not be compressed in order to allow adequate respiratory excursion. This also prevents engorgement of the epidural veins that may increase intraoperative bleeding.
  - When the patient is in the prone position, re-check to make sure that the ETT has not been misplaced.

— Autologous blood transfusion
  - Intraoperative cell salvage may be utilized to reduce the need for allogeneic blood transfusion. However, the efficiency of the autotransfusion device, used

intraoperatively, may be relatively low in relation to the total extravasation, as the postoperative blood loss can be substantial.
  - The acute normovolaemic haemodilution technique has also been successfully employed in selected patients.
- Maintenance of anaesthesia
  - Maintain adequate oxygenation and normocarbia; prevent vasodilatation caused by hypercarbia.
  - Controlled hypotension is useful in reducing intraoperative blood loss but formal hypotensive anaesthetic techniques are usually not necessary.
- Wake-up test
  - If wake-up test is utilized, the anaesthesiologist should be alerted approximately 20 minutes before the test.
  - At this juncture, administer a bolus dose of fentanyl and withhold infusion or further bolus doses of neuromuscular blocking drug, so that its effect would have worn off by the time the test is performed. Turn off the volatile anaesthetic after 10 minutes and maintain anaesthesia with oxygen-nitrous oxide.
  - During the test, turn off nitrous oxide and administer 100% oxygen.
  - Check that the train of four (TOF) count on the peripheral nerve stimulator has returned to 4. It is not necessary to reverse the neuromuscular blockade.
  - Speak to the patient and get him/her to grip your hand. This is to make sure that the patient is conscious enough to understand and follow your commands. Then ask the patient to move his/her toes.
  - At the end of the wake-up test, administer a dose of neuromuscular blocking drug and a long-acting opioid such as morphine. Maintain anaesthesia with nitrous oxide-oxygen-volatile anaesthetic.
  - If the TIVA technique is used, withhold the propofol infusion and reduce remifentanil infusion to 0.05 μg/kg/min before the test. After the test, re-commence propofol infusion, administer a dose of neuromuscular blocking drug and increase the infusion rate of remifentanil.
  - A dose of IV midazolam may be administered for its amnesic properties.
  - There are many disadvantages and limitations to the wake-up test, such as:
    - It is a "once only" test and cannot detect spinal cord injury as and when it occurs, or ensure that no injury occurs after the test has been performed.
    - It is not applicable to small children, the intellectually impaired or patients who are unwilling or unable to cooperate with the anaesthesiologist.
    - It is stressful to the patient and tends to create preoperative anxiety.

- — It is only practical to test the motor function of the spinal cord while the sensory function is not tested.
- — A positive test is reassuring, but a negative test may or may not be attributable to spinal cord injury.

— Spinal cord monitoring

- Some other means of monitoring the spinal cord function during scoliosis surgery have been used. This includes monitoring of somatosensory evoked potential (SSEP) and motor evoked potential (MEP), which test the sensory and motor pathways of the spinal cord respectively.
- Simultaneous monitoring of both pathways is desirable.

— Postoperative management

- Reversal of neuromuscular blockade and extubation are along the usual guidelines.
- Postoperative ICU management is indicated for patients with respiratory impairment, those undergoing thoracotomy and anterior fusion, and those with complicated intraoperative course associated with massive blood loss and haemodynamic instability.
- Effective postoperative analgesia facilitates early chest physiotherapy and breathing exercises. This is especially important following thoracotomy and anterior spinal instrumentation. Intravenous PCA is the method of analgesia most commonly employed.

FURTHER READING

1. Singelyn FJ, Capdevila X. Regional anaesthesia for orthopaedic surgery. Curr Opin Anaesthesiol 2001;14:733–40.
2. Borgeat A, Ekatodramis G. Orthopaedic surgery in the elderly. Best Prac Res Clin Anaesthesiol 2003;17:235–44.
3. Rodgers A, Walker N, Schug S, et al. Reduction of postoperative mortality and morbidity with epidural or spinal anaesthesia: Results from overview of randomized trials. Br Med J 2000;321:1493–1510.
4. Urwin SC, Parker MJ, Griffiths R. General versus regional anesthesia for hip fracture surgery: A meta-analysis of randomized trials. Br J Anaesth 2000;84:450–5.
5. Parker MJ, Urwin SC, Handoll HH, Griffiths R. General versus spinal/epidural anaesthesia for surgery for hip fractures in adults (Cochrane Review). Cochrane Database Syst Rev 2000;4:CD000521.

6. Nuwer MR. Spinal cord monitoring with somatosensory techniques. J Clin Neurophysiol 1998;15:183–93.
7. McCann ME, Brustowicz RM, Bacsik J, et al. The bispectral index and explicit recall during the intraoperative wake-up test for scoliosis surgery. Anesth Analg 2002;94:1474–8.

Chapter 47

Anaesthesia for Long Surgical Procedures

INTRODUCTION

Advances in surgical techniques and instruments enable more complex and time-consuming surgical procedures to be performed. The parallel advances in anaesthesia in patient monitoring and availability of newer anaesthetic agents mean that patient safety is not compromised even after long hours of surgery and anaesthesia. Examples of such protracted procedures include plastic and reconstructive surgery (re-implantation of limbs or digits, free flaps), ENT surgery (laryngectomy, tracheal resection), radical neck dissection for tumour excision, hepatic surgery and major vascular, cardiothoracic and neurosurgical procedures.

There are a host of problems which are commonly encountered in patients undergoing prolonged surgical procedures. These include:

— Intraoperative hypothermia.
— Haemodynamic instability.
— Problems with fluid and electrolyte balance.
— Massive blood loss with multiple transfusion of blood and/or blood products.
— Cumulative effects of anaesthetic agents.
— Problems associated with positioning of the patient.
— Intraoperative and postoperative analgesia.
— Postoperative management.

Another real problem among the operating team would be staff fatigue, boredom and inattention. This should be addressed and appropriately managed in order to minimize surgical and anaesthetic risks that the patient may be subjected to.

PREOPERATIVE ASSESSMENT

— Carry out routine assessment with particular attention to cardiovascular, respiratory, metabolic and airway problems.
— Ensure that patient's medical condition is optimized before surgery. This is obviously not possible in emergency procedures such as re-implantation of severed limb or digits.
— Explain to the patient the anaesthetic plan and postoperative management, such as ICU admission, methods of pain relief, presence of intravenous cannulae, drains or indwelling urinary catheter.
— Prescribe appropriate premedication for the case. Include night sedation if indicated.
— GXM blood and/or blood products according to nature of the surgery and the amount of anticipated blood loss.
— Thromboprophylaxis is indicated for all patients. The specific method of thromboprophylaxis depends on the patient factors and nature of surgery. Options include SC standard heparin or low molecular weight heparin (LMWH), graduated compression stockings and intermittent calf compression during the surgical procedure (see Chapter 24).

ANAESTHETIC MANAGEMENT

These are pertinent aspects of management.

— **Monitoring**
- Standard monitoring of ECG, non-invasive BP, pulse oximetry and capnography.
- Invasive haemodynamic monitoring of intraarterial BP and CVP for major surgery with significant blood loss or fluid shifts.
- Urine output measurement via indwelling urinary catheter.
- Core temperature monitoring.
- Peripheral nerve stimulator to monitor degree of neuromuscular blockade.
- Others: oxygen analyzer, anaesthetic agent concentration monitor, airway pressure, ventilator disconnect alarm.

The maxim that "*the best monitor is a vigilant anaesthesiologist*" is even more apt in this scenario.

— **Temperature control**
- Take active measures to prevent intraoperative hypothermia (see Chapter 6) but avoid overheating the patient.
- Patients who develop hypothermia despite all measures are likely to experience delayed recovery from anaesthesia, and postoperative management may need to be tailored accordingly.

— **Positioning**
- Avoid nerve traction or compression due to improper positioning, e.g., lower brachial plexus injury due to overabduction of shoulder, compression of the common peroneal nerve and stretching of the sciatic nerve in lithotomy position.
- Bony prominences and pressure areas should be well-padded with cotton wool or towels.
- Make sure that structures such as the head and neck, the hips are supported to avoid ligamentous injury or muscle strain.
- Avoid venous congestion at the surgical site to reduce intraoperative blood loss, e.g., 15–20° reverse Trendelenburg position for head and neck surgery, avoid abdominal compression in spine surgery.

— **Anaesthetic techniques**
- Choice of anaesthetic technique for induction depends on the patient's preoperative status and in particular the state of the airway.
  - Prepare for difficult intubation if the patient has intraoral or laryngeal tumour: consider options of awake fibreoptic intubation or tracheostomy under local anaesthesia.

— Preoxygenation followed by rapid sequence induction and intubation with cricoid pressure is required for the patient with "full stomach" presenting for emergency re-implantation surgery.

- A balanced anaesthetic technique with opioid, volatile anaesthetic, neuromuscular blocking drug, oxygen and/or nitrous oxide is usually employed.
- Low-flow anaesthesia using circle system with carbon dioxide absorbent is preferred.
- Use a combined regional and general anaesthesia technique in suitable patients, e.g., general anaesthesia combined with epidural or plexus blocks for the upper or lower limb. By means of the catheter technique, satisfactory analgesia can be extended far into the postoperative period.
- Neuromuscular blockade may be maintained by intermittent bolus doses or continuous infusion (e.g., atracurium 0.3–0.5 mg/kg/hr or vecuronium 0.05–0.1 mg/kg/hr). The degree of neuromuscular blockade should be monitored especially in elderly patients or those with significant hepatic or renal disease.
- Controlled hypotension may be required to reduce blood loss especially during the initial period of dissection for tumour surgery.
- Maintain adequate oxygenation, normocarbia and stable haemodynamic parameters. This is particularly important for free flap and re-implantation surgery to ensure graft viability.
- Check ABG, blood glucose, serum electrolytes, haematocrit 4-hourly or more often if indicated. Correct any metabolic derangement detected.

— **Fluid management and blood transfusion**

- Ensure adequate vascular access with at least 2 large-bore intravenous cannulae for fluid replacement and/or transfusion of blood and blood products. Set up rapid infusion device if massive blood loss or fluid shifts are likely.
- Fluid management is guided by the patient's haemodynamic status (CVP in particular), estimated fluid and blood loss, urine output and intraoperative measurements of ABG, haematocrit, glucose and electrolyte concentrations.
- Maintain urine output > 0.5 ml/kg/hr. Refer to Chapter 73 for management of oliguria.
- Avoid undertransfusion which compromises the patient's cardiovascular status, or overtransfusion which results in fluid overload and tissue oedema.
- Consider autologous blood transfusion by means of acute normovolaemic haemodilution or intraoperative cell salvage in suitable patients.
- Replace blood according to the magnitude and speed of blood loss, clinical manifestations and haemodynamic parameters.

- Consider blood component therapy in massive blood transfusion associated with signs of coagulopathy.

— **Miscellaneous issues**
- Ensure that the eyes are closed and covered with eye-pads to avoid exposure keratitis.
- Securely fasten the ETT and its connections to prevent accidental extubation or disconnection, particularly important in head and neck surgery or in positions other than supine.
- Nitrous oxide diffuses into the ETT cuff and increases the cuff pressure. This should be regularly checked and adjusted accordingly so that the cuff does not exert excessive pressure on the tracheal mucosa.
- Note the tourniquet time if a limb tourniquet is used. Remind the surgeon if this exceeds the recommended time (1–1.5 hours for upper limb, 2 hours for lower limb). Most pneumatic tourniquet sets have timers with alarms incorporated, which can be activated at preset intervals.
- It is important to have proper documentation on the anaesthesia record. This is especially so if the patient's intraoperative course has been stormy and problematic.
- If possible, have regular breaks by getting a relief anaesthesiologist to take over temporary management of the patient from time to time. All necessary information should be passed over systematically to your colleague, and you should be readily contactable if needed.

SPECIAL CONSIDERATIONS

Free Flap Surgery

— In free flap surgery, tissue from the donor site is transferred and attached to a distant recipient site by means of microvacular anastomosis. In contrast, a pedicle or rotational flap is one which is raised and rotated to fill a neighbouring defect while the arteriovenous connections remain intact.

— The free flap is usually used to provide tissue cover following trauma or after resection of malignancy. Similar considerations apply for re-implantation for severed limbs or digits since the re-implanted parts are in essence "free flaps".

— The ultimate result of graft survival depends not only on surgical expertise but also on the state of the microcirculation in the graft. Anaesthetic management should strive towards ensuring graft survival by optimizing oxygen flux and tissue perfusion. This can be provided by:

- Smooth induction with attenuation of sympathetic responses to intubation, avoiding hypertension and tachycardia.
- Stable haemodynamic parameters, with good cardiac output, adequate vasodilation, wide pulse pressure.
- Adequate oxygenation and normocarbia.
- Optimal haematocrit levels at 30–35%: avoid extremes of haemoconcentration with increased blood viscosity, or haemodilution with inadequate oxygen-carrying capacity.
- Sympathetic blockade by means of regional anaesthetic technique, e.g., epidural anaesthesia, brachial plexus blocks.
- Prevention of hypothermia which causes peripheral vasoconstriction and postoperative shivering.
- Use of dextran solution which reduces platelet adhesiveness and improves microcirculation. Usual regime for adult patient consists of 500 ml, commenced intraoperatively and infused over 6 hours, followed by 500 ml over 12 hours for 1 day.
- Smooth emergence and adequate analgesia in the immediate postoperative period.

— Postoperative management includes oxygen supplementation, analgesia, haemodynamic monitoring and hourly observation of the flap to monitor the temperature, colour and arterial pulses.

Laryngectomy with Radical Neck Dissection and Flap Reconstruction

— This illustrates a long surgical procedure in a patient who is likely to be elderly, with concomitant medical conditions and some degree of upper airway obstruction.

— There are three parts to this procedure.

- In laryngectomy, the larynx is resected and a permanent tracheostomy is fashioned. Partial laryngectomy with laryngeal reconstruction and temporary tracheostomy may be performed for early laryngeal tumours as an alternative to radiotherapy.
- Radical neck dissection involves excision of the sternomastoid muscle, the jugular veins and associated lymph nodes.
- Flap reconstruction is required if the defect in radical neck dissection is large; usually a rotational flap is harvested from the pectoralis major muscle. Simple closure and split skin graft are other alternatives for closing the defect.

— Airway management options depend on the degree of airway obstruction, the potential airway difficulty anticipated, the indirect laryngoscopy findings regarding the site and size of laryngeal tumour. Options include direct laryngoscopy and endotracheal intubation, an awake fibreoptic laryngoscopy or tracheostomy under local anaesthesia. Endotracheal intubation is preferred because the presence of a tracheostomy tube often hinders surgical dissection.

— Central venous cannulation is usually performed at the antecubital fossa since the jugular route is not possible and the subclavian route is too near to the surgical field.

— Blood loss may be substantial during tumour resection and radical neck dissection, especially if the patient has received radiotherapy prior to surgery. The blood may seep under the drapes, accumulate at the back of the neck and become apparent only after removal of the drapes at the end of the surgery.

— Some degree of controlled hypotension may be useful to reduce intraoperative blood loss. This should be carried out with caution if the patient has significant cardiopulmonary disease or hypertension (see Chapter 51).

— Beware of venous air embolism during neck dissection, manifested by sudden decrease in end-tidal CO_2; and be prepared for prompt management of this complication (see Chapter 77). Other important structures at the neck may also be damaged, such as the vagus, hypoglossal, phrenic and branches of the facial nerve leading to cranial nerve palsies and respiratory embarrassment. Bradycardia may result from manipulation of the carotid body during neck dissection.

— The ETT cuff is deflated and the ETT partially withdrawn to the upper trachea when the surgeon is creating the tracheostomy. When the surgeon has fashioned the tracheostomy stoma, a long J-shaped flexometallic tube (e.g., Laryngoflex®) is inserted into the stoma. Disconnect the breathing system from the ETT and reconnect at the flexometallic tube via a sterile catheter mount. Manually ventilate to ensure that chest expansion and breath sounds are equal bilaterally. Pass a suction catheter down the tube to remove blood and secretions that may have tracked down into the trachea.

— Take precautions to ensure optimal conditions for flap survival, as highlighted on pages 627–628.

— Depending on the patient's co-morbid conditions and intraoperative events, the patient may be managed in the ICU, HDU or general ward.

— Head and neck oedema usually occur postoperatively because venous drainage from the head and neck is markedly impaired following neck dissection.

POSTOPERATIVE MANAGEMENT

— Postoperative ICU management is indicated in patients with significant concomitant cardiovascular, respiratory or airway problems, unstable haemodynamic status or hypothermia, or if the surgical procedure has been long and complicated.

— If the patient is to be managed in HDU or general ward, ensure that he/she is awake, comfortable, relatively pain-free, haemodynamically stable and breathing well before being discharged from PACU. The patient may need to be observed for a longer period in PACU. An elective tracheostomy may be a safer option for patients with head and neck surgery, particularly those involving the oral cavity and the airway.

— Continue oxygen therapy for 24 hours postoperatively for patients with significant risk factors for hypoxia, namely poor general health status (ASA III or above), obesity, advanced age, severe cardiac or respiratory disease and major thoracic or upper abdominal surgery. Monitor oxygen saturation by means of pulse oximetry.

— Closely monitor the haemodynamic and fluid status. Send blood samples for biochemical and haematological tests. Correct electrolyte abnormalities and consider blood transfusion if haematocrit < 30%.

— Options for postoperative analgesia include:
  - Regional analgesia: epidural or brachial plexus block.
  - Intravenous patient-controlled analgesia.
  - Intravenous infusion of morphine for ICU patient.
  - SC or IM morphine.

  Supplement with oral or rectal non-steroidal antiinflammatory drug (NSAID) if its use is not contraindicated.

— Effective postoperative analgesia facilitates early and effective chest physiotherapy and breathing. Continue thromboprophylaxis and encourage early ambulation to prevent DVT.

— Resume oral or enteral feeding as soon as the patient's condition permits. Consider early total parenteral nutrition (TPN) for patients who are likely to have delayed resumption of enteral feeding.

— Prophylactic antibiotic treatment, usually started in the OT after induction of anaesthesia, should be continued postoperatively in view of long hours of exposure and tissue trauma which is often extensive. Watch for signs of sepsis, send relevant samples for culture and sensitivity testing and adjust antibiotic regimen if necessary.

FURTHER READING

1. MacDonald DJF. Anaesthesia for microvascular surgery: A physiological approach. Br J Anaesth 1985;57:904–12.
2. Waters JH, Miller LR, Clack S, Kim JV. Cause of metabolic acidosis in prolonged surgery. Crit Care Med 1999;27:2142–6.

Chapter 48

Anaesthesia for Plastic and Reconstructive Surgery

INTRODUCTION

Plastic and reconstructive surgery has made great advances in surgical technique as well as perioperative care and rehabilitation of patients. As a result, more complex surgical procedures are being performed on patients who may have been previously thought to be too difficult. More patients at the extremes of age group are also accepted for surgery. There are also many types of aesthetic surgery performed solely for cosmetic purposes, such as liposuction, abdominoplasty, breast augmentation or reduction.

Types of procedures performed under plastic and reconstructive surgery include these.

- Cleft lip and cleft palate surgery.
- Craniofacial surgery.
- Tumour resection and reconstructive surgery, including free flap or rotational flap.
- Microvascular surgery, including re-implantation of severed limbs or digits (see Chapter 47).
- Surgical management of burns: debridement, escharotomy, skin grafting, release of burns contracture (see Chapter 27).
- Aesthetic surgery.

CLEFT LIP AND CLEFT PALATE SURGERY

Cleft lip and cleft palate may co-exist or exist separately; they may be unilateral or bilateral, complete or incomplete. Surgical correction for cleft lip is usually performed at 3–6 months of age while cleft palate repair is usually delayed until the child is at least 9 months old but preferably before speech development. This is one of the commonest procedures in plastic surgery but is certainly not something to be taken lightly. The anaesthesiologist should be conversant with airway management as well as paediatric anaesthesia in order to provide optimal anaesthetic management for these patients.

The anaesthetic concerns include:

- Management of paediatric anaesthesia and its associated problems.
- Possibility of difficult intubation which exists not only in patients with dysmorphic features but in those with large defects as well.
- Presence of associated congenital anomalies, more so in patients with cleft palates, such as:
  - Pierre-Robin syndrome: micrognathia, macroglossia, congenital heart disease.
  - Treacher-Collins syndrome: mandibulofacial dysostosis characterized by deafness, hypoplasia of facial bones, auricular abnormalities, cardiovascular malformations.
  - Goldenhar syndrome: oculo-auriculo-vertebral dysplasia characterized by eye and ear abnormalities, micrognathia, maxillary hypoplasia, cleft or high-arched palate, cervical synostosis, congenital heart disease.

  Those pertaining to the airway and cardiovascular system are of concern to the anaesthesiologist.
- Requirement for the patient to be awake, quiet, relatively pain-free and with adequate airway protection at the end of surgery.

Anaesthetic Management

Premedication

- The patient is assessed and any anaesthetic problems identified prior to surgery. A thorough airway assessment should be made to rule out possible airway problems.
- A runny nose is fairly common and should not contraindicate surgery unless it is accompanied by purulent secretion, recent respiratory tract infection or fever and other systemic manifestations.
- Premedication is omitted in small children and those with potential airway problems; older children may be given oral premedication.
- Antisialogogue in the form of atropine or glycopyrrolate is not routinely given as premedication. It is administered intravenously at induction of anaesthesia and only if indicated.

Induction of anaesthesia

- The commonest method of induction is inhalational anaesthesia with nitrous oxide, oxygen and sevoflurane.
- If there is potential airway difficulty, the patient is gently ventilated to assess whether mask ventilation is possible. It may be difficult to obtain an adequate seal with the face mask particularly in the patient with micrognathia or prominent premaxilla.
- Ventilation is assisted until the patient is adequately anaesthetized. If no intubation problem is anticipated, a dose of non-depolarizing neuromuscular blocking drug is administered after venous access is established. If the ability for intubation is in doubt, a gentle laryngoscopy is performed to attempt to visualize the vocal cords and glottis.
- In a patient with cleft lip, intubation may be aided by inserting a roll of gauze into the cleft so that the laryngoscope blade would not be lodged there, making it difficult to manoeuvre the endotracheal tube to the correct place.
- An oral RAE tube of appropriate size is used. The ETT is securely anchored in the midline so that it would be situated in the groove of the mouth-gag used by the surgeon.
- A moist pharyngeal pack is inserted to absorb blood that trickles into the pharynx. This may be inserted either by the anaesthesiologist or the surgeon. Remember to remove the pharyngeal pack at the end of the operation.

— The patient is positioned supine with the neck hyperextended by putting a "sand-bag" or rolled towel under the shoulders. The head end of the operating table is tilted upwards slightly to reduce venous congestion and hence blood loss. Re-auscultate the chest after positioning to make sure that the endotracheal tube is still in place.

— Intra- and postoperative analgesia is provided using a multi-modal analgesic regimen of intravenous short-acting opioid (e.g., fentanyl), rectal paracetamol or diclofenac and infiltration of local anaesthetic at the surgical site.

Maintenance of anaesthesia

— Take over ventilation manually when the surgeon inserts the mouth-gag to make sure that the ETT is not obstructed or accidentally dislodged.

— Closely monitor the patient's clinical signs and amount of blood loss especially in cleft palate repair. Blood loss during cleft palate repair may be large enough to warrant blood transfusion.

Emergence from anaesthesia

— A tongue stitch may be required to pull the tongue forward to prevent or relieve airway obstruction in the postoperative period.

— At the end of the surgery, remove the pharyngeal pack, suction any residual blood in the pharynx under direct vision and look for the return of airway reflexes. Reverse the neuromuscular blockade, position the child on his/her side and remove the ETT in this position.

— Ensure that postoperative analgesia is adequate so that the patient will not be struggling and crying in pain while awake. This also helps to prevent postoperative bleeding.

CRANIOFACIAL SURGERY

This form of surgery aims to correct the complex deformities of the cranium, orbit and face. The abnormalities necessitating craniofacial surgery may be congenital or acquired, the latter often secondary to trauma or following extensive surgery for removal of tumours.

Congenital anomalies predominate in craniofacial procedures in the younger age group. These include craniosynostosis, in which one or more of the skull sutures become prematurely fused; and craniofacial synostosis, in which there is premature suture ossification associated with abnormalities of the skull base and upper face. Examples are facial clefts involving the orbit, midline fronto- or nasoencephalocele, craniostenosis, Crouzon's syndrome, Pfeiffer's syndrome, Apert's syndrome and Treacher-Collins syndrome.

These clinical features may be present.

— Central nervous system: intracranial hypertension, visual failure, squints, cranial nerve palsies, mental deterioration, general hypotonia, obstructive sleep apnoea.
— Face: maxillary hypoplasia, malocclusion, airway abnormality, upper airway obstruction (some severe enough to require tracheostomy).
— Eyes: hypertelorism (increased distance between orbits), shallow orbits, exorbitism, corneal ulceration, keratitis.

Surgery is performed in these patients to prevent or reduce intracranial hypertension. Fronto-orbital advancement is carried out as soon as possible to increase the intracranial volume, thus allowing brain growth and halting mental retardation. The surgical procedure is usually long and complex as it involves total reconstruction of the mid-face, orbits and cranium.

Optimal management of these patients demands a multi-disciplinary approach involving the plastic surgeon, neurosurgeon, ophthalmologist, oral surgeon, paediatrician as well as the anaesthesiologist. The anaesthesiologist should be experienced in paediatric anaesthesia, neuroanaesthesia and airway management.

These are the anaesthetic concerns.

— Paediatric anaesthesia and its problems.
— Presence of intracranial hypertension and the need to prevent further increases in ICP.
— Associated congenital anomalies particularly in the cardiovascular system.
— Potential airway problems, in terms of intubation difficulty at induction, maintenance of airway patency and integrity during surgery and possibility of postoperative airway obstruction secondary to bleeding, oedema or secretions.
— Blood loss is usually massive and difficult to quantify.
— Problems associated with long surgical procedures (see Chapter 47).

Anaesthetic Management

— The child is assessed and potential problems identified prior to surgery. Arrangement is made for postoperative management in ICU. Blood and plasma are reserved for the procedure.

— Anaesthesia is induced with nitrous oxide, oxygen and sevoflurane. The approach to airway management is the same as for cleft lip/cleft palate surgery outlined earlier. Endotracheal tube should be securely anchored or stitched in position.

— Venous access is extremely important in anticipation of massive blood loss and transfusion requirements. There should be at least 2 free-running peripheral lines: one for infusion of intravenous fluids, the other for transfusion of blood and blood products.

— Monitors include these.
  - ECG, non-invasive BP, pulse oximetry, capnography, temperature, urine output via an indwelling urinary catheter.
  - Invasive haemodynamic monitors of intraarterial BP and CVP (central venous catheterization is usually via the femoral vein).

— Take measures to conserve heat and prevent hypothermia in the child (see Chapter 6).

— Maintain anaesthesia and muscle relaxation. Adjust ventilation to produce $PaCO_2$ 30–35 mmHg. Ensure adequate oxygenation. Send blood samples for baseline ABG, serum electrolyte concentration and haematocrit.

— To minimize brain retraction and postoperative cerebral oedema, brain bulk is reduced by moderate hyperventilation and intraoperative frusemide or mannitol.

— Fluid therapy is guided by clinical signs of colour, pulse rate, blood pressure, CVP, urine output and haematocrit measurement. Be prepared for early blood transfusion.

— Postoperative ICU management is essential and the patient is electively ventilated until clinical condition is stabilized and effects of prolonged anaesthesia are dissipated.

TUMOUR RESECTION AND RECONSTRUCTION

The patient is likely to be elderly with associated medical conditions which should be assessed and optimized. The actual site of the tumour, the extent of tumour involvement, the nature of the surgical procedure and the plans for postoperative management are important considerations in the anaesthetic management.

These are the anaesthetic concerns.

— The patient is often elderly with multiple co-morbidities.

— Potential airway problems exist as a result of limitations in mouth opening or head and neck mobility, distorted airway anatomy by tumour, oedema, previous surgery or radiotherapy, or fixation of tissues by tumour, surgical scars or radiation fibrosis.

— As a result of tumour infiltration and inability to eat, the patient is usually cachexic and malnourished. He/she may be anaemic, dehydrated and may have electrolyte imbalance.
— The surgical procedure is lengthy with major blood loss and haemodynamic changes.
— There is risk of venous air embolism during neck dissection.
— Graft viability in microvascular surgery is subject to various factors, some of which can be modified by anaesthesia.

Anaesthetic Management

— Careful preoperative assessment and optimization of the medical conditions is essential. The patient may be put on partial or total parenteral nutrition to improve the nutritional status. Anaemia, electrolyte imbalance and dehydration should be corrected before the patient is scheduled for surgery.
— There is a delicate balance between taking time to optimize the patient's conditions and the problem of undue delay that allows further spread of the tumour. Urgent surgical intervention is clearly indicated if the tumour encroaches on the airway and produces respiratory difficulty.
— Airway management is a major component of the anaesthetic plan. The options are:
  - Intravenous induction and suxamethonium if no difficulty is anticipated.
  - Examination of the airway under sedation and topical anaesthesia before anaesthetic induction if airway is doubtful.
  - Awake fibreoptic intubation under topical anaesthesia and/or sedation.
  - Tracheostomy under local anaesthesia.
— The reader is referred to Chapter 47 for details on intraoperative and postoperative management.
— Postoperative ICU or HDU management is usually indicated. Decision whether to ventilate the patient depends on the general status of the patient, intraoperative haemodynamic stability, site, extent and duration of surgery, and presence of airway oedema with risk of airway obstruction if the patient is extubated. This problem is obviated if an elective tracheostomy is performed during the surgery.

AESTHETIC SURGERY

Aesthetic surgery is a rapidly expanding specialty both in terms of the number of patients seeking treatment and the techniques and approaches available. Patients who request for such surgery are usually normal individuals but with a heightened consciousness about their looks, who view aesthetic surgery as a means to enhance their self-esteem and reduce self-consciousness.

Aesthetic surgery usually falls under three categories:

- Correction of abnormal feature (e.g., prominent ears, large nose, breasts which are too big or too small).
- Reversal of signs of ageing (e.g., facial wrinkles, thinning hair, drooping breasts or buttocks).
- Treatment of health-related problems (e.g., obesity, cellulite, chronic skin problems).

As the realms of aesthetic surgery are subjective, it is not uncommon to find a proportion of the patients seeking treatment to correct a seemingly unsatisfactory appearance; or a far-from-obese individual insisting on liposuction (suction lipoplasty) or abdominoplasty to get rid of excess fat tissue in the body. Doctors differ in their attitude to surgery for purely cosmetic reasons – some feel it is justified given the patient's psychological make-up, others feel it puts a strain on the existing health resources and deprive other more "deserving" patients of valuable surgical time. Whatever the doctor's personal attitude may be, anaesthetic management for such patients should be approached in the same professional and empathic manner as patients with clinical disorders.

Anaesthetic management of such patients is usually straightforward, with attention to intra- and postoperative pain relief being the main concern. A combination of general anaesthesia with locoregional block is the usual anaesthetic technique.

Many procedures are performed under local anaesthesia administered by the surgeons themselves – the use of large volumes of dilute local anaesthetic for liposuction being a prime example. This has resulted in reports of morbidity and even mortality when practitioners who are not specifically trained in anaesthesiology and resuscitation are confronted with systemic toxicity caused by local anaesthetic overdose. Guidelines for sedation and analgesia by non-anaesthesiologists have been drawn up by various professional organizations in the USA, UK and Australia. These should be complied with in order to safeguard the well-being of patients seeking aesthetic surgery.

FURTHER READING

1. Sculerati N, et al. Airway management in children with major craniofacial anomalies. Laryngoscope 1998;108:1806–12.
2. Mason RA, Fielder CP. The obstructed airway in head and neck surgery. Anaesthesia 1999;54:625–8.
3. Dougherty TB, Nguyen T. Anesthetic management of the patient scheduled for head and neck cancer surgery. J Clin Anesth 1994;6:74–82.
4. Practice Guidelines for sedation and analgesia by non-anesthesiologists. A report by the American Society of Anesthesiologists Task Force on Sedation and Analgesia by Non-anesthesiologists. Anesthesiology 1996;84:459–71.

Anaesthesia for Day-Care Surgery

INTRODUCTION

Day-care surgery, also known as day-case, ambulatory or outpatient surgery, has become an integral part of the services provided by the anaesthetic and surgical units. After a day-care procedure, the patient is expected to be discharged from the hospital later on the same day itself. Advances in anaesthetic and surgical techniques, along with escalating healthcare costs, have resulted in an ever-increasing number of surgical procedures being performed on a day-care basis. This is expected to increase even further as outcome data confirming the safety of day-care surgery become widely accepted.

The numerous advantages of day-care surgery have been emphasized time and again. These include cost-effectiveness, reduced inpatient workload and increased hospital efficiency, patient convenience and psychological benefits with reduced socio-psychological stresses, reduced incidence of hospital-acquired infection and early mobilization. These advantages have been replicated in many studies and practical experiences worldwide.

Appropriate selection of both patients and procedures is the key to safe and effective day-care surgery. Optimal anaesthetic management also plays an important role in providing rapid and smooth postoperative recovery. The various aspects of day-care anaesthesia, namely patient selection criteria, anaesthetic drugs and techniques, postanaesthesia management, discharge criteria and postdischarge instructions are highlighted here.

GUIDELINES FOR DAY-CARE SURGERY

Specific guidelines for patient inclusion criteria, types of surgical procedures and recommended anaesthetic techniques may vary from hospital to hospital. Here are some general guidelines to be considered.

— **Screening**
- There should be a sequential pathway with clear-cut guidelines to follow in order to select the patients suitable for day-care surgery. These guidelines should be widely available to surgeons and anaesthesiologists, and should be reviewed from time to time in case any modification in selection criteria is necessary.
- The surgeon usually screens patients during clinic visits. The screening process can be made easier by getting the patients to fill out health/anaesthesia questionnaires and delegating the task of preliminary assessment to specially trained nurses at the clinics.
- The surgeon may refer the patient to the anaesthesiologist if doubt arises as to the patient's suitability for day-care surgery.

— **Information**
- The patient should receive verbal and written information in simple understandable format with these details.
  - — General information about day-care surgery.
  - — Fasting instructions on solid food, clear fluids and breast milk for young children.
  - — Specific instructions about medications which should be continued or omitted on the day of surgery.

  - Postdischarge instructions.
- The patient should also be informed about the date and time of the scheduled surgery, and the time of expected arrival to the Day-Care Unit on the day of surgery.

— **Patient selection**
- These patients are acceptable for day-care surgery.
  - Physical status ASA I and II (some centres accept medically stable ASA III or IV patients but only after consultation with the anaesthesiologist).
  - Body mass index < 35.
  - Willingness to have the procedure performed as day-care and ability to follow discharge instructions.
  - Small children aged ≥ 6 months, post-conceptual age ≥ 60 weeks with no previous history of ventilation or apnoea. Younger children may be accepted after prior consultation with the anaesthesiologist; arrangements should be made for longer postoperative observation.
- Note that most centres do not impose an upper age limit. Patients should be selected according to their physical fitness rather than the chronological age *per se*.
- In all cases, the ultimate decision on the suitability of a patient for day-care surgery is made by the anaesthesiologist.

— **Social considerations**
- The patient or parents should understand the postanaesthetic care instructions and comply with them particularly with regard to public safety.
- A responsible adult should be available to take the patient home in a suitable vehicle, either a car or a taxi (bus or train is not suitable).
- There should be a responsible adult to care for the patient at home for at least overnight. The person should be physically and mentally capable of making decisions for the patient's welfare where appropriate.
- The distance from the house to the hospital should not be more than 20 km or within an hour's travelling time.
- Access to a telephone should be readily available at all times.

— **Types of surgery**
- These surgical criteria should be fulfilled.
  - Short, simple procedure which is not expected to last more than 1½ hours.
  - Minimal risk of postoperative complications such as haemorrhage or airway compromise.

— Minimal postoperative pain which is controllable by simple analgesics.
— No special postoperative nursing requirements.
— No period of prolonged immobility after the procedure.
— A rapid return to normal fluid and food intake.

- Examples of surgical procedures suitable for day-care
  a) In children
     — Herniotomy, circumcision, hydrocele excision, cystoscopy.
     — Myringotomy with grommet insertion.
  b) In adults
     — Dilatation and curettage, hysteroscopy, gynaecological laparoscopic procedure: diagnostic laparoscopy, laparoscopic sterilization.
     — Excision of breast lumps, lipoma, herniorrhaphy, haemorroidectomy.
     — Simple orthopaedic procedures: closed manipulation and reduction (CMR) of fractures/dislocations, carpal tunnel release, excision of ganglions, knee arthroscopy.

— There should, ideally, be dedicated day-care surgery lists. If the OT list is shared between inpatients and outpatients, priority on OT list sequence should be given to day-care surgery patients. The last case should be completed by 2 pm.

— Postoperative pain can be controlled with oral analgesics or rectal suppositories. No intravenous opioid is used unless the pain is not controllable with oral or rectal medication, in which case a short-acting opioid analgesic such as fentanyl is often used.

— After being observed for 4 hours postoperatively in the Day-Care Unit, the patient is to be reviewed by the anaesthesiologist and surgeon before discharge.

— The patient should be sent home in a private vehicle or taxi. If the patient is a child being transported in a private vehicle, one other responsible person besides the driver should be present to look after the child during transport.

PREOPERATIVE PREPARATION

— The patient reports to the Day-Care Unit on the morning of surgery. Initial assessment is done by the nurses before the patient is seen by the anaesthesiologist.

— Assessment should include:
- Features of respiratory tract infection or fever.
- Time of last meal.

  - Presence of responsible person to accompany the patient postoperatively.
  - Means of transport home.
  - Patient's weight, height, vital signs, relevant findings on physical examination.
- If the patient is a child, eutectic mixture of local anaesthetic (EMLA) cream is applied to the dorsum of the hand in preparation for venepuncture.
- No premedication is necessary unless the patient is extremely anxious, in which case oral midazolam may be prescribed. Small doses of anxiolytics or short-acting opioids are not expected to prolong recovery time.

ANAESTHETIC MANAGEMENT

- Top priorities for successful day-care surgery are the four As: alertness, ambulation, analgesia and alimentation. The anaesthetic technique should enable the patient to achieve the above in the shortest possible time during the postoperative period. Desirable features in anaesthetic agents include rapid onset and offset, excellent analgesia and amnesia, provision of good surgical conditions and early recovery.
- The use of general anaesthesia with spontaneous ventilation supplemented with individual nerve blocks or wound infiltration is encouraged. Short-acting anaesthetic drugs used for induction and maintenance of general anaesthesia include propofol, remifentanil, alfentanil or fentanyl, sevoflurane or desflurane. The recovery characteristics of propofol – rapid and clear-headed emergence, lack of residual psychomotor effects, antiemesis – are well suited to the requirements of day care anaesthesia.
- The total intravenous anaesthesia (TIVA) technique is advocated by some anaesthesiologists, in which inhalational anaesthetic agents are omitted and oxygen-enriched air is administered instead. The technique utilizes propofol infusion (either manually adjusted or target-controlled) and an opioid, either remifentanil infusion or bolus doses of alfentanil or fentanyl. The use of neuromuscular blockade is dictated by surgical requirements.
- There is no contraindication to endotracheal intubation. However, extra care should be taken to be gentle during airway manipulation in order to minimize trauma and postoperative sore throat. Cases which do not need muscle relaxation or airway protection are best done under spontaneous ventilation via face mask or laryngeal mask airway. The use of LMA ProSeal™ is also suitable for day-care procedures especially if intermittent positive pressure ventilation is indicated.

— If neuromuscular blockade is necessary, suitable neuromuscular blocking drugs include mivacurium and atracurium. Mivacurium is a short-acting non-depolarizing neuromuscular blocking drug that is metabolized by plasma cholinesterase. Other than the short duration of action, its advantage in the day-care setting lies in the fact that it is unnecessary to antagonize its effects with neostigmine. Suxamethonium is best avoided because postoperative myalgia is common and this may delay the resumption of normal activity.

— The patient should be well hydrated in order to reduce the problems of post-operative nausea and vomiting (PONV). Provide antiemetic prophylaxis in high-risk patients undergoing procedures associated with high incidence of PONV. (see Chapter 61).

— Adjuncts for postoperative pain relief:
  - Rectal paracetamol 20 mg/kg per dose, or diclofenac 1 mg/kg per dose for children.
  - Non-steroidal antiinflammatory drug (NSAID) such as ketorolac in adults in the absence of contraindications.
  - Cyclooxygenase-2 (COX-2) inhibitors such as parecoxib, etoricoxib.

  These reduce opioid requirement and hence the problem of opioid-induced PONV.

Regional Anaesthesia in Day-Care Surgery

— The use of regional anaesthesia in day-care surgery is controversial. The advantages gained by avoiding GA and reducing incidence of PONV are counter-balanced by the longer time required for RA to wear off, and the risk of sending the patient home with the surgical site still partially anaesthetized. Special instructions must be given to the patient before discharge to avoid inadvertent damage to the anaesthetized part of the body.

— Spinal anaesthesia, if desired, should be performed early on the list to maximize time for recovery. Incidence of post-spinal headache is reduced by using fine pencil-point spinal needles (e.g., 25–27G Whitacre™ needle). The use of 5% lignocaine, a short-acting local anaesthetic, has been set back by reports of transient neurologic syndrome (TNS) associated with its use. Use of a lower concentration of lignocaine, 2% instead of 5%, has been advocated; the suggested dose being 40–70 mg (2–3.5 ml of 2% lignocaine) for most cases. An alternative is the use of 0.25% rather than 0.5% bupivacaine, which gives a similar onset time but shorter duration of block. The anaesthesiologist should ensure that the patient has made full recovery of motor power and proprioception before discharge to allow safe ambulation. The patient should also be able to pass urine before discharge.

— Epidural anaesthesia is not suitable because of a longer time needed to perform the block, slower onset, and the advantage of provision for extending the block is irrelevant in the setting of day-care surgery. It is also not advisable to use epidural or intrathecal opioids for day cases.
— Caudal anaesthesia is especially suitable for children presenting for bilateral inguinal hernia repair, since ilioinguinal nerve blocks for both sides may render the dose of local anaesthetic excessive. This provides excellent postoperative analgesia but may be associated with delayed voiding of urine.
— Brachial plexus block via the axillary and infraclavicular approaches are more suitable for day-care surgery compared to other approaches because of their relative lack of complications, such as intravascular or intrathecal injection and pneumothorax associated with the interscalene approach and supraclavicular approach respectively. These blocks are technically simple to perform and provide prolonged postoperative analgesia, but precautions should be taken about care of the partially anaesthetized limb. An arm sling should be provided for the patient before discharge.
— Lower extremity blocks such as femoral and sciatic blocks are less useful compared to brachial plexus blocks because mobilization is difficult following these blocks.
— Field blocks in the form of ilioinguinal block and penile block are often used for hernia repair and circumcision respectively in the paediatric patient. These offer good intra- and postoperative analgesia so that the child is comfortable during emergence from general anaesthesia and during the early postoperative period.

RECOVERY

— The patient is observed in the PACU with heart rate, BP and pulse oximetry monitoring until fully conscious. Requirements for the facilities and staffing of PACU are fully applicable to day-care units. The patient is discharged from the OT by the anaesthesiologist according to the Post-Anaesthetic Recovery Score (PARS) chart. This is the same procedure as for inpatients.
— Postoperative pain relief is usually adequate with a multi-modal analgesic therapy consisting of intravenous opioid, local anaesthetic nerve block or wound infiltration, and NSAID or COX-2 inhibitor. If more analgesia is required it should be treated early with intravenous bolus doses of fentanyl 25–50 μg. Simple oral analgesics may be of help later when the patient resumes oral intake.

— The patient is transferred to the Day-Care Unit for the second stage of recovery. This area should be adequately supervised by nursing staff and should have ready access to resuscitation equipment, oxygen and suction. The area should also be provided with comfortable reclining chairs for patients, who must not leave this area unaccompanied. Various criteria should be fulfilled before the patient is deemed to have regained street fitness for discharge. The patient should be reviewed by both the anaesthesiologist and the surgeon prior to discharge.

— If there is an anaesthetic or surgical problem postoperatively, the anaesthesiologist or surgeon should be notified immediately. The patient may have to be admitted for further management or observation. Causes for unscheduled postoperative admission include:

- Slow recovery from anaesthesia.
- Unstable haemodynamic status.
- Uncontrolled pain or PONV.
- Surgical problems: unexpectedly extensive surgery, bleeding from surgical site, need for repeat surgery.
- Inadequate social circumstances not previously known.

CRITERIA FOR DISCHARGE

— The patient should be awake, alert and oriented to person, place and time.

— The patient is not in any respiratory difficulty.

— Vital signs are within the normal range, and stable for at least an hour.

— The patient is able to move within the limits imposed by age and the procedure.

— Ability to dress and walk should be equivalent to preoperative standards.

— The patient should be comfortable and relatively pain-free.

— The patient is not vomiting or dehydrated and is able to take and retain a small amount of clear fluid.

— There should be minimal bleeding or drainage from the operation site.

— The ability to void, previously considered a strict discharge criterion, is no longer considered to be compulsory before discharge. The patient or guardian should, however, be instructed to contact the hospital if he/she remains unable to void for more than 12 hours. Patients at significant risk of urinary retention (central neural blockade, pelvic and other surgery) must have voided before discharge.

POSTDISCHARGE INSTRUCTIONS

— Written and verbal instructions for all relevant aspects of postanaesthetic and surgical care must be given to the patient and the accompanying adult. Include relevant phone numbers for emergency medical care.

— The patient must be accompanied by a responsible person during the trip home as well as within the house for at least the first night after discharge.

— Suitable analgesics should be provided for at least the first day after discharge. Advice on any other regular medication is also necessary.

— Due to the residual effects of the anaesthetic, these activities are strictly prohibited within the 24-hour postoperative period.
  - Consuming alcohol.
  - Operating machinery.
  - Driving a vehicle.
  - Making important decisions.

— The patient should be followed up the next day with a telephone enquiry.

FURTHER READING

1. Troy AM, Cunningham AJ. Ambulatory surgery: An overview. Curr Opin Anaesthesiol 2002;15:647–57.
2. Rawal N. Analgesia for day-case surgery. Br J Anaesth 2001;87:73–87.
3. Ghatge S, Lee J, Smith I. Sevoflurane: An ideal agent for adult day-case anesthesia? Acta Anaesthesiol Scand 2003;47:917–31.
4. Liu SS. Optimizing spinal anesthesia for ambulatory surgery. Reg Anaesth 1997;22:500–10.

Chapter 50

Anaesthesia for Oral and Maxillofacial Surgery

INTRODUCTION

Oral and maxillofacial (OMF) surgery encompasses a wide range of procedures, from simple dental extractions to complex reconstructive craniofacial procedures that involve multi-disciplinary approach and require skilled anaesthetic management.

As in upper airway surgical procedures in ENT surgery, airway considerations are paramount in OMF surgery. The patient may have preexisting anatomical abnormalities that complicate airway management, airway patency may be compromised intraoperatively or the surgical procedure itself (e.g., intraoral maxillary–mandibular fixation) may pose problems in the postoperative period.

Surgical procedures in OMF surgery include:

- Surgical extractions of impacted teeth.
- Orthognathic surgery: maxillary or mandibular osteotomy, craniofacial surgery.
- Surgery for maxillofacial trauma: reduction of fractures in maxilla, mandible or the zygomatic complex.
- Drainage procedures for odontogenic infections: dental abscess, Ludwig's angina.
- Resection of maxillofacial tumours and reconstructive surgery.

GENERAL CONSIDERATIONS

- Patients undergoing OMF surgery belong to a wide range of age groups, e.g., children or the mentally subnormal who require general anaesthesia because they cannot cooperate with dental procedures under local anaesthesia, children or young adults for orthognathic surgery and elderly patients with maxillofacial tumours for resection.
- A thorough preoperative airway assessment should be performed to identify patients with potential airway management difficulties. Patients with maxillofacial trauma, tumours and infection are likely to be problematic, and careful planning of airway management options is required.
- In the absence of airway problems, general anaesthesia is induced using an opioid and an intravenous induction agent. Endotracheal intubation is facilitated by use of a non-depolarizing neuromuscular blocking drug, and anaesthesia is maintained with volatile anaesthetic, opioid, nitrous oxide and oxygen in a balanced anaesthetic technique.
- Depending on the nature and severity of airway problems, other airway management options include inhalational induction, blind nasal intubation, awake fibreoptic intubation and surgical airway by means of tracheostomy or cricothyrotomy.
- Nasotracheal intubation is frequently used in OMF surgery. For unilateral intraoral procedures, an oral ETT secured on the opposite side of the mouth may be acceptable. If any doubt exists it is best to discuss the options with the surgeon.
- For nasotracheal intubation, the patency of the nostril should be checked beforehand. A nasal vasoconstrictor (e.g., phenylephrine) may be used in an attempt to reduce nasal trauma during intubation. A preformed nasal ETT, e.g., nasal RAE of size 6.0 to 7.5 is often used, with 6.0 for adult female and 7.0 or 7.5 for adult

male. The ETT should be placed in warm water before use to soften the material and lubricated with lignocaine gel or KY Jelly prior to insertion.

— After intubation, the ETT and its connector to the breathing system should be securely fastened to avoid accidental extubation or disconnection, as the anaesthesiologist's access to the airway is severely restricted during surgery.
— A moist pharyngeal pack is inserted to prevent blood and debris from contaminating the airway, and removed at the end of the surgery. If possible, it is advisable to perform a direct laryngoscopy prior to reversal of neuromuscular blockade to confirm removal of the pharyngeal pack and absence of active bleeding at the surgical site.
— Proper eye care is important to avoid corneal abrasions or exposure keratitis. The eyes should be closed and protected with eyepads, and care should be taken not to allow iodine-based prepping solutions to come in contact with the eyes.
— A dose of IV dexamethasone should be administered at induction to reduce postoperative oedema, particularly of the airway and surrounding soft tissue.
— Most OMF surgical procedures are short or medium-length procedures. Orthognathic surgery and tumour resection tend to be long and complicated. Aspects of anaesthetic management for long surgical procedures are discussed in Chapter 47.

MAXILLOFACIAL TRAUMA

— Maxillofacial trauma can result from a blunt injury (e.g., motor vehicle accident, sports injuries, fights or thermal injury) or a penetrating injury (e.g., knife or gunshot wounds).
— Management of maxillofacial trauma includes the ABCs of resuscitation, which may include immediate endotracheal intubation if the airway or breathing is compromised. It is advisable to intervene early in the case of severe facial trauma, before swelling and obstruction develop to make endotracheal intubation a difficult if not impossible proposition. Airway management can be extremely challenging because of soft tissue oedema, active bleeding, presence of foreign bodies or regurgitation of gastric contents. Associated injuries, head, cervical spine and chest injuries in particular, may impact airway management options; these should be sought and actively excluded.
— In the acute situation, airway management options include:

- Endotracheal intubation by direct laryngoscopy.
- Use of supraglottic airway adjuncts, e.g., LMA, oesophageal-tracheal Combitube (ETC).
- Cricothyrotomy with transtracheal jet ventilation.
- Tracheostomy under local anaesthesia.

Note that fibreoptic intubation may not be feasible in the presence of blood and secretions. Insertion of LMA or ETC is often performed by paramedics in the pre-hospital setting. This can be life-saving in the face of difficult or failed intubation.

— Midface fractures are often classified under LeFort.
  - LeFort I: horizontal fracture which separates maxillary alveolus from midface.
  - LeFort II: a pyramidal fracture around the nose which separates maxilla from zygoma.
  - LeFort III: complete dislocation of facial from cranial skeleton which runs parallel to skull base.

— It has been the traditional teaching that nasotracheal intubation is contraindicated in LeFort III fractures or when there is evidence of basal skull fractures with CSF rhinorrhoea, due to the risks of possible disruption of the cribriform plate, cranial intubation or meningitis. However, several reports have described the successful placement of a nasotracheal tube over a fibreoptic bronchoscope without cranial intubation or other complications.

— The precise nature of maxillofacial injury should be noted and understood. Clinical examination may be limited by trismus and soft tissue swelling; exact diagnosis often depends on radiographic findings.

— Trismus or soft tissue swelling may limit the mouth opening. This can usually be overcome when the patient is under anaesthesia. However, mechanical restriction of temporomandibular joint (TMJ) movement may be caused by a zygomatic arch fracture impacting on coronoid process of the mandible. It is important for the anaesthesiologist to rule out the mechanical causes because these will be unresolved even under anaesthesia. Tracheostomy under local anaesthesia would then be the safest option to secure the airway.

— An isolated mandibular fracture usually poses no problem for intubation but the anaesthesiologist should be aware of the possibility of avulsion and aspiration of loose teeth during airway manipulation. Bimandibular fractures with postero-inferior displacement of the flail segment may lead to acute airway obstruction and require airway intervention. Under anaesthesia, the anterior jaw movement is increased and intubation is usually straightforward.

— Emergency surgery for maxillofacial trauma may be indicated for immediate control of haemorrhage or exploration and repair of trauma from a penetrating injury. Most other surgery can be delayed for 5–7 days to allow facial swelling to subside. This obviates the risks of the full stomach, allows time for management of other associated injuries and optimization of associated medical conditions.
— Endotracheal intubation is indicated for emergency surgery in view of aspiration risks and the need for reliable means of airway control. Use of airway adjuncts in the form of laryngeal mask airway has been described for less urgent surgery involving the zygomatic complex because the aspiration risks are reduced and the surgical approach is often extra-oral (usually via a temporal approach).
— Intra-oral maxillary–mandibular fixation and occlusion of the teeth may be required to facilitate the alignment and internal fixation of fracture fragments. Extubation should only be done when the patient is fully awake and demonstrating adequate breathing efforts. Wire-cutters should be available by the patient's bedside in case acute airway intervention and re-intubation becomes a necessity.

ORTHOGNATHIC SURGERY

— This involves correction of musculoskeletal, dento-osseous, soft tissue deformities of the jaws and surrounding structures. Surgery is complex and often involves maxillary and/or mandibular osteotomy to realign the facial skeleton. These are major surgical procedures and may involve the plastic surgeon, ENT surgeon, neurosurgeon and ophthalmologist.
— The patients are usually adolescents and young adults who present for surgery with the aim to improve facial aesthetics. Other than cosmesis, some surgery may be indicated to correct malocclusion, reduce pain related to TMJ movement, correct respiratory dysfunction due to obstructive sleep apnoea and improve speech patterns. Patients presenting for craniofacial surgery are often children with congenital syndromes such as Crouzon, Pfeiffer or Apert. These are discussed in Chapter 48.
— The surgery is often long and blood loss may be substantial. Aspects of management for long surgical procedures (Chapter 47), thromboprophylaxis (Chapter 24), maintenance of normothermia (Chapter 6) and blood conservation strategies to reduce the use of allogeneic transfusion (Chapter 5) are pertinent here.

— Postoperative management in ICU is often necessary in view of the prolonged and extensive nature of surgery. The degree of oedema in the face and airway structures is likely to be substantial, so overnight sedation and mechanical ventilation are often indicated.

ODONTOGENIC INFECTIONS

— Infections in the oral and maxillofacial region range from an infected tooth with dental abscess to extensive soft tissue involvement of the head and neck with significant airway compromise. Example of the latter is Ludwig's angina, an infection involving the sublingual, submandibular and submental spaces bilaterally that often arises from poor dentition or unclean dental procedures. The most feared complication of Ludwig's angina is airway obstruction leading to hypoxaemia and death. Patients at greatest risk of sudden airway obstruction are those presenting with oedema and elevation of the floor of the mouth, swelling and limited mobility of the tongue, oedema and deviation of the uvula, excessive salivation, trismus and neck pain with limited mobility. The patient may also present with intracranial extension, mediastinitis and overwhelming sepsis.

— Surgery may be indicated for incision and drainage of the infected area under appropriate antibiotic cover. Given the significant anaesthetic risks involved, it is best that the procedure be done under local anaesthesia or nerve blocks. However, general anaesthesia is often required because local anaesthesia is often inadequate in the presence of infected tissue. The anaesthesiologist may also be consulted for emergency airway management in a patient presenting with acute airway obstruction.

— The patient often feels more comfortable remaining in the upright position. He/she should be allowed to do so during transport and induction of anaesthesia, as airway obstruction is likely to occur in the supine position.

— Options of airway management include:
- Inhalational induction followed by gentle laryngoscopy and intubation.
- Awake fibreoptic intubation.
- Elective tracheostomy in severe cases.

— The surgeon should be scrubbed and ready at the time of intubation in case a surgical airway is urgently needed.

— The possibility of rupturing the abscess and aspirating the infected material into distal airways should be borne in mind. Blind intubation techniques are not advisable, and any airway manipulation should be done gently and cautiously to avoid trauma and bleeding to the swollen and friable airway structures. A suction device with rigid Yaunkeur suction catheters should be ready in case the abscess ruptures.

POSTOPERATIVE MANAGEMENT

— Most OMF procedures have uneventful intra- and postoperative courses and do not pose problems for postoperative management.

— Postoperative pain following dental procedures is usually mild to moderate. The use of nerve blocks or local infiltration is useful to reduce postoperative analgesic requirements. Major surgery with extensive dissection may require intravenous patient-controlled analgesia for postoperative analgesia.

— Postoperative airway management can sometimes be just as challenging as during induction of anaesthesia. The decision whether to leave the ETT *in situ* depends on many factors, namely preoperative airway compromise, length and complexity of the surgical procedure, anticipated airway changes following surgery (including the use of intermaxillary fixation). Other factors such as haemodynamic stability, level of consciousness, co-morbid conditions and return of airway reflexes are important considerations as well.

— If doubt exists regarding the ability to maintain airway patency or adequate ventilation, it would be prudent to leave the ETT *in situ* until the clinical condition improves. In certain cases it may be advisable to perform an elective tracheostomy.

— A trial of extubation can be carried out with the aid of an airway exchange catheter, which allows insufflation of oxygen and subsequent re-intubation should the need arises. The patient is observed at PACU for signs of airway obstruction, respiratory distress or desaturation. The catheter is removed after 30–60 minutes if the patient's condition is satisfactory.

— The patient should be monitored for evidence of bleeding in the immediate postoperative period. Bleeding may present as slow ooze leading to formation of a haematoma, which may cause airway obstruction and necessitates urgent airway intervention.

FURTHER READING

1. Krohner RG. Anesthetic considerations and techniques for oral and maxillofacial surgery. Int Anesthesiol Clin 2003;41:67–89.
2. Mayhew JF. Airway management for oral and maxillofacial surgery. Int Anesthesiol Clin 2003;41:57–65.
3. Goodisson DW, Shaw GM, Snape L. Intracranial intubation in patients with maxillofacial injuries associated with base of skull fractures. J Trauma 2001;50:363–6.
4. Neff SPW, Merry AF, Anderson B. Airway management in Ludwig's angina. Anaesth Intens Care 1999;27:659–61.
5. Marple BF. Ludwig's angina: A review of current airway management. Arch Otolaryngol Head Neck Surg 1999;125:596–600.

D

Issues in Anaesthesia

Chapter 51

Controlled Hypotensive Anaesthesia

INTRODUCTION

Controlled hypotension, also referred to as deliberate or induced hypotension, has been variously defined as a reduction of systolic blood pressure to 80–90 mmHg, a reduction of mean arterial pressure (MAP) to 50–65 mmHg or a 30% reduction of baseline MAP.

Controlled hypotensive anaesthesia is an anaesthetic technique employed as part of the blood conservation strategies to limit intraoperative blood loss, and in so doing, reduce the need for transfusion of allogeneic blood. This reduction in blood usage is especially relevant for specific groups: patients with rare blood groups or antibodies for whom it is difficult to obtain compatible blood and Jehovah's Witnesses who do not accept any transfusion of blood or its derivatives.

In addition, controlled hypotension may be utilized for the benefit of the surgeon. Visualization of the surgical field is improved as a result of decreased intraoperative bleeding. This gives rise to better operating conditions and facilitates surgery, particularly procedures done under the operating microscope. This technique has been employed in major plastic, head and neck, ENT, vascular, orthopaedic and microsurgical procedures.

PROBLEMS OF CONTROLLED HYPOTENSIVE ANAESTHESIA

Controlled hypotensive anaesthesia is not without risks, and questions remain regarding its safety, the duration and extent ("how low can you go?") of hypotension. Controversies continue to exist regarding indications and degree of "safe" and allowable hypotension.

These are the problems of controlled hypotensive anaesthesia.

- Adequacy of regional perfusion, especially to vital organs such as the brain, heart and kidneys, may be compromised in susceptible individuals or if the degree of hypotension is excessive.
- Rebound hypertension may occur after effects of the hypotensive agents have worn off.
- Postanaesthetic recovery may be prolonged if adjuncts such as opioids and volatile anaesthetic agents have been extensively used during the procedure.
- The risk of intraoperative awareness under general anaesthesia may be increased if high FiO_2 has been used during controlled hypotensive anaesthesia without ensuring that an adequate depth of anaesthesia has been maintained.

CONTRAINDICATIONS

This anaesthetic technique is not advisable in these patient categories and clinical situations.

- Patients in extremes of age group – the very young and the very old – because of limited physiological reserves to compensate for decreased organ perfusion during hypotension, even though no specific age-related limits have been established as absolute contraindications.
- Pregnant patients, as hypotension may compromise the uteroplacental circulation and hence the fetal well-being.
- Patients with significant cardiovascular disease such as coronary artery disease and uncontrolled hypertension, as hypotension may compromise myocardial perfusion even further.

- — Patients with significant cerebrovascular disease where maintenance of adequate cerebral perfusion is a concern.
- — Patients with autonomic neuropathy, e.g., diabetic patients, where hypotension is poorly compensated and may worsen silent myocardial ischaemia.
- — Patients with significant pulmonary disease and compromised respiratory function, because of the risk of hypoxaemia associated with increased dead space ventilation, V/Q mismatch and intrapulmonary shunting caused by some hypotensive agents.
- — Patients with significant hepatic and renal disease, because the preexisting disease condition may be worsened by a further reduction in organ blood flow.
- — Clinically unstable patients, physical status ASA III and above.
- — Patients with hypovolaemia due to whatever cause, severe anaemia or sickle cell disease.

ANAESTHETIC MANAGEMENT

Smooth conduct of anaesthesia is just as important as the use of specific agents to achieve hypotension. The choice of anaesthetic technique may also play a role. The use of central neuraxial blockade reduces sympathetic outflow, blunts surgical stress response and provides surgical anaesthesia, even though the degree of hypotension may be difficult to control.

These aspects of anaesthetic management for controlled hypotensive anaesthesia should be noted.

- — Preoperative considerations
  - This includes adequate premedication to prevent tachycardia and hypertension prior to induction of anaesthesia.
  - Option for regional anaesthesia in suitable cases.
  - Consider pretreatment with α_2-agonists (e.g., clonidine, dexmedetomidine) for their sedative, anxiolytic and haemodynamic stabilizing properties.
  - Pretreatment with angiotensin-converting enzyme (ACE) inhibitors (e.g., captopril, elanapril) has also been advocated by some anaesthesiologists. These drugs attenuate the reflex sympathetic response seen with direct-acting vasodilators and limit their dose requirements.
- — Intraoperative monitoring
  - ECG: lead II and CM_5 for detection of myocardial ischaemia.
  - Intraarterial BP monitoring if profound hypotension is required.

- CVP monitoring if large blood losses are anticipated.
- Pulse oximetry and capnography.
- Urine output, peripheral nerve stimulator and temperature monitoring for long cases.
- Bispectral index (BIS) as a guide to monitoring depth of anaesthesia.

— Smooth induction and intubation
- Allow adequate time for neuromuscular blocking drug to act before attempting intubation; monitor the degree of neuromuscular blockade using peripheral nerve stimulator.
- Obtund sympathetic reflexes associated with airway manipulation using IV lignocaine or esmolol.
- Avoid coughing and bucking on endotracheal tube.

— Proper positioning
- For head and neck surgery, place the patient in reverse Trendelenburg position with a 15–20° tilt; avoid kinking of the neck veins, which results in venous congestion.
- For lumbar spine surgery, ensure that the chest and pelvis are supported while the abdomen is not compressed, because abdominal compression results in epidural venous congestion and increases intraoperative blood loss.

— Adequate ventilation and depth of anaesthesia
- Ensure adequate oxygenation and normocarbia, as hypercarbia causes vasodilatation and increases operative blood loss while hypocarbia causes vasoconstriction that may compromise regional blood flow.
- Maintain adequate depth anaesthesia with volatile anaesthetic agents (isoflurane, sevoflurane) and opioids (fentanyl, morphine). In contrast with halothane, the newer volatile anaesthetics decrease mean arterial pressure predominantly through decreased peripheral resistance, with cardiac output being well maintained over the normal anaesthetic maintenance range.

— Use of hypotensive agents
- Commonly used hypotensive agents include β-adrenergic blockers (labetalol, esmolol) and vasodilators (nitroglycerin, sodium nitroprusside, hydralazine). Calcium channel blockers such as diltiazem and nicardipine have also been used. Other drugs include adenosine, trimetaphan and diazoxide. Some of the hypotensive agents are listed in Table 51–1.
- A combination of labetalol or esmolol and sodium nitroprusside is often used. Heart rate changes are attenuated since reflex tachycardia associated with

Table 51–1. Hypotensive agents used in controlled hypotensive anaesthesia

Drug	Mechanism of Action	Advantages	Disadvantages
β-blockers (esmolol, labetalol)	β-adrenergic blockade; negative inotropy and chronotropy	▪ Rapid onset and offset (esmolol) ▪ Decrease myocardial O_2 consumption	▪ Decrease cardiac output ▪ Heart block ▪ Bronchospasm
Sodium nitroprusside (SNP)	Direct vasodilator (resistance vessels); nitric oxide production	▪ Rapid onset and offset ▪ Easily titratable	▪ Cyanide toxicity ▪ Increase ICP ▪ Increase intrapulmonary shunt ▪ Reflex tachycardia ▪ Rebound hypertension ▪ Risk of coronary steal
Nitroglycerin (GTN)	Direct vasodilator (capacitance vessels); nitric oxide production	▪ Rapid onset and offset ▪ Easily titratable ▪ No coronary steal, useful in myocardial ischaemia	▪ Less efficacious compared with SNP ▪ Increase ICP ▪ Increase intrapulmonary shunt ▪ Methaemoglobinaemia
Calcium channel blockers (nicardipine)	Decreased transmembrane calcium movement; vasodilatation	▪ Rapid onset ▪ Increase cardiac output	▪ Prolonged duration of action ▪ Increase ICP ▪ Increase intrapulmonary shunt

Table 51–1. *(continued)*

Drug	Mechanism of Action	Advantages	Disadvantages
Adenosine	Vasodilatation; negative chronotropy	▪ Rapid onset and offset ▪ No reflex tachycardia ▪ Increase coronary flow ▪ No tachyphylaxis	▪ Limited efficacy when used alone ▪ Decrease cardiac output ▪ Heart block ▪ Bronchospasm ▪ Detrimental effects on renal blood flow
Hydralazine	Vasodilatation		▪ Delayed onset ▪ Low efficacy ▪ Reflex tachycardia

sodium nitroprusside is counterbalanced by the bradycardic effect of β-blockers. In this manner smaller doses of both drugs are employed to achieve the same pharmacological effect compared to single agent therapy. Risks of their side-effects are correspondingly reduced. For example, the duration and magnitude of postoperative rebound hypertension associated with sodium nitroprusside is often reduced by concomitant use of β-blockers.
- For healthy, normotensive individuals, MAP may be maintained at 50–65 mmHg. In hypertensive patients, MAP should be maintained at a higher value as the lower limit of autoregulation is shifted upwards. As a rule of thumb, a safe target to follow is a 30% reduction of baseline MAP.

— Other measures
- Increase FiO_2 to 0.5 to prevent hypoxaemia as a result of increased dead space and V/Q mismatching secondary to hypotension. Many of the direct-acting vasodilators and calcium channel blockers cause increased intrapulmonary shunting by interfering with hypoxic pulmonary vasoconstriction. Clinical consequences are minimal in patients with normal respiratory function but may be significant in patients with preexisting pulmonary disease.
- Increase concentration of volatile anaesthetic or administer a dose of opioid to maintain depth of anaesthesia. Bispectral index is a useful monitor for depth of anaesthesia even though it is not totally foolproof against occurrence of awareness under anaesthesia.
- Check ABG to monitor oxygenation and acid-base status. Monitor lactate concentration especially when sodium nitroprusside is used.
- Monitor for signs of myocardial ischaemia. Abandon the hypotensive anaesthesia technique if myocardial ischaemia is detected.

At the end of the hypotensive anaesthesia technique, discontinue the hypotensive agents and allow BP to return to normal. The patient's haemodynamic status should be closely monitored at the PACU. Patients may exhibit persistent hypotension or rebound hypertension. Both should be treated accordingly.

APPENDIX

SODIUM NITROPRUSSIDE

1. **Dose and administration**

   — Dilute 50 mg in 500 ml of dextrose 5% and protect the solution from light.

— Administer the drug as intravenous infusion via syringe pump, with starting dose 0.5–1.5 μg/kg/min, average dose 3 μg/kg/min.
— Do not exceed 3 mg/kg. Consider alternative or additional drugs to reduce total dose.

2. **Signs of cyanide toxicity**
   — Tachyphylaxis: increased infusion requirements over time.
   — Increased mixed venous oxygen tension.
   — Central nervous system dysfunction: change in mental status, headache, seizures, coma (not detected in anaesthetized, paralyzed patients!).
   — Cardiovascular instability: cardiac arrhythmias, ST segment changes on ECG.
   — Increasing metabolic acidosis: increasing base deficit, plasma lactate concentration > 10 mmol/L.

3. **Treatment of suspected cyanide toxicity**
   — Withhold SNP infusion and administer 100% oxygen (despite normal O_2 saturation).
   — Administer amyl nitrite inhalations for 15–30 seconds each minute until 3% sodium nitrite can be prepared for intravenous administration. This should be given slowly at a dose of 5 mg/kg.
   — Administer IV sodium thiosulphate 150–200 μg/kg over 15 minutes.
   — Commence or continue mechanical ventilation.
   — Correct metabolic acidosis with sodium bicarbonate.
   — Consider infusion of hydroxocobalamin (vitamin B_{12a}) at 25 mg/hr.

FURTHER READING

1. Testa LD, Tobias JD. Pharmacologic drugs for controlled hypotension. J Clinical Anesth 1995;7:326–37.
2. Tobias JD. Controlled hypotension in children: A critical review of available agents. Paediatric Drugs 2002;4:439–53.
3. Hack H, Mitchell V. Hypotensive anaesthesia. Br J Hosp Med 1996;55:482–5.

Chapter 52

Monitored Anaesthesia Care

GENERAL CONSIDERATIONS

Monitored anaesthesia care refers to continued observation of the patient during diagnostic or therapeutic procedure by a healthcare provider. The responsibility of the healthcare provider is specific – that of monitoring the patient's level of sedation, vital signs and respiratory effort by clinical means and aided by monitoring devices. This practice aims to improve patient care and safety during minor procedures under local anaesthesia and/or sedation.

Examples of procedures best done under monitored anaesthesia care include:

— Endoscopic procedures such as gastro-duodenoscopy, colonoscopy, sigmoidoscopy.

— Minor surgical procedures performed under local anaesthesia.

— Painful diagnostic or treatment procedures such bone marrow aspiration, trephine biopsy, change of burns dressing.
— Special situations such as intravascular administration of X-ray contrast medium in a patient considered to be susceptible to anaphylaxis.

The term *conscious sedation* is often mentioned in the context of monitored anaesthesia care. This refers to a minimally depressed level of consciousness that retains the patient's ability to maintain an unobstructed airway continuously and independently. The patient is able to respond appropriately to physical stimulation and verbal commands.

Although anaesthesiologists, by virtue of their training and experience, are best qualified to provide sedation services, their availability remains somewhat limited by primary commitments to the OT, ICU or pain service. As such, it is common practice that surgeons and physicians themselves provide sedation during many of these procedures without the assistance of the anaesthesiologist. To ensure safe conduct of sedation, guidelines for sedation by non-anaesthesiologists have been drawn up by various professional organizations in the USA, UK and Australia.

The National Confidential Enquiry into Patient Outcome and Death (NCEPOD) is a form of mortality audit carried out in the United Kingdom. The 2004 NCEPOD report "Scoping Our Practice" focused on inpatient deaths occurring within 30 days of interventional gastrointestinal endoscopy. These are some of the findings on sedation and monitoring.

— In 14% of mortality cases the sedation was thought to be inappropriate and mainly due to excessive dosages.
— Combined intravenous sedation and topical oropharyngeal local anaesthesia might have contributed to aspiration pneumonia in some patients.
— Monitoring was deficient in 23% of mortality cases.

Here are some of the recommendations proposed by the NCEPOD Committee.

— Pulse oximetry should be used in all patients.
— Supplemental oxygen should be given to all patients undergoing therapeutic endoscopy.
— There should always be a person with defined responsibility for patient observation and record keeping.
— After a therapeutic endoscopy all patients should be nursed in an area with equipment and staff similar to that recommended for a recovery facility.

— Clear protocols for the administration of sedation should be available and implemented.

The guidelines provided in this chapter are meant for the anaesthesiologists since certain drugs described here may cause respiratory depression or excessive sedation. These drugs should only be administered by trained personnel who are skilled in resuscitation and airway maintenance. Drugs for sedation, anaesthesia and resuscitation should also be prepared. The availability of equipment for monitoring, anaesthesia and resuscitation should be checked prior to commencement of monitored anaesthesia care.

DRUGS USED FOR PROCEDURES

Local anaesthetic drugs that are frequently used include lignocaine 1% or 2% with or without adrenaline, bupivacaine 0.5% and ropivacaine 0.75%. Prilocaine 0.5% or lignocaine 0.5% can be used for intravenous regional anaesthesia or Bier's block. The local anaesthetic drug may be the sole anaesthetic during the procedure, or administered together with some form of intravenous sedation. Recommendations for maximum dosage should be followed in order to avoid local anaesthetic toxicity and its systemic manifestations. If large volumes of local anaesthetics are required for the nerve block or local infiltration, these should be administered in dilute solutions so that the maximum dose is not exceeded.

The nature and amount of sedative drugs administered depend on the nature of the procedure as well as the general condition of the patient. These must be individualized and the doses titrated to the response of the patient. Some procedures are more stimulating, evoke more pain and discomfort than others, while pain threshold and anxiety levels differ from one patient to another. Combinations of benzodiazepine (e.g., midazolam, diazepam) and opioid (e.g., pethidine, fentanyl, nalbuphine) are frequently used. Drugs with shorter duration of action (e.g., alfentanil, remifentanil) have also been used.

In paediatric patients, drugs such as chloral hydrate, paraldehyde and syrup preparations of diazepam or trimeprazine have been used to provide sedation. However, the dose requirements and onset of action of these drugs are often unpredictable and unreliable.

Low-dose ketamine (0.5–1 mg/kg), by virtue of its potent analgesic effect, is useful for patients undergoing painful treatment procedures (e.g., change of burns dressing). However, ketamine should not be used by non-anaesthesiologists or in areas where equipment for resuscitation and airway management is not readily available.

Intravenous propofol is fast gaining popularity in providing sedation during monitored anaesthesia care. As propofol itself does not possess analgesic properties, analgesia is provided by means of local anaesthetic infiltration of the surgical wound or small doses of opioid analgesic. The initial propofol bolus dose of 0.5 mg/kg is much lower than doses used to induce general anaesthesia. The patient is then given intermittent bolus doses of 10 mg per dose as and when necessary. Alternatively, propofol can be administered in the form of continuous infusion at a rate of 4 mg/kg/hr. More sophisticated methods of drug administration include patient-controlled sedation (PCS) which is similar to patient-controlled analgesia (PCA), variable-rate infusion and target-controlled infusion (TCI). In the latter technique, the target plasma concentration is usually maintained within 0.5–1.5 μg/ml, titrating to response. Again this is a much lower dose compared to doses used during total intravenous anaesthesia (TIVA).

Together with propofol infusion in its various forms, remifentanil may also be administered at a rate of 0.01–0.05 μg/kg/min, titrating to response. Its extremely short half-life is ideal for providing analgesia and sedation in this context, as prolonged analgesic effect is neither necessary nor desired.

MONITORED ANAESTHESIA CARE: RECOMMENDATIONS

Even though some procedures are done within the OT complex, many others are done elsewhere in the hospital, for example the endoscopy clinic or treatment room in general wards. The problems faced by the anaesthesiologist are similar to those encountered while anaesthetizing patients in the Radiology Department and the psychiatric ward.

— All patients due to receive sedation should be fasted according to general anaesthesia guidelines, as loss of protective airway reflexes following excessive sedation may occur.

— Preprocedure assessment should be just as thorough as for any patient coming for anaesthesia. Co-existing medical problems and potential anaesthetic problems should be identified. Care should be taken while providing sedation for the elderly or medically compromised patients. Patients with obstructive sleep apnoea may develop airway obstruction while supine and under sedation.

- Facilities, equipment and anaesthetic assistance should be adequate. This should include patient monitors, resuscitation drugs and equipment, facilities to administer general anaesthesia if necessary, and facilities to observe the patient in a designated recovery area after the procedure.
- Minimum monitors include continuous ECG, non-invasive BP and pulse oximetry. These should be available for all patients.
- The patient's level of sedation should be assessed from time to time. Maintain verbal communication with the patient to detect signs of oversedation. An example of sedation scores used is the Observer's Assessment of Alertness/ Sedation Scale (see Appendix). The composite sedation score should be maintained at 3 or 4.
- Venous access should be established in the patient before the start of the procedure. The intravenous cannula can be flushed with heparinized saline and stoppered. Infusion of intravenous fluid is not necessary unless clinically indicated.
- All patients should receive oxygen by clear mask or nasal prongs. It has been demonstrated that significant desaturation often occurs in patients undergoing endoscopic procedures without oxygen supplementation.
- There should be an area dedicated for observation of the patient after the procedure. The patient should be reviewed before discharge from the recovery area.
- If the procedure is done as a day-case procedure, there should be provision for the patient to be admitted for further observation and subsequent management if the patient's condition warrants it.
- The clinical observation, types and doses of drugs administered and any intra-procedural events should be documented clearly and the record kept together with the patient's case notes.

SUMMARY

Surgical procedures done under monitored care by the anaesthesiologist should not be regarded lightly. The patients should receive the same standard of care and monitoring during the procedure and recovery as any other patient would receive. It is the combined responsibility of the surgeon and the anaesthesiologist to ensure patient comfort and safety during and after such procedures.

APPENDIX

OBSERVER'S ASSESSMENT OF ALERTNESS/SEDATION SCALE

Responsiveness	Speech	Facial expression	Eyes	Composite score level
Responds readily to name spoken in normal tone	Normal	Normal	Clear, no ptosis	5
Lethargic response to name spoken in normal tone	Mild slowing or thickening	Mild relaxation	Glazed or ptosis (less than half the eye)	4
Responds only after name is called loudly and/or repeatedly	Slurring or prominent slowing	Marked relaxation	Glazed and marked ptosis (half the eye or more)	3
Responds only after mild prodding or shaking	Few recognizable words			2
Does not respond to mild prodding or shaking				1

FURTHER READING

1. Hatch DJ, Sury MRJ. Sedation of children by non-anaesthetists. Br J Anaesth 2000;84:713–4.
2. Holzman RS, Cullen DJ, Eichhorn JH, Philip JH. Guidelines for sedation by non-anesthesiologists during diagnostic and therapeutic procedures. J Clin Anesth 1994;6:265–76.
3. "Scoping our practice". The 2004 Report of the National Confidential Enquiry into Patient Outcome and Death. NCEPOD. London, 2004.

Chapter 53

Awareness and Depth of Anaesthesia Monitoring

INTRODUCTION

Memory can be classified into 2 types: explicit (or conscious) memory, and implicit (or unconscious) memory. Explicit memory refers to the conscious recollection of previous experiences, equivalent to "remembering". In contrast, implicit memory refers to changes in behaviour that are produced by previous experiences but without any conscious recollection of those experiences.

The term "awareness" is often used to describe explicit memory during anaesthesia, while "recall of awareness" refers to the ability to remember the episode of awareness.

It is important to distinguish the two because awareness can occur without subsequent recall.

The incidence of awareness with recall in non-obstetric and non-cardiac surgical cases is estimated to be 0.2–0.3%. The incidence is similar in total intravenous anaesthesia (TIVA) as in conventional inhalational anaesthesia. It is higher when light anaesthesia is used, for example, in cardiac surgery (1.1–1.5%), caesarean section (0.4%) and major trauma cases (11–43%!). Patients who have experienced awareness during anaesthesia report the perception of paralysis, conversations and surgical manipulations, accompanied by feelings of helplessness, fear and impending doom. Approximately 0.01% of patients report suffering from pain while being awake.

Awareness during anaesthesia is a distressing experience that may result in serious emotional injury and posttraumatic stress disorder. Patients may suffer from repetitive nightmares, anxiety, a preoccupation with death and a concern with sanity, which may make them reluctant to discuss their symptoms. In terms of medico-legal consequences, claims for awareness during anaesthesia account for 2% of all claims in the American Society of Anesthesiologists Closed Claims Project.

CAUSES OF AWARENESS

Anaesthetic requirement is a balance between the amount of anaesthetic administered and the state of consciousness of the patient. The intensity of stimulation varies markedly during any surgical procedure, while cardiovascular effects of anaesthetic drugs may limit the amount that can be safely administered to the patient, especially one who is haemodynamically unstable. Thus critical imbalances between anaesthetic requirement and delivery may occur.

The main causes of awareness include:

— *Light anaesthesia:* common examples are caesarean section, cardiac surgery, bronchoscopy, hypovolaemic or critically ill patients presenting for trauma or other emergency surgery. In all these cases the patient may be given minimal anaesthetic with neuromuscular blockade as part of the balanced anaesthetic technique.

— *Increased anaesthetic requirement:* some patients may be more "resistant" to the effects of anaesthetics than others and require higher doses to produce unconsciousness. These include the younger patients, smokers and long-term users of certain substances (alcohol, opioids and recreational drugs).

— *Equipment malfunction or failure:* this results in delivery of inadequate anaesthetic to the patient. Examples include empty or incorrectly mounted vaporizers, failure

of nitrous oxide supply, entrainment of air in breathing system or ventilator, malfunctioning syringe pump, or disconnection, kinking or blockage of the perfusor tubing resulting in failure of delivery of intravenous anaesthetic agent.
- *Other anaesthetic mishaps:* examples are drug error (wrong drug, wrong dilution), failure to deepen the anaesthetic during attempts at intubation or resuscitation.

DEPTH OF ANAESTHESIA MONITORING

Depth of anaesthesia monitoring is employed in an attempt to reliably predict adequacy of anaesthetic delivery, and in so doing it is hoped that the occurrence of awareness can be prevented. These methods are proposed.
- Clinical signs.
- CNS monitoring: electroencephalography (EEG), cerebral function monitor (CFM), bispectral index (BIS), evoked responses, e.g., somatosensory, visual, middle latency auditory evoked response (MLAER).
- Isolated forearm technique.
- Lower oesophageal contractility.
- Others: skin conductance, electromyography.

Many of these methods are imprecise, lacking in sensitivity and specificity. Autonomic responses to noxious stimuli during light anaesthesia – tachycardia, hypertension, sweating, lacrimation and pupillary dilatation – are unreliable indicators of anaesthetic depth. With current anaesthetic techniques that are largely relaxant- and opioid-based, periods of intraoperative awareness may not be heralded by haemodynamic changes or accompanied by muscle movements.

Some methods (e.g., EEG monitoring) require expert interpretation and are affected by the type of anaesthetic agents used, while others (e.g., isolated forearm technique) may be limited by the length of surgery. Two methods – BIS and MLAER – appear to be most promising although the latter is less frequently used.

BISPECTRAL INDEX (BIS)

Bispectral analysis is a technique of mathematical signal processing that quantifies the degree of phase coupling between different frequency components of an EEG signal. The BIS monitor records and processes the EEG to calculate a single, dimensionless number that is designed to help the anaesthesiologist adjust dosage of anaesthetic drugs. It has gained considerable popularity because it is non-invasive and simple to use.

The claimed usefulness of BIS monitors include:

— BIS as a guide to anaesthetic administration in order to reduce doses and hasten recovery.
— BIS as a monitor for depth of anaesthesia to reduce incidence of awareness during anaesthesia.

However, these claims have not been fully substantiated, for these reasons.

— Detailed cost analysis actually revealed that the EEG electrodes used in BIS monitoring more than offset any cost savings on drug use.
— The applicability of BIS monitoring to "real world" multi-drug anaesthetic regimen requires further evaluation because the development of the BIS algorithm was based mainly on single anaesthetic agent studies.
— BIS is not 100% foolproof in preventing intraoperative awareness. There are well-documented case reports of preserved consciousness even with BIS values of 50–65 (values recommended for general anaesthesia), and a case of awareness with explicit recall has even occurred with a BIS reading of 47.

Certain artefacts can affect the BIS reading. These include:

— Muscle activity: patient movement, shivering, twitching, blinking, rolling the head.
— Mechanical device which generates high frequency activity in close proximity (e.g., intravenous fluid and patient warming devices).
— Incorrect placement of electrodes.
— Output from cardiac pacemakers.
— Paradoxical delta waves, noted during anaesthetic maintenance and emergence.

The recommended BIS ranges are 65–85 for sedation, and 40–65 for general anaesthesia. Values < 40 reflect burst suppression, a pattern associated with deep anaesthesia. There is a low probability of explicit recall with BIS ≤ 70 (Table 53–1). It should be remembered that clinical judgement should always be used when interpreting BIS in conjunction with other available clinical signs. Reliance on BIS alone for intraoperative anaesthetic management is not recommended since artefacts and poor signal quality may lead to inappropriate BIS values.

Table 53–1. Bispectral index range guidelines

<table>
<tr><th>BIS</th><th>Clinical State</th><th>Implication</th></tr>
<tr><td>100</td><td>Awake</td><td></td></tr>
<tr><td></td><td>Light/moderate sedation</td><td rowspan="2">Light hypnotic state</td></tr>
<tr><td>70</td><td>Deep sedation, with low probability of explicit recall</td></tr>
<tr><td>60</td><td>General anaesthesia, with low probability of consciousness</td><td>Moderate hypnotic state</td></tr>
<tr><td>40</td><td>Deep hypnotic state</td><td></td></tr>
<tr><td>0</td><td>Flat line EEG</td><td></td></tr>
</table>

ANAESTHETIC MANAGEMENT GUIDELINES TO REDUCE RISK OF AWARENESS

These measures are useful in our attempts to prevent awareness during anaesthesia.

— Use amnesic drugs (e.g., benzodiazepines) for premedication or intraoperatively, especially if light anaesthesia is anticipated.

— Regular maintenance and checking of the anaesthetic machine and drug delivery systems.

— Clearly label all drug syringes and double check to ensure that correct drugs and doses are administered to the patient.

— Ensure that anaesthetic agents (inhalational and intravenous agents) are delivered to the patient.
  - Inhalational agent: flowmeters, level of anaesthetic in vaporizers, anaesthetic agent concentration monitoring.
  - Intravenous agent: preferably a dedicated cannula for drug infusion, volume and pressure alarms on infusion pumps, vigilance with the amount of drug infused and integrity of the delivery system.

— Administer an adequate dose of induction agent. Remember to give supplemental doses if there is a delay in inserting an endotracheal tube or other airway device.

— Avoid muscle paralysis unless absolutely necessary since voluntary movements or movement responses to noxious stimuli are suppressed under neuromuscular blockade.
— Supplement nitrous oxide and opioids with volatile anaesthetic and ensure that the end-tidal concentration of the volatile anaesthetic is at least 0.6 MAC, and at least 0.8–1 MAC when used alone.
— Somatic and autonomic signs of insufficient anaesthesia should be treated with anaesthetic agents, not with neuromuscular blocking drugs, β-blockers or vasodilators.
— Be mindful of the potential for awareness in hypovolaemic patients under light anaesthesia. Deepen the anaesthetic level with hypnotic, opioid or volatile anaesthetics as soon as is feasible.
— Discuss the potential for awareness with patients in whom the risks are relatively high, consider intraoperative auditory masking with earplugs or headphones.
— Utilize a means of monitoring anaesthetic depth (e.g., BIS monitor) particularly in high-risk cases.
— Clinical assessment always takes precedence over the BIS value if there is a disparity between the two: *blind reliance on BIS to rule out awareness should be discouraged.*

WHAT IF AWARENESS HAS OCCURRED?

Management of a patient who has experienced awareness should be precise, detailed and compassionate. The different aspects of management should be clearly documented as this may be of medico-legal interest.

Suggested measures include these.

— See the patient at the earliest opportune time.
— Verify the patient's account on the events during which awareness is alleged to have occurred.
— Give possible explanation to the occurrence of awareness.
— Offer sympathy and reassurance but do not apportion blame to any specific individual or event.
— Arrange for psychological support; do not delay referral to a psychologist or psychiatrist.

— Document the interview in the patient's case notes and keep a photocopy for future reference.
— Inform the surgeon, nursing staff and medical defence body.
— Follow up the patient.

FURTHER READING

1. Ghoneim MM, Block R. Learning and memory during general anesthesia: An update. Anesthesiology 1997;87:387–410.
2. Ghoneim MM, Weiskopf RB. Awareness during anesthesia. Anesthesiology 2000;92:597–602.
3. Ranta OVS, et al. Awareness with recall during general anesthesia: Incidence and risk factors. Anesthesiology 1998;86:1084–9.
4. Mychaskiw G, et al. Explicit intraoperative recall at a bispectral index of 47. Anesth Analg 2001;92:808–9.
5. Rampil IJ. Monitoring depth of anesthesia. Curr Opin Anaesthesiol 2001;14:649–53.
6. Kumar A, Bhattacharya A, Makhija N. Evoked potential monitoring in anaesthesia and analgesia. Anaesthesia 2000;55:225–41.
7. Thornton C, Sharpe RM. Evoked responses in anaesthesia. Br J Anaesth 1998;81:771–81.
8. Johansen JW, Sebel PS. Development and clinical application of electroencephalographic bispectrum monitoring. Anesthesiology 2000;93:1336–44.
9. Plourde G. BIS EEG monitoring: What it can and cannot do in regard to unintentional awareness. Can J Anesth 2002;49:R1–R4.
10. O'Connor MF, Daves SM, Tung A, Thisted R, Apfelbaum J. BIS monitoring to prevent patient awareness during general anesthesia. Anesthesiology 2001;94:520–2.

Chapter 54

Brain Death and Organ Donation

INTRODUCTION

The subject of death often evokes emotions of grief, helplessness and despair not only among the patient's relatives but also among the healthcare providers. This is particularly so if the event has been sudden, violent or unexpected, or if the victim were of a young age. The concept of *brain death means death* may not be accepted by grieving relatives still in the stage of denial, and it is important that we should be able to empathize and counsel them during their period of impending bereavement.

Death is the permanent cessation of the coordinated function of the organism as a whole, while brain death (or brainstem death) is defined as the irreversible cessation of brainstem function. A person certified to be brain dead is dead, and adults with brain death will develop asystole within a week regardless of the treatment being given.

The brain death concept is relevant both in terms of proper utilization of ICU facilities and the procurement of organs for transplantation. It is morally and economically unjustifiable to continue ventilating brain dead patients in ICU and potentially deprive other patients of ICU facilities. As for organ donation, it is important to start the mechanism of organ procurement as early as possible, since organ survival is jeopardized when it is retrieved from a brain dead patient already in circulatory collapse.

TESTS TO CONFIRM BRAIN DEATH

The diagnosis of brain death is a clinical one. Various bedside tests are carried out to demonstrate the absence of reflexes which indicate the existence of brainstem activity. These preconditions should be met and other derangements excluded or corrected before the tests can be carried out.

Preconditions

- The patient is in apnoeic coma for at least 12 hours and requires full mechanical ventilation.
- The cause of the coma is fully established and sufficient to explain the status of the patient.
- Brain damage is irremediable and is of known structural cause.

Exclusions

- Significant hypothermia (core temperature < 32°C).
- Centrally depressant drugs or neuromuscular blocking drugs.
- Acid-base abnormality.
- Metabolic or endocrine disease such as uncontrolled diabetes mellitus, uraemia, hyponatraemia, hepatic encephalopathy, Addison's disease, thyrotoxicosis.
- Markedly elevated $PaCO_2$.
- Severe hypotension.

- Presence of abnormal posturing such as decerebrate posture, as this indicates the presence of some brainstem activity.

Tests

- Pupillary light reflex: absence of papillary response to light; pupils at midposition with respect to dilatation (4–6 mm).
- Corneal reflex: no response to lightly touching the cornea with a cotton wool.
- Oropharyngeal (gag) and tracheobronchial (cough) reflex: no response to oropharyngeal suction or passage of suction catheter through the endotracheal tube to carina and beyond.
- Motor response in cranial nerve distribution: no grimacing in response to noxious stimuli.
- Oculocephalic reflex (Doll's eye sign)
  - The head is moved rapidly from side to side.
  - If the brainstem is dead the eyes remain in a fixed position within the orbit.
  - If the brainstem is intact the eyes appear to move to the opposite side and then realign with the head.
- Vestibulo-ocular reflex (caloric test)
  - Do an auroscopy to exclude tympanic membrane perforation or presence of excessive wax.
  - Irrigate the external auditory meatus with 30 ml of ice cold water on each side and look for nystagmus during or after the test.
  - The test is negative when no eye movement is observed.
- Apnoea test
  - Ventilate with 100% oxygen for 10 minutes (or 20 minutes in the presence of severe lung disease), adjust ventilator setting to maintain $PaCO_2$ above 40 mmHg.
  - Disconnect ventilator and insufflate oxygen at 6 L/min via a tracheal catheter.
  - Monitor oxygen saturation with pulse oximetry.
  - Measure $PaCO_2$ at 5-minute intervals until $PaCO_2$ exceeds 55 mmHg.
  - Re-ventilate after the apnoea test.
  - Disconnection from the ventilator should not exceed 10 minutes at any time.
  - The test is abandoned if cyanosis or desaturation ($SpO_2 < 90\%$) occurs, blood pressure decreases by more than 10%, ECG abnormalities (ventricular arrhythmias, ST-segment depression) are observed or if spontaneous respiratory movement occurs.

The medical practitioners (preferably anaesthesiologists, physicians, neurologists or neurosurgeons) carrying out the tests should be experienced in diagnosing brain death and should not be members of the transplant team. Two sets of tests should be carried out with an interval of at least 6 hours to reduce observer error. Further investigations, such as electroencephalography, brainstem auditory evoked potentials, cerebral angiography, transcranial Doppler or radioisotope studies, are not necessary for the confirmation of brain death.

For children less than 2 years old, the guidelines are modified in 2 areas:

— EEG is required for brain death diagnosis
— Interval between two examinations is longer compared to adults:
  - term – 2 months: at least 48 hours apart
  - 2 months – 1 year: at least 24 hours apart
  - 1–18 years: at least 12 hours apart

When brain death is confirmed after the tests, the findings should be conveyed to the relatives in a sympathetic manner. Subsequent care of the brain dead patient is dictated by the wishes of the relatives and the potential for organ donation. If organ donation is not an option, ventilatory and cardiovascular support can be withdrawn at a time acceptable to all parties concerned. If organ donation is agreed upon, steps should be taken to maintain normal parameters to maximize organ viability while the mechanisms for organ donation are set into motion.

ORGAN DONATION

These are the steps in the process of organ procurement from brain dead donors.

— Identification of the suitable organ donor.
— Referral for organ donation by the primary care team.
— Explanation to family about prognosis and possibility of brain death.
— Verbal family interest for donation.
— Tests to confirm brain death.
— Written family consent for donation following the declaration of death.
— Referral to organ transplant team for identification of suitable transplant recipients.

NON-HEART-BEATING DONATION

In non-heart-beating donation (NHBD), death is declared when the patient goes into asystole and procedures for organ procurement are instituted. Again the physician declaring death should not be a member of the transplant team in order to avoid a conflict of interest.

There is a clear transition from the care of a patient to the recovery of the organs (usually the lungs, liver and kidneys) from a cadaver. The time interval between complete cessation of circulatory function and declaration of death varies in different centres (range of 2–10 minutes). The longer it takes, the less opportunity exists for multiple organ procurement since the absence of cardiorespiratory function adversely affects the suitability of organs for successful transplantation.

PATHOPHYSIOLOGICAL CHANGES ASSOCIATED WITH BRAIN DEATH

The anaesthesiologist should have a working knowledge of the pathophysiological changes following brainstem death in order to provide optimal conditions for organ survival. These changes are summarized here.

- Cardiovascular system
  - Initial "sympathetic storm": massive catecholamine release following brainstem infarction, leading to tachycardia, hypertension, increased cardiac output and peripheral vascular resistance.
  - Later loss of sympathetic activity leading to peripheral vasodilatation, hypotension, asystole and death, usually within 72 hours.
- Respiratory system: neurogenic pulmonary oedema is common.
- Endocrine system: reduction in antidiuretic hormone leading to diabetes insipidus; hypothyroidism and hypoadrenalism contribute to cardiovascular collapse.
- Loss of thermoregulatory function, leading to poikilothermia and usually hypothermia.
- Coagulopathy caused by release of thromboplastin and other mediators from ischaemic brain tissue.

MANAGEMENT OF THE BRAIN DEAD FOR ORGAN PROCUREMENT

This is a complex and dynamic process directed towards maintenance of end-organ function and viability. Optimum management of different organ systems can be in conflict, for example, fluid resuscitation to improve organ perfusion may worsen pulmonary oedema. This can be resolved by identifying which organs are being considered for transplantation.

— One should strive to maintain the "Rule of 100" – systolic BP > 100 mmHg, urine output > 100 ml/hr, PaO_2 > 100 mmHg, haemoglobin concentration > 100 g/l (or 10 g/dl) – to ensure adequate organ perfusion and oxygen carriage.

— Cardiovascular instability with hypotension and cardiac arrhythmias frequently occur. Haemodynamic management aims to achieve normovolaemia, maintain a normal afterload and optimize cardiac output without relying on high doses of inotropes. The latter tend to increase myocardial oxygen demand and deplete the myocardial adenosine triphosphate (ATP), decreasing its suitability for heart transplantation.

— In view of lower carbon dioxide production in the brain dead patient, the minute ventilation should be reduced to 60–70% of the previous value to avoid alkalosis with consequent reduction in oxygen availability to tissues. Tidal volume should be maintained at 6–8 ml/kg to prevent volutrauma by overinflation, or atelectasis by underinflation. PEEP is set to 5–10 cmH_2O and FiO_2 is adjusted to maintain SpO_2 at 95%.

— Other aspects of management include:
  - Means to achieve normothermia.
  - Correction of coagulopathy.
  - Treatment of diabetes insipidus with vasopressin or desmopressin (DDAVP).
  - Correction of acid-base, electrolyte and endocrine abnormalities.

— In the OT, movements and haemodynamic responses to noxious stimuli can still occur during the process of organ retrieval. These responses occur from a spinal reflex arc that involves the adrenal medulla. These can be rather disconcerting to the personnel not familiar with brain death and are best controlled using neuromuscular blockade and opioids/volatile anaesthetic agents.

— Low-dose inotropic support and fluid therapy are maintained. Normocarbia and SpO_2 95–97% should be achieved throughout the procedure. The large incision required for multiple organ retrieval can lead to a rapid and undesired decline in the core temperature, which may predispose the heart to ventricular fibrillation. The OT temperature should be increased and measures should be taken to prevent hypothermia.

— Ventilation is stopped once the organs have been harvested. The whole process is often distressing to all concerned especially if the donor is a child or young adult. The psychological trauma to the medical team should be acknowledged and addressed.

FURTHER READING

1. Randell TT. Medical and legal considerations of brain death. Acta Anaesthesiol Scand 2004;48:139–44.
2. Wijdicks EFM. The diagnosis of brain death. N Engl J Med 2001;344:1215–21.
3. Settergren G. Brain death: An important paradigm shift in the 20th century. Acta Anaesthesiol Scand 2003;47:1053–68.
4. Smith CR, Lowell JA. Ethical considerations in organ donation and transplantation. J Intensive Care Med 2000;15:231–6.
5. Truog RD, Robinson WM. Role of brain death and the dead-donor rule in the ethics of organ transplantation. Crit Care Med 2003;31:2391–6.
6. Young PJ, Matta BF. Anaesthesia for organ donation in the brainstem dead – Why bother? (Editorial) Anaesthesia 2000;55:105–6.
7. Van Norman GA. Another matter of life and death: What every anaesthesiologist should know about the ethical, legal, and policy implications of the non-heart-beating cadaver organ donor. Anesthesiology 2003;98:763–73.
8. Van Norman GA. Ethical issues and the role of anesthesiologists in non-heart-beating organ donation. Curr Opin Anaesthesiol 2003;16:215–9.

Chapter 55
Autologous Blood Transfusion

INTRODUCTION

Blood transfusion is not without risks even though it has undoubted benefits. Concerns about the safety of allogeneic transfusion include transmission of infectious agents such as HIV or hepatitis virus, intravascular haemolysis, electrolyte and metabolic disturbances and circulatory overload in susceptible individuals. Allogeneic transfusion is also thought to induce immunomodulation in the recipient, giving rise to increased incidence of postoperative infections and risk of cancer recurrence.

The decision to transfuse blood or blood components must be based on careful assessment and clear indication that the transfusion is necessary to save life or prevent a major morbidity. It is *NOT* advisable to transfuse blood indiscriminately in order to "top up" the haemoglobin value to 10 g/dl. Similarly, an average healthy patient can tolerate an intraoperative blood loss of 500 ml without requiring blood transfusion.

Autologous blood transfusion (ABT), or autotransfusion in short, means, "transfusing the patient with his/her own blood". This technique of blood conservation has been shown to be safe and effective in reducing the need for allogeneic transfusion. It has the added advantages of eliminating the problems of disease transmission and red cell allo-immunization.

While it is not necessary to obtain specific written consent for autologous transfusion procedures in OT, the patient should be informed about the proposed procedure and its benefits. The patient should understand that even though ABT reduces the likelihood of allogeneic blood transfusion, this does not obviate its need altogether. Allogeneic transfusion would still be given if the clinical situation warrants its usage.

INDICATIONS FOR ABT

ABT is particularly useful in these clinical situations.

- Major surgery with significant blood loss or sustained venous oozing.
  - Cardiothoracic surgery.
  - Vascular surgery such as aortic aneurysm surgery.
  - Liver transplantation or resection.
  - Total joint replacements.
  - Extensive spinal instrumentation such as scoliosis surgery.
- Patients with rare blood groups and multiple red cell antibodies because of the problem of blood compatibility.
- Immuno-compromised patients; to prevent immunological effects of allogeneic transfusions such as allo-immunization or graft-versus-host disease.

CONTRAINDICATIONS TO ABT

ABT is unsuitable for these patient groups.

- Patients at extremes of age group are not suitable candidates because of limitation in body reserves.
- Patients with significant cardiovascular, respiratory or cerebral disease are unsuitable for predonation and acute normovolaemic haemodilution techniques but may benefit from intraoperative cell salvage.
- For patients in whom the surgical field is contaminated by bacterial flora (e.g., bowel contents), malignant tumour cells, fat or amniotic fluid, intraoperative cell

salvage is not suitable because of risks of septicaemia, dissemination of malignant disease, embolism and disseminated intravascular coagulation (DIC) respectively.

— Certain religious groups such as the Jehovah's Witnesses will not accept a transfusion of blood or its derivatives.

In the case of Jehovah's Witnesses, note that perioperative cell salvage may be acceptable provided that the equipment is arranged in a closed circuit that is constantly linked to the patient's circulation and without storage of the patient's blood. Similarly, some Jehovah's Witnesses may accept acute normovolaemic haemodilution provided that the blood withdrawn remains in contact with the patient's circulation and is re-infused when necessary. These preferences should be specifically discussed prior to anaesthesia and documented clearly in the patient's case notes.

METHODS OF BLOOD COLLECTION

Four main techniques are described here.

— Predonation or preoperative autologous donation.

— Acute normovolaemic haemodilution.

— Intraoperative cell salvage.

— Postoperative cell salvage.

Predonation

Predonation, or preoperative autologous donation, is particularly useful for patients with rare blood groups scheduled for elective major surgery since it may be difficult to obtain compatible blood for such patients.

Careful selection of appropriate patients is important to ensure a safe and successful predonation programme. Predonation is not suitable in these situations:

— The scheduled surgery is intermediate and blood usage is not definite: ABT should only be considered if the likelihood of transfusion exceeds 50%.

— Patients who are infected with HIV, hepatitis or any active bacterial infections.

— Anaemic patients with haemoglobin < 10 g/dl.

— Children and pregnant patients.

— Patients with significant medical problems such as severe cardiac or respiratory disease.

Blood is collected over a period of a few weeks, up to 1 week before the scheduled operation. Up to 4 units can be collected in this manner. The blood collected is clearly labelled with the patient's particulars and stored separately in the Blood Bank. The patient is given haematinics (oral iron and folate) in the mean time.

This system is labour-intensive but has low cost-effectiveness. Suitable patients must be motivated to travel to the Blood Bank repeatedly before their scheduled operation. This may be inconvenient, stressful and may decrease their productivity at work. It also requires close cooperation among the surgeon, the anaesthesiologist and the Blood Bank. Clear guidelines must be drawn up regarding selection of suitable patients as well as the logistics of blood collection and storage. In addition, operating lists need to be coordinated to ensure guaranteed operating dates for patients involved in such a programme.

Acute Normovolaemic Haemodilution

Acute normovolaemic haemodilution (ANH) entails removal of blood from a patient immediately before surgery, either before or shortly after induction of anaesthesia, with simultaneous fluid replacement using colloid and/or crystalloid solution in order to maintain the circulating volume. This method should be considered in situations where the potential blood loss is likely to exceed 20% of the blood volume. Suitable patients are those with a preoperative haemoglobin > 11 g/dl and without severe cardiac disease such as moderate to severe left ventricular impairment, unstable angina, severe aortic stenosis or critical left main stem coronary artery disease.

The responsibility for the ANH procedure itself often rests with the anaesthesiologist. Appropriate blood collection bags are used to ensure a standard anticoagulant/blood ratio. Venesection of a central or large peripheral vein is undertaken using either a large-bore intravenous cannula or needle attached to the blood collection bag. The volume of blood removed depends on the patient's estimated blood volume (EBV) and haematocrit (Hct). A rough guide is based on the formula:

$$\textbf{Volume} = \textbf{EBV} \times \frac{\textbf{(Initial Hct − Final Hct)}}{\textbf{Average Hct}}$$

where EBV = 70 ml/kg in adults; 80 ml/kg in children

The final haematocrit may be targeted at 30% in healthy patients with no significant cardiovascular or respiratory disease. Either a crystalloid or a colloid solution is infused as blood is removed so that normovolaemia is maintained. The volume to be infused per ml of blood removed is 3 ml for crystalloid solution and 1 ml for colloid solution.

Each unit of autologous blood must be clearly labelled as "UNTESTED BLOOD: FOR AUTOLOGOUS USE ONLY" together with the patient's name, registration number, date and time, and the order of collection (if more than one pack is collected). If the anticipated time interval between blood collection and re-infusion is 6 hours or more, the blood bags must be stored at –4°C in the blood fridge; otherwise they can be kept at OT temperature of approximately 18–20°C.

Blood is transfused once major blood loss has ceased, and earlier if necessary. The units are re-infused in the reverse order of removal so that the one with the highest haematocrit and the greatest concentration of coagulation factors is administered last. Any unused autologous blood is to be disposed of as hazardous waste, preferably in OT. No autologous blood should be transferred to the general blood supply.

The ANH technique is a widely-available, low-cost option with the potential advantages of reduced red cell loss during surgery (secondary to reduced haematocrit) and improved oxygen delivery (secondary to reduced blood viscosity). Of theoretical benefit is the availability of fresh autologous blood with normal clotting factor concentrations and functioning platelets at the end of the surgery. However, its efficacy in reducing transfusion requirements has been questioned.

Introoperative Cell Salvage

This procedure entails the collection and re-infusion of autologous red cells lost during surgery.

There are 3 main types of red cell salvage devices.

1. **Centrifugal processor (automated cell saver)**
   — Shed blood is aspirated into a collection reservoir via heparinized tubing.
   — Cells are separated by haemoconcentration and differential centrifugation.
   — Unwanted components – fibrin, debris, plasma, leukocytes, microaggregates, complement, platelets, free haemoglobin, most of the heparin – are removed by washing in saline.
   — The final product consists of a packed red cell-saline mixture with Hct 50–60%.
   — This has an excellent long-standing safety record and becomes more cost-effective with large volume losses.

2. **Haemofiltration processor**
   - Shed blood is suctioned, anticoagulated and collected in a reservoir with a disposable liner.
   - When the liner is full or at the end of the procedure, the liner is removed and the blood is washed in a red cell washer before it is re-infused.
   - This is less efficient than centrifugal processors and has a longer processing time.

3. **Single re-infusion device**
   - Shed blood is anticoagulated and collected in a canister.
   - The blood is filtered and reinfused without washing with saline.
   - This method is relatively simple, involves no specialized equipment other than the filter, and suitable for low volume losses.
   - Its safety and efficacy is not tested; reinfusion of activated clotting factors may increase risks of DIC and postoperative bleeding in patients who received unwashed blood during cell salvage.

Major drawbacks of the cell salvage technique include high cost of the machinery and requirement for trained personnel. The main side-effects consist of air embolism, coagulation abnormalities and DIC-like syndrome ("salvaged blood syndrome"). Limitations of the suitability of this technique remain; contraindications include the presence of bacteria, malignant cells, fat, amniotic fluid, and the use of topical clotting agents (collagen, cellulose, thrombin) or other foreign material at the operative field.

Postoperative Cell Salvage

This technique, similar to intraoperative cell salvage, should be considered when the postoperative blood loss is sufficient to require blood transfusion. Blood may be salvaged from the body cavity or joint spaces, collected into a receptacle and reinfused with or without processing.

Even though this technique is most often used in cardiac surgical patients, it has also been used in selected orthopaedic procedures such as total knee replacements. Following cardiac surgery, shed mediastinal blood (if more than 200 ml/h) is drained into the cardiotomy reservoir, collected into a blood bag and reinfused to the patient. The procedure is stopped when drainage is less than 100 ml/h, if the patient develops haematuria, allergic reactions or high fever. The safety and benefit of the use of unwashed blood remains questionable, as the blood recovered is often dilute, partially haemolyzed and defibrinated, may contain high concentrations of cytokines and activated clotting factors which increase the risk of DIC.

FURTHER READING

1. Vanderlinde ES, Heal JM, Blumberg N. Autologous transfusion. Br Med J 2002;324:772–5.
2. Spahn DR, Leone BJ, Reves JG, Pasch T. Cardiovascular and coronary physiology of acute isovolemic hemodilution: A review of nonoxygen-carrying and oxygen-carrying solutions. Anesth Analg 1994;78:1000–21.
3. Napier JA et al. Guidelines for autologous transfusion II. Perioperative haemodilution and cell salvage. Br J Anaesth 1997;78:768–71.
4. Wells PS. Safety and efficacy of methods for reducing perioperative allogeneic transfusion: A critical review of the literature. Am J Ther 2002;9:377–88.

Chapter 56

Low-Flow Anaesthesia

INTRODUCTION

Low-flow anaesthesia, coupled with the use of rebreathing systems, has been in existence for a long time. In the last few decades, however, it has been superseded by high-flow, non-rebreathing anaesthetic techniques. Lately, concerns of cost, environmental pollution and development of more comprehensive monitoring and safety features have prompted a renewed interest in low-flow anaesthesia.

Even though the cost of anaesthesia constitutes only a small percentage of the total healthcare costs, the anaesthesiologist should still be involved in cost containment efforts by attempting to reduce anaesthetic drug expenditures. Low-flow anaesthesia is a simple but highly effective method of cost minimization by reducing fresh gas flow (FGF) during inhalational anaesthesia. Knowledge of the pharmacokinetic behaviour of inhalational anaesthetics, coupled with the use of modern anaesthetic equipment and monitoring technology, renders low-flow anaesthesia to be a safe and cost-effective technique.

DEFINITION

Various definitions in the context of low-flow anaesthesia have been proposed. Some of these definitions are summarized here.

Rebreathing refers to inhalation of some or all of previously exhaled gases. This is of no adverse physiological consequence unless the rebreathed gas contains carbon dioxide that re-enters the patient's alveoli, which results in carbon dioxide retention and hypercarbia.

Low-flow anaesthesia is defined as a technique which, using a rebreathing system, results in at least 50% of the exhaled air being returned to the lungs after carbon dioxide absorption. If modern rebreathing systems are used, this degree of rebreathing is achieved only if FGF is reduced to about 2 L/min.

In practical terms, low-flow anaesthesia often means a total FGF of 1 L/min or less. This can be subdivided into low-flow (0.5–1.0 L/min), minimal flow (0.25–0.5 L/min) and metabolic flow (< 0.25 L/min).

Closed system anaesthesia is a form of low-flow anaesthesia in which the maintenance FGF is just sufficient to replace the volume of gas and vapour taken up by the patient. The system must be leak-proof and no excess gas is vented through the relief valve.

ADVANTAGES AND DISADVANTAGES

Some of the advantages of low-flow anaesthesia have already been alluded to earlier. These include:

- Economical use of anaesthetic gases and vapours, which is especially relevant for expensive volatile anaesthetics such as desflurane and sevoflurane.
- Reduction in OT and environmental pollution.
- Conservation of heat and humidity with improved "climate" of anaesthetic gases
    - Reduced heat loss by latent heat of vaporization.
    - Preservation of mucociliary clearance at respiratory tract.

An indirect benefit of low-flow anaesthesia is that it promotes greater understanding of the function of the anaesthetic equipment and the pharmacokinetics of inhalational anaesthesia.

Some of the claimed disadvantages of low-flow anaesthesia include:

- Unfamiliarity with the technique.
- Inability to rapidly alter the composition of inspired gases.
- Increased risk of hypoxia or hypercarbia.
- Increased risk of over- or underdosage of inhalational anaesthetics.
- Accumulation of potentially toxic trace gases such as methane, carbon monoxide, acetone.
- Production of carbon monoxide when desiccated carbon dioxide absorbent reacts with volatile anesthetic agents especially desflurane, isoflurane and enflurane.
- Interaction of sevoflurane with carbon dioxide absorbent resulting in its degradation to produce compound A, which causes nephrotoxicity in rats.

Of the above-perceived disadvantages, unfamiliarity with the technique is the most often quoted reason and probably the biggest stumbling block faced by the anaesthesiologist. However, complexity and the alleged need for mathematical calculations should not be reasons to avoid the technique. These problems can be overcome by proper training, regular usage and understanding of the uptake kinetics of the anaesthetic gases. It can be a safe technique provided that there are suitable monitoring devices and also efficient means of carbon dioxide absorption.

The compound A issue concerning sevoflurane in low-flow anaesthesia has been the subject of numerous investigations. The US Food and Drug Administration (FDA) had earlier prohibited the use of sevoflurane in rebreathing systems with flow rates less than 2 L/min. It subsequently permitted a change in the sevoflurane labelling, from a recommended lower limit of 2 to 1 L/min, but with a 2 MAC-hour maximum exposure. This conservative recommendation has been challenged, because low-flow sevoflurane is considered to be as safe as low-flow isoflurane, even at long exposures. Studies have consistently shown no effects of compound A formation on postoperative renal function after moderate to long-duration low-flow sevoflurane anaesthesia, when assessed by serum creatinine, blood urea nitrogen and urinary excretion of protein and glucose.

Desflurane, enflurane and isoflurane can be degraded to carbon monoxide by carbon dioxide absorbents, and there have been case reports of carbon monoxide poisoning associated with the use of desflurane with or without low-flow anaesthesia. The amount of carbon monoxide formation is greater with drier absorbent, and with barium hydroxide, than with soda lime.

The solution to the compound A and carbon monoxide issues could lie in the nature of carbon dioxide absorbents and not the anaesthetic technique itself. Absorbents that do not contain either sodium hydroxide or potassium hydroxide, both of which appear to enhance the production of compound A and carbon monoxide, are being marketed. Examples of such absorbents include calcium hydroxide (Amsorb®) or lithium hydroxide. The widespread application of such absorbents in the future would eliminate any potential hazard from these toxic compounds.

Low-flow anaesthesia is only practical in surgical procedures of intermediate to long duration, since high flows are required during anaesthetic induction and emergence to allow rapid uptake and removal of anaesthetic gases respectively.

This anaesthetic technique is also not suitable in patients who may have increased levels of acetone, ethanol and carbon monoxide, such as:

- Decompensated diabetes mellitus.
- Prolonged starvation.
- Chronic alcohol abuse.
- Acute alcohol intoxication.
- Heavy smoker.

REQUIREMENT FOR LOW-FLOW ANAESTHESIA

- Proper anaesthetic equipment
  - Anaesthetic machine fitted with flowmeters that have smaller graduations for low-flow rates < 1L/min.
  - Circle system with functioning CO_2 absorber.
  - Calibrated vaporizers with accurate flow compensation: existing vaporizers can be used.
  - Leak-proof anaesthetic system and breathing circuit.
  - A ventilator with rising bellows during the expiration phase: this enables easier detection of leaks and avoids problem of air entrainment if the gas inflow is insufficient.
- Adequate and functioning monitoring devices
  - Pulse oximetry.
  - Disconnect or low pressure alarm for ventilator.
  - Respiratory monitor with airway pressure and spirometry.
  - Multi-gas analyzers which continuously measure the inspired and end-tidal concentrations of oxygen, carbon dioxide, nitrous oxide (if this is used) and

volatile anaesthetic agents.

- The use of an oxygen analyzer is mandatory when nitrous oxide is administered, in order to prevent delivery of hypoxic mixtures to the patient.

— Gas extracted through the multi-gas analyzer should be returned to the circuit just prior to the CO_2 absorber. The nipple at the back of the gas analyzer for collection of extracted gas is connected via a length of tubing to a T-piece attached to the breathing circuit.

PRACTICAL GUIDELINES

1. **Knowledge:** Be familiar with the low-flow technique.

2. **Patient and case selection:** Rule out patients and surgical procedures unsuitable for this technique.

3. **Checking**
   - — As with high-flow anaesthesia, proper checking of anaesthetic equipment and monitoring devices prior to anaesthesia is essential.
   - — Checking for leaks specific for low-flow anaesthesia
     a. Leak test for the anaesthetic machine
        - Completely deflate a rubber suction bulb (this may be modified from the bulb used in a sphygmomanometer) and attach it to the common gas outlet.
        - Observe for 10 seconds.
        - The bulb should not re-inflate. Re-inflation indicates entrainment of air from the atmosphere through a leak in the anaesthetic machine.

     b. Leak test for the breathing system
        - Pressurize the breathing system to 50 cmH_2O by pressing on the oxygen bypass button while completely closing the expiratory valve and occluding the patient end.
        - Check FGF required to maintain this pressure.
        - The FGF should be less than 0.1 L/min for low-flow anaesthesia.
   - — Check that the disconnect alarm of the ventilator is functioning.

4. **Induction of anaesthesia**
   - — Standard induction sequence and gas flows are used.

- Initial high gas flows are required to assist in denitrogenation of patient and breathing system, as well as hastening uptake of volatile anaesthetic agents.

5. **Maintenance of anaesthesia**
   - Reduce the gas flows after an interval of 10–15 minutes on high flows to achieve equilibrium, once the intended end-tidal concentration of the anaesthetic agent has been achieved. Usual initial settings: oxygen 0.5 L/min, nitrous oxide 0.5 L/min and isoflurane or sevoflurane 2–3%. Air may be used instead of nitrous oxide in selected cases.
   - Adjust the vaporizer setting to achieve the desired inspired concentration as measured by the multi-gas analyzer. Note that there may be a significant difference between the inspired anaesthetic concentration and the concentration delivered from the vaporizer when the fresh gas inflow is less than 1 L/min. For example, when the total fresh gas flow is 0.75 L/min (0.25 L/min O_2 with 0.5 L/min N_2O) the dialled concentration is approximately twice that of the actual inspired concentration.
   - Uptake of nitrous oxide decreases with time as the body gets more saturated. Reduce the nitrous oxide flow stepwise by 0.1 L/min each time to 0.2 L/min.
   - Maintain oxygen flow at a level adequate for basal oxygen consumption. This usually means a flow of 0.25 L/min or more, as it may not be safe to go below this value. The inspired oxygen concentration should be kept at 0.35 or higher if necessary.
   - Intermittent high flows (e.g., 5 minutes every hour) are necessary to flush out waste gases such as methane, carbon monoxide and acetone.
   - Use high flows for 3–5 minutes at any time after the breathing system integrity is breached (e.g., tracheal suctioning through the endotracheal tube) or when a rapid increase or decrease in the anaesthetic depth is desired.

6. **Emergence from anaesthesia**
   - Turn off nitrous oxide flow and vaporizer earlier than with conventional high-flow technique.
   - Use high oxygen flow to wash out residual anaesthetic gases from the patient and breathing system.

As familiarity with the low-flow anaesthetic technique grows, the anaesthesiologist will be able to "fine-tune" his/her technique so that the conduct of anaesthesia will be as smooth and straightforward as the conventional technique. The advantages in terms of cost savings and reduced environmental pollution can then be better appreciated.

FURTHER READING

1. Coetzee JF, Stewart LJ. Fresh gas flow is not the only determinant of volatile agent consumption: A multi-centre study of low-flow anaesthesia. Br J Anaesth 2002;88:46–55.
2. Baxter AD. Low and minimal flow inhalational anaesthesia. Can J Anaesth 1997;44:643–52.
3. Mapleson WW. The theoretical ideal fresh-gas flow sequence at the start of low-flow anaesthesia. Anaesthesia 1998;53:264–72.
4. Baum JA, Aitkenhead AR. Low-flow anaesthesia. Anaesthesia 1995;50:S37–S44.
5. Suttner S, Boldt J. Low-flow anaesthesia. Does it have potential pharmacoeconomic consequences? Pharmacoeconomics 2000;17:585–90.
6. Baum JA. Low-flow anaesthesia: The theory and practice of low flow, minimal flow and closed system anaesthesia, 4th Ed. Oxford: Butterworth-Heinemann, 2000.
7. Meakin GH. Low-flow anaesthesia in infants and children. Br J Anaesth 1999;83:50–7.
8. Berry PD, Sessler DI, Larson MD. Severe carbon monoxide poisoning during desflurane anesthesia. Anesthesiology 1999;90:613–6.

Chapter 57

Total Intravenous Anaesthesia

INTRODUCTION

As the name implies, total intravenous anaesthesia (TIVA) is delivery of the anaesthetic agents entirely by the intravenous route, and in doing so avoid the use of inhalational anaesthetic agents. Contrary to popular belief, TIVA is not a new anaesthetic technique.

The practice of using intravenous anaesthetics as sole anaesthetic agents has been in existence for a long time. The technique was previously used for short and minor procedures since accumulation of intravenous agents in long procedures resulted in prolonged psychomotor effects and unsatisfactory recovery characteristics. The anaesthetic agents in use included ketamine, thiopentone, methohexitone, etomidate, althesin and diazepam.

TIVA as we know today took off in a big way with the introduction and widespread usage of propofol. Tremendous progress has been made both in terms of knowledge of pharmacokinetics and hence "fine-tuning" of the anaesthetic technique, as well as development in infusion technology for accurate and reliable drug delivery. Further refinements have produced computer-controlled infusion systems in the form of target-controlled infusion (TCI).

The pharmacologic profile of propofol – a short distribution phase, short elimination half-life and high clearance rate – is ideally suited for TIVA. Anaesthesia with propofol is characterized by rapid, clear-headed recovery without hangover effects frequently associated with other intravenous anaesthetic agents. The non-emetogenic effect of propofol (regarded as antiemetic by some) also results in decreased incidence of postoperative nausea and vomiting (PONV).

INTRAVENOUS VERSUS INHALATIONAL ANAESTHESIA

For most anaesthesiologists, inhalational agents remain the routine choice for maintenance of anaesthesia in spite of introduction of new intravenous agents. One of the reasons is the fact that most, if not all, anaesthesiologists have been brought up using inhalational rather than intravenous agents, and old habits certainly die hard.

Problems of inhalational agents are summarized here.

— Environmental concerns such as effects of fluorinated hydrocarbons and ethers on the ozone layer.

— The need for expensive scavenging systems for waste gases.

— Possible effects of long-term occupational exposure to subanaesthetic doses of inhalational agents: teratogenesis, carcinogenesis, increased risk of abortions.

— Known triggering agents for malignant hyperthermia.

— Myocardial depression, arrhythmogenicity.

— Respiratory depression, laryngo- or bronchospasm during transitional zone of anaesthesia.

- Inhibition of hypoxic pulmonary vasoconstriction.
- Risk of halothane hepatitis (halothane) and nephrotoxicity (methoxyflurane).
- Increase in cerebral blood flow and intracranial pressure.
- Interaction with carbon dioxide absorbent: degradation of sevoflurane to produce compound A; carbon monoxide production with desflurane, isoflurane and enflurane.
- Problems peculiar to nitrous oxide
  - Risk of diffusion hypoxia.
  - Increased pulmonary vascular resistance.
  - Diffusion into enclosed air cavities worsening pneumothorax, air embolism, intestinal obstruction, pneumoencephalocele, middle-ear pressure, intraocular pressure.
  - Depression of bone marrow function.
  - Interference with DNA synthesis.
  - Nitrous oxide is a potent greenhouse gas, as the medical proportion of nitrogen oxide emission is a significant amount of the global total.

On the other hand, due consideration should be given to the potential for toxicity of the intravenous agents or their carrier solutions.

- Anaphylactoid and anaphylactic reactions to intravenous agents occur more frequently than serious renal or hepatotoxicity with volatile anaesthetics.
- In the ICU setting when high infusion rates of propofol are used for prolonged periods, one must make allowance for the lipid and osmotic loads imposed on susceptible patients.
- Propofol infusion syndrome – lactic acidosis, myocardial failure, renal failure and hypertriglyceridaemia – has been reported in critically ill children undergoing prolonged propofol infusion at high doses (> 48 hr and > 4 mg/kg/hr respectively).
- Microbial growth and potential for infection of infusion solutions, particularly propofol, is another issue that needs to be addressed. The propofol formulation has been supplemented with ethylene diamine tetraacetic acid (EDTA) or sulphite in order to overcome bacterial contamination. However, that does not obviate the need for drug preparation using a proper sterile technique and adherence to recommended guidelines.

WHAT ABOUT VIMA?

Intravenous agents are commonly used for induction of anaesthesia followed by inhalational agents for maintenance. The transition phase from induction to maintenance could lead to light anaesthesia if the intravenous agent undergoes rapid redistribution and before an adequate anaesthetic depth is attained with the inhalational agent. This has promoted the interest in "single agent" anaesthesia to eliminate such a transition phase. Volatile induction and maintenance of anaesthesia (VIMA) is popularized following the introduction of sevoflurane into clinical practice. The favourable pharmacologic profile of sevoflurane makes it ideal to be used for both induction and maintenance of anaesthesia.

Among the claimed advantages of VIMA using sevoflurane are:

— Smooth induction of anaesthesia due to minimal airway irritation, coughing or breath-holding

— Rapid induction, rapid adjustment and control of anaesthetic depth throughout the procedure, rapid emergence and quick return of psychomotor skills. All these are possible because of its low blood: gas partition coefficient of 0.69.

— Stable heart rate at concentrations less than 2 MAC.

ADVANTAGES AND PROBLEMS OF TIVA

Many of the advantages of TIVA are closely linked to the favourable pharmacologic profile of propofol, such as rapid, clear-headed recovery and reduced incidence of PONV. The TIVA technique is environmentally friendly and avoids problems of inhalational anaesthetic agents. Patients at risk of malignant hyperthermia can be safely anaesthetized using TIVA. Certain ENT procedures such as endoscopic laryngoscopy and microsurgery (ELMS), laser airway surgery and bronchoscopy are better managed using TIVA rather than inhalational anaesthesia. Similarly, TIVA is more suitable in certain thoracic and neurosurgical procedures because it does not inhibit hypoxic pulmonary vasoconstriction or cause an increased cerebral blood flow relevant in such procedures.

The TIVA technique is not without problems. Among them are:

— Unfamiliarity and hence reluctance to use the technique.

— Uncertainty in assessment of the depth of anaesthesia with risk of intraoperative awareness.

— Possible error during drug dilution or calculation of infusion rate, resulting in under- or overdosage.

- Inadequate anaesthesia due to problems in drug delivery, e.g., problems with intravenous access (occlusion or extravasation), infusion tubing (occlusion or disconnection) or malfunction of infusion pump.
- Inability to monitor drug delivery in TIVA with the risk of interruption being unrecognized, unlike inhalational anaesthesia, which can be assessed by ventilation and expired gas analysis.
- Large interindividual variation of pharmacokinetics and pharmacodynamics that may result in overdosage in some and inadequate anaesthesia in others.
- Cost: initial capital outlay for infusion pumps (TCI infusion devices in particular), syringes specific for TCI, drugs and disposables; this is somewhat counterbalanced by sophisticated agent-specific vaporizers (e.g., for desflurane) and expensive new volatile anaesthetics.

REQUIREMENTS OF TIVA

- It is essential to have a basic understanding of the pharmacokinetics of the intravenous agents used in TIVA.
- Desirable features of infusion pumps
  - Simplicity and user-friendliness.
  - Ability to change infusion rate rapidly and conveniently.
  - Facility for "purge" or bolus.
  - Ability to deliver high infusion rates for induction and maintenance of anaesthesia.
  - Accurate and reliable drug delivery.
  - Compatibility with various sizes and makes of syringes.
  - Clear legible display even in dim light conditions.
  - Distinctive audible warning for occlusion, low volume, low battery power.
  - Physical features: lightweight, compact and robust, equipped with battery as back-up power.
- One should be familiar with the operation of the infusion pump, particularly the newer ones with more sophisticated functions incorporated into the pump.
- Venous access
  - The intravenous cannula should be 20G or larger to permit high infusion rates without excessive pressure build-up.
  - Separate, dedicated tubing for drug infusion is highly desirable. If this is not possible, use a 3-way tap and an antireflux valve on the fluid infusion line.

— Monitors
  - As in inhalational anaesthesia, extent of monitoring is dictated by the condition of the patient and nature of surgery.
  - It is important to monitor the integrity of venous access, infusion line and infusion pump to ensure accurate drug delivery.
  - There is no direct or reliable monitor for depth of anaesthesia.

PRACTICAL GUIDELINES

— Although TIVA, by definition, does not use any inhalational anaesthetics, changing from totally inhalational to totally intravenous anaesthesia is a significant change in practice. It is recommended, therefore, that nitrous oxide may be used during the transition stage of "PIVA" or *partial intravenous anaesthesia* until the anaesthesiologist gains confidence with the technique. When nitrous oxide is dispensed with later, the dose of opioid should be increased to ensure adequate depth of anaesthesia.

— Again, be familiar with the drugs used during intravenous anaesthesia. Various drugs are used for their specific actions: hypnosis, muscle relaxation, analgesia, anxiolysis and antiemesis. These are shown in Table 57–1.

Table 57–1. Drugs used during TIVA*

Drug Class	Examples
Hypnotic	**Propofol**, etomidate, thiopentone, methohexitone, ketamine
Opioid analgesic	**Remifentanil**, **fentanyl**, alfentanil, sufentanil, morphine
Muscle relaxant	**Atracurium**, **vecuronium**, **rocuronium**
Anxiolytic	**Midazolam**, diazepam
Antiemetic	**Ondansetron**, dexamethasone, promethazine

*Drugs in common usage are listed in bold.

— Establish appropriate monitoring for the condition of the patient and nature of surgery.

— Carefully dilute and label the intravenous agents.
  - Have a fixed system of dilution to avoid unnecessary confusion, e.g., propofol (undiluted): 10 mg/ml; atracurium; 5 or 10 mg/ml; vecuronium; 1 mg/ml.
  - Modify dilution for small children, or use 1 ml ("insulin") syringe.

— A bolus dose of fentanyl or other opioid analgesic is administered at induction of anaesthesia. Subsequent doses can be administered as intermittent bolus doses or continuous infusion. Recommended doses are:
  - Fentanyl: 1–4 μg/kg bolus, 1–5 μg/kg/hr infusion.
  - Alfentanil: 5–20 μg/kg bolus, 30–50 μg/kg/hr infusion.
  - Sufentanil: 0.5–1.0 μg/kg bolus, 0.2–1.0 μg/kg/hr infusion.
  - Remifentanil: 0.5 μg/kg/min at induction, 0.25 μg/kg/min after tracheal intubation then stepwise adjustment by 0.05 μg/kg/min according to haemodynamic status

— Manual infusion regime for propofol
  - Induction dose 1 mg/kg over 20 seconds, followed by 10 mg/kg/hr for 10 minutes, 8 mg/kg/hr for 10 minutes and 6 mg/kg/hr thereafter, the "10–8–6" rule.
  - A smaller bolus dose of 1 mg/kg, given over 20 seconds, causes a smaller reduction in blood pressure compared to the conventional 2–2.5 mg/kg bolus.

— If neuromuscular blockade and intubation are required, a dose of neuromuscular blocking drug (atracurium, vecuronium or rocuronium) is administered to facilitate tracheal intubation. The patient is given oxygen or oxygen-air mixture as appropriate and guided by pulse oximetry. FiO_2 is usually maintained at 0.3.

— As in conventional anaesthesia, there may be wide interpatient variability in terms of dose requirement and response. The infusion rate must be titrated according to surgical stimulus and patient response, with increases in maintenance infusion during periods of stimulation such as skin incision or sternotomy. Different types of surgery may require different infusion regimens. If anaesthesia is inadequate, a bolus dose should be administered followed by an increase in infusion rate.

— Careful adjustment and fine-tuning of infusion rate towards the end of surgery will serve to hasten recovery. Reduce the infusion rate stepwise as surgery comes to the end; the actual rate of reduction depends on the nature of surgery and the speed of the surgeon. Generally, infusion of propofol can be terminated at skin closure. If remifentanil has been used during TIVA, administer a dose of long-acting opioid analgesic to provide adequate analgesia for the patient during the immediate postoperative period.

TIVA IN CHILDREN

— The use of TIVA in children is less popular compared to inhalational anaesthesia, because of inhalational induction being the usual method of anaesthetic induction, and uncertainties about pharmacokinetic and pharmacodynamic variations in the paediatric age group.

— Compared to adults, children tend to have a large central compartment volume and rapid clearance of intravenous anaesthetics and opioids. On the other hand, immaturity of hepatic enzyme systems and renal function causes significant impairment in the clearance of intravenous agents and their metabolites in the neonate, especially if preterm.

— In clinical terms, higher bolus doses are required to reach a given blood concentration and higher infusion rates are required to maintain a steady blood concentration in children. For example, the induction dose of propofol is 2.5–4 mg/kg in children instead of 2 mg/kg in adults.

— This is the proposed manual infusion regime in children 3–11 years to achieve a target concentration of 3 μg/ml (as extrapolated from the "10–8–6" rule in adults).
  - Loading dose of 2.5 mg/kg, followed by
  - L15 mg/kg/hr for 15 minutes; 13 mg/kg/hr for 15 minutes; 11 mg/kg/hr for 30 minutes; 10 mg/kg/hr for 1 hour; 9 mg/kg/hr for 2 hours.

— After prolonged infusions in children, recovery may be relatively slow because of the slow washout of this lipophilic drug from poorly perfused tissues especially fat. This is reflected by a comparatively larger context-sensitivity halftime (*vide infra*) in children.

— The role of TIVA is increasing in paediatric cardiac surgery, day-care surgery, ENT and ophthalmic surgery. It is also advantageous in diagnostic and therapeutic procedures such as imaging studies in radiology, bone marrow sampling, lumbar puncture, dressing changes and radiotherapy.

THE PROBLEM OF "AWARENESS"

Awareness implies wakefulness with or without recall of events during the period when the patient is thought to be under anaesthesia. The sensations recalled can be auditory, tactile, or worse of all, pain and the feeling of doom. It is an extremely traumatic experience for the patient, and in medico-legal terms it can also be extremely costly for the anaesthesiologist.

The stages of anaesthesia defined by Guedel in 1920 were observed when inhalational agents were the sole anaesthetics used. When the technique of balanced anaesthesia with muscle paralysis was popularized, several of the signs that defined the stages of anaesthesia could not be observed. Even though various methods have been proposed for the measurement of anaesthetic depth, these were often indirect and imprecise. Until now there is no reliable monitor to guarantee that the patient is adequately anaesthetized and that no awareness occurs under anaesthesia.

This problem became more acute when TIVA was introduced and the inhalational anaesthetics – nitrous oxide and volatile anaesthetic agents – were omitted. There is no definite end-point to decide whether the amount of intravenous anaesthetics administered is "not enough", "just enough" or "too much". Measurements of blood concentrations are impractical in the clinical setting and furthermore these values may not correlate directly with anaesthetic depth.

Even though it has been claimed that the incidence of awareness is no higher in TIVA than inhalational anaesthesia, this is an important issue that needs to be addressed if TIVA were to have a great impact in revolutionizing the practice of anaesthesia.

TARGET-CONTROLLED INFUSION

Instead of manually altering the infusion rates of intravenous anaesthetic agents such as propofol, a new and sophisticated infusion technique called target-controlled infusion (TCI) has been developed. This is a computer-controlled infusion system that makes use of pharmacokinetic models of drug distribution and elimination, together with patient information (age and weight), to perform the necessary complex calculations to achieve a set target concentration. It delivers the required amount of drug and maintains this calculated target value until the anaesthesiologist alters it. In doing so, the anaesthesiologist is able to achieve and maintain the desired blood concentration of the drug appropriate for any individual patient and level of surgical stimulation at any time. Since drug effect is more closely related to blood concentration than to infusion rate, drug delivery via TCI is capable of creating stable blood concentrations of intravenous anaesthetic agents.

Minimum infusion rate is the intravenous equivalent of minimum alveolar concentration (MAC) of an inhalational anaesthetic. Effective blood concentration of an intravenous agent is another term that is indicative of the potency of the intravenous anaesthetic. Target blood concentrations are determined by studies that define EC_{50} and EC_{95} (effective blood concentrations required to prevent movement in response to a painful stimulus in 50% and 95% of the population respectively) for a given intravenous anaesthetic. Context-sensitive halftime, the time required for the effector site concentration to decline by 50% after terminating the infusion, is used to predict time to awakening after the infusion is discontinued. This is of relevance because the fall in concentration of drug at the effector site depends upon how long the effector site has been exposed to the drug, how rapidly redistribution away from the effector site occurs and the rate of metabolism and excretion of the drug.

Based on the pharmacokinetic profile of the drug, the TCI system determines the initial loading dose needed to achieve the target concentration and the infusion rate needed to maintain it, and controls the infusion automatically. This is done without the need for complex mathematical calculations by the anaesthesiologist. Propofol has been studied extensively and the population pharmacokinetic profiles have been incorporated into the Diprifusor® system, which is the only commercially available TCI system thus far. At present there is no TCI system developed specifically for children as they require a different set of pharmacokinetic variables, and the Diprifusor® is not licensed for use in patients less than 16 years old. The "Paedfusor", a prototype paediatric TCI system, is conceptually similar to the adult Diprifusor® but with software appropriate for children down to age of 6 months and weighing 5 kg. This is being developed and is not yet commercially available.

In view of interpatient variability in pharmacokinetics and pharmacodynamics, the target propofol concentration should be titrated against the patient's response in order to achieve the depth of anaesthesia required. A young, healthy, unpremedicated patient obviously requires a higher concentration compared to an elderly, ill or premedicated patient. In ASA I and II patients, the target blood concentration for propofol is in the range of 6–7 μg/ml when used with oxygen-enriched air, and 4–5 μg/ml with 67% nitrous oxide in oxygen. Low-dose TCI (at 0.5–2.0 μg/ml) can also be used for sedation during surgery performed under loco-regional block.

Induction of anaesthesia can be achieved with either slow titrated intravenous bolus injection of propofol or infusion from the TCI system itself. In adult patients below 55 years, start with an initial target of 4 μg/ml in premedicated patients and 6 μg/ml in unpremedicated patients. Induction time with these targets is in the range of 60–120 seconds. Higher targets allow more rapid induction of anaesthesia but may be associated with greater haemodynamic disturbance and respiratory depression.

A lower initial target concentration should be used in patients above 55 years and those in ASA III or IV. The target concentration can be increased by 0.5–1 μg/ml at 1–minute intervals to achieve a gradual induction of anaesthesia.

The target concentrations for propofol during maintenance of anaesthesia should be varied accordingly. Satisfactory anaesthesia can be achieved in the range of 3–6 μg/ml during the maintenance phase. The predicted propofol concentration on awakening is in the region of 1–2 μg/ml depending on the analgesic administered.

Supplementary analgesia is usually required since propofol does not possess analgesic properties. Remifentanil is ideally suited for use in conjunction with propofol because of its rapid onset of action, short elimination half-life, and a context-sensitive halftime of approximately 3 minutes that remains constant regardless of duration of infusion. The recommended target concentration for remifentanil is 4 ng/ml; stepwise adjustments of 1 ng/ml each time can be made depending on haemodynamic parameters. TCI system for remifentanil ("Remifusor") was recently licensed in Europe, but published studies have so far failed to demonstrate clear-cut superiority of TCI over manually controlled infusions. There is uncertainty as to whether such a system would simply increase equipment cost without demonstrable patient benefits.

SUMMARY

Total intravenous anaesthesia offers an attractive alternative to inhalational anaesthesia. Many of the problems of inhalational anaesthesia can be circumvented by TIVA. On the other hand, the drawbacks of TIVA are mainly related to concerns about occurrence of awareness under intravenous anaesthesia and the reluctance of anaesthesiologists to experiment with new techniques.

It must be remembered that both intravenous and inhalational anaesthetic techniques are not mutually exclusive. They are both useful tools at the disposal of the anaesthesiologist. The introduction of TIVA does not mean that inhalational anaesthesia has no place in modern anaesthesia. The role of inhalational anaesthesia in paediatrics and in difficult airway management cannot, and certainly will not, be replaced by TIVA.

FURTHER READING

1. Viviand X, Leone M. Induction and maintenance of intravenous anaesthesia using target-controlled infusion systems. Best Prac Res Clin Anaesthesiol 2001;15:19–33.
2. Rowan KJ. Awareness under TIVA: A doctor's personal experience. Anaesth Intens Care 2002;30:505–6.

3. Morton NS. Total intravenous anaesthesia (TIVA) in paediatrics: Advantages and disadvantages. Paed Anaesth 1998;8:189–94.
4. McFarlan CS, Anderson BJ, Short TG. The use of propofol infusions in paediatric anaesthesia: A practical guide. Paed Anaesth 1999;9:209–16.
5. Eyres R. Update on TIVA. Paed Anaesth 2004;14:374–9.
6. Varveris DA, Morton NS. Target controlled infusion of propofol for induction and maintenance of anaesthesia using the Paedfusor: An open pilot study. Paed Anaesth 2002;12:589–93.
7. Sneyd JR. Recent advances in intravenous anaesthesia. Br J Anaesth 2004;93:725–36.

Chapter 58

Acute Pain Management

INTRODUCTION

Pain, one of the sequelae of acute injury, may initiate a whole host of physiological changes termed "stress response" which, if left unchecked, may adversely affect the cardio-respiratory function. The impact of effective analgesia on postoperative morbidity has been the subject of numerous studies. It is now recognized that optimal pain management plays an important role in hastening postoperative recovery and reducing the incidence of morbidity related particularly to the cardiovascular and respiratory systems.

Effective pain management begins even before commencement of surgery. Adequate opioid premedication and preemptive analgesia in various forms are postulated to reduce postoperative analgesic requirement and possibly reduce the risk of chronic pain development. Similarly, good surgical skills, meticulous haemostasis and gentle tissue handling by the surgeon are just as important in reducing tissue trauma and the severity of postoperative pain.

Even though postoperative patients form the majority of patients under acute pain management, they are by no means the only group benefiting from such management. Other categories of patients include those suffering from burns, chest trauma such as rib fractures and painful conditions such as acute pancreatitis.

The concept of a team of healthcare providers dedicated to acute pain management is well established in many parts of the world. The Acute Pain Service (APS) team comprises the anaesthesiologist, nursing staff – both APS nurses and ward nurses – surgeons and pharmacists. The setting up of APS in hospitals, headed by anaesthesiologists, is indeed timely and essential.

In any APS set-up, procedure protocols for the medical and nursing staff should be clearly written and individualized to the needs and availability of equipment, manpower and training in any particular hospital. Observation charts incorporating the APS treatment, patient's haemodynamic and respiratory parameters (BP, pulse rate, respiratory rate), pain scores, sedation scores and side-effects should be used. There should be regular audit and continuing medical education programme to ensure that the doctors and nurses concerned have the necessary knowledge and skills to assess and manage postoperative pain.

PRINCIPLES OF APS MANAGEMENT

Prior Planning and Patient Information

— The APS technique appropriate for the patient and surgery should be planned preoperatively and discussed with the patient during the premedication visit. This is particularly important for patient-controlled analgesia by means of intravenous or epidural route: ivPCA or PCEA respectively.

— In the absence of contraindications, a multi-modal approach to pain management, comprising an opioid, local anaesthetic and a non-steroidal antiinflammatory drug (NSAID), is more effective than therapy using a single modality.

— Analgesics should be administered preemptively when pain is anticipated and before it is experienced; and they should be prescribed on a regular rather than on demand ("PRN") basis.

Communication with Surgical and Nursing Staff

— There should be adequate communication between the anaesthesiologist and the surgeon so that postoperative analgesic orders are not duplicated.

— The APS instructions to ward nurses should be written clearly in the patient's case notes and APS forms.
— At no time during APS management should parenteral opioids be administered in addition to APS orders without prior consultation with the anaesthesiologist.
— The anaesthesiologist in charge of APS should be contacted if pain relief is unsatisfactory or should complications to the treatment arise. The anaesthesiologist should review the patient promptly so that appropriate remedial measures may be taken.
— There should be round-the-clock APS coverage. An appropriate mechanism – APS pagers, names and contact numbers of specific doctors – should be implemented such that the anaesthesiologist can be easily contacted at all times.

Pain Assessment

— This should be done regularly and systematically, at least every 4 hours and more frequently if additional treatment has been administered or if complication arises.
— The patient should be taught simple pain scores such as verbal rating scale, numerical rating scale or visual analogue scale (VAS). Obtain pain scores at rest as well as on movement, deep breathing or coughing. The values of these scores should be documented in the observation chart.

Management of Breakthrough Pain

— Unexpected pain or increasing pain should be investigated since this may be associated with significant surgical complication. Its cause should be identified and rectified as soon as possible.
— When additional analgesic is administered, monitor the patient closely for its effect and possible complications.

APS TECHNIQUES

Postoperative pain management is an evolving field with innovations in the use of systemic and neuraxial opioids, regional anaesthetic techniques (e.g., brachial plexus blocks), patient-controlled intravenous or epidural analgesia and co-analgesic therapies using NSAIDs. The latter are often useful in reducing analgesic requirements and improving the quality of pain relief. These can be given parenterally (IV or IM ketorolac), rectally (diclofenac, paracetamol in children) and orally when the patient resumes oral intake.

The newer selective cyclooxygenase-2 or COX-2 inhibitors (rofecoxib, celecoxib, parecoxib) have comparatively fewer gastrointestinal and haematological side-effects. However, deterioration of renal function continues to be of concern even in the COX-2 inhibitors, and any preoperative evidence of renal dysfunction should preclude their use at least until further evidence appears. Rofecoxib has been withdrawn from the market worldwide following reports of increased relative risk for confirmed cardiovascular events such as myocardial infarction, sudden cardiac death and stroke. The safety of other COX-2 inhibitors awaits further study.

Common APS techniques include epidural analgesia, intravenous patient-controlled analgesia (ivPCA), regional blocks and subcutaneous morphine. Selection of technique is influenced by the site and extent of surgery, the patient's age, general health status, education level, ability to cooperate and follow instructions, and practical issues such as the availability of PCA pumps and infusion devices. For example, the epidural technique is unsuitable for head and neck surgery while the PCA technique is unsuitable for those who are unable or unwilling to follow instructions on PCA use.

Other routes of analgesic administration include continuous subcutaneous infiltration of local anaesthetic, intranasal and transdermal fentanyl (transdermal patch or even a fentanyl patient-controlled transdermal system). These techniques are still being developed and are not widely available as yet.

1. **Epidural Analgesia**

Epidural analgesia is useful following major abdominal, thoracic, vascular and orthopaedic surgery. In addition to its analgesic effects, epidural analgesia may decrease the incidence of deep vein thrombosis following orthopaedic surgery and improve lower limb circulation following vascular surgery. A combination of local anaesthetic and opioid is frequently used because the two drugs act synergistically to improve analgesic efficacy and reduce incidence of side-effects.

Many hospital pharmacies provide premixed syringes prepared under sterile conditions. These are preferred to diluting and mixing the epidural solutions in OT or in the ward. Usual epidural infusion regimen consists of bupivacaine 0.1% with fentanyl 2 µg/ml, infusion at 5–12 ml/hr for lumbar epidural or 3–8 ml/hr for thoracic epidural.

Alternatives to epidural bupivacaine/fentanyl infusion include:

— 0.1% ropivacaine with 2 μg/ml fentanyl.
— Plain bupivacaine 0.125%.
— Opioid-only solution, e.g., pethidine 2 mg/ml, given by continuous infusion at 5–8 ml/hr, or bolus doses of pethidine 50 mg (5 mg/ml) every 4-hourly.

Patient-controlled epidural analgesia may be used instead of continuous infusion or intermittent bolus doses. This is the usual regimen.

— Solution: bupivacaine 0.1% with fentanyl 2 μg/ml.
— PCEA bolus: 5 ml.
— Lockout interval: 10–15 minutes.
— Background infusion: 5 ml/hr.
— 4-hour limit: usually not set since this is limited by the lockout interval itself.

2. Intravenous Patient-Controlled Analgesia

Suitable patients for ivPCA should be identified and briefed about this technique of analgesia, ideally during the premedication visit. The information can be reinforced in the OT before induction of anaesthesia. The patient is further instructed in the postoperative period when the PCA machine is set up and ready for use. The anaesthesiologist or APS nurse should ensure that the patient understands the instruction and uses it correctly. It should be emphasized to the patient that nobody else should activate the demand bolus on the PCA.

Prior to commencement of PCA, ensure that the patient has reasonably adequate analgesia by administering IV bolus doses of an opioid if necessary, titrating to effect. It is desirable to have a separate, dedicated intravenous cannula for PCA. If sharing is unavoidable due to limited venous access, an antireflux valve should be fitted to the fluid infusion tubing to prevent accumulation of the opioid there should the intravenous cannula become blocked.

Morphine is the drug of choice for ivPCA. The usual settings for PCA morphine are:

— Concentration: 1 mg/ml.
— PCA bolus: 1 mg (1 ml), or 0.5 mg (0.5 ml) for patients > 60 years.
— lockout interval: 5 minutes.
— background infusion: usually none.
— 4-hour limit: usually not set since this is limited by the lockout interval itself.

Patients with significant renal impairment require special attention since opioids have prolonged duration of action in such patients. The lockout interval should be extended to 10–15 minutes and the patients should be closely monitored for risks of oversedation, respiratory depression and oxygen desaturation.

Pethidine may be used in place of morphine, the equivalent dose being 10 mg pethidine for 1 mg morphine. Prolonged usage is not advisable as norpethidine (active metabolite of pethidine) may accumulate and cause toxicity manifested as convulsions.

Nausea and vomiting associated with ivPCA can be troublesome and distressing to some patients. An antiemetic may be prescribed on a regular basis, or given concomitantly with intravenous PCA morphine (2.5 mg of droperidol added to 10 mg of morphine in PCA pump).

Monitoring for patients on ivPCA should include checking the PCA pump for amount of drug delivery. Most PCA machines incorporate the drug history function in terms of total drug used, number of demands and number of successful delivery. If the number of demands far exceeds drug delivery, it is possible that the patient does not understand the proper usage of the demand button and needs further explanation and instruction, or the PCA settings may be inappropriate for the patient's analgesic requirements.

3. Peripheral Nerve Blocks

The benefits of peripheral nerve blocks can be extended to the postoperative period with the catheter technique, for example, in brachial plexus, sciatic, femoral and intrapleural blocks. Continuous infusion technique similar to epidural analgesia is utilized, typically with 0.2% ropivacaine or 0.125% bupivacaine at a rate of 5–10 ml/hr. Patient-controlled analgesia can be used instead of continuous infusion, with a bolus dose of 3–5 ml, lockout interval 30 minutes and background infusion rate of 5 ml/hr. Unlike central neuraxial blockade where opioids act on the opioid receptors in the substantia gelatinosa, opioids are not useful in peripheral nerve blocks.

The insertion site should be regularly inspected for erythema and swelling. The extent of motor and sensory blockade should also be documented. If the patient complains of breakthrough pain, the extent of blockade should be checked first, followed by injecting a bolus of local anaesthetic (e.g., 10–15 ml of 0.5% ropivacaine) to reactivate the catheter. Note that analgesia is unlikely to improve only by increasing the infusion rate alone. If the bolus dose fails to result in blockade after 30 minutes, the catheter could have migrated and should be removed. An alternative pain management technique, such as ivPCA, should be offered instead.

4. Subcutaneous Morphine

This is a cheap and simple means of achieving reasonable postoperative analgesia even though absorption is not as reliable as the intravenous or epidural routes. An indwelling catheter (e.g., 25G "butterfly" needle) is placed subcutaneously just below the clavicle. The deadspace of the tubing is primed with undiluted morphine and a stopper is attached to its end. The catheter is covered with a transparent dressing so that the insertion site can be inspected for swelling, redness or infection.

The recommended dose of morphine is 5–10 mg 4-hourly for patients between 18–60 years, and 2.5–5 mg 4-hourly for patients above 60 years. Undiluted morphine is injected slowly to lessen the likelihood of pain on injection. As the needle has been primed with morphine, the needle should not be flushed with saline either before or after drug administration.

The first dose of subcutaneous morphine can be administered in PACU if the patient complains of pain. However, if the patient is in severe pain, intravenous bolus doses of opioid (fentanyl, pethidine) should be given to achieve rapid pain relief.

MONITORING

These parameters should be monitored.

- BP, pulse rate, respiratory rate.
- Pain score* at rest and on movement or coughing.
- Sedation score**.
- Side-effects: nausea, vomiting, pruritus, urinary retention, motor block.

*Pain assessment can be done in various ways.

- Verbal rating scale: 0 = no pain; 1 = slight pain; 2 = moderate pain; 3 = severe pain; 4 = worst pain imaginable.
- Numerical rating scale: scoring between 0 and 10, where 0 = no pain and 10 = worst pain imaginable.
- Visual analogue scale (VAS): the patient is asked to score on a 10-cm line with "no pain" at one end and "worst pain ever" at the other end; this is then measured by the observer to give a score of 0–10 or 0–100.

**Sedation score: 0 = none (awake, alert); 1 = mild (dozing intermittently); 2 = moderate (frequently drowsy, easily arousable); 3 = severe (difficult to arouse); S = sleeping.

Initial monitoring is done every hour for 4 hours, and subsequently every 4 hours if the patient is stable. Repeat the same if a bolus dose has been administered. The insertion site of catheter or intravenous cannula should be regularly inspected for redness or swelling, to rule out problems of inflammation and extravasation respectively.

The ward staff should be instructed to contact the APS team if this occurs.

- Inadequate pain relief.
- Sedation score of 3.
- Respiratory rate < 10/min.
- Hypotension: systolic BP < 100 mmHg or > 20% reduction in the normal BP.
- Excessive nausea, vomiting, pruritus.
- High sensory block, unilateral numbness or excessive motor block in patients receiving epidural analgesia.

Oxygen and naloxone should be available in the ward. A good practice is to attach an ampoule of naloxone to the infusion pump or PCA machine so that one does not have to search for the drug during an emergency.

COMPLICATIONS

If any of these complications occur, some resuscitative measures may be necessary while attempts are made to contact the APS team.

1. **Hypoventilation and/or oversedation**
   - Stop epidural infusion or PCA.
   - Check pupil size and conscious level.
   - Administer oxygen by mask, assist ventilation via self-inflating bag and face mask if necessary.
   - Administer IV naloxone 0.1 mg bolus doses up to 0.4 mg until the patient's condition improves.

2. **Nausea and/or vomiting**
   - Administer antiemetics: IV ondansetron 1 mg, IV or IM metoclopramide 10 mg or IV droperidol 1.25–2.5 mg.
   - Prescribe antiemetic to be administered on a regular basis.

3. **Pruritus**
   - Most patients require nothing further than reassurance.
   - Antihistamine may be useful in some patients but may cause increased sedation.
   - If pruritus is troublesome, a small dose of IV naloxone 0.05–0.1 mg can be administered but this runs the risk of reversing the analgesic effect of the opioid.
   - Consider switching to pethidine instead. The incidence of pruritus is lower with pethidine than morphine.

4. **Hypotension**
   - Quick assessment of the patient's general status: re-check BP, feel for peripheral pulses, check CVP if available.
   - Establish and treat the likely cause of hypotension, such as hypovolaemia due to bleeding or fluid restriction, myocardial event and sepsis.
   - If high epidural block is suspected
     - Check the level of sensory and motor blockade.
     - Stop the epidural infusion.
     - Infuse 200 ml of Ringer's lactate solution then reassess.
     - Administer bolus doses of ephedrine 5–10 mg each dose.
     - Consider migration of epidural catheter into the subdural or subarachnoid space.
   - If you are satisfied that the epidural catheter is correctly sited and the BP has returned to normal after resuscitation, you may re-commence epidural infusion at a lower rate.
   - If there is any doubt about the correct placement of the epidural catheter, it would be wiser to remove the catheter and utilize other means of analgesia.

5. **Excessive sensory or motor block**
   - Establish the extent and level of sensory and motor block.
   - Consider the possibility of epidural catheter migration into the subdural or subarachnoid space.
   - Observe the patient for hypotension or respiratory difficulty; take resuscitative measures if necessary.
   - Administer oxygen; closely monitor BP, pulse rate, SpO_2, respiratory rate, sedation and pain scores. Observe for regression of sensory or motor block.
   - Stop the epidural infusion and use an alternative means of pain relief.

6. **Urinary retention**
   - This usually does not warrant termination of epidural analgesia especially if the patient derives excellent pain relief from the technique.
   - Look for other causes of urinary retention and treat accordingly.
   - Encourage the patient to void. If unsuccessful and in the presence of a full bladder, perform bladder catheterization (either in-and-out or continuous bladder drainage).

7. **Inadequate pain relief**
   - Ensure that the drug has been delivered to the patient.
     - Check insertion site for swelling to indicate drug extravasation to the subcutaneous tissue.
     - Check marking on the epidural catheter at skin to exclude catheter migration.
     - Check the integrity of the infusion tubing to rule out disconnection, occlusion or kinking.
     - Ensure that the infusion devices are in good working order; check that an appropriate amount of drug remains in the syringe.
   - Administer a bolus dose of an appropriate drug and volume. Mechanical causes of kinking or occlusion are ruled out if the drug can be injected easily.
   - Observe the patient for evidence of pain relief, and give additional doses if necessary until the patient is comfortable. Review and modify the dose regimen if necessary.
   - Consider the use of NSAIDs in suitable patients.
     - Oral naproxen, etoricoxib, celecoxib, meloxicam.
     - Or rectal diclofenac if oral intake has not been re-established.
   - Consider alternative means of analgesia if there is no pain relief after a sufficient amount of drug has been given and sufficient time has elapsed.

The APS coverage for postoperative patients usually lasts for 72 hours. By then most patients would have re-commenced oral intake and would have been prescribed some form of oral analgesic. Ill patients and those recovering from bowel surgery will require a longer period of APS management. There should be a period of overlap between starting oral analgesic and terminating APS treatment to ensure that the postoperative pain management is optimal.

FURTHER READING

1. Werner MU, Soholm L, Rotboll-Nielsen P, Kehlet H. Does an acute pain service improve postoperative outcome? Anesth Analg 2002;95:1361–72.
2. Kehlet H, Holte K. Effect of postoperative analgesia on surgical outcome. Br J Anaesth 2001;87:62–72.
3. Joshi GP, White PF. Management of acute and postoperative pain. Curr Opin Anaesthesiol 2001;14:417–21.
4. Wheatley RG, Schug SA, Watson D. Safety and efficacy of postoperative epidural analgesia. Br J Anaesth 2001;87:47–61.
5. Moiniche S, Kehlet H, Dahl JB. A qualitative and quantitative systematic review of preemptive analgesia for postoperative pain relief. Anesthesiology 2002;96:725–41.
6. Kissin I. Preemptive analgesia. Anesthesiology 2000;93:1138–43.
7. McCrory CR, Lindahl SGE. Cyclooxygenase inhibition for postoperative analgesia. Anesth Analg 2002;95:169–76.
8. Buttar NS, Wang KK. The "aspirin" of the new millennium: Cyclooxygenase-2 inhibitors. Mayo Clin Proc 2000;75:1027–38.
9. Gilron I, Milne B, Hong M. Cyclooxygenase-2 inhibitors in postoperative pain management: Current evidence and future directions. Anesthesiology 2003; 99:1198–1208.
10. Romsing J, Moiniche S. A systematic review of COX-2 inhibitors compared with traditional NSAIDs, or different COX-2 inhibitors for post-operative pain. Acta Anaesthesiol Scand 2004;48:525–46.

Chapter 59
Chronic Pain Management

INTRODUCTION

Chronic pain management is a specialized field that is involved in the treatment of pain and its related problems. The chronic pain conditions may be oncologic or non-oncologic, both of which should be taken seriously as the non-oncologic pain may be no less severe or debilitating to the patient.

While acute pain conditions are usually straightforward and fairly easy to manage, it may not be the case in chronic pain management. It is essential to understand the pathophysiology of the underlying pain process and the psychological overtones in order to appropriately manage the chronic pain condition. Optimal management of such patients requires a multi-disciplinary approach that may involve some or all of these specialists: the primary care physician, anaesthesiologist, psychiatrist, neurologist, orthopaedic surgeon, oncologist, physiotherapist, occupational therapist and social worker.

Chronic pain management is a highly specialized field in anaesthesiology. Some basic principles and available treatment options will be outlined here.

TERMINOLOGY

— *Pain* is defined as an unpleasant sensory and emotional experience associated with the actual or potential tissue damage.
— *Acute pain* is pain following injury to the body, which generally disappears when the healing process is complete. It is often associated with objective physical signs and symptoms of autonomic system activity such as sweating, tachycardia and nausea.
— *Chronic pain* is pain which persists past the time when healing is expected to be complete. Time frame for healing varies for different disease conditions but is usually between 1 to 6 months. Chronic pain may be associated with depression and changes in personality, lifestyle and functional abilities.

PATHOPHYSIOLOGY

Pain may be classified as:

— **Nociceptive pain:** pain produced by activation of normal pain fibres. It may be either somatic (e.g., back pain) or visceral (e.g., chronic pancreatitis).
— **Neuropathic pain:** pain resulting from abnormalities in, or damage to, the nervous system. Examples include postherpetic neuralgia ("shingles"), reflex sympathetic dystrophy, phantom limb pain, central poststroke pain, tic doloureux.
— **Psycho-behavioural pain:** pain resulting from anxiety, depression, neurosis, hysteria and communicated in behaviour such as limping, grimacing, complaining, going to doctors or reluctance to work.

Chronic pain is often a complex multi-dimensional problem. Sometimes 2 or even all 3 of the abovementioned components may be seen in a single patient.

TYPES OF CHRONIC PAIN

- *Cancer pain* is associated with the underlying malignancy. Pain may result from local tumour infiltration, widespread metastases to bones and pleura or nerve entrapment and compression.
- *Benign chronic pain* is non-oncologic in nature. Examples include:
    - Herpes zoster neuralgia.
    - Trigeminal neuralgia.
    - Chronic postsurgical pain.
    - Complex regional pain syndrome.
    - Phantom limb pain.
    - Low back pain.
    - Primary fibromyalgia.
    - Intermittent claudication or pain of ischaemic origin.
- *Chronic postsurgical pain* is said to occur when these criteria are satisfied.
    - The pain developed after a surgical operation.
    - The pain is of at least 2 months' duration.
    - Other causes for the pain have been excluded (e.g., continuing malignancy or chronic infection).
    - The possibility that the pain is continuing from a preexisting problem must be explored and excluded.
- *Complex regional pain syndrome* is a disorder characterized by pain and dysfunction of the sympathetic nervous system. It encompasses a great heterogeneity of symptoms. Diagnostic criteria defined by the International Association for the Study of Pain (IASP) include:
    - The presence of an initiating noxious event or cause of immobilization (not present in 5–10% of patients).
    - Continuing pain, allodynia or hyperalgesia in which the pain is disproportionate to any known inciting event.
    - Evidence at some time of oedema, changes in skin blood flow or abnormal sudomotor activity in the region of pain.
- Note that the presence of other conditions to account for the degree of pain and dysfunction would exclude the diagnosis of complex regional pain syndrome.

MANAGEMENT OF CHRONIC PAIN

This is a vast field and is beyond the scope of the manual. Interested readers are advised to refer to textbooks and recent journals on this topic.

General Principles of Management

— No blanket ruling is applicable for all patients as individualization is essential and desirable.

— A multi-disciplinary team approach is again emphasized.

— The patient should be thoroughly investigated to exclude conditions that may be medically or surgically treatable. This will be more effective than symptomatic relief of pain alone.

— A combination of treatment modalities – e.g., use of analgesics, adjuvant drugs and physiotherapy – usually works better than a single treatment modality.

Treatment may be pharmacological or non-pharmacological. Available treatment options are listed here.

— **Pharmacological**
- Opioids.
- Non-steroidal antiinflammatory drugs (NSAIDs).
- Steroids.
- Psychoactive drugs for adjuvant therapy: antidepressants, anxiolytics, sedatives, anticonvulsants.
- Local anaesthetic: individual nerve blocks, sympathetic blocks, epidural, spinal.
- Intrathecal clonidine.
- Guanethidine, reserpine in intravenous regional anaesthesia (IVRA).
- Neurolytics such as phenol, absolute alcohol.

— **Non-pharmacological**
- Transcutaneous electrical nerve stimulation (TENS).
- Biofeedback.
- Trigger point injection.
- Acupuncture, acupressure.
- Infrared, ultrasound therapy.
- Cryotherapy.
- Hypnosis, relaxation exercises.
- Physiotherapy for rehabilitation programmes, strengthening exercises.
- Surgery.

OPIOIDS

Treatment with opioids will be elaborated further since this is the mode of therapy most frequently encountered. Commonly used drugs are morphine or its derivatives, such as codeine, dihydrocodeine, pethidine and methadone.

Principles of Treatment

— Individualize dose and route of administration of opioids
  - Various routes of administration are available but some are not suitable for outpatients. The most suitable route of administration for the patient should be selected.
    — Oral: the most convenient and well-accepted route, with morphine available in syrup and slow release formulations.
    — Parenteral: intramuscular; subcutaneous; intravenous (bolus doses, infusion or patient-controlled analgesia).
    — Rectal.
    — Intrathecal, epidural.
    — Transdermal (for fentanyl).
  - Note that the optimal analgesic dose varies widely among patients and even in the same patient during different stages of the disease.

— Give each analgesic an adequate trial by dose titration before abandoning the drug and switching to another drug. Do not use placebo to assess the nature of pain.

— Administer the drug regularly to achieve steady drug plasma levels. Do not administer on PRN basis to avoid the "peak and trough" effect, i.e., periods of possible overdosage alternating with underdosage.

— Be familiar with the dose and time-course of several strong opioids. Note that the patient may respond differently to different opioids.

— Recognize and treat opioid side-effects, e.g., sedation, nausea and/or vomiting, respiratory depression, constipation.

— Watch for *tolerance*, manifested by an increased dose requirement to maintain the original analgesic effect. This is usually associated with physical dependence. Steps to delay development of tolerance include the use of combination of opioids and non-opioids; and switching to an alternative opioid since there may be incomplete cross tolerance.

— *Physical dependence* is said to occur when abrupt cessation of treatment leads to withdrawal syndrome. This is an expected occurrence in the presence of continuous use of opioids and does not necessarily imply addiction. Signs and symptoms include anxiety, irritability, salivation, lacrimation, rhinorrhoea, sweating, piloerection ("goose bumps"), chills and hot flushes, nausea, vomiting, abdominal cramps.

— *Psychological dependence or addiction* refers to the pattern of compulsive drug use where there is continued craving for an opioid and the need to use the opioid for effects other than pain relief, such as mood elevation and euphoria. This may be associated with drug-seeking behaviour.

— Most patients develop some tolerance and physical dependence but risk of iatrogenic addiction is small. Opioids should *not* be withheld from patients, particularly from terminally ill cancer patients, for fear of inducing addiction.

FURTHER READING

1. Macrae WA. Chronic pain after surgery. Br J Anaesth 2001;87:88–98.
2. Harden RN. Complex regional pain syndrome. Br J Anaesth 2001;87:99–106.
3. Nikolajsen L, Jensen TS. Phantom limb pain. Br J Anaesth 2001;87:107–16.
4. Collett BJ. Chronic opioid therapy for non-cancer pain. Br J Anaesth 2001;87:133–43.
5. Eccleston C. Role of psychology in pain management. Br J Anaesth 2001;87:144–52.
6. Gralow I. Cancer pain: An update of pharmacological approaches in pain therapy. Curr Opin Anaesthesiol 2002;15:555–61.
7. Nurmikko TJ, Eldridge PR. Trigeminal neuralgia – pathophysiology, diagnosis and current treatment. Br J Anaesth 2001;87:117–32.

Chapter 60

Quality Assurance in Anaesthesia

DEFINITIONS

Quality of anaesthetic care can be defined as the degree to which patient care services increase the probability of desired patient outcome and reduce the probability of undesired outcome, given the current state of knowledge.

Quality assurance (QA) is an audit process in which the existing system of patient care services is studied, and through which recommendations are made to achieve or further improve quality of care.

There are three main areas of QA studies, namely mortality review, critical incident reporting or morbidity review, and morbidity and mortality case presentations. These are further elaborated below.

MORTALITY REVIEW

Mortality reviews study cases with a definite end-point – death – and the circumstances leading to it, whether any preventive measures or modifications in management could have averted the outcome. Examples of mortality reviews include:

— Confidential Enquiry into Maternal and Child Health (CEMACH) in the UK, which encompasses deaths in expectant mothers and children up to the age of 16 years.
— National Confidential Enquiry into Patient Outcome and Death (NCEPOD) in the UK.
— Perioperative Mortality Review (POMR) in Malaysia.
— American Society of Anesthesiologists (ASA) Closed Claims Project for both mortality and morbidity reviews.
— Anaesthesia-related Mortality Review in Australia: triennial reports since 1985, coordinated by the Australian and New Zealand College of Anaesthetists (ANZCA).

Confidential Enquiry into Maternal and Child Health (CEMACH)

The Confidential Enquiries into Maternal Deaths (CEMD), started in 1952, is a triennial report on maternal mortality in the UK. In the report, maternal death is defined as "the death of a woman while pregnant or within 42 days of termination of pregnancy, from any cause related to or aggravated by the pregnancy or its management, but not from accidental or incidental causes". Deaths are further subdivided into direct, indirect, late and fortuitous, each with its specific definition that is elaborated in the report.

Maternal mortality has decreased dramatically over the decades as a result of improved obstetric and anaesthetic care. Among the anaesthesia-related deaths, the leading causes identified include failed intubation leading to hypoxia and/or aspiration of gastric contents in general anaesthesia, and local anaesthetic overdose in regional anaesthesia. The consistent finding in the majority of these triennial reports has been the fact that general anaesthesia is associated with a higher risk of mortality compared to regional anaesthesia. This same conclusion was arrived at in an audit report on anaesthesia-related deaths during obstetric delivery in the US.

In 2003 the mortality reviews for maternal deaths, stillbirths and deaths in infancy were merged as part of a strategy for the development of the national confidential enquiries in the UK. These are now known as the Confidential Enquiry into Maternal and Child Health (CEMACH) and this includes mortality in children up to 16 years of age.

National Confidential Enquiry into Patient Outcome and Death (NCEPOD)

National Confidential Enquiry into Patient Outcome and Death is another form of mortality review carried out in the UK. NCEPOD, the organization responsible for the audit, operates under the umbrella of the National Institute of Clinical Excellence (NICE) as an independent confidential enquiry. Through this organization, medical clinical practices are reviewed by means of confidential surveys, and evidence-based recommendations are made with the aim to improve the quality and safety of patient care.

Its precursor, the National Confidential Enquiry into Perioperative Deaths, was established in 1988 and its first report was published in 1990. Sixteen reports have been published by NCEPOD on various aspects of health care in the UK. Samples for study have ranged from a percentage of all deaths within 30 days of surgery, to those deaths within a specific age range or specific procedures. The 2004 report "Scoping Our Practice" focused on inpatient deaths occurring within 30 days of interventional gastrointestinal endoscopy.

Perioperative Mortality Review (POMR)

This form of mortality reporting, started in 1992, is an on-going project undertaken by the Ministry of Health of Malaysia. It involves confidential voluntary reporting of all deaths associated with surgical intervention. Initially the time period studied covered 7 postoperative days; it has now been extended to include deaths that occur during or after surgery within the duration of hospital stay.

This project aims to audit the quality of surgically related health services provided by the Ministry of Health. The areas of emphasis include:

- Operating facilities.
- Anaesthetic expertise.
- Availability of HDU/ICU.
- Supportive facilities such as radiology, laboratory, Blood Bank services.

Both surgeons and anaesthesiologists are required to complete the POMR report after a perioperative death has occurred. This is then forwarded to the POMR Committee, which comprises consultant surgeons, gynaecologists and anaesthesiologists. Two independent assessors from the Committee assess the report. Based on the expert opinion, final decisions and recommendations are made at the Committee meeting.

Deaths are classified under 6 categories.

Category 1: Anaesthesia is the main contributory factor.

Category 2: Death is due to both anaesthetic and surgical factors.

Category 3: Surgery is the main contributory factor.

Category 4A: High-risk death where management was substandard.

Category 4B: High-risk death where management was satisfactory.

Category 5: Unexpected deaths where patient was expected to make a full recovery, for example, postoperative myocardial infarction.

Category 6: Causes cannot be ascertained either due to insufficient data or otherwise.

MORBIDITY REVIEW

Morbidity in anaesthesia can be classified into 3 groups:

— *Minor:* the problem causes moderate distress but no prolongation of hospital stay or permanent sequelae.

— *Intermediate:* the problem causes serious distress or prolongation of hospital stay, or both, but no permanent sequelae.

— *Major:* the problem causes permanent disability or disfigurement.

Contrary to death as the definite end-point in mortality studies, morbidity reviews are hampered by lack of clear definition as to what constitutes morbidity in anaesthesia. Some cases are simply not reported because these are felt by the anaesthesiologists involved to be "too trivial" for reporting.

Reporting of morbidity cases is usually carried out in a confidential and voluntary manner rather than by compulsion. However, despite repeated assurances of anonymity and confidentiality, fears of medico-legal consequences or punitive measures are certainly factors that contribute to underreporting of cases. If the extent of underreporting is significant, the whole study process would be an exercise in futility as any conclusion or recommendation derived therein would be meaningless.

Incident Reporting in Anaesthesia

A critical incident is defined as any untoward event that causes, or has the potential to cause, life-threatening injury or permanent disability to the patient. The incident may or may not be preventable.

The aims of critical incident reporting are manifold. Assessment of such reports may be used for these purposes.

1. **Educational purpose**
   - Cases can be presented to colleagues in morbidity reviews held at regular intervals in the Department of Anaesthesia.
   - Relevant historical reports can be retrieved and reviewed to combine a single case report into a series of case studies.

2. **Documentation of rare conditions**
   - Examples of such conditions include atypical pseudocholinesterase, malignant hyperthermia, halothane hepatitis, anaphylaxis, rare congenital syndromes.
   - This may be of great relevance if the same patient, or, in the case of an inheritable condition, if a member of the patient's family presents for anaesthesia.

3. **Identification of causes of critical incidents and development of preventative clinical strategies**
   - Clinical strategies were developed as a result of morbidity reports associated with the conditions. These were then modified and adopted as standard anaesthetic practice over the years.
   - Examples include fluid preloading prior to central neuraxial blockade, preoxygenation for patients at risk of difficult intubation and cricoid pressure for patients at risk of gastric aspiration.

4. **Monitoring and management of complications**
   - Complications such as inadvertent dural puncture or difficult intubation can be identified, their incidence established and relevant management protocols developed.

5. **Use in decision-making analysis**
   - Incident reporting forms the basis of decision-making for staffing and facilities.
   - Examples include allocation of different categories of staff in various locations of patient care, appropriate training of medical, nursing and paramedic personnel, purchase and allocation of new anaesthetic and monitoring equipment, establishment of anaesthesia-based services such as Acute Pain Service.

Anesthetic Incident Monitoring

An example for anaesthetic incident reporting is the Australian Anaesthetic Incident Monitoring Study (AIMS) started in 1987 by the Australian Patient Safety Foundation. The study is designed to find out the nature of the incident ("*What happened*" – equipment, pharmacological or airway problems), factors contributing and minimizing the incident ("*Why it happened*"), and any suggested corrective strategies that the respondent feels is necessary. Collected data includes the patient age group, ASA status, procedure category, anaesthetic technique, monitors in use, time, place and phase of anaesthesia when the incident occurred, as well as the outcome of the incident (both immediate and long term).

Airway problems constitute the largest proportion of incidents reported. These include problems concerning proper placement of endotracheal tube (difficult, failed, endobronchial or oesophageal intubation), non-ventilation (obstruction due to bronchospasm, blood, secretion or vomitus) and problems associated with the endotracheal tube (kinking, disconnection, accidental extubation).

Pharmacological incidents include allergic phenomenon, side-effect, under- or overdosage of drug, wrong drug administration, inappropriate drug, drug interaction or contamination.

Equipment incidents are mainly due to breathing system problems such as leak, disconnection, misconnection, rebreathing and overpressure. Problems involving other equipment used in airway management and conduct of anaesthesia are also reported.

As in other incident reports, human error is found to be the commonest factor attributed to anaesthetic incidents. A host of factors have been identified; these include distraction or inattention, fatigue or illness, lack of training, fault of anaesthetic technique, error of judgement, haste, pressure to proceed and failure to check equipment before proceeding with the case. Other reasons include inadequate assistance or supervision, lack of communication between the surgeon and anaesthesiologist, and inadequate preoperative assessment and/or preparation of patient. There are also other causes such as lack of monitor or problem with monitor, failure of facility or equipment, unfamiliar equipment or environment, sick patient or contribution by the surgical team.

Factors thought to minimize the severity and duration of incident include initial detection of the incident by monitor (pulse oximeter, in particular, has been found to be useful), healthy patient, high awareness via QA activity, prior experience or training, skilled assistance and supervision, and detection of equipment malfunction by re-checking.

Selected cases can be discussed during department meetings as a form of QA exercise, and findings from the study can be analyzed and presented on a regular basis.

MORBIDITY AND MORTALITY CASE PRESENTATION

This is another form of QA activity that is beneficial to all concerned. Cases that result in morbidity or mortality can be collected and presented during Department of Anaesthesia meetings at regular intervals.

The M&M presentations should be conducted in a non-threatening, non-punitive manner. The aims of these sessions are to analyze the circumstances leading to adverse outcomes, look for possible preventive measures and discuss how these problems can be recognized and properly managed in future.

If properly conducted, M&M presentations can serve as a powerful learning tool because such "real life" experiences tend to be better remembered than knowledge gathered from books or journals. Such sessions should never be turned into "witch-hunts", as it defeats the purpose of learning and open discussion if the person involved in the case is bombarded and humiliated in front of his/her colleagues.

CLINICAL PRACTICE GUIDELINES

Clinical practice guidelines are systematically developed statements that assist in decision-making about appropriate health care for specific clinical situations. These are based on scientific evidence of the effectiveness of healthcare interventions, and in the absence of such evidence are supplemented by expert opinion. Recommendations are made based on the best evidence among all available information.

However, not all institutions adopt the key elements recommended in the guidelines, while some physicians and anaesthesiologists may not wish to comply with the recommendations. Therefore, although the evidence supporting most guideline recommendations is impressive, the impact that these guidelines have on anaesthesia safety and quality remains unknown. Specific protocol developments, taking into account the characteristics and constraints of a particular institution, may result in better compliance and hence greater effectiveness.

PROTOCOLS

Protocols are developed to address specific problems and to ensure that steps are taken in a logical sequence for diagnosis and management purposes. The anaesthesiologist should be familiar with the protocols, so that when actual problems arise precious time is not wasted in trying to figure out what the next step in the management sequence should be. Familiarity also instils confidence so that the anaesthesiologist is in control of the crisis situation and is able to make clear-headed, logical decisions. Examples of protocols include the American Heart Association (AHA) Emergency Cardiac Care Committee for cardiac arrest situations, the ASA practice guidelines for difficult airway management, failed intubation protocol in caesarean section and crisis management protocol "COVER ABCD – A SWIFT CHECK".

"COVER ABCD – A SWIFT CHECK" is a mnemonic system presented in a study coordinated by the Australian Patient Safety Foundation. The first part – "COVER ABCD" – covers 95% of the incidents, 3% of which are cardiac arrests. This should be memorized so that actions can be carried out quickly and thoroughly. The second part – "A SWIFT CHECK" – handles the remaining 5% of the incidents. It calls for a quick review based on a checklist that does not have to be memorized.

C **C**irculation and Colour (saturation)
O **O**xygen Supply and Oxygen Analyzer
V **V**entilation (intubated patient) and Vaporizers
E **E**ndotracheal Tube and Eliminate Machine
R **R**eview Monitors and Review Equipment

A **A**irway (with face mask or laryngeal mask)
B **B**reathing (with spontaneous ventilation)
C **C**irculation (in more detail than above)
D **D**rugs (consider all given or not given)

A Be **A**ware of **A**ir and **A**llergy

SWIFT CHECK of patient, surgeon, process and responses.

WAYS TO REDUCE ANAESTHETIC INCIDENTS

Based on the morbidity and mortality reports, ways to reduce anaesthetic incidents or accidents would necessarily be numerous and diverse. Here is a list.

1. **Equipment**
    — Thorough checking of anaesthetic, airway and resuscitation equipment at the start of each anaesthesia session.
    — Quick abbreviated check immediately before commencement of each anaesthetic.

— Regular servicing and maintenance.
— Improvement in equipment design based on feedback from end-users.
— Conduct of procedures at appropriate areas, e.g., cardiac procedures at cardiac-protected areas.

2. **Personnel**
   — Adequate training and supervision of various categories of hospital staff: anaesthesiologists, anaesthetic assistants, nursing staff at PACU, technicians and ward staff particularly in ICU, HDU, A&E Department and surgical ward.
   — Early referral and consultant involvement in management of complex cases.
   — Improvement in work conditions:
     - Adequate number of medical and nursing staff per working shift.
     - Limit working hours to decrease fatigue, as this has been demonstrated to impair vigilance and accuracy of response, and may contribute to adverse events and critical incidents.
   — Back-up facilities and support staff in radiology, laboratory, Blood Bank.

3. **Recognition of risk factors and adequate preoperative preparation**
   — Optimization of medical condition before elective surgery.
   — Proper preoperative assessment and resuscitation in patients presenting for emergency surgery.
   — Multi-disciplinary team approach for difficult and complex cases.
   — Adequate preoperative fasting, with acid aspiration prophylaxis for patients at risk of regurgitation and aspiration of gastric contents.
   — Management plan for patients with potential airway problems, and back-up options if the initial attempt fails.
   — Resuscitation drugs and equipment available and ready for use.

4. **Monitors**
   — Vigilant anaesthesiologist at all times – *most important monitor!*
   — Properly calibrated and functioning equipment.
   — Logical, evidence-based selection of monitoring in specific cases particularly over the use of invasive monitors, which requires consideration of risks versus benefits.
   — Awareness regarding uses, limitations and complications of specific monitors.
   — Monitor alarms with these desirable features.

- Both audio and visual, with distinctive sound that is easily identifiable.
- Default alarm limits which can be adjusted for individual cases.
- Presence of silence and disable function, but the alarm should not be permanently disabled.

5. **Good anaesthetic practices**
   - Appropriate dilution of drug and clear labelling of drug syringes.
   - Universal precaution and aseptic technique for all invasive procedures.
   - Appropriate anaesthetic technique based on patient's condition and nature of surgery.
   - Careful titration of anaesthetic drugs to clinical effect, particularly important in elderly, debilitated patients.
   - Anticipation, early recognition and aggressive management of anaesthetic mishaps.

6. **Adequate postoperative care**
   - Particular emphasis on airway management, ventilation, cardiovascular support and acute pain management.
   - Well-trained, experienced staff with adequate monitoring and resuscitation facilities in PACU.
   - Availability of HDU and ICU for perioperative management of high-risk patients.
   - Availability of support staff for postoperative chest physiotherapy and limb exercises; adequate postoperative pain control by the Acute Pain Service.

7. **Continuing medical education**
   - Implementation of audit and QA activities.
   - Morbidity and mortality case discussions.
   - Use of simulator as training aids for airway and crisis management.
   - Clinical practice guidelines and specific protocol development.
   - Regular discussion sessions with surgeons with the aim for improved communication and decision-making.

FURTHER READING

1. Lagasse RS. Indicators of anesthesia safety and quality. Curr Opin Anaesthesiol 2002;15:239–43.

2. Katz RI, Lagasse RS. Factors influencing the reporting of adverse perioperative outcomes to a quality management program. Anesth Analg 2000;90:344–50.

3. Confidential Enquiry into Maternal and Child Health. Why Mothers Die 2000–2002: The Sixth Report of the Confidential Enquiries into Maternal Death in the United Kingdom. London: RCOG Press, 2004.

4. "Scoping Our Practice": The 2004 Report of the National Confidential Enquiry into Patient Outcome and Death. London: NCEPOD, 2004.

5. Fletcher GCL, McGeorge P, Flin RH, Glavin RJ, Maran NJ. The role of non-technical skills in anaesthesia: A review of current literature. Br J Anaesth 2002;88:418–29.

6. Arbous MS, et al. Mortality associated with anaesthesia: A qualitative analysis to identify risk factors. Anaesthesia 2001;56:1141–53.

E

Problems in Anaesthesia

Chapter 61

Common Problems in Anaesthesia

INTRODUCTION

This section deals with some of the common problems encountered in anaesthesia. Although these problems may be regarded as trivial when compared to life-threatening complications such as hypoxaemia or cardiac arrest, they are by no means less distressing to the patient concerned. Some not so common but serious problems (e.g., intraarterial injection of drugs) have been included in this chapter as well.

POSTOPERATIVE NAUSEA AND VOMITING

Postoperative nausea and vomiting (PONV) is one of the most common complications following surgery, with an incidence of 60–70% in high-risk patients. While PONV is rarely fatal, many patients consider it as one of the most unpleasant postoperative symptoms. It can lead to increased time spent in PACU, extended nursing care and unanticipated hospital admission for day surgery patients – all factors resulting in an increase in healthcare costs. Besides causing distress and discomfort to the patient, potential morbidity associated with PONV includes increases in intraocular and intracranial pressures, suture dehiscence, oesophageal rupture, haematoma formation and aspiration pneumonitis.

Strategies for the management of PONV encompass these aspects.

— Identification of patients at risk.
— Reduction in baseline risk factors for PONV.
— Antiemetic therapy for prophylaxis of PONV.
— Treatment of PONV.

Risk Factors for PONV

It is important to identify risk factors for PONV because it is not cost-effective to adopt a policy of universal PONV prophylaxis. This is unlikely to benefit patients at low risk for PONV and would put them at risk from the potential side-effects of antiemetic agents.

These factors are associated with increased risks for PONV.

— **Patient-specific factors**
  - Females and children.
  - Non-smoking status.
  - History of PONV or motion sickness.

— **Anaesthetic factors**
  - Inhalational anaesthesia with the use of volatile anaesthetic agents and nitrous oxide.
  - Intraoperative and postoperative use of opioids.
  - Hypotension and intraoperative dehydration.
  - Gastric dilatation from overzealous mask ventilation.

— **Surgical factors**
  - Duration of surgery: each 30-minute increase in duration increases PONV risk by 60%.

- Nature of surgery: increased risk in laparoscopy, ENT surgery, neurosurgery, breast surgery, strabismus surgery, laparotomy, plastic surgery.

Reduction of Baseline Risk Factors for PONV

— A multi-modal antiPONV approach should be adopted similar to the multi-modal analgesic regimens for acute pain management.

— Preoperative fasting to avoid full stomach in elective cases. However, the hydration status of the patient should be adequate since dehydration itself can promote PONV.

— Selection of anaesthetic agents or techniques
  - Regional anaesthesia instead of general anaesthesia wherever possible.
  - Propofol for induction and maintenance of anaesthesia in the form of total intravenous anaesthesia (TIVA).
  - Avoid emetogenic agents such as nitrous oxide and volatile anaesthetics.
  - Use multi-modal analgesic regimens to minimize the use of opioids: combination of local anaesthetic, non-steroidal antiinflammatory drug (NSAID) and small dose of short-acting opioids.
  - Minimize dose of neostigmine (< 2.5 mg) or omit its use altogether.

— Avoid prolonged mask ventilation to prevent gastric distension. Consider inserting a nasogastric tube to decompress the stomach if this is excessive.

— Prevent hypotension perioperatively.
  - Fluid preloading prior to performing central neuraxial blockade especially subarachnoid block.
  - Aggressive treatment of hypotension with intravenous fluids and/or vasopressor if it occurs.

— At completion of laparoscopic surgery, get the surgeon to release as much carbon dioxide as possible from the peritoneal cavity.

— Gentle handling of the patient during transfer from operating room to PACU. Avoid sudden jolts and changes in position.

Antiemetic Therapy for Prophylaxis of PONV

- Serotonin (5-HT$_3$) receptor antagonists, e.g., ondansetron, granisetron.
  - Adult dose: IV ondansetron 4–8 mg; paediatric dose: ondansetron 50–100 μg/kg up to 4 mg.
  - Greater efficacy in the prevention of vomiting than nausea.
  - Most effective when administered at the end of surgery.
  - Note that a smaller dose is used for treatment of PONV, e.g., ondansetron 1 mg rather than 4–8 mg for prophylaxis.
- Dexamethasone
  - Adult dose: 5–10 mg IV; paediatric dose: 150 μg/kg up to 8 mg.
  - Most effective when administered before induction of anaesthesia.
- Droperidol
  - Adult dose: 0.625–1.25 mg IV; paediatric dose: 50–75 μg/kg up to 1.25 mg.
  - Efficacy is equivalent to ondansetron for PONV prophylaxis with very good effect against nausea.
  - Most effective when administered at the end of surgery.
  - Case reports of prolonged QT interval and cardiac dysrhythmias led to this drug being withdrawn from the market in some countries.
  - May be given concomitantly with intravenous PCA morphine (2.5 mg of droperidol added to 10 mg of morphine in PCA pump).
- Other antiemetics
  - Examples: promethazine, haloperidol, prochlorperazine, transdermal scopolamine.
  - Side-effects include dizziness, dry mouth, sedation.
  - Use of phenothiazines is limited in day-care surgery because of sedation.

Note

- Prophylactic PONV therapy in high-risk patients is more cost-effective than placebo because of the increased costs associated with PONV.
- Metoclopramide is ineffective for PONV prophylaxis.

— Combination therapy using drugs with different mechanisms of action is superior to monotherapy: drug combinations with proven efficacy are 5-HT_3 antagonist plus droperidol and 5-HT_3 antagonist plus dexamethasone. Triple therapy with 5-HT_3 antagonist, droperidol and dexamethasone has also been described for high-risk patients.

Treatment of PONV

— Exclude contributing factors to PONV, for example:
- Drug causes such as concomitant use of opioids (e.g., morphine in PCA).
- Mechanical causes such as blood or secretions at the oropharynx, intestinal obstruction resulting in vomiting.

— Choice of antiemetics depends on prior PONV prophylaxis.
- No prophylaxis: administer small dose of 5-HT_3 antagonist (e.g., ondansetron 1 mg IV).
- Prophylaxis with 5-HT_3 antagonist plus a second agent: administer drug from a different class.
- Triple therapy within 6 hours postsurgery: do not repeat initial therapy. Use alternative drugs: droperidol 0.625 mg IV; dexamethasone 2–4 mg IV or promethazine 12.5 mg IV.
- Triple therapy more than 6 hours after surgery: repeat 5-HT_3 antagonist and droperidol.

Figure 61–1 summarizes the different aspects of management of PONV.

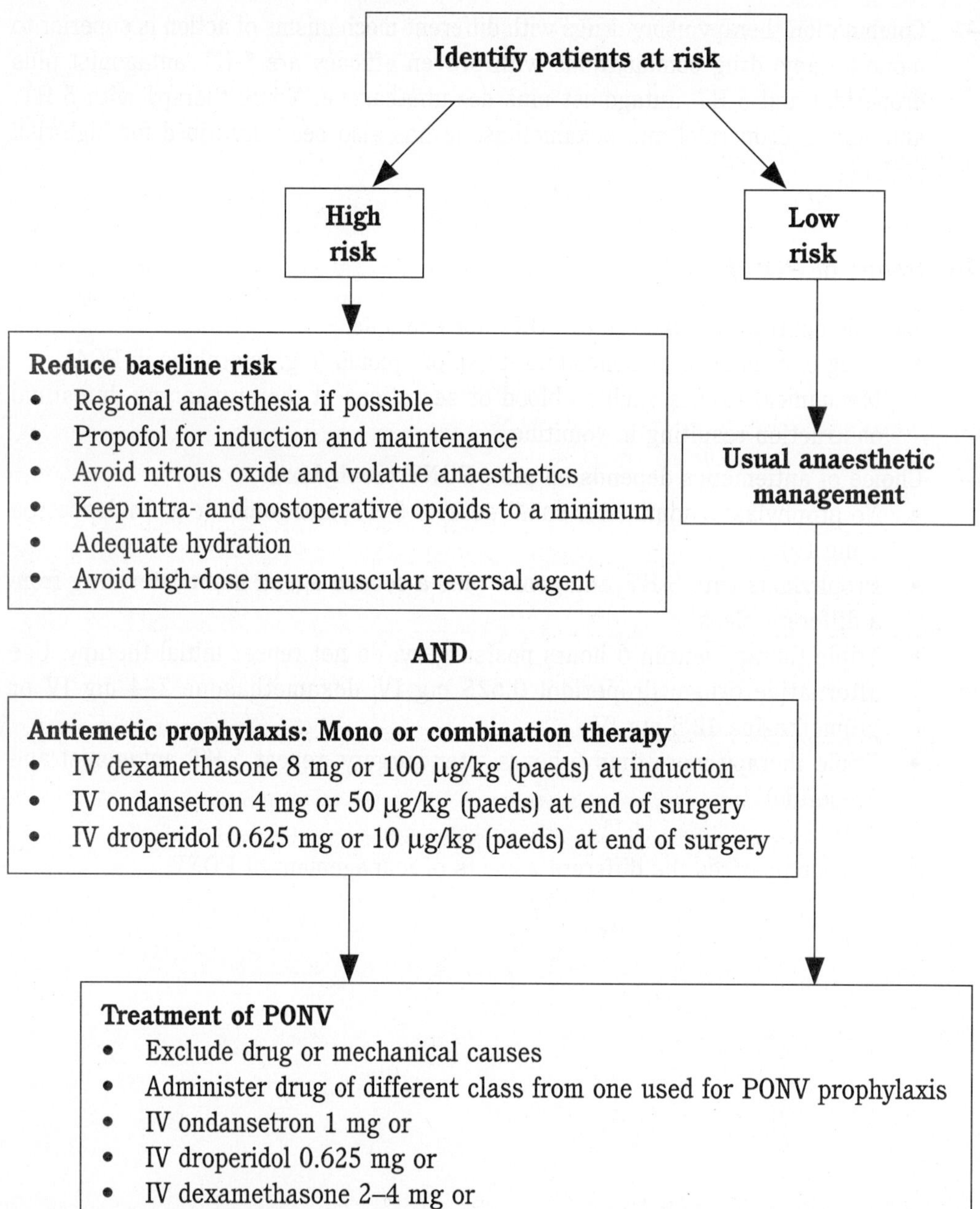

Figure 61–1. Management of postoperative nausea and vomiting

which causes intense chemical arteritis throughout the blood vessel wall resulting in severe ischaemia. Large doses of propofol can lead to transient reduction in blood flow, but limb morbidity remains unlikely and specific management is probably not required.

Prevention

— Prominent labels and colour coding should be displayed on the arterial transducer-infusion system. Do not attach yellow injection ports ("yellow stoppers") on the arterial line 3-way connector in case this is mistaken to be a venous cannula.

— Always verify the correct injection port or intravenous infusion set before injecting the drug.

— Re-site the intravenous cannula if its correct placement is in doubt.

— Administer intravenous drug in small titrating doses and observe for response; ask specifically for any pain experienced.

— It is a good practice to palpate for the radial artery pulse while injecting the drug into an intravenous cannula on the dorsum of the hand.

Signs and Symptoms

— There may be backflow of blood in the infusion tubing even though this is an unreliable sign especially if the patient's perfusion state is compromised.

— The conscious patient complains of intense burning pain that radiates down the area of perfusion by the artery.

— Further changes include these.
  - Distal blanching or blistering of the skin.
  - Absence of arterial pulse.
  - Oedema, hyperaesthesia, motor weakness (within 2 hours).
  - Deep purple discolouration followed by gangrene (late).

Immediate Management

— Stop injection immediately but leave the cannula or needle *in situ.*

— Institute measures to minimize damage by diluting the irritant drug, reverse vasospasm and prevent thrombosis.

— Flush the artery with heparinized saline to dilute the drug.
— Administer 10 ml of 1% lignocaine into the artery to reduce vasospasm and pain.
— Administer drugs with vasodilatory action.
  - Tolazoline (noradrenaline antagonist) 5 ml of 1% solution.
  - Papaverine 40–80 mg in 10–20 ml normal saline.
  - Procaine 10–20 ml of 0.5% solution.
— Check the arterial pulse, keep the hand warm, keep hourly circulation chart.
— If the immediate measures have managed to reverse vasospasm and perfusion returns, remove the cannula and apply pressure to the puncture site to prevent haematoma formation.

Subsequent Management

— Perform sympathetic blockade to promote vasodilation and reduce risk of thrombosis.
  - Stellate ganglion block or brachial plexus block; the former is more effective than the latter.
  - Intravenous regional anaesthesia (IVRA) using guanethidine if available.
— Consider anticoagulation with heparin (after establishing sympathetic blockade) to prevent further intraarterial thrombosis.
— Surgical embolectomy may be indicated in selected cases of documented extensive thrombosis in an attempt to prevent irreversible ischaemia and gangrene.

FURTHER READING

1. Gan TJ, et al. Consensus guidelines for managing postoperative nausea and vomiting. Anesth Analg 2003;97:62–71.
2. Habib AS, Gan TJ. Evidence-based management of postoperative nausea and vomiting: A review. Can J Anesth 2004;51:326–41.
3. Tramer MR. Strategies for postoperative nausea and vomiting. Best Prac Res Clin Anaesthesiol 2004;18:693–701.
4. Gupta A, et al. Does the routine prophylactic use of antiemetics affect the incidence of postdischarge nausea and vomiting following ambulatory surgery? Anesthesiology 2003;99:488–95.

5. Henzi, I, Sonderegger J, Tramer MR. Efficacy, dose-response, and adverse effects of droperidol for prevention of postoperative nausea and vomiting. Can J Anesth 2000;47:537–51.
6. White PF. Droperidol: A cost-effective antiemetic for over thirty years (Editorial). Anesth Analg 2002;95:789–90.

Chapter 62

Crisis Management: General Principles

INTRODUCTION

All anaesthesiologists must deal with crises of varying degrees of severity at one time or another in their careers. The more severe cases may deteriorate rapidly and result in major morbidity or death, this can be an extremely traumatic experience for all concerned. In the majority of cases, an anaesthetic mishap may manifest as an unforeseeable problem that is immediately recognized and rectified, and no adverse sequelae are demonstrable on the patient.

Various algorithms have been designed to address specific problems encountered, such as the management of cardiac arrest by the American Heart Association (AHA) Emergency Cardiac Care Committee, and the management of difficult airway by the American Society of Anesthesiologists (ASA). Whatever the situation may be, it is important that the anaesthesiologist should have a general plan that he/she can adhere to when a crisis arises, so that rapid diagnosis and management steps can be instituted immediately to minimize damage to the patient.

PRINCIPLES OF CRISIS MANAGEMENT

When a crisis arises, the immediate response should always be active resuscitation to support the airway, breathing and circulation. The anaesthesiologist should immediately declare a crisis situation and enlist the help of more personnel for resuscitation. In the meantime a quick assessment should be performed to evaluate the severity of the disorder and the possible underlying causes. Further action depends on the underlying causes and the response of the patient to the initial resuscitation.

Initial Response to a Serious Event

— Begin immediate life-support measures.

— Withhold all anaesthetic agents in use and administer 100% oxygen (double check with oxygen analyzer that the gas delivered is indeed oxygen).

— Check the patient's pulse, BP, SpO_2 and $ETCO_2$.

— Commence cardiopulmonary resuscitation (CPR) if there is no palpable carotid pulse or recordable BP.

Take Command as Team Leader

— The anaesthesiologist, because of his/her resuscitation skills and technical knowledge, is usually the best person to take over the leadership role during resuscitation and with assistance from the surgeon and OT nurses.

— The team leader should decide on the tasks that need to be carried out, prioritize them and assign specific tasks to specific individuals.

— It is important for the team leader to remain calm and organized in order to maintain control of the crisis situation. A nervous and panicky leader does not instil confidence among the team members and will only make the situation worse.

Early Declaration of an Emergency Situation

— The anaesthesiologist is sometimes reluctant to acknowledge that a crisis situation is at hand, either because of a sense of denial (*"This can't be happening to me!"*), or for fear of upsetting the surgical routine. However, it should be stressed that it is always better to mobilize help early before the crisis escalates out of control.

— Inform the surgeon that a crisis is developing, call for assistance and ask for other colleagues to help with resuscitation. The appropriate sense of urgency should be conveyed without inducing undue panic.
— Distribute the workload by assigning specific tasks to individuals according to their skills, such that the more experienced individuals would perform the more critical tasks.
— There should be good communication among team members to avoid duplication of the same action.

Reassessment and Re-Evaluation

— Keep thinking ahead and mentally review the possible underlying causes that may lead to the crisis.
— Reassess the patient's condition at frequent intervals to look for improvement or deterioration, and new clinical signs that may have developed to confirm or refute the initial diagnosis.
— Encourage the others to contribute. A second person with a fresh approach may detect missed clues and clinch the correct diagnosis.
— Send for relevant investigations; establish more venous access and invasive means of monitoring if necessary.
— If not already involved, the supervising consultant should be contacted as soon as possible if the crisis is life-threatening, or if death on the OT table is a distinct possibility.

Further Action to be Taken

— Decision whether to proceed with surgery depends on these factors.
  - The nature, extent and severity of the crisis.
  - The most likely underlying diagnosis.
  - The patient's response to resuscitation and subsequent therapy.
  - The urgency of the surgery.

— It is important to communicate with the surgeon and come to a mutual agreement on a further course of action to be undertaken, the options being:
  - To allow the surgery to proceed if the crisis has been quickly controlled, if the patient's condition is stable, if the surgery is emergent or if the procedure has started.
  - To limit the extent and complexity of the procedure if possible.
  - To abandon the procedure if the crisis has been severe, the patient remains unstable and/or the procedure is elective in nature

— Arrange for admission to ICU or HDU as indicated.

Documentation of Crisis

— The primary task of the anaesthesiologist is always to attend to the patient first rather than record-keeping.

— Documentation is often done retrospectively, a task made easier by automated recording of vital signs incorporated in the newer monitors. Alternatively, one of the assistants (usually the junior most!) can be assigned to the task of record-keeping if enough skilled personnel are available during the crisis.

— Accurate documentation is important for quality assurance purposes and also as a defence against possible litigation in future.

Follow-Up After a Major Crisis

— After a serious perioperative event, the responsibility of the anaesthesiologist does not end when the patient is transferred to the ICU or HDU. The patient should be followed up and the anaesthesiologist concerned should stay involved in the patient's subsequent care.

— It will be necessary to speak with the patient's immediate family or guardian in the event of a major crisis that has led to an adverse outcome. This is best done together with the surgeon initially to avoid different representation of events and course of action.

— Relevant information to be conveyed to the family includes the facts pertaining to the case (rather than speculations of what might have happened), possible diagnosis and cause of the crisis, and steps currently taken to care for the patient.

— Be prepared to answer questions and clarify any misconceptions the family may have about the situation.
— The anaesthesiologist him/herself may need stress management after a perioperative catastrophe since it can be extremely traumatic and demoralizing for the individual. It may be necessary for another colleague to take over the anaesthesia session if the anaesthesiologist is too psychologically affected to continue.

DEALING WITH DEATH ON THE TABLE

— In most cases death in a moribund patient is expected and the high risks of perioperative mortality would have been conveyed and accepted by the patient and immediate family during the preoperative period. Even then, it is still distressing for all concerned when death actually occurs on the OT table.
— An unexpected death on the table can be a harrowing experience that can have considerable psychological and professional consequences. This is especially so when the death is due to anaesthetic factors such as human error or equipment failure. It is psychologically devastating to the OT staff as well as the patient's relatives. Added to this stress is the reaction of the relatives on learning the news and the potential for litigation.
— Being a coroner's case, the necessary notification must be made and in most cases a postmortem would be required. All cannulation lines and tubes must be left *in situ* because in some cases the postmortem diagnosis would hinge on the clues that these would provide.
— The anaesthetic equipment should be decommissioned until its safety has been formally re-certified. Drug ampoules should be kept aside and checked by a senior colleague, preferably someone who did not participate in the initial resuscitation. Drug checks should include the identity, dose, batch number and expiry date as printed on the drug ampoule.
— One of the most difficult tasks at hand is breaking the news to the relatives and dealing with their subsequent reaction. This should be done in a sympathetic manner and together with the surgeon so as to avoid misrepresentation and further misunderstanding. Brief facts of the case should be conveyed to the relatives who would often be too distraught to absorb more information. Further interviews with the relatives would be necessary at a later date and time.

— Again stress management – through counselling and debriefing – for the anaesthesiologist concerned is of utmost importance. Both informal debriefing with other members of the operating team and sympathetic peer review in the form of departmental mortality and morbidity meeting may help to overcome the sense of distress and failure. It often helps to know that other colleagues would probably have conducted the anaesthetic in a similar fashion under the circumstances. On the other hand, it would be an expensive lesson learned if death had resulted from gross mismanagement on the part of the anaesthesiologist, who should learn not to commit the same error again.

— Incidents leading to the death should be clearly and accurately documented after the event, preferably with the assistance of a senior colleague who can help with the composition and editing process. This should be carried out as soon as feasible when details are still fresh in the mind. Copies of the report should be forwarded to the head of department, hospital director and the medical defence union.

— Other than the official records, the anaesthesiologist should also compile a detailed account of the case – preoperative assessment and discussion with the patient, intraoperative events leading to death, efforts at resuscitation including names of personnel involved and details of subsequent interviews with the relatives. This is kept for reference and serves as a personal reminder if future legal proceedings become necessary.

FURTHER READING

1. Cooper JB, Cullen DJ, Eichhorn JH, et al. Administrative guidelines for response to an adverse anesthesia event. J Clin Anesth 1993;5:79–84.
2. Gaba DM, Fish SK, Howard SK. *Crisis Management in Anesthesiology*. New York: Churchill Livingstone, 1994.
3. Kumar V, Barcellos WA, Mehta MP, Carter JG. An analysis of critical incidents in a teaching department for quality assurance: A survey of mishaps during anaesthesia. Anaesthesia 1998;43:879–83.
4. White SM. "Death on the table". (Editorial) Anaesthesia 2003;58:515–8.
5. Aitkenhead AR. Anaesthetic disasters: Handling the aftermath. Anaesthesia 1997; 52:477–82.

Chapter 63

Anaphylaxis/Anaphylactoid Reactions

DEFINITION

These are definitions of commonly used terms in relation to drug allergy and anaphylaxis:

— *An adverse drug reaction* is the occurrence of any drug effect that is not of therapeutic, diagnostic or prophylactic benefit to the patient.

— *Drug allergies* are adverse reactions resulting from immunologic responses to drugs or their metabolites. These reactions result in organ-specific or systemic hypersensitivity that usually recur on subsequent exposure to the same drug.

— *Anaphylaxis* is an exaggerated response to a substance to which an individual has become sensitized. The hypersensitivity reaction is IgE-mediated and results in release of histamine, serotonin and other vasoactive substances from basophils and mast cells.

— An *anaphylactoid reaction* occurs by a different, non-immune mechanism (not mediated by IgE) but is clinically indistinguishable from anaphylaxis. The clinical presentation and management of both are identical, even though life-threatening reactions are more likely to be immune-mediated.

TRIGGERING AGENTS

The incidence of anaphylaxis ranges from 1:10,000 to 1:20,000, with a mortality rate of 3.5–4.7%. The most likely offending agents are neuromuscular blocking drugs (60% of the cases), latex and antibiotics (15% each). It is important to emphasize that a previous history of drug exposure is not necessary, particularly for neuromuscular blocking drugs, due to occurrence of cross-reactivity.

The following agents have been implicated.

Anaesthetic Agents

— Neuromuscular blocking drugs: more common in suxamethonium and benzylisoquinolones (atracurium, mivacurium, cisatracurium) than aminosteroids (pancuronium, vecuronium, rocuronium) even though *all* neuromuscular blocking drugs have been implicated.

— Intravenous induction agents (thiopentone, propofol): Cremophor EL was implicated in earlier preparations of propofol.

— Local anaesthetics (amino-esters)
- The occurrence of anaphylaxis to local anaesthetic *per se* is extremely rare.
- most "reactions" are caused by inadvertent intravascular injection or systemic absorption of local anaesthetic rather than true allergy.

— Opioids (morphine, pethidine): it is not always easy to distinguish between anaphylaxis and histamine release.

Other Drugs and Substances

— Latex.

— Colloids: especially gelatin solutions and dextrans.

— Antibiotics: penicillin, cephalosporins, vancomycin.

— Radiographic contrast media such as fluorescein.
— Intravenous dyes such as methylene, isosulphan blue.
— Protamine, aprotinin.
— Methylmethacrylate (bone cement).
— Chlorhexidine.

MANIFESTATIONS

— Reactions may occur at any time during anaesthesia but more than 90% of cases occur immediately or soon after induction of anaesthesia.
— Clinical manifestations are highly variable both in features and severity. Reactions may be mild and confined to the skin, or sudden and catastrophic. The severity can be classified into mild, moderate and severe.
  - *Mild:* sensation of warmth, flushing, pruritus, rhinorrhoea, scattered urticaria, brief retching, diaphoresis.
  - *Moderate:* persistent vomiting, diffuse urticaria, headache, facial oedema, mild bronchospasm or dyspnoea, palpitations, abdominal cramps, hypotension.
  - *Severe:* tachycardia or bradycardia, arrhythmias, overt bronchospasm, laryngeal oedema, pulmonary oedema, cardiorespiratory collapse, death.
— Many of the above symptoms are masked when the patient is under anaesthesia, and the various signs may not manifest all at once. Hence there must be a high index of suspicion especially if these systems are involved, either singly or in combination.
  - *Skin:* generalized flush, rash, urticaria, angio-oedema.
  - *Respiratory:* bronchospasm, stridor, laryngeal oedema.
  - *Cardiac:* hypotension, cardiovascular collapse, arrhythmia, pulmonary oedema.
— Differential diagnoses include these.
  - *Skin:* non-allergic flush.
  - *Respiratory:* acute exacerbation of asthma or chronic obstructive pulmonary disease, pulmonary aspiration, tension pneumothorax, pulmonary embolism, airway obstruction due to any cause.
  - *Cardiac:* anaesthetic drug overdose, cardiogenic shock, vasovagal reaction, venous air embolism, cardiac tamponade.

MANAGEMENT

Initial Treatment

— **Stop exposure to antigen**
- Stop administration of the likely offending agent.

— **Declare crisis**
- If a serious reaction is taking place, *call for help*.
- Inform the surgeon that an anaphylactic reaction is occurring so that he/she can be prepared to terminate the procedure if the patient is not responsive to initial treatment.

— **Airway management and positioning**
- Administer 100% oxygen, consider early endotracheal intubation if the patient has not been intubated, as further development of angio-oedema may compromise airway patency later.
- Lay the patient flat with the legs elevated if hypotension occurs.

— **Discontinue anaesthetic agents**
- Reduce or discontinue administration of volatile anaesthetic if blood pressure is low.
- Volatile anaesthetic may be used for its bronchodilatory properties in isolated bronchospasm with normotension.
- Note that volatile anaesthetics are also myocardial depressants and some may be arrhythmogenic by sensitizing the myocardium to catecholamines administered for therapy.

— **Intravascular volume expansion**
- Commence rapid infusion of crystalloid solution (10–25 ml/kg) over 20 minutes, repeat if necessary.
- Consider colloid infusion when the volume of crystalloid solution infused exceeds 30 ml/kg, but be aware that colloids themselves may cause histamine release and worsen any on-going reaction.
- Large volumes up to 2–4 litres may be needed since vasodilatation occurs and up to 40% of intravascular volume may be lost into the interstitial space.

— **Adrenaline**
- *Adrenaline is the drug of choice for anaphylaxis*, as its α-adrenergic action causes vasoconstriction and reverses hypotension; and β-adrenergic action causes positive inotropy, bronchodilation and reduction of mediator release.

- The dose of adrenaline depends on the patient's haemodynamic status: doses given for cardiovascular collapse will cause extreme hypertension and tachycardia if administered to normotensive or mildly hypotensive patients.
  - For hypotension: 0.5–1 ml increments of 1:10,000 dilution (50–100 μg).
  - For cardiovascular collapse: 1 mg bolus doses (10 ml of 1:10,000 dilution) or more.
  - Undiluted adrenaline 1:1,000 should never be given intravenously.
- Administer bolus doses of adrenaline every 1–2 minutes until clinical response is satisfactory as shown by improvement in blood pressure, reductions in airway resistance and angio-oedema.
- If the patient remains hypotensive, commence adrenaline infusion at 0.05 μg/kg/min and titrate dose to response.

— **Monitors**
- Insert cannulae for invasive BP and CVP monitoring.
- Insert an indwelling urinary catheter to monitor urine output.

— **Subsequent management**
- All patients who have a serious reaction should be managed in ICU, as the reaction may be protracted with persistent arterial hypotension, pulmonary hypertension, right ventricular dysfunction, non-cardiogenic pulmonary oedema, respiratory obstruction or laryngeal oedema.

Secondary Treatment

— **Antihistamines**
- Administer IV diphenhydramine 0.5–1 mg/kg or chlorpheniramine 10–20 mg by slow intravenous infusion.
- H_1 receptor antagonists counter the adverse effects mediated by histamine but should be injected slowly as they have antidopaminergic effects and may cause hypotension.
- The role of H_2 receptor antagonists in acute reactions remains unproven, but IV ranitidine 50 mg is often administered.

— **Corticosteroids**
- Consider IV hydrocortisone 100–300 mg or IV methylprednisolone 1–2 g.
- Steroids are not useful in the initial management because of their delayed onset of action, but can be beneficial in preventing or reducing the severity of delayed symptoms.

— **Others**
- Administer β_2 agonists (salbutamol or terbutaline) for persistent bronchospasm.
- Check ABG for acidosis and consider sodium bicarbonate 0.5–1 mEq/kg.

— **Airway evaluation prior to extubation**
- In the presence of laryngeal oedema, the endotracheal tube should be left *in situ* until oedema subsides: deflate the cuff and check for air leak around the endotracheal tube during positive pressure ventilation at 20 cmH_2O peak inflation pressure.
- Consider trial of extubation with the aid of Cook™ airway exchange catheter in borderline cases; re-intubate by railroading an endotracheal tube down the exchange catheter if necessary (see Chapter 25).
- Admit to ICU for observation and/or ventilation if the reaction is severe and protracted.

— **Immediate investigations**
- Serum mast cell tryptase concentration
  - This is a neutral protease released from mast cell granules during degranulation in an anaphylactic or anaphylactoid reaction.
  - Samples should be taken as soon as practicable after the onset of reaction, after 1 hour and again after 6–24 hours.
  - Levels greater than 15 ng/ml are likely to indicate an IgE response (basal level < 1 ng/ml).
- Estimation of other substances are not useful because these are either non-specific (complement C_3,C_4) or the levels are only transiently elevated (histamine).
- These tests may confirm the occurrence of anaphylactic or anaphylactoid reaction but they do not identify the causative agent.

Follow-Up Management

— **Documentation and explanation**
- Document the incident clearly in the case notes: likely causative agent, clinical manifestations, management and response.
- Any patient who has a suspected anaphylactic reaction associated with anaesthesia should be fully investigated.
- Advise the patient on the need to investigate and identify the agent responsible for the reaction; make arrangements to ensure that the tests are performed and interpreted adequately.

- Inform the patient the likely substance causing the reaction, provide a detailed letter recounting the circumstances so that the next anaesthesiologist can be alerted to the problem.
- A Medic Alert bracelet is encouraged especially if the offending agent has been identified.

— **Further investigations**

- The patient should be referred to an allergy centre for specialist investigation by a trained allergist.
- The test is carried out 6 weeks after the acute episode; the patient should not be on steroids or antihistamines which may mask the skin reaction at the time of the skin test.
- Ensure that full resuscitation equipment is available: oxygen, airway equipment, adrenaline (diluted and drawn up in a syringe, with more ampoules available).
- Establish intravenous access before testing.
- The allergist uses either a skin prick test or an intradermal test using fresh diluted solutions of likely agent, with dilutions from 1:10 to 1:10,000 depending on the specific agent tested.
- In the intradermal test, 0.1 ml of the test solution is injected at the surface of forearm intradermally and saline (control) is injected on another site.
- A positive reaction occurs when flare and wheal greater than 10 mm diameter appear less than 10 minutes and persist longer than 30 minutes.

— **Future anaesthetic**

- Details of the causative agent, severity of the previous reaction and response to treatment should be obtained if feasible.
- Consider alternative anaesthetic options.
  - — Use regional anaesthesia instead of general anaesthesia in appropriate cases.
  - — Use inhalational rather than intravenous induction if the latter agent is implicated.
  - — Omit the use of neuromuscular blocking agents if these are the likely offending agents.
- Consider pretreatment to reduce the severity of reactions.
  - — Oral prednisone 50 mg or IV hydrocortisone 200 mg 6 hourly for 3 doses (at 13 and 7 hours and 1 hour before anaesthesia).
  - — Oral diphenhydramine 50 mg 1 hour before anaesthesia.
  - — Oral ranitidine 150 mg 1 hour before anaesthesia.

- Establish full monitoring and intravenous access of at least 18G cannula in an adult. Ensure that resuscitation equipment and drugs, including adrenaline (drawn up and diluted), are available prior to induction of anaesthesia.
- If the drug responsible for reaction cannot be identified, avoid drugs which are known to cause hypersensitivity reactions. Appropriate drugs with low potential for hypersensitivity and histamine release include volatile anaesthetics, etomidate, fentanyl, benzodiazepines.
- Administer the drugs slowly and be vigilant about the possibility of anaphylactic reaction; treat early and aggressively if this occurs.

LATEX ALLERGY

— "Latex" refers either to the natural sap of the rubber tree *Havea brasiliensis*, or to products made from the sap. Latex-containing medical products include gloves, urinary catheters, tourniquets, rubber plunger of syringes, intravenous tubing, haemodialysis and ventilator equipment.

— The use of universal precautions, widely implemented in the 1980s in response to the human immunodeficiency virus (HIV) epidemic, led to dramatic increases in the use of latex gloves and the incidence of latex anaphylaxis.

— Two types of reactions are associated with latex allergy.
  - Irritant contact dermatitis, Type IV hypersensitivity reaction (delayed, cell-mediated).
  - Immediate Type I IgE-mediated hypersensitivity reaction or anaphylaxis.

— These are some typical clinical scenarios of latex allergy.
  - Children with myelomeningocele (spina bifida) for multiple surgical procedures.
  - Patients with congenital genitourinary abnormalities or multiple reconstructive surgical procedures.
  - Healthcare workers or other workers with occupational exposure to latex.
  - Individuals with history of atopy or allergy to fruits such as kiwi-fruit, avocado, mango, passion fruit, banana.

— Unlike reactions due to anaesthetic agents, latex allergy reactions typically begin 30–60 minutes into the procedure rather than at induction of anaesthesia.

— Methods of prevention
  - Obtain careful history of previous allergic reactions, atopy or asthma.
  - Schedule the patient to be first on the operating list in the morning.

- Inform all OT personnel regarding the patient's allergy to latex, and clearly label "Latex Allergy" on all doors leading into the operating room.
- Drugs for treatment of anaphylaxis should be diluted and drawn up.
- Establish a latex-free environment: avoid contact with latex-containing devices, such as urinary catheters, anaesthetic reservoir bags and face masks, intravenous infusion sets, drug vials with latex stoppers, elastic in disposable OT caps.
- Latex-free kit should contain these items:
    - Disposables: non-latex gloves, latex-free intravenous infusion sets, syringes, intravenous cannulae.
    - Anaesthetic equipment: plastic masks and airways, laryngeal mask airway, polyvinyl chloride (PVC) endotracheal tubes, neoprene reservoir bags, silicon self-inflating bags, plastic breathing circuit tubings.

FURTHER READING

1. Hepner DL, Castells MC. Anaphylaxis during the perioperative period. Anesth Analg 2003;97:1381–95.
2. Plaud B, Donati F, Debaene B. Anaphylaxis during anaesthesia. Br J Anaesth 2002;88:604–6.
3. Mertes PM, Laxenaire MC. Allergic reactions occurring during anaesthesia. Eur J Anaesth 2002;19:240–62.
4. deShazo RD, Kemp SF. Allergic reactions to drugs and biologic agents. JAMA 1997;278:1895–1906.
5. Hepner DL, Castells MC. Latex allergy: An update. Anesth Analg 2003;96:1219–29.
6. Kam PC, Lee MS. Latex allergy: An emerging clinical and occupational health problem. Anaesthesia 1997;52:570–5.
7. Ellis AK, Day JH. Diagnosis and management of anaphylaxis. Can Med Assoc J 2003;169:307–12.
8. Payne V, Kam PCA. Mast cell tryptase: A review of its physiology and clinical significance. Anaesthesia 2004;59:695–703.
9. Association of Anaesthetists of Great Britain and Ireland. Suspected anaphylactic reactions associated with anaesthesia. London, 2003. www.aagbi.org/pdf/Anaphylaxis.pdf

Chapter 64

Aspiration of Gastric Contents

INTRODUCTION

Pulmonary aspiration occurs when there is inhalation of gastric contents into the tracheobronchial tree. This can be caused by passive regurgitation or active vomiting when the patient is unable to protect the airway.

The danger of pulmonary aspiration was recognized in obstetric anaesthesia in the 1930s and its aetiology was established by Mendelson in 1946. The often quoted "critical" though arbitrary values (pH 2.5, volume 25 ml or 0.4 ml/kg) give rise to clinically significant chemical pneumonitis and increased morbidity, classically described in obstetric patients as *Mendelson's syndrome*. The presence of food particles gives rise to additional problems of acute airway obstruction, atelectasis and hypoxaemia.

Perioperative pulmonary aspiration, with an estimated incidence ranging from 1:2,000 to 1:14,000 anaesthetics in the general surgical population, is an infrequent event. The incidence in obstetric patients is at least twice that of the general surgical population. Other associated factors include emergency after-hour procedure, extremes of age, gastrointestinal and abdominal procedures, impaired consciousness, obesity and the lithotomy position during surgery.

Despite the infrequent occurrence of pulmonary aspiration, its impact on individual patients can be devastating. The reported mortality rates from pulmonary aspiration range from 5–62%, those who are ill (ASA III or more) and elderly being more susceptible.

The incidence of aspiration associated with the use of laryngeal mask airway (LMA) has been estimated at 0.02%. The primary limitation of the LMA and other supraglottic devices is that they do not reliably protect the lungs from regurgitated gastric contents. An assessment of aspiration risk is critical to determining the suitability of an LMA. The use of LMA variants in the form of intubating LMA or LMA ProSeal™ may provide additional protection against aspiration. However, based on evidence at present, these devices cannot be recommended for use in patients with known risk for pulmonary aspiration.

PREDISPOSING FACTORS

Factors that predispose patients to increased risks of pulmonary aspiration of gastric contents can be classified into three areas.

1. **Patient factors**
   - Increased gastric content
     - Gastric hypersecretion: pregnancy, obesity.
     - Lack of fasting: emergency surgery.
     - Delayed gastric emptying: pregnancy, obesity, gastric stasis following trauma or parenteral opioids, gastrointestinal tract (GIT) pathology (intestinal obstruction, gastric outlet obstruction, bleeding from upper GIT), diabetic autonomic neuropathy, renal failure.
   - Increased tendency to regurgitate
     - Decreased lower oesophageal sphincter tone: pregnancy, obesity, hiatus hernia.
     - Gastro-oesophageal reflux: hiatus hernia, GIT pathology.
     - Oesophageal pathology: stricture, carcinoma, previous surgery.
     - Extremes of age.

- Laryngeal incompetence
    - Depressed level of consciousness.
    - Anatomical abnormalities of the larynx.
    - Neuromuscular disorders with bulbar or pseudobulbar palsy.

2. **Surgical factors**
    - Upper abdominal surgery: gastric contents may be extruded proximally by surgical manipulation.
    - Laparoscopic surgery: increase in intraabdominal pressure in the presence of pneumoperitoneum.
    - Lithotomy and Trendelenburg position during surgery: promotes passive regurgitation.

3. **Anaesthetic factors**
    - Local anaesthetic block of laryngeal apparatus.
    - Inadequate reversal of neuromuscular blockade or persisting effects of anaesthetic agents.
    - Inappropriate anaesthetic technique
        - Laryngoscopy before adequate depth of anaesthesia and muscle relaxation has been attained, resulting in coughing, regurgitation and vomiting.
        - Premature extubation before reflexes have fully returned to protect the airway against regurgitation and aspiration.
        - Use of laryngeal mask airway or other supraglottic airway adjuncts instead of endotracheal intubation in patients at risk.
    - Difficulty in airway management
        - Gastric distension following difficulty with or prolonged intermittent positive pressure ventilation via face mask.
        - Ineffective cricoid pressure or premature release of cricoid pressure before endotracheal tube (ETT) placement has been confirmed.
        - Delay in insertion of ETT: problems with tracheal intubation, oesophageal intubation (especially if unrecognized).

PREVENTION

Given the problems associated with regurgitation and aspiration of gastric contents under anaesthesia, these preventive measures should be undertaken.

1. **Prophylactic measures**
   - Preoperative fasting
     - Fasting should be at least 6 hours for solids, up to 2 hours for clear fluids in elective surgery; and at least 6 hours of fasting in emergency surgery (if feasible).
     - This does not guarantee an empty stomach especially in emergency cases, patients in pain, or those who have been given opioids for pain relief.
   - Drugs to reduce gastric acidity or volume
     - Non-particulate antacids 0.3M sodium citrate 30 ml.
     - H_2 receptor antagonists, e.g., ranitidine, cimetidine orally or intravenously.
     - Prokinetics, e.g., metoclopramide.
     - Proton pump inhibitors, e.g., omeprazole.
   - Insertion of nasogastric tube
     - This does not guarantee complete stomach emptying, as solid particles may not be totally removed even with large-bore stomach tubes.
     - The presence of nasogastric tube itself during induction of anaesthesia may impair competency of lower oesophageal sphincter (LOS) and predispose to regurgitation and aspiration.
   - Apomorphine-induced emesis is very unpleasant to the patient and is rarely, if at all, used now.

2. **Anaesthetic techniques**
   - Avoid general anaesthesia in high-risk cases; opt for regional anaesthetic technique if possible.
   - Avoid depression of laryngeal reflexes: do not use local anaesthetic spray or injection at glottic and subglottic levels.

3. **Preventive measures under general anaesthesia**
   - If the nasogastric tube is *in situ*, suction this prior to induction of anaesthesia. Some anaesthesiologists prefer to withdraw the nasogastric tube slightly so that the tip of the catheter is above LOS.
   - The standard anaesthetic technique is preoxygenation followed by rapid sequence induction, application of cricoid pressure and intubation using a cuffed ETT.
   - Cricoid pressure should be applied by a trained anaesthetic assistant from the time the patient loses consciousness until ETT is inserted, the cuff inflated

and its correct placement checked and confirmed. It should be maintained if difficulty is encountered during intubation.

— If active vomiting occurs, release cricoid pressure immediately and turn the patient's head to the side. Place the patient in Trendelenburg position and suction the oropharynx to clear the vomitus.
— At the end of the surgery, do not remove the ETT until the patient is fully conscious and with demonstrable return of protective laryngeal reflexes.

MANIFESTATIONS

Although aspiration may occur at any time (including immediately before induction of anaesthesia), most cases appear to occur during tracheal intubation and extubation. Gastric contents may be visualized in the oropharynx during or after intubation, or may be suctioned out of the ETT.

Have a high index of suspicion; always consider the possibility of pulmonary aspiration if this occurs:

— When tracheal intubation has been difficult or established only after multiple attempts.
— When there are unexpected difficulties with oxygenation or ventilation.
— When there is evidence of bronchospasm with high airway pressures, wheeze or reduced air entry.
— When the patient requires unexpectedly frequent tracheal suctioning for secretions.

Chest X-ray findings depend on the volume, pH and nature of pulmonary aspirate. These may be unremarkable in 15–20% of cases or show pneumonic infiltrates, atelectasis, ARDS (acute respiratory distress syndrome) picture in full-blown cases. There may be evidence of collapse consolidation if airways are blocked by solid food particles.

MANAGEMENT

— If gastric contents and/or pulmonary aspiration are recognized at intubation:
  - Immediately tilt the OT table to a 30° Trendelenburg position.
  - Quickly clear the oropharynx of gastric contents.
  - Intubate and perform tracheal suctioning through the ETT before mechanical ventilation.
  - Avoid prolonged efforts at suctioning the trachea especially if SpO_2 is falling.

— If there are problems with oxygenation, increase FiO_2 up to 1.0 and maintain positive pressure ventilation with positive end-expiratory pressure (PEEP).
— Aspiration of particulate material with persistent hypoxaemia warrants immediate bronchoscopic suctioning and removal.
— Inform and discuss the problem with the surgeon. Elective surgical procedures should be postponed if there is significant aspiration giving rise to problems with oxygenation and/or ventilation. Emergency surgery should be kept to the minimum procedure consistent with patient safety.
— Supportive care includes these measures.
  - Use bronchodilators to treat bronchospasm.
  - Frequent chest physiotherapy and suctioning.
  - Appropriate monitoring: SpO_2, serial ABG.
  - Cardiovascular support if indicated.
— Antibiotics
  - Prophylactic antibiotics are not generally given, as the choice of antibiotics should be based on clinical manifestations as well as results of Gram stain, culture and sensitivity.
  - Prophylaxis is indicated for aspiration of faeculent or infected material.
— Corticosteroids
  - The role of corticosteroids in management of aspiration has been disputed.
  - They may modify the inflammatory response but have not been shown to be beneficial during acute hypoxaemia.
  - They do not alter the clinical outcome and may in fact impair healing process by interfering with the normal immune response.
— Mild cases may be managed in the ward and followed up daily (more frequently if necessary).
  - Continue oxygen therapy with SpO_2 monitoring.
  - Serial ABG, CXR.
  - Regular chest physiotherapy and suctioning.
  - Early intervention if the patient's condition deteriorates: consider respiratory support in the form of continuous positive airway pressure (CPAP), biphasic positive airway pressure (BIPAP) and ICU admission for ventilatory support.
— Severe cases with significant hypoxaemia or bronchospasm require admission to ICU for elective ventilation using IPPV with PEEP and supportive measures outlined above. Note that hypoxaemia may be relatively resistant to treatment with PEEP in patients with ARDS.

FURTHER READING

1. Asai T. Who is at increased risk of pulmonary aspiration? (Editorial) Br J Anaesth 2004;93:497–500.
2. Kalinowski CPH, Kirsch JR. Strategies for prophylaxis and treatment for aspiration. Best Prac Res Clin Anaesthesiol 2004;18:719–37.
3. Warner MA. Is pulmonary aspiration still an important problem in anesthesia? Curr Opin Anaesthesiol 2000;13:215–8.
4. Petroz GC, Lerman J. Pulmonary aspiration and lung injury. Curr Opin Anaesthesiol 2000;13:291–7.
5. Schneck H, Scheller M. Acid aspiration prophylaxis and cesarean section. Curr Opin Anaesthesiol 2000;13:261–5.
6. Engelhardt T, Webster NR. Pulmonary aspiration of gastric contents in anaesthesia. Br J Anaesth 1999;83:453–60.
7. Kluger MT, Short TG. Aspiration during anaesthesia: A review of 133 cases from the Australian Anaesthetic Incident Monitoring Study (AIMS). Anaesthesia 1999;54:19–26.

Chapter 65

Bronchospasm

INTRODUCTION

Bronchospasm refers to the reversible narrowing of medium and small airways due to smooth muscle contraction. It describes a clinical manifestation and not a diagnosis, as there are many underlying causes that may lead to bronchospasm, such as the ones listed here.

- Acute exacerbation of asthma.
- Chronic obstructive pulmonary disease (COPD) with reversible component of airway narrowing.
- Recent or on-going respiratory tract infection.
- Medications such as β-blockers, histamine-releasing drugs, anticholinesterases.
- Various forms of airway irritation
  - Chemical: smoke inhalation, aspiration of gastric contents.
  - Mechanical: airway manipulation or tracheal intubation at light planes of anaesthesia, carinal irritation secondary to endobronchial intubation.
  - Physical: temperature, cold dry gases.

- Pulmonary aspiration of gastric contents.
- Acute pulmonary oedema from whatever cause.
- Pneumothorax.
- Anaphylaxis or anaphylactoid reactions.
- Pulmonary embolism due to gas, air, thrombus or amniotic fluid.

MANIFESTATIONS

Clinical manifestations of bronchospasm occur as a result of bronchoconstriction as well as the effects of hypercarbia and/or hypoxaemia.

Clinical features include:

- Decreased lung compliance with high peak inspiratory pressure.
- Prolonged expiratory phase with expiratory rhonchi or wheeze.
- Upward sloping of expiratory capnograph tracing.
- Reduced air entry or chest movement which may be localized or generalized depending on underlying pathology.
- Decreased SpO_2 and cyanosis in severe cases.
- Sympathetic overactivity secondary to hypercarbia and/or hypoxaemia, manifested as sweating, hypertension, bounding pulse, tachyarrhythmias.
- Restlessness in a conscious patient.

Differential diagnosis of bronchospasm includes mechanical problems to the endotracheal tube (ETT) and breathing system due to various causes.

- ETT problems: kinking; obstruction with secretions, blood, vomitus or foreign body; endobronchial intubation; cuff herniation with partial occlusion of ETT lumen.
- Breathing system or ventilator problems: kinked tubing, malfunctioning unidirectional valves or other components of the circuit or ventilator.

MANAGEMENT

1. **Ensure adequate oxygenation and ventilation**
   - Increase FiO_2 to 1.0 if oxygenation is compromised.
   - Manually ventilate the lungs to assess compliance.

2. **Ensure that the problem is truly "bronchospasm"**
   — Quick inspection of the breathing system and ventilator to rule out mechanical problems.
   — Confirm the position and patency of the ETT
   - Pass a suction catheter down the ETT to check if this is possible; remove bronchial secretions if present.
   - Deflate the pilot balloon of the ETT cuff to exclude cuff herniation as a cause of the problem (deflation would allow easier ventilation if the problem is due to cuff herniation); re-inflate after testing.
   - Consider removal of ETT and re-intubation in doubtful cases.

   — Auscultate the chest to assess breath sounds and adventitious sounds.

Mild Bronchospasm

— Diagnose and remove the source of the problem, such as oropharyngeal or ETT suction to remove secretions, re-adjust the depth of ETT in the case of endobronchial intubation.

— Increase the depth of anaesthesia with a volatile anaesthetic. Sevoflurane is the least irritant and arrhythmogenic in the presence of hypercarbia.

— These measures are usually adequate to abort the bronchospasm.

Moderate to Severe Bronchospasm

— Administer 100% oxygen while maintaining depth of anaesthesia with volatile anaesthetic and/or propofol.

— Bronchodilator therapy using β_2-adrenergic agonists, administered via ETT or parenterally.
- Administration via ETT: 4–8 puffs of terbutaline or salbutamol from metered dose inhaler (MDI), followed by 2 puffs every 10 minutes according to heart rate. This is not a very reliable method since most of the aerosol may be deposited along the ETT or larger airways.
- Administration via ETT: salbutamol 2.5 mg by nebulizer attached to the breathing system via a T-piece connector and with a separate oxygen source for nebulization. This is more reliable and is the preferred method of administration.
- Parenteral administration: IV or SC salbutamol 250 μg.

— Use of other drugs:
  - Corticosteroids, in the form of IV methylprednisolone 1–2 mg/kg or IV hydrocortisone 200 mg, may be administered even though its antiinflammatory action is not immediate and takes effect only after a few hours.
  - Ipratropium bromide, a parasympatholytic antagonist, may be administered in addition to β_2-adrenergic agonists via the ETT: 6 puffs, followed by 2 puffs every 10 minutes.
  - Small doses of IV adrenaline 10 μg (0.1 ml of 1:10,000 dilution) may be considered, especially if anaphylactic reaction cannot be definitely excluded. The dose of adrenaline may be repeated if the patient responds to the initial doses. Note that the initial dose (10 μg) is one-tenth to one-fifth the dose used when anaphylaxis is suspected (50–100 μg).
  - IV ketamine 2 mg/kg may be useful for its bronchodilator action in refractory cases.
  - Similarly, magnesium sulphate may be used for its effect on smooth muscle relaxation. The adult dose is 2 g administered by slow IV injection. Observe for hypotension and muscle relaxation.
  - IV lignocaine 1.5–2 mg/kg may be considered.
  - The use of aminophylline is decreasing because of its toxic effects, particularly tachyarrhythmias. This is given as a slow 5 mg/kg loading dose IV, followed by continuous infusion at 0.6 mg/kg/hr.

— Systematically consider the possible underlying causes for bronchospasm and treat accordingly.
  - Pulmonary aspiration of gastric contents: suction, bronchodilators, consider rigid bronchoscopy if particulate material is aspirated.
  - Acute pulmonary oedema: diuretics, inotrope support.
  - Pneumothorax: needle aspiration, chest tube insertion.
  - Anaphylaxis or anaphylactoid reactions: adrenaline bolus doses and infusion, stop administration of offending agent.
  - Pulmonary embolism due to gas, air, thrombus or amniotic fluid: supportive measures.

— Watch for cardiac arrhythmias, especially tachyarrhythmias.

— Send blood sample for ABG. Consider arranging for CXR on OT table, but this should not delay chest tube insertion if tension pneumothorax is clinically suspected.

— A high-performance ventilator (such as an ICU ventilator) may be required for optimal ventilation and oxygen delivery: use slow rate, prolonged expiration, accept moderate degrees of hypercapnia provided oxygenation is not compromised.

— Inform the surgeon if bronchospasm remains unresolved. Stop the surgical procedure as soon as possible. Transfer to ICU for further management of bronchospasm.

FURTHER READING

1. Gal TJ. Bronchial hyperresponsiveness and anesthesia: Physiologic and therapeutic perspectives. Anesth Analg 1994;78:559–73.
2. Pinto P, Lexley M, Orrett FA, Balbirsingh M. Physiologic perspectives of therapy in bronchial hyperreactivity. Can J Anaesth 1996;43:700–13.

Chapter 66

Intraoperative Hypoxia

INTRODUCTION

Intraoperative hypoxia is an anaesthetic crisis that demands immediate action to identify the possible underlying cause(s) and institute corrective measures. Causes are often obvious but in some cases the precise cause of the oxygen desaturation may remain elusive. One must be vigilant and have a definitive management plan that allows systematic consideration and elimination of potential causes while ensuring that the problem of hypoxia is corrected in the shortest possible time.

CAUSES

Hypoxaemia results in failure of oxygen delivery to the tissue, so every step of the oxygen cascade – from oxygen supply, through the respiratory, cardiovascular, and haematological systems, to the mitochondrial level – should be considered to be potentially at fault.

These causes should be considered.

— **Hypoxic inspired gas**
- Oxygen supply failure.
- Incorrect flowmeter settings.
- Malfunction of anaesthetic machine.

— **Problems with ventilation**
- Intubation problems: failed intubation, misplacement of ETT (oesophageal, endobronchial).
- ETT problems: disconnection, kinking, obstruction, cuff herniation.
- Pharyngeal obstruction in unintubated patients: tongue falling back, improperly positioned laryngeal mask airway or other devices.
- Breathing system problems: disconnection, leak, obstruction, malfunctioning uni-directional valves in circle system.
- Laryngo- or bronchospasm: anaphylaxis, light anaesthesia, pulmonary aspiration, acute exacerbation of asthma or COPD.
- Decreased functional residual capacity (FRC): tension pneumothorax, diaphragmatic splinting as a result of pneumoperitoneum, fat or gravid uterus.
- Hypoventilation while on spontaneous ventilation or on IPPV: inappropriate ventilator settings, problems with ventilator.
- Respiratory depression in a spontaneously breathing patient: excessive level of central neuraxial blockade, overdose of opioids or other respiratory depressants.
- Preexisting severe pulmonary disease.
- One-lung ventilation, either accidentally or intentionally.

— **Intracardiac or intrapulmonary shunts**
- Atelectasis.
- Pulmonary oedema.
- Right-to-left shunt: cyanotic heart disease, Eisenmenger's syndrome.

— **Reduced pulmonary blood flow (dead space ventilation)**
- Embolism involving air, gas, thrombus, fat or amniotic fluid.
- Cardiac arrest or severe hypotension.

— **Inadequate oxygenation at end-organ**
- Shock due to any cause.
- Carbon monoxide poisoning.

— **Increased oxygen demand**
- Malignant hyperthermia.
- Severe sepsis.

— **Spurious causes** (low pulse oximeter readings rather than actual hypoxaemia)
  - Methaemoglobinaemia: interpreted as deoxyhaemoglobin by pulse oximeter; hence underreading may occur.
  - Intravascular dyes, e.g., methylene blue, indocyanine green.
  - Vasoconstriction leading to inadequate signal for SpO_2 estimation: hypotension, hypothermia, peripheral vascular disease, e.g., Raynaud's phenomenon, sickle cell disease.
  - Ischaemia or venous congestion at the limb.
  - Movement artefacts.

PREVENTION

Various preventive measures can be undertaken to reduce the risk of hypoxia:

— Identify patients at risk
  - Potential difficulty for mask ventilation and/or intubation.
  - Severe lung disease.
  - Presence of intracardiac shunts: watch for reversal of shunt.
  - Morbid obesity.
  - Pregnancy.
  - Malignant hyperthermia susceptibility.
  - Likelihood of pulmonary aspiration.

— Prior checking of anaesthetic machine and monitors
  - Central supply and back-up cylinders for oxygen supply.
  - Properly calibrated oxygen analyzer.
  - Functioning oxygen failure warning device.

— Means of reducing pulmonary aspiration risks
  - Preoperative fasting.
  - Acid aspiration prophylaxis.
  - Rapid sequence induction with cricoid pressure.
  - Use of cuffed ETT.

— Preoxygenation before induction of anaesthesia for patients at risk.

— Prevention of problems related to ETT
  - Confirm ETT placement by clinical means and routine use of capnography.
  - Reconfirm ETT placement after changing the patient's position.
  - Proper securing of ETT and its connection to prevent accidental disconnection or extubation.

— Use of monitors
  - Equipment monitors: oxygen analyzer, ventilator disconnect alarm.
  - Patient monitors: capnography, pulse oximetry, haemodynamic monitors, temperature, airway pressure and spirometry.

— Increase FiO_2 in patients at risk
  - Poor pulmonary status.
  - Surgery likely to be associated with hypoxia, such as bronchoscopy.

— Measures to prevent bronchospasm
  - Smooth induction and intubation.
  - Avoidance of histamine-releasing drugs.
  - Ensure adequate depth of anaesthesia before airway instrumentation.

— Ensure stable haemodynamic status
  - Intravenous fluids for volume replacement.
  - Early transfusion of blood and/or blood products.

MANAGEMENT

This demands urgent resuscitative measures with simultaneous checking and evaluation to identify underlying causes.

— Quick overall assessment
  - Anaesthetic machine: oxygen source, flowmeter reading, oxygen analyzer, confirm FiO_2.
  - Breathing circuit: rule out obstruction, kinking or disconnection.
  - Patient's colour: pallor, central cyanosis (may not be apparent in gross anaemia with haemoglobin < 5 g/dl).
  - Monitors: capnograph tracing, airway pressure, spirometry, BP, heart rate, ECG, temperature, SpO_2.
  - Adjust pulse oximeter probe if the SpO_2 tracing is not satisfactory.

— Disconnect from the ventilator and ventilate manually
  - Initial 3–4 large breaths to recruit collapsed alveoli.
  - Assess compliance and ease of ventilation.

— Increase FiO_2 to 1.0 if SpO_2 remains low
  - Maintain anaesthesia by administering an intravenous anaesthetic or increasing concentration of volatile anaesthetic in the absence of severe hypotension or cardiac arrest.

- Use a separate oxygen source (e.g., from oxygen cylinder) if there is any doubt about oxygen supply from the anaesthetic machine.
- Use a different breathing system, or a self-inflating bag, if there is problem with breathing system integrity or function which cannot be identified quickly.

— Rule out ETT problems
- Reconfirm proper placement of ETT: chest expansion, auscultation, capnograph tracing, direct laryngoscopy to confirm passage of ETT through the vocal cords.
- Pass a suction catheter down the ETT to confirm patency and to remove secretions.
- Partially deflate and re-inflate ETT cuff to rule out problem of cuff herniation.
- If the position of the ETT is in doubt and the patient is rapidly desaturating, the safest approach is to remove the ETT and manually ventilate the patient with a face mask.

— Examine the lungs
- Look for bilateral and equal chest expansion.
- Auscultate for breath sounds, crepitations, rhonchi.
- Percuss for hyper-resonance if pneumothorax is suspected.
- Consider possibilities of tension pneumothorax, pulmonary aspiration, pulmonary oedema, anaphylaxis, atelectasis. Look for other clinical features to support or refute your diagnosis.

— Look at the surgical field to rule out these problems
- Excessive pneumoperitoneum causing reduced FRC, worsened by Trendelenburg position.
- Inadvertent pneumothorax.
- Excessive surgical bleeding.
- Embolism involving air, CO_2, thrombus, fat, cement or amniotic fluid.

— Correct haemodynamic derangements
- Volume resuscitation with intravenous fluids, blood and/or blood products.
- Inotrope support for patients with decreased myocardial contractility.
- Vasoconstrictor for patients in septicaemic shock.
- Maintain systemic vascular resistance and reduce pulmonary vascular resistance in patients with intracardiac shunts to minimize right-to-left shunting.

— Attempts to improve oxygen delivery
- Adjust ventilatory pattern: mode of ventilation, tidal volume, respiratory rate, I:E ratio.

- Consider using PEEP to prevent atelectasis.

— Send blood samples for ABG analysis and haemoglobin estimation.

— Treat underlying causes accordingly.

— Watch for complications of prolonged hypoxia
  - ECG changes suggestive of myocardial ischaemia.
  - Consider possibility of hypoxic encephalopathy if the patient fails to regain consciousness following general anaesthesia.
  - Acute tubular necrosis following prolonged hypotension.
  - Lactic acidosis secondary to anaerobic metabolism.

FURTHER READING

1. Bamber I. Airway crises. Curr Anaesth Crit Care 2003;14:2–8.

Chapter 67

Postoperative Stridor

DEFINITION

Stridor is a high-pitched inspiratory sound caused by upper airway obstruction, usually at laryngeal level. This is in contrast with bronchospasm, which refers to airway obstruction at the medium and small airways due to smooth muscle contraction.

CAUSES

Stridor may be attributable to many causes.

— Laryngospasm
  - Laryngospasm is caused by acute glottic closure of the vocal cords due to various causes.

- This may occur during airway manipulation or extubation in the "transitional zone", when the patient is neither fully awake nor well anaesthetized.
- It may be triggered off by secretions within or near the larynx.
- Patients with reactive airway disease associated with asthma, COPD, chronic smoking and active or recent respiratory tract infection are especially at risk.

— Laryngeal oedema
- This may occur following laryngeal surgery or instrumentation.
- It may complicate major fluid resuscitation especially if the patient is placed in the Trendelenburg position for prolonged periods.
- In obstetric patients, laryngeal oedema may be present in parturients with preeclampsia or following prolonged and repeated Valsalva attempts at delivery during second stage of labour.

— Extrinsic or intrinsic compression of the airway
- Extrinsic causes include haematoma following neck surgery or injury to blood vessels in the necks, huge goitre or anterior mediastinal mass.
- Intrinsic causes include laryngeal tumour in various forms (carcinoma, polyp, papilloma); inhaled foreign body in the airway.

— Paralysis of one or both vocal cords
- Vocal cord palsy may be secondary to a preexisting pathology of recurrent laryngeal nerve, or following neck surgery with inadvertent damage to the recurrent laryngeal nerve.
- Unilateral nerve palsy results in hoarseness of voice, ineffective cough, and increase risk of aspiration.
- Bilateral nerve palsy causes stridor which may mimic laryngospasm but does not improve with standard airway manoeuvres.

— Presence of mass, fluid or blood in the airway
- This may be due to foreign body inhalation, blood or secretions following airway surgery, excessive secretions in heavy smoker or presence of lesion (e.g., laryngeal tumour, papilloma) in preexisting airway pathology.

— Congenital or acquired airway pathology
- Laryngomalacia in infants is associated with stridor due to infolding of the laryngeal wall during inspiration.
- Tracheomalacia, often caused by long-standing goitre or tumour, causes softening and partial collapse of the tracheal wall during inspiration.

— Residual effect of anaesthetic agents
  - Hypoventilation and incoordinate respiratory muscle function occur when the patient is not fully awake.
  - Inadequate respiratory excursion resulting from inadequate reversal of neuromuscular blockade can give rise to stridor.
  - Decreased conscious state with the tongue falling back may cause airway obstruction.

PREVENTION

The patients at risk of developing postoperative stridor should be identified and measures should be taken to minimize the likelihood of its occurrence.

Some measures are listed here.

— Use steroids such as IV dexamethasone to minimize airway oedema following trauma, instrumentation or surgery of the airway.

— Remove all foreign bodies from the airway at the end of surgery.

— Ensure adequate reversal of neuromuscular blockade.

— Delay extubation if airway oedema is strongly suspected.

— Aggressively clear secretions before extubation and as necessary afterward.

— Extubate either when the patient is fully awake or while deeply sedated enough to ablate airway reflexes.

— Maintain airway support (chin lift, oropharyngeal airway) in a patient who is not fully conscious to ensure a patent airway and prevent the tongue from falling back.

MANIFESTATIONS

Patients with stridor are often in respiratory distress with these clinical features.

— Noisy, high pitched inspiration.

— Reduced inspiratory volume.

— Use of accessory muscles of respiration.

— Paradoxical chest/abdominal movements.

— Restlessness, “air hunger”.

- Secretions in mouth, nose, pharynx.
- Falling SPO_2, cyanosis.
- Inability to excrete CO_2, resulting in hypercarbia with low $ETCO_2$.
- Signs of sympathetic overactivity: hypertension, tachyarrhythmias, ventricular premature contractions.
- Bradycardia leading to cardiac arrest – ominously late sign!

Note that standard airway support manoeuvres may not result in much improvement, and measures to relieve upper airway obstruction should be instituted early.

MANAGEMENT

Urgent management is indicated because hypoxaemia will set in if early measures are not taken to rectify the problem. These include:

- Immediate management
  - Deliver high flows of oxygen (10–15 L/min) by face mask.
  - Apply standard airway support using chin lift, jaw thrust; insert oro- or nasopharyngeal airway.
  - Assess the depth and adequacy of respiration.
  - Assist ventilation with continuous positive airway pressure (CPAP).
  - Encourage the patient to take slow, steady breaths.
  - Suction the oropharynx to remove secretions.
  - Consider administering an additional dose of anticholinesterase (half the initial dose) if inadequate reversal of neuromuscular blockade is strongly suspected: be wary of cholinergic crisis in susceptible individuals such as patients with myasthenia gravis.
  - Closely monitor the patient's oxygen saturation and review the haemodynamic status.
- If stridor does not resolve or falling SpO_2/cyanosis sets in
  - Call for help; ask for difficult intubation trolley; prepare for emergency re-intubation.
  - Use a smaller sized endotracheal tube in case of laryngeal oedema.

- Remember that laryngeal mask airway may not overcome airway obstruction if the obstruction occurs at the glottic or subglottic level.
- If tracheal intubation is difficult and SpO_2 remains low, perform an immediate cricothyrotomy and begin transtracheal jet ventilation.

— If this occurs after neck surgery, and neck haematoma is suspected
- Call for the surgeon immediately.
- Remove dressings from the wound.
- Remove the wound sutures if haematoma is found. Surgical exploration of wound, haemostasis and re-suture will be required.
- Re-intubation if there is no improvement.

— If this occurs after airway surgery, and airway oedema is suspected
- Call for the surgeon immediately.
- Administer intravenous dexamethasone if not given previously.
- Thoroughly suction the mouth and pharynx.
- Consider the possibility of retained gauze, pharyngeal pack or other foreign body in the airway.
- Consider nebulization with racemic adrenaline after the presence of foreign body has been ruled out: dose of adrenaline 0.05 ml/kg (maximum 5 ml of 1:1,000 solution) administered via the nebulizer.
- Prepare for direct examination of airway and/or re-intubation.

— Options after re-intubation
- Trial of extubation if the underlying cause has been identified and corrected.
  — Laryngospasm has resolved.
  — Foreign body in the airway has been removed.
  — Neck haematoma has been drained.
  — Neuromuscular blockade has been fully reversed.
- Full or assisted ventilation in ICU if the underlying cause is not immediately correctable.
  — Tracheomalacia.
  — Recurrent laryngeal nerve palsy.
  — Laryngeal oedema.
- Consider tracheostomy in patients with severe tracheomalacia or bilateral recurrent laryngeal nerve palsy which is unlikely to resolve with conservative management.

— Reassessment after the airway has been secured. These complications may be encountered.

- Pulmonary aspiration.
- Postobstructive pulmonary oedema.
- Airway trauma.
- Myocardial ischaemia.

Appropriate management should be instituted for each complication.

FURTHER READING

1. Rose DK, Chen MM, Wigglesworth DF, DeBoer DP. Critical respiratory events in the postanesthetic care unit. Anesthesiology 1994;81:410–8.
2. Hartley M, Vaughan RS. Problems associated with tracheal extubation. Br J Anaesth 1993;71:561–8.
3. McConkey PP. Postobstructive pulmonary oedema: A case series and review. Anaesth Intens Care 2000;28:72–6.

Chapter 68

Perioperative Cardiac Arrhythmias

INTRODUCTION

Benign cardiac arrhythmias are common in the perioperative period and may occur in 60–80% of patients. Most of these are transient bradyarrhythmias and premature atrial and ventricular depolarizations. Even though heart rhythm other than sinus is listed as one of the risk factors in Goldman's Multi-factorial Risk Index, newer guidelines do not consider haemodynamically insignificant arrhythmias to result in postoperative cardiac complications. However, the occurrence of perioperative arrhythmias may unmask the presence of previously undiagnosed cardiopulmonary disease, and should prompt the anaesthesiologist to search for predisposing factors and correct them as far as possible.

Tachyarrhythmias can be classified according to the morphology of the QRS complex on ECG.

— Narrow QRS complex or supraventricular tachycardia (SVT).
  - Sinus tachycardia.
  - Atrial fibrillation (AF).
  - Atrial flutter.
  - Atrial tachycardia (ectopic and re-entrant).
  - Multi-focal atrial tachycardia.
  - Atrioventricular (AV) nodal re-entry tachycardia.
  - Junctional tachycardia.
  - Accessory pathway-mediated tachycardia.

— Wide QRS complex tachycardia.
  - Ventricular tachycardia (VT).
  - Ventricular fibrillation (VF).
  - SVT with aberrant conduction (bundle-bunch block, intraventricular conduction defect).

Bradyarrhythmias and conduction disorders may also be seen. Sinus bradycardia is usually benign, while various degrees of conduction disorders may be of concern in the perioperative setting. Patients at risk of developing complete heart block should have prophylactic transvenous pacing wire inserted before surgery, and transcutaneous pacing units should be readily available during the perioperative period.

Serious cardiac arrhythmias leading to cardiac arrest are highlighted in Chapter 69.

PREDISPOSING FACTORS

These factors should be considered and corrected as far as possible.

— Preexisting cardiac arrhythmias.
— Myocardial ischaemia or infarction.
— Hypotension of various causes.
— Hypoxaemia, hypercarbia, acidosis, electrolyte imbalance.
— Extreme hypothermia.
— Mechanical irritation, such as central venous catheter, pulmonary artery catheter, chest drain.
— Micro- or macro-shock.
— Drug toxicity, e.g., digitalis.
— Total spinal (severe bradycardia may be more likely than cardiac arrest).

PRINCIPLES OF MANAGEMENT

— **Diagnosis of arrhythmia**
  - Distinguish between supraventricular and ventricular rhythms; note that most wide-complex tachycardias are ventricular in origin.
  - If possible, obtain an ECG tracing before and during pharmacological interventions, and after conversion to a regular rhythm. A 12-lead ECG is preferred to tracing from a single lead on the monitor. This is often not feasible in the OT setting while the patient is on the OT table and surgery is on-going.

— **Assessment of haemodynamic status**
  - Assess whether the patient is haemodynamically stable.
  - Look for evidence of tissue hypoperfusion or impaired consciousness in an unanaesthetized patient.

— **Initiation of treatment measures**
  - Haemodynamically unstable patients require immediate cardioversion.
  - Stable patients are treated pharmacologically with the aim of achieving ventricular rate control.
  - Efforts to convert rhythm back to sinus by means of antiarrhythmic agents are more controversial. For recent-onset perioperative SVT, more than 50% revert to sinus rhythm spontaneously within 24 hours, and most of the antiarrhythmic agents have limited efficacy for successful chemical cardioversion.

— **Reassessment**
  - Re-check haemodynamic status, prepare for immediate cardioversion if the patient becomes unstable at any stage.
  - Correct predisposing factors that might have triggered the event.
  - In the OT setting, discuss with the surgeon and decide whether it is safe to commence or proceed with surgery.
  - Arrange for admission to ICU, CCU or HDU for postoperative observation and management. Arrange for cardiology consult.

SYNCHRONIZED CARDIOVERSION

— A direct current (DC) shock is administered in synchronized cardioversion in an attempt to covert arrhythmia to sinus rhythm.

— This is indicated in haemodynamically unstable patients with SVT.

— If the patient is conscious, administer midazolam, fentanyl or a small dose of intravenous induction agent such as etomidate (preferred over propofol in unstable patients).

- If not already intubated, the patient may require endotracheal intubation if the risk of gastric aspiration is high; otherwise achieve airway maintenance by means of face mask or laryngeal mask airway.
- Monitor the patient's ECG, blood pressure and oxygen saturation during the procedure.
- The defibrillator is engaged on synchronized mode and energy level selected according to the type of arrhythmia.
  - Paroxysmal SVT and atrial flutter often respond to lower energy levels (start with 50 J).
  - AF requires a starting energy level of 100 J, escalating to 200 J, 300 J, 360 J for each subsequent attempt.
- Reset the synchronization mode after each attempt because most defibrillators default back to unsynchronized mode.
- If delays in synchronization occur and the clinical condition is critical, go immediately to unsynchronized shocks.

MANAGEMENT OF SUPRAVENTRICULAR TACHYCARDIA

- In a patient who suddenly develops SVT, attempts should be made to rule out potential causes unless the patient exhibits extreme haemodynamic instability.
- In less urgent cases, initial vagal manoeuvres such as carotid massage may be performed. IV adenosine 6 mg can be administered as a rapid bolus and repeated at 12 mg after 1–2 minutes if no response is seen.
- Stable SVT can be treated with either β-blockers or calcium channel blockers to slow down the ventricular rate. IV esmolol is suitable and easily titratable because of its short duration of action.
- Calcium channel blockers may be used with caution in patients with compromised cardiac function, diltiazem being preferable to verapamil in this context because it has less negative inotropic action. However, hypotension may necessitate discontinuation of diltiazem treatment.
- For patients with congestive cardiac failure, digoxin and amiodarone are recommended for rate control of SVT. Digoxin has a slow onset of action and should be used in conjunction with another agent until it starts to take effect.
- Paroxysmal SVT secondary to accessory pathways such as the Wolff-Parkinson-White (WPW) syndrome merits a special mention. Patients with WPW are at risk

of developing VF if they are treated with AV-nodal blocking agents such as digoxin, β-blockers, calcium channel blockers or adenosine, as a result of enhanced conduction along the accessory pathway. Procainamide should be used instead.

MANAGEMENT OF VENTRICULAR TACHYCARDIA

- Therapeutic approach to VT depends on its morphology (monomorphic or polymorphic) as well as whether it is sustained or non-sustained.
- In the absence of cardiac disease, asymptomatic non-sustained VTs do not require antiarrhythmic drug therapy although serum potassium, magnesium and calcium concentrations should be checked and corrected if abnormal. Patients with known cardiac disease should be treated with lignocaine.
- Antiarrhythmic drug therapy for sustained monomorphic VT includes lignocaine, procainamide, amiodarone and β-blockers.
- In the presence of polymorphic VT with prolonged QT interval (torsades de pointes), treatment is focused on reversal of the QT prolongation. Treatment includes IV magnesium sulphate (2–4 g), potassium supplement and manoeuvres aimed at increasing the heart rate (atropine, isoprenaline, temporary overdrive pacing). Lignocaine and phenytoin are suitable antiarrhythmic agents.

FURTHER READING

1. Thompson A, Balser JR. Perioperative cardiac arrhythmias. Br J Anaesth 2004;93:86–94.
2. Shammash JB, Ghali WA. Preoperative assessment and perioperative management of the patient with nonischemic heart disease. Med Clin N Am 2003;87:137–52.
3. American Heart Association. Guidelines 2000 for cardiopulmonary resuscitation and emergency cardiovascular care. Circulation 2000;102 (suppl I).

Chapter 69

Cardiac Arrest

Felicia Lim and C.Y. Lee

INTRODUCTION

Many cardiac arrhythmias that occur during anaesthesia are fortunately benign, transient and require little intervention. However, serious and life-threatening dysrhythmias can occur and require urgent treatment. Successful management includes identification of the patients at risk, early diagnosis and treatment, and correction of the underlying abnormalities which precipitate the cardiac arrhythmia.

Cardiac arrest occurs when there is absence of effective cardiac mechanical activity, while electrical activity of the heart may or may not be present during the arrest.

These conditions are included.

— Asystole.

— Ventricular tachyarrhythmias.

    - Pulseless ventricular tachycardia (pulseless VT).
    - Ventricular fibrillation (VF).
- Pulseless electrical activity (PEA), including:
    - Electromechanical dissociation (EMD).
    - Pseudo-EMD.
    - Idioventricular rhythms.
    - Ventricular escape rhythms.
    - Bradyasystolic rhythms.
    - Postdefibrillation idioventricular rhythms.

PATIENTS AT RISK

These are predisposing factors to serious and life-threatening cardiac arrhythmias.

- Patients with preexisting cardiac arrhythmias.
- Myocardial ischaemia or infarction.
- Hypovolaemia and shock state, such as major trauma with cardiac tamponade, tension pneumothorax, ruptured great vessels.
- Hypoxaemia, hypercarbia acidosis, electrolyte imbalance.
- Drug toxicity, e.g., digitalis.

PREVENTION

These are preventive measures to reduce the occurrence of cardiac arrhythmias.

- Preoperative stabilization or correction of arrhythmia and any precipitating factors; optimize and continue antiarrhythmic therapy during the perioperative period.
- Avoidance of elective surgery after recent myocardial infarction.
- Prophylactic transvenous pacemaker insertion for patients with high-grade atrioventricular block; ensure proper functioning of pacemaker prior to surgery.
- Adequate intravascular volume replacement in hypovolaemia.
- Early recognition and appropriate management of total spinal block.
- Close monitoring of the cardiovascular system: continuous ECG and invasive pressures as indicated.
- Availability of defibrillator, transcutaneous pacemaker and cardiac resuscitation drugs for patients at risk.

MANAGEMENT

1. **Verify that there is no pulsatile flow**
   — Feel for the carotid or femoral pulse.
   — Look at monitors.
   - Unable to measure non-invasive BP.
   - Flat invasive arterial waveform with MAP < 20 mmHg without CPR.
   - Absence of pulse oximeter waveform.
   - Fall in end-tidal CO_2 on capnograph.
   - Absent or abnormal rhythm on ECG.

2. **Call for help**
   — Alert the surgeon, ask him to stop surgery and help resuscitate the patient.
   — Call for more assistants and anaesthetic colleagues.
   — Ask for the resuscitation trolley and defibrillator.
   — Get assistants to draw up resuscitation drugs such as atropine and adrenaline.

3. **Turn off all anaesthetics and administer 100% oxygen at high flow rate**

4. **Begin basic life support**
   — *Airway:* The patient may have been intubated and ventilated, if not apply head tilt and chin lift to maintain airway patency.
   — *Breathing*
   - Ventilate manually at 12 breaths/min until the patient is intubated.
   - Commence or continue mechanical ventilation if the patient is intubated so that other tasks can be attended to.

   — *Circulation*
   - Begin chest compressions at 80–100/min in adults with compression: ventilation ratio of 5:1.
   - Ensure proper compression technique, check arterial waveform during compression if intraarterial cannulation is available.

5. **Diagnose and treat arrhythmias**
   Follow American Heart Association (AHA) Advanced Cardiac Life Support (ACLS) recommendations.

— **Ventricular arrhythmias: Ventricular fibrillation (VF), pulseless ventricular tachycardia (VT).**
- Defibrillate 3 times in a row: 200, 300, 360 J.
- Check rhythm after the first three shocks.
- If persistent or recurrent VF/VT:
  — Secondary ABCD survey for more advanced assessment and treatment.*
  — Adrenaline 1.0 mg, repeat every 3–5 minutes.**
  — Attempt defibrillation at 360 J.
  — Consider antiarrhythmic agents: amiodarone, lignocaine, magnesium sulphate, procainamide.
  — Consider sodium bicarbonate (1 mEq/kg initial dose, check ABG and correct accordingly).
  — Resume attempts to defibrillate.

The sequence should be "drug-shock, drug-shock" pattern

* Secure airway by endotracheal intubation or insertion of airway adjunct (if this has not been done earlier), confirm effective oxygenation and ventilation, establish venous access, identify cardiac rhythm, treat identified reversible causes.

** In the 2000 edition of the ACLS recommendations, it is advocated that IV vasopressin 40 IU should be administered as a single, one-time dose in persistent or recurrent VF/VT after three defibrillation attempts. Vasopressin is a powerful vasoconstrictor and duplicates the positive effects of adrenaline without the adverse effects of the latter.

— **Asystole**
- Check the lead and cable connections, verify asystole in another lead, increase amplitude of tracing.
- Consider possible causes.
  — Hypoxia
  — Hyper- or hypokalaemia
  — Preexisting acidosis
  — Drug overdose
  — Hypothermia

- Transcutaneous pacing if considered, perform immediately.
- Adrenaline 1 mg, repeat every 3–5 minutes.
- Atropine 1 mg, repeat every 3–5 minutes up to a total of 0.04 mg/kg.

— **Pulseless electrical activity**

- Consider possible causes using *mnemonic "PATHO"* and treat accordingly.

  P (tension) **p**neumothorax, **p**ulmonary embolism
  A **a**cute myocardial infarct, **a**cidosis
  T (cardiac) **t**amponade
  H **h**ypovolaemia, **h**ypoxia, **h**ypothermia, **h**yperkalaemia
  O (drug) **o**verdose: tricyclic antidepressants, digitalis, β-blockers, calcium channel blockers

- Adrenaline 1 mg, repeat every 3–5 minutes.
- Atropine 1 mg if bradycardia occurs, repeat every 3–5 minutes to a total of 0.04 mg/kg.

— **Bradycardia**

- Atropine 0.5–1 mg, repeat every 3–5 minutes up to a total of 0.04 mg/kg.
- Transcutaneous pacing if available.
- Dopamine 5–20 μg/kg/min.
- Adrenaline 0.1–1 μg/kg/min.
- Prepare for transvenous pacing.
- *Note:* Isoprenaline should be used with extreme caution; it may be harmful at higher doses.

6. **Consider aetiology of cardiac arrest**

— Review drugs administered, actions or therapeutic manoeuvres taken prior to the arrest.
— Correct any obvious underlying causes.

7. **Secure intravenous access and other monitors**

— Insert large-bore intravenous cannulae and central venous catheter for administration of drugs, but *remember that CPR takes priority over intravenous cannulation.*
— Many drugs used during resuscitation (e.g., adrenaline, atropine, lignocaine) can be given via the endotracheal tube if no venous access is available.
— Check ABG and correct acid-base abnormalities.

— Intraarterial cannulation if peripheral pulses can be felt.
— Bladder catheterization to monitor urine output.

8. **Other aggressive measures in selected cases**
   — Open chest with internal cardiac massage.
   — Institute cardiopulmonary bypass with intraaortic balloon pump.

9. **Subsequent management**
   — Abandon or complete the surgical procedure in the shortest possible time.
   — Arrange for ICU bed and admit patient for ventilation and cardiovascular support.
   — Review by the cardiologist for subsequent therapy.

PAEDIATRIC RESUSCITATION

These guidelines are the recommendations by Paediatric Life Support Working Party based on "Guidelines 2000 for Cardiopulmonary Resuscitation and Emergency Cardiovascular Care" issued by the International Liaison Committee on Resuscitation and American Heart Association. A number of major changes have been introduced.

Important Points to Note in Paediatric Resuscitation

— Cardiopulmonary arrest in infants and children is usually not a sudden event but is the result of prolonged deterioration in respiratory and cardiopulmonary function.
— Commonest underlying cause of cardiac arrest in children is respiratory failure. Second commonest cause is circulatory failure due to loss of fluid or sepsis. Cardiac arrests of primarily cardiac origin are uncommon in children.
— Most important aspect of resuscitation is early recognition of impending arrest and swift intervention.
— Most important intervention is providing an airway and ensuring adequate ventilation.

Paediatric resuscitation is classically divided into basic life support (Figure 69–1) and advanced life support (Figure 69–2). This division is artificial, as both should run concurrently with the advanced procedures providing more definitive treatment.

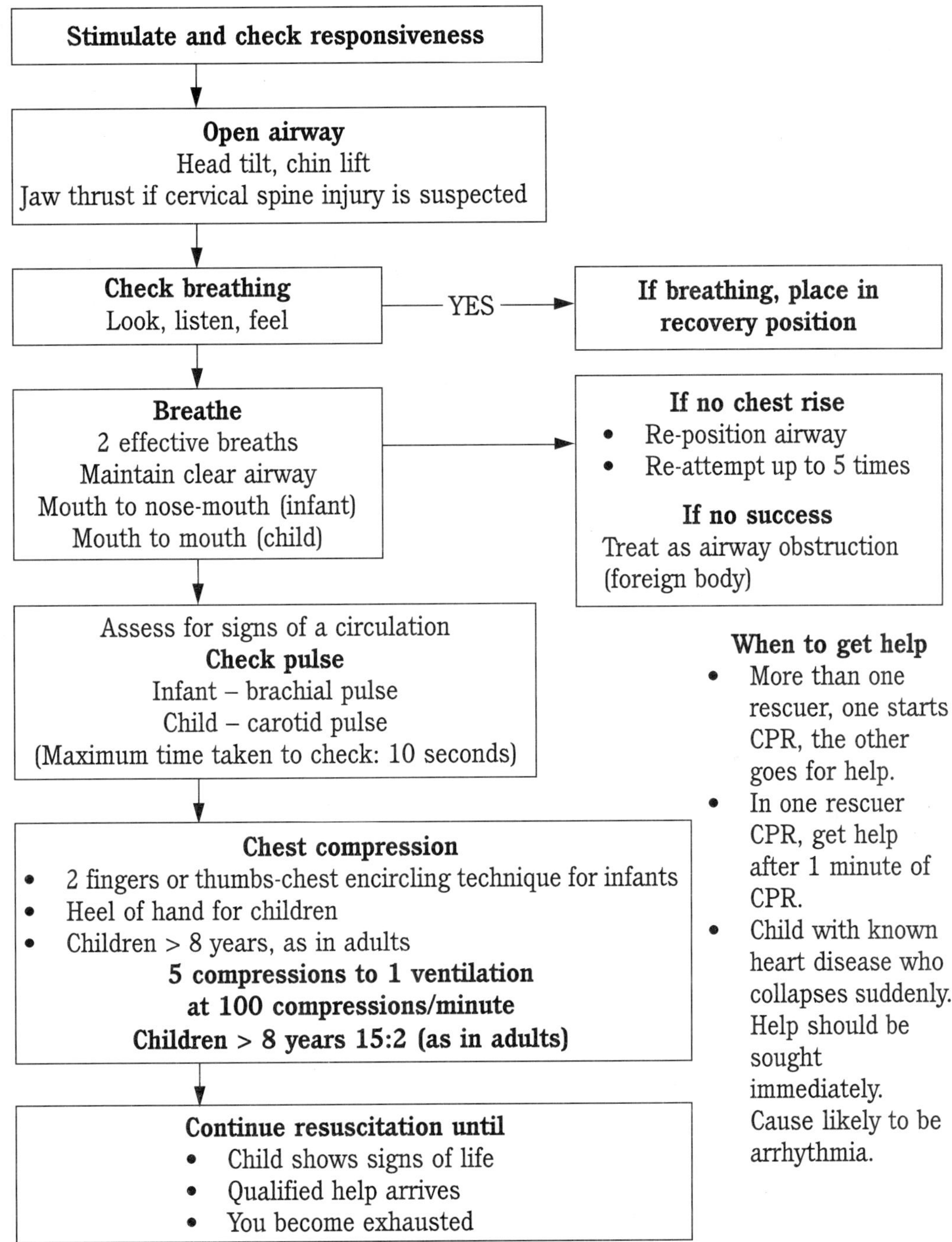

Figure 69–1. Paediatric basic life support

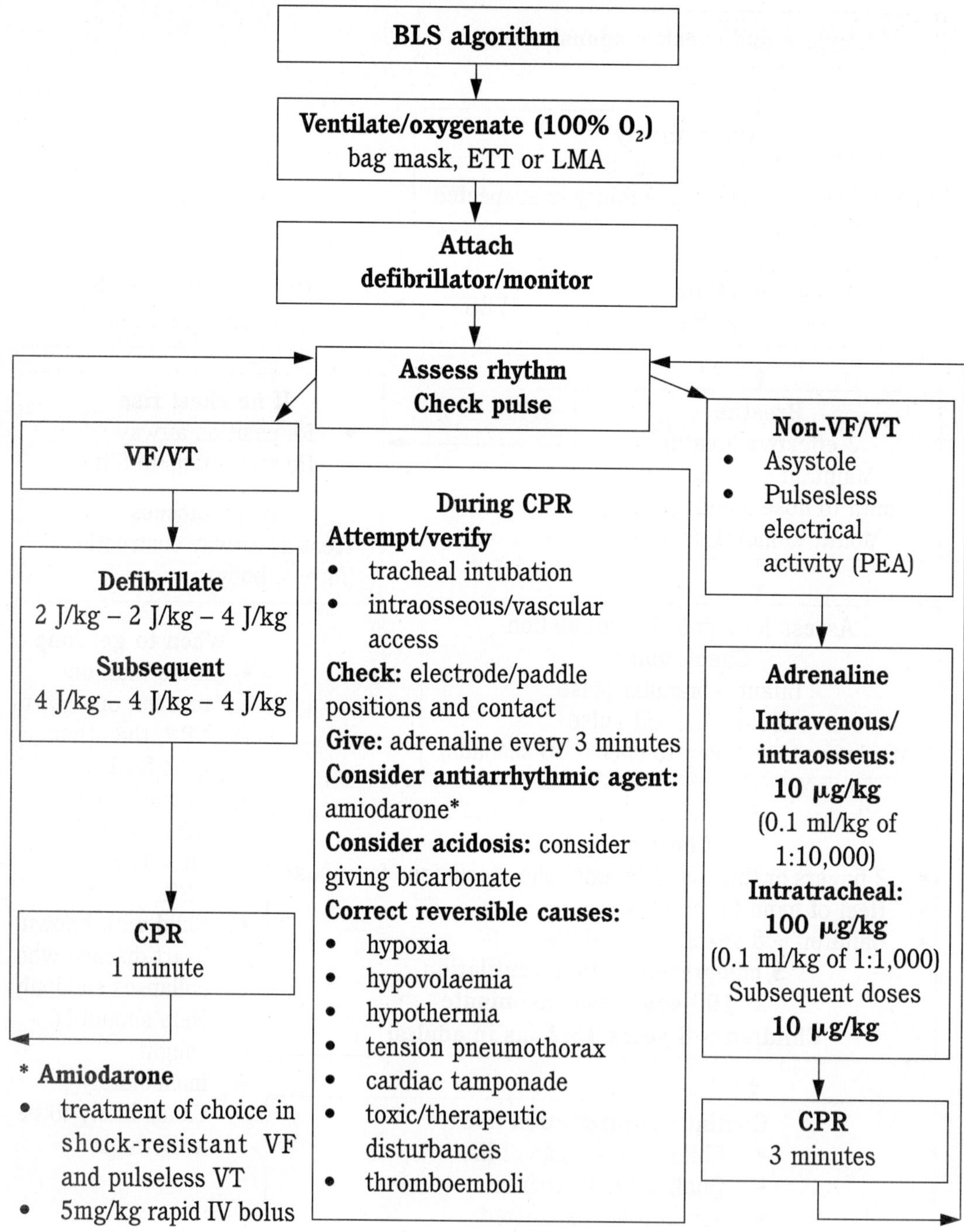

Figure 69–2. Paediatric advanced life support

FURTHER READING

1. Atlee JL. Cardiac arrhythmias: Drugs and devices. Curr Opin Anaesthesiol 2001;14:3–9.
2. Dorian P, et al. Amiodarone as compared with lidocaine for shock-resistant ventricular fibrillation. N Engl J Med 2002;346:884–90.
3. Kern KB, Halperin H, Field J. New guidelines for cardiopulmonary resuscitation and emergency cardiac care: Changes in the management of cardiac arrest. JAMA 2001;285:1267–9.
4. American Heart Association. Guidelines 2000 for cardiopulmonary resuscitation and emergency cardiovascular care. Circulation 2000;102 (suppl I).
5. Pauli H, McKeague H. Sudden haemodynamic collapse and dysrhythmias. Curr Anaesth Crit Care 2003;14:15–23.

Chapter 70

Intraoperative Hypotension

DEFINITION

Hypotension is a reduction in arterial blood pressure greater than 20% below the baseline value. For an average non-hypertensive adult, this usually means a systolic blood pressure ≤ 90 mmHg, or a mean arterial pressure (MAP) ≤ 60 mmHg.

CAUSES

Hypotension may be caused by reductions in preload, myocardial contractility, systemic vascular resistance (SVR), either singly or in combination. The causes can be classified into five areas.

— **Drug causes**
  - Overdosage or overrapid administration of anaesthetic agents.
  - Anaphylaxis or anaphylactoid reaction.
  - Excessive use of antihypertensive agents.

- Drug interaction: certain antihypertensives such as, angiotensin converting enzyme (ACE) inhibitors, angiotensin II receptor antagonists, may potentiate hypotensive effects of anaesthetic agents.
- Drug errors: wrong drug, wrong drug dilution, wrong dose.

— **Anaesthetic technique**
- Central neuraxial blockade especially subarachnoid block.
- Inadequate intravenous fluid preload or use of vasopressor.
- Inadvertent intrathecal injection of local anaesthetic (LA) resulting in high spinal or total spinal.
- Inadvertent intravascular injection of LA resulting in systemic LA toxicity.
- Deliberate hypotension under controlled hypotensive anaesthesia.
- Increase in mean intrathoracic pressure under controlled ventilation with positive end-expiratory pressure (PEEP).

— **Cardiovascular causes**
- Hypovolaemia due to any cause: dehydration, bleeding or third space losses.
- Shock syndromes: hypovolaemic, cardiogenic, anaphylactic or septicaemic shock.
- Pulmonary embolism secondary to thrombus, air, CO_2, amniotic fluid, fat or bone cement.
- Blood transfusion reaction.
- Cardiac pathology
  - — Myocardial ischaemia or infarction.
  - — Cardiac arrhythmias.
  - — Heart failure, acute pulmonary oedema.
  - — Cardiac tamponade.
- Abrupt changes in patient position
  - — From supine to sitting position: sudden reduction in effective blood volume.
  - — From lithotomy to supine position when the legs are lowered too abruptly, especially when the patient is hypovolaemic.
  - — Lateral position with kidney bridge in place: venous return may be impeded by compression of inferior vena cava.

— **Respiratory causes**
- Tension pneumothorax.
- Hypoxaemia due to any cause (late sign).

— **Surgical manoeuvres**
- Vagal reflex by traction or dilatation of viscera (usually associated with bradycardia).

- Oculocardiac reflex (associated with bradycardia).
- Abdominal packs or retractors impeding venous return.
- Pneumoperitoneum impeding venous return during laparoscopic surgery.
- Rapid removal of aortic cross-clamps during aortic surgery.

MANAGEMENT

— *Quickly verify* the blood pressure reading by re-checking.

— *Look at the patient's colour* for pallor or cyanosis: this may be misleading in the presence of hypothermia and extreme anaemia (Hb < 5 g/dl) when cyanosis may be absent. Also look for skin changes such as flushing, rashes, urticaria, oedema that may point to the diagnosis of anaphylaxis.

— *Feel for the peripheral pulse*, note the volume, rate, rhythm, regularity, character of pulse.

- **Strong pulse**
  - — Consider measurement error or transient hypotension.
  - — Repeat blood pressure measurement, palpate the distal pulse manually and check the reading at which pulsation returns.
  - — Move the BP cuff to another site if necessary.
  - — For invasive BP monitoring: check the height of pressure transducer and recalibrate if necessary, ensuring that no damping of the arterial trace occurs.
- **Weak pulse** appropriate to BP reading as indicated on the monitor
  - — Start treatment immediately.
  - — Look for underlying cause of hypotension while resuscitative measures are being carried out.
- **No pulse**
  - — Feel for the carotid pulse.
  - — If the carotid pulse is not palpable, inform the surgeon and immediately commence cardiopulmonary resuscitation (CPR).
  - — *Call for help* to assist in resuscitation.

— **Look at the monitors**

- Check ECG for arrhythmias and ST segment T-wave changes indicative of myocardial ischaemia or infarct.
- Check pulse oximeter for SpO_2 and pulse rate: the signal is likely to be poor or absent because of decreased peripheral perfusion.

- Check capnography for end-tidal CO_2 tracings: $ETCO_2$ may be low or absent due to reduced pulmonary perfusion in the low-flow or cardiac arrest situation; a precipitous drop in $ETCO_2$ is indicative of significant pulmonary embolism.
- Check CVP reading and look at arterial waveform if these are available.

— **Look at the surgical field**

- Assess the amount and rate of blood loss: this may be difficult to estimate in some cases.
- Inform the surgeon if hypotension is due to vagal reflex or abdominal packs/retraction impeding venous return.
- Consider the possibility of pulmonary embolism secondary to thrombus, air, CO_2, amniotic fluid, fat or bone cement in relevant surgical procedures.
- Get the surgeon to re-apply aortic cross-clamp (aortic surgery) until more fluids and/or vasopressors have been administered.
- Elevate the patient's legs above the level of the heart or place the patient in the Trendelenburg position.

— **Ensure adequate ventilation and oxygenation**

- Administer 100% oxygen if SpO_2 is low or hypotension is severe.
- Cut down or withhold administration of volatile anaesthetic if hypotension is severe.
- Do a quick check to ensure that there are no problems with the anaesthetic machine, breathing system, endotracheal tube and cuff.
- Disconnect from the ventilator and manually ventilate the lungs to assess its compliance.
- Auscultate the chest for breath sounds, adventitious sounds (rhonchi or crepitations), heart sounds and murmurs to look for signs indicative of tension pneumothorax, bronchospasm, cardiac tamponade or pulmonary oedema.
- Excessively high block following central neuraxial blockade which affects cardiovascular and respiratory functions requires intubation and ventilation.

— **Expand circulating blood volume**

- Rapid infusion of intravenous fluids; use pressure bags or rapid infusion devices if necessary.
- Insert additional wide-bore intravenous cannulae.
- Consider giving colloids or blood for rapid volume expansion.
- Send blood samples for group and cross match if more blood is likely to be needed.
- Liaise with the Blood Bank, request for blood products (cryoprecipitate, fresh frozen plasma, platelets) if there is clinical evidence of disseminated intra-

vascular coagulation (DIC) such as prolonged ooze from surgical field or venepuncture site or failure of blood to clot.

— *Ask for help* if hypotension is severe or if blood loss is massive. You will need assistance to resuscitate the patient.

— *Vasopressors or inotropes* may be necessary if hypotension is severe
- Ephedrine 5–10 mg increments.
- Phenylephrine 50–100 μg increments.
- Dopamine infusion 5–10 μg/kg/min.
- Adrenaline 1:10,000 0.5–1 ml (50–100 μg) increments.

— **Reassessment**
- Check BP, pulse, CVP, SpO_2 in response to therapy.
- *Remember: hypovolaemia is a very common, but NOT the only, cause of hypotension!*
- Look for specific cause for hypotension and treat accordingly.
- Consider inserting cannulae for invasive arterial BP and CVP monitoring if these are not in place.
- Check urine output, fluid balance, haematocrit, ABG.
- Correct acidosis to improve myocardial contractility and myocardial response to inotropes.
- A return of pulse oximeter tracing is a reassuring sign that resuscitative measures are effective.
- Evaluate cardiac status: myocardial ischaemia or infarction can be the cause or effect of prolonged hypotension in susceptible individuals.
- It may be necessary to infuse vasopressors or inotropes in addition to intravenous fluids to maintain blood pressure close to the baseline value.

FURTHER READING

1. Stainsby D, MacLennan S, Hamilton PJ. Management of massive blood loss: A template guideline. Br J Anaesth 2000;85:487–91.

Chapter 71

Intraoperative and Postoperative Hypertension

INTRODUCTION

Hypertension is defined as an elevation of systolic, diastolic or mean arterial pressure ≥ 20% over baseline value or above age-corrected absolute limits (i.e., systolic blood pressure = age + 100 mmHg).

Hypertension is a common occurrence in the perioperative setting. In the immediate period before induction of anaesthesia, an anxious patient may have markedly elevated BP, which often settles to its normal value once the patient is under anaesthesia. It can also occur intraoperatively and postoperatively, the latter being one of the most common cardiovascular events in PACU.

If left unchecked, intraoperative and postoperative hypertension can precipitate cardiovascular and cerebrovascular events. It can also lead to increased intra- and postoperative blood loss (especially if haemostasis is not well secured) and hence should be diagnosed and treated expediently.

CAUSES OF HYPERTENSION

Intraoperative Hypertension

The causes for intraoperative hypertension are summarized here.

— **Patient factors**
- Preexisting hypertension, especially if poorly controlled.
- Raised intracranial pressure (Cushing's reflex), associated with reflex bradycardia.
- Endocrinopathies: phaeochromocytoma, thyrotoxicosis, carcinoid tumour.
- Autonomic dysreflexia.
- Malignant hyperthermia.

— **Surgical factors**
- Systemic absorption of adrenaline used for infiltration of surgical wounds.
- Aortic cross-clamping with sudden increase in systemic vascular resistance.
- TURP syndrome, associated with hypervolaemia.

— **Anaesthetic factors**
- Inadequate levels of anaesthetic depth, neuromuscular blockade or analgesia.
- Hypercarbia and/or hypoxia due to various causes.
- Acute fluid overload.
- Pharmacological effects of drugs such as ketamine, ergometrine, vasoactive drugs (e.g., adrenaline, ephedrine, phenylephrine).
- Drug interaction, e.g., monoamine oxidase inhibitor (MAOI) with pethidine leading to hypertensive crisis.
- Drug error: wrong drug, wrong drug dilution, wrong dose.

— **Spurious hypertension**

Equipment malfunction or measurement error, such as:
- Wrong calibration of pressure transducer for intraarterial BP measurement.
- Use of BP cuff that is too narrow for the arm circumference.

Postoperative Hypertension

Additional causes of hypertension relevant in the postoperative setting include:

- Inadequate pain relief, anxiety.
- Hypothermia, shivering.
- Hypoxaemia, hypercarbia.
- Anaesthesia emergence, excitement, delirium.
- Restlessness due to bladder distension.
- Hypervolaemia.
- Increased intracranial pressure.
- Drug-induced causes: vasopressor therapy, rebound hypertension following controlled hypotensive anaesthesia on cessation of hypotensive agents.
- Surgical factors: postoperative hypertension is often associated with cardiothoracic, vascular (e.g., carotid endarterectomy, aortic surgery), head and neck and neurosurgical procedures.

MANIFESTATIONS

Hypertension is diagnosed when there is more than one elevated BP readings. An isolated reading should be re-checked in case there is an error in BP measurement.

- Signs of sympathetic activity:
  - Tachypnoea in patients with spontaneous respiration.
  - Tachycardia, bounding pulse.
  - Sweating, lacrimation, pupillary dilatation.
- Bradycardia may be present if the underlying cause is raised intracranial pressure or autonomic dysreflexia.
- Secondary manifestations of severe hypertension include:
  - Altered level of consciousness in awake patient.
  - Myocardial ischaemia or infarction.
  - Cardiac dysrrhythmias.
  - Acute heart failure, pulmonary oedema.

MANAGEMENT OF INTRAOPERATIVE HYPERTENSION

The more common causes of hypertension should be excluded before considering the rarer ones.

— **Verify that the hypertension is real**
- Repeat BP measurement, feel for the distal pulse on the occluded arm and check the reading at which pulsation returns.
- Move the BP cuff to another site if necessary.
- For invasive BP monitoring: check the height of pressure transducer and re-calibrate if necessary, ensuring that the arterial trace is not underdamped.
- *Do not spend too long checking and re-checking:* precious time may be wasted on this while measures should be taken to diagnose the cause and treat the underlying pathology.

— **Ensure adequate oxygenation and ventilation**
- It is important to rule out hypoxia and hypercarbia as the cause of intra-operative hypertension.
- Check the pulse and colour of the patient.
- Look at the monitors: ECG, SpO_2, end-tidal CO_2.
- Check anaesthetic equipment: oxygen analyzer, breathing circuit, soda lime, valves, ventilator connection, endotracheal tube and cuff.
- Manually ventilate the patient to feel for compliance, watch bilateral chest expansion and auscultate the lungs for breath sounds.

— **Assess depth of anaesthesia**
- Inhalational anaesthesia: check anaesthetic agent concentration and MAC reading on monitor.
- Intravenous anaesthesia: rule out problems with infusion pump, infusion tubing or intravenous cannula to make sure that intravenous anaesthetic is being delivered to the patient.
- Administer volatile anaesthetic, opioid analgesic or intravenous anaesthetic if depth of anaesthesia is deemed inadequate.
- Administer an additional dose of neuromuscular blocking drug if neuromuscular blockade is wearing off and in the presence of adequate anaesthetic depth.

— **Review fluid management**
- Consider administration of frusemide 10–20 mg if overtransfusion is suspected.

- Raised intracranial pressure may require urgent therapy with mannitol and/or frusemide.
- Check for distended bladder; relieve this if present.

— **Specific antihypertensive drug therapy**

The following antihypertensive agents may be used if specific treatment is necessary. This is summarized in Table 71–1.

- Beta blockade (particularly useful in the presence of tachycardia).
  - Esmolol (short-acting β-adrenergic blocker): 10–20 mg increments, dose 0.5–1 mg/kg.
  - Labetalol (α- and β-adrenergic blocker): 5–10 mg increments.
- Vasodilator (may cause further tachycardia).
  - Hydralazine: 5 mg slow IV every 15 minutes.
  - Sodium nitroprusside infusion.*
  - Nitroglycerin infusion.*
  - Nicardipine (calcium channel blocker): 5 mg/hr initially, increase by 2.5 mg/hr every 15 minutes, maximum 15 mg/hr.

* Needs invasive haemodynamic monitoring.

Table 17–1. Antihypertensive agents for management of hypertensive emergencies

Clinical Scenario	Drug of Choice
Severe acute hypertension	Sodium nitroprusside, often in combination with β-blocker (esmolol) or α- and β-blocker (labetalol)
Hypertension with no cardiac compromise	Vasodilator (hydralazine) Calcium channel blocker (nicardipine)
Hypertension with myocardial ischaemia	Nitroglycerin infusion
Hypertension with tachycardia and ischaemia ischaemia	β-blocker (esmolol) or α- and β-blocker (labetalol) in combination with nitroglycerin infusion
Hypertension with heart failure	ACE inhibitor Inodilator Vasodilator

— Review blood pressure after excluding and treating the more common causes. Think of the rarer conditions if blood pressure remains elevated despite treatment.
— Close monitoring of blood pressure intra- and postoperatively. Inform the surgeon if blood pressure control is a problem. Start the patient on antihypertensive therapy postoperatively.

MANAGEMENT OF POSTOPERATIVE HYPERTENSION

Treatment should be individualized. The underlying causes of hypertension – pain, anxiety, hypothermia, hypoxaemia, inadequate ventilation leading to hypercarbia, distended bladder – should be identified and treated. When the underlying problem has been solved, it is often unnecessary to institute specific antihypertensive therapy.

Short-term administration of antihypertensive drugs is recommended when there is no identifiable, treatable cause of hypertension. Intravenous agents are commonly recommended since most cases occur shortly after surgery when the patient is recovering from the effects of anaesthesia.

Treatment options (after ruling out the other causes of hypertension):

- IV labetalol 5–10 mg.
- IV esmolol 0.5–1 mg/kg.
- IV hydralazine 5 mg.
- IV infusion of potent vasodilators such as sodium nitroprusside, nitroglycerin can be used especially following cardiac surgery but the haemodynamic parameters must be invasively monitored.

The use of sublingual nifedipine in the immediate postoperative period is not advisable. Absorption from the sublingual route is difficult to control, reduction of BP may be excessive, and tachycardia may facilitate development of myocardial ischaemia.

The treatment goal is based on the patient's preoperative BP, a conservative target being approximately 10% above that baseline value.

FURTHER READING

1. Skarvan K. Perioperative hypertension: New strategies for management. Curr Opin Anaesthesiol 1998;11:29–35.
2. Rose DK, Cohen MM, DeBoer DP. Cardiovascular events in the postanesthesia care unit. Anesthesiology 1996;84:772–81.
3. Haas CE, LeBlanc JM. Acute postoperative hypertension: A review of therapeutic options. Am J Health-Syst Pharm 2004;61:1661–73.

Chapter 72

Malignant Hyperthermia

SOME FACTS ABOUT MALIGNANT HYPERTHEMIA

Malignant hyperthermia (MH), also known as malignant hyperpyrexia, is an inherited myopathic disorder of fulminant hypermetabolic crisis precipitated by certain triggering agents. Exposure to these agents results in an abnormal release of calcium into the cytoplasm causing myofibrillar contraction, accelerated metabolic rate and increased carbon dioxide and heat production. Increase in skeletal muscle metabolism and subsequent rhabdomyolysis may lead to acute renal failure.

The incidence of MH is reported to be 1:10,000–1:200,000 with a male preponderance. Hereditary pattern is autosomal dominant with incomplete penetrance. Mortality rate of a full-blown MH is 60–75%. With better knowledge, early recognition as well as the use of dantrolene and other forms of resuscitative measures, the mortality rate from MH reactions in the past 10 years is approximately 2–3%. The time of presentation ranges from immediately postinduction (25% cases), intraoperative (50% cases) to postoperative period (25% cases).

Suxamethonium and volatile anaesthetic agents are well-known triggers for MH. Patients at risk are those with past or family history of MH. The incidence is higher in the paediatric and young adult populations compared to older patients. Two conditions – central core disease and King-Denborough syndrome – have definite associations with MH. Certain congenital abnormalities (e.g., strabismus, musculoskeletal deformities) and other neuromuscular diseases have been linked with MH even though no definite causal relationship has been established.

CLINICAL MANIFESTATIONS

Clinical manifestations of full-blown MH are listed here.

— Sustained jaw rigidity (masseter spasm) following suxamethonium may be an early sign.

— Increased carbon dioxide production resulting in rapidly increasing end-tidal CO_2, rapid utilization and increased heat production in CO_2 absorber and tachypnoea in a spontaneously ventilating patient.

— Cardiovascular instability with labile BP; ECG abnormalities such as sinus tachycardia, tachyarrhythmia, multiple ventricular ectopics, peaked T-waves; cardiovascular collapse.

— Falling SpO_2 despite increase in FiO_2; cyanosis.

— Rapid rise of core temperature of > 2°C/hr, sometimes as much as > 1°C every 10 minutes; hyperthermia is not an early sign and is usually apparent only after hypercarbia and tachycardia.

— Marked generalized skeletal muscle rigidity.

— Metabolic and respiratory acidosis from excessive production of CO_2 and lactic acid.

— Rhabdomyolysis leading to hyperkalaemia, myoglobinuria.

— Renal tubular damage and acute renal failure.

— Disseminated intravascular coagulation (DIC).

Differential diagnoses include:

— Inadequate anaesthetic depth with awareness during anaesthesia.
— Endocrine disorders: thyrotoxic crisis, phaeochromocytoma.
— Neurolept malignant syndrome (NMS): hyperthermia, acidosis, hyperkalaemia and myoglobinuria following use of neuroleptics particularly haloperidol.
— Drugs causing tachycardia or hyperthermia, such as atropine, scopolamine.
— Recreational drug overdose: cocaine or ecstasy.
— Pyrexia of other causes, sepsis.
— Hypercarbia due to hypoventilation, re-breathing, exhaustion of CO_2 absorbent in circle circuit.
— Faulty equipment for measuring temperature or CO_2.
— Iatrogenic overheating.

MANAGEMENT

Successful outcome in MH hinges on its early diagnosis and expedient management on recognition of a reaction. Several modes of treatment must be instituted simultaneously and with emphasis on the urgency of the situation.

— *As soon as the diagnosis is made, inform the surgeon and declare an MH emergency. Get help. Ask for the MH trolley.*
— **Initial measures**
  - Stop all possible triggering agents.
  - Administer 100% oxygen; increase fresh gas flows and hyperventilate at 2–3 times the minute ventilation.
  - Use a fresh breathing circuit and "volatile anaesthetic-free" anaesthetic machine if possible, but do not waste time doing so at the expense of other more urgent measures.
  - Get a self-inflating bag and a separate oxygen source to ventilate the patient while waiting for the anaesthetic machine to be changed.
  - Maintain anaesthesia with intravenous anaesthetic agents (opioids, sedatives) and non-depolarizing neuromuscular blocker as needed.

— **Dantrolene sodium: The definitive treatment for MH**
  - Dantrolene sodium acts by depressing the intrinsic mechanism of excitation-contraction coupling in skeletal muscle.

- It is a yellow/orange powder stored in a vial of 20 mg with 3 gm of mannitol and sodium hydroxide. It should be protected from light. Each vial is reconstituted with 60 ml of water. The resultant solution should be injected into a large vein or a fast running infusion because it is alkaline (pH 9.5) and highly irritating to peripheral veins.
- Get an assistant to prepare dantrolene solution, as this takes some time to reconstitute.
- Administer an initial dose of 2.5 mg/kg over 5 minutes. Further 1 mg/kg bolus doses can be given at 5–10 minute intervals until normalization of the hypermetabolic state and disappearance of all MH symptoms, usually at a total dose of 10 mg/kg or less. Reconsider diagnosis of MH if > 20 mg/kg dantrolene is not successful.

— **Initiate cooling by various measures**
- Withhold the use of heating devices, remove garments or blankets, reduce OT temperature.
- Surface cooling with ice packs or cold water.
- Cold intravenous solutions.
- Cold gastric lavage via nasogastric tube.
- Cold peritoneal lavage if the peritoneal cavity is opened.

Monitor core temperature to assess response to treatment and *avoid overcooling*. Stop active cooling measures when temperature decreases to 38°C. Avoid peripheral vasoconstriction as this prevents heat loss.

— **Establish monitoring**
- Insert urinary catheter, intraarterial and central venous cannulae (if not present).
- Send these samples for investigations.
  — Blood for ABG, urea and electrolytes including calcium concentration, creatine kinase (CK) concentration, coagulation screen.
  — Urine for myoglobin assay.

— **Management of cardiac arrhythmias, acidosis, hyperkalaemia**
- Hypoxia, hypercarbia, acidosis and hyperkalaemia all contribute to tachyarrhythmias and ectopics. Therapy should aim at correction of the underlying causes.
- Administer IV lignocaine 1 mg/kg or IV procainamide 200 mg for persistent ventricular arrhythmia. Avoid calcium channel blockers as they may interact with high-dose dantrolene and may precipitate severe hyperkalaemia and cardiac arrest.

- Acidosis in a ventilated patient can be initially treated with sodium bicarbonate 1–2 mEq/kg and then as indicated by serial ABG estimations.
- Treat hyperkalaemia with insulin 10 U administered together with glucose 50 g.

— **Management of renal function and coagulopathy**
- Maintain urine output > 1–2 ml/kg/hr with intravenous fluids and diuretics as guided by serial CVP measurements.
- Use normal saline instead of potassium-containing intravenous fluids.
- Consider further doses of mannitol (in addition to the mannitol contained in the dantrolene solution) or frusemide to promote diuresis.
- Cryoprecipitate, platelets and fresh frozen plasma may be required to correct coagulation abnormalities if DIC occurs.

— **ICU management**
- Recrudescence occurs in 25% of cases; hence close monitoring is required for at least 24 hours.
- Administer further doses of dantrolene if rigidity, rhabdomyolysis, elevated temperature or hypercarbia persist. Further doses of dantrolene (approximately 1 mg/kg every 4–6 hours) may be necessary for at least 24 hours after control of episode. Watch for muscle weakness, a side-effect of dantrolene.
- Repeat ABG and biochemical tests frequently as indicated.
- Monitor haemodynamic parameters and urine output. Watch for cardiovascular instability, renal failure and coagulopathy.
- The patient may be extubated 8–12 hours later if the general condition is satisfactory.

SUBSEQUENT MANAGEMENT

— Complete and thorough documentation is essential. Information includes description of the MH episode, personnel involved, measures instituted and the patient's response to treatment. This should be done at the earliest available opportunity and should be recorded clearly in the patient's case notes and anaesthesia record.

— Inform the patient and family members regarding the disorder. If facilities are available, arrange for muscle biopsy (for *in vitro* halothane-caffeine contracture test) for the patient 3 months after the episode. If the diagnosis of MH-susceptibility is confirmed, immediate family members should be investigated in the same manner.

— Counsel the patient and family members regarding future anaesthetics and encourage the use of Medic Alert bracelet or any other form of warning.

FUTURE ANAESTHETIC MANAGEMENT

— The surgery should be performed under regional anaesthesia where appropriate.

— If general anaesthesia is necessary, anaesthetic agents known for triggering MH should be avoided.

— An anaesthetic machine free of volatile anaesthetic agent should be used. This can be prepared by removing the vaporizers and flushing through the machine and ventilator with 100% oxygen at maximal flows for 20–30 minutes.

— Oral preanaesthetic dantrolene prophylaxis is no longer recommended. The necessity of prophylactic IV dantrolene 2 mg/kg at induction has also been questioned as long as the anaesthetic is trigger-free and dantrolene is available at the OT.

— Establish intraoperative monitoring. Mandatory monitoring include ECG, blood pressure, capnography, pulse oximetry and core temperature. Further monitors may be established as appropriate to the patient's condition and nature of surgery.

— These drugs are considered safe for MH patients: all intravenous induction agents including ketamine, non-depolarizing neuromuscular blocking drugs, nitrous oxide, opioids, local anaesthetics, benzodiazepines, metoclopramide, atropine, glycopyrrolate, and neostigmine. The use of total intravenous anaesthesia (TIVA) is recommended.

— Avoid calcium channel blockers because they can produce marked cardiac depression in combination with dantrolene.

— Have a high index of suspicion for early diagnosis and intervention if MH occurs.

— The patient should be closely monitored in ICU or HDU for 24–48 hours postoperatively as MH may occur during this period.

APPENDIX

SUGGESTED CONTENTS ON MH TROLLEY

Drugs

— Dantrolene sodium: 36 vials.

— 8.4% sodium bicarbonate: 10 ampoules.

— 50% dextrose solution: 2 ampoules.
— Insulin 100 U/ml: 1 vial (kept in refrigerator).
— 10% calcium chloride: 2 ampoules.
— 2% lignocaine hydrochloride: 5 ampoules.
— 20% mannitol: 500 ml × 2 bottles.
— Frusemide 20 mg/2 ml: 4 ampoules.
— Heparin 5,000 U/ml: 1 vial.
— Sterile water for injection: 500 ml × 5 bottles.

Others

— Intravenous catheters/cannulae of various sizes for adult and paediatric patients.
— Syringes × 5 each at 2 ml, 5 ml, 10 ml, 50 ml.
— Urinary catheters of various calibres.
— Temperature probes: nasopharyngeal, rectal.
— Orogastric/nasogastric tubes of various calibres.
— Clear plastic bags (for making ice packs) × 10.
— Laboratory request forms (haematology, electrolytes, clotting screen, urine for myoglobin).
— Blood investigation bottles (FBC, electrolytes, calcium, CK, clotting studies).
— Urine specimen containers.

FURTHER READING

1. Finsterer J. Current concepts in malignant hyperthermia. J Clin Neuromusc Dis 2002;4:64–74.
2. Hopkins PM. Malignant hyperthermia: Advances in clinical management and diagnosis. Br J Anaesth 2000;85:118–28.
3. Adnet PJ, Gronert GA. Malignant hyperthermia: Advances in diagnostics and management. Curr Opin Anaesthesiol 1999;12:353–8.
4. Krause T, et al. Dantrolene – A review of its pharmacology, therapeutic use and new developments. Anaesthesia 2004;59:364–73.
5. Ali SZ, Taguchi A, Rosenberg H. Malignant hyperthermia. Best Prac Res Clin Anaesthesiol 2003;17:519–33.

Chapter 73
Oliguria

INTRODUCTION

Oliguria is generally defined as urine output of less than 0.5 ml/kg/hr, or a daily urine output of less than 400 ml in an adult. The patient is considered to be anuric if the daily urine output decreases to less than 100 ml/24 hr.

Acute renal failure (ARF) is defined as an abrupt decline in renal function associated with retention of nitrogenous waste and disruption of fluid and electrolyte homeostasis. There is no consensus regarding a quantifiable definition of ARF. The origin of ARF is usually classified as prerenal (35% of cases), intrarenal (50–55%) and postrenal (10%).

Commonly ARF follows renal hypoperfusion of varying degrees. Mild renal hypoperfusion can be compensated by local mechanisms which preserve renal blood flow and glomerular filtration rate (GFR). Moderate renal hypoperfusion results in a loss of GFR and prerenal ARF, but may be reversible if circulation is adequately restored. Severe renal hypoperfusion results in persistent renal ischaemia and intrarenal ARF; and is often associated with histological evidence of acute tubular necrosis (ATN).

Oliguria can be an ominous sign since oliguric ARF carries mortality as high as 80% despite improvements in dialysis therapies. It is, therefore, important that the underlying cause should be identified and appropriate treatment instituted early to avoid development of renal failure.

CAUSES OF OLIGURIA

Mechanical causes

- Blocked, dislodged or disconnected urinary catheter: *easiest to treat, need to rule out first!*
- Ureteral obstruction due to stones, stricture or tumour.
- Surgical factors (especially during pelvic surgery): compression of bladder by retractors, unintentional cystotomy or ligation of one or both ureters.

True reduction of urine volume

- Renal hypoperfusion, secondary to
  - Hypovolaemia.
  - Congestive heart failure.
  - Aortic cross-clamp during aortic surgery.
  - Increased intraabdominal pressure with compression of renal vasculature.
  - Shock arising from any cause.
- Intrinsic renal disease.
- Excessive secretion of antidiuretic hormone (ADH).

"AT RISK" SITUATIONS FOR THE KIDNEY

Predisposing factors to the development of perioperative ARF can be considered under factors related to the patient, anaesthesia and surgery, as well as events during resuscitation and intensive care management.

Patients at risk

— Advanced age.
— Diabetes mellitus.
— Preexisting renal insufficiency.
— Renovascular disease such as renal artery stenosis.
— Cardiac failure.
— Hepatic dysfunction with jaundice.
— Pregnancy-induced hypertension.
— Excessive preoperative fluid restriction.
— Abnormal fluid losses with inadequate replacement.

Anaesthesia and surgery

— Lengthy or extensive surgery with large fluid shifts.
— Surgery of the aorta or renal vessels.
— Cardiopulmonary bypass.
— Major biliary tree surgery, liver transplantation.
— Kidney transplantation.

Intensive care and resuscitation

— Prolonged hypotension or hypovolaemia.
— Rhabdomyolysis and myoglobinuria from trauma, crush injury, malignant hyperthermia.
— Massive transfusion or transfusion of mismatched blood with resultant haemoglobinuria.
— Septicaemia especially secondary to intraabdominal sepsis.
— Obstetric complications such as abruptio placentae.
— Nephrotoxic drugs and substances (Table 73–1).

Table 73–1. Nephrotoxic drugs and substances

Category	Example
Analgesic	Aspirin, NSAIDs
Antimicrobial agent	Aminoglycosides, amphotericin B, vancomycin, sulphonamides, rifampicin
Antipsychotic drug	Lithium
Anticancer drug	Cisplatinum, methotrexate
Immunosuppressant	Cyclosporin
Others	Radiocontrast agents, pigments (haemoglobin, myoglobin), calcium, uric acid, heavy metals, ACE inhibitors, diuretics

PREVENTION

— **Identify patients at risk and preoperative optimization**
- Be aware of patient and surgical factors (listed above) which predispose to perioperative development of ARF.
- Optimize hydration and consider invasive haemodynamic monitoring in the perioperative period to guide fluid therapy and use of vasoactive drugs.
- Consider timing of elective surgery in relation to diagnostic procedures which require administration of intravenous radiocontrast media: time given for optimization of renal function and for kidneys to "recover" before surgery.

— **Monitoring of renal function**
- Bladder catheterization and hourly urine output measurement is the only practical means of monitoring renal function during anaesthesia and surgery, even though urine output *per se* is not a reliable indicator of renal function.
- Hourly urine output should be maintained at 0.5–1 ml/kg or greater.
- A decline in urine output should trigger an evaluation of the patient's haemodynamic and intravascular status, and steps to rule out mechanical causes of oliguria.

— **Modification of surgical technique**
- Use of endovascular technique of aortic aneurysm repair reduces aortic manipulation and renal ischaemia compared to open surgery. This is associated with lower incidence of postoperative renal injury.

- Aortic cross-clamp time is the strongest predictor of postoperative renal dysfunction, especially if the time exceeds 50 minutes.
- Other preventive measures suggested include hypothermic renal perfusion, intermittent arterial blood renal perfusion.

— **Maintenance of stable haemodynamic parameters**
- Optimize circulating blood volume, cardiac output and mean arterial pressure to ensure adequate renal perfusion.
- Early and aggressive intravenous fluid or blood replacement to maintain haemodynamic stability.

— **Use of inotropes**
- These are indicated in patients with low cardiac output despite adequate intravascular volume status.
- The inotropes have minimal direct effect on the renal vasculature. They act by optimizing cardiac output, increasing mean arterial pressure, improving systemic circulation and indirectly renal perfusion.
- The speed and extent in which renal perfusion is re-established bears greater importance than the precise nature of inotropes used to achieve it.

— **Use of diuretics**
- Mannitol has been used in a variety of clinical situations for renal protection, such as abdominal aortic aneurysm surgery, major biliary tree surgery and prevention of nephropathy secondary to radiocontrast agents or rhabdomyolysis. However, the only setting where mannitol has been shown to be of benefit is renal transplantation.
- High-dose diuretics may convert oliguric ARF to the non-oliguric form which carries a better prognosis (mortality rates of 50–80% for oliguric ARF versus 10–40% for non-oliguric ARF).
- Prophylactic administration of loop diuretics may have a deleterious effect on renal function. Maintenance of preload, cardiac output and blood pressure remains the mainstay of prevention of ARF.
- No beneficial effects have been demonstrated by loop diuretics on renal function in the treatment of established ARF. However, the increase in urine output may facilitate fluid management and improve compromised cardiorespiratory function.

— **Other agents**
- Fenoldopam, a selective dopaminergic (DA_1) agonist, causes natriuresis and renal vasodilation with minimal effect on blood pressure at a dose of 0.02–0.05 μg/kg/min. Studies are still inconclusive about its potential nephroprotective role.

MANAGEMENT

- Ensure that the urinary catheter is patent and in place.
  - Palpate the bladder, or get the surgeon to inspect for distended bladder if the abdomen is open.
  - Rule out the surgical factors mentioned above.
  - Check the course of the reservoir tubing for kinks, leaks, displacement or disconnection.
  - Inspect the collection reservoir for amount and colour of urine, and the presence of blood clots or debris which may cause mechanical obstruction and prevent urine flow.
  - Irrigate the bladder with saline through the catheter to rule out obstruction. Replace catheter if necessary.
- Assess the patient's haemodynamic and intravascular volume status.
  - Check the state of hydration, BP, heart rate, CVP (insert central line if not in place).
  - Maintain systolic BP > 100 mmHg and CVP 5–10 mmHg.
  - Check haemoglobin and haematocrit; transfuse if necessary.
  - Administer 200–300 ml of intravenous fluids then check response to fluid challenge.
  - Consider inotrope support if cardiac output remains low despite optimizing the volume status.
- If the intravascular volume is adequate:
  - Administer a dose of IV frusemide 0.5–1 mg/kg and observe for response.
  - Consider regular doses of frusemide if there is a positive response.
  - Consider dopamine infusion 2.5–5 μg/kg/min (see below).
- Send for investigations (Table 73–2):
  - Urine: urinalysis (pH, specific gravity, glucose, protein and bilirubin content, microscopic examination of urinary sediment for red or white blood cell, bacteria, casts, crystals), urinary electrolytes and osmolality.
  - Blood: urea, creatinine and electrolytes, serum osmolality, ABG, haemoglobin concentration, haematocrit.
- Consult the nephrologist if patient remains oliguric or shows signs of renal failure. Consider early renal replacement therapy in the form of haemofiltration, peritoneal dialysis or haemodialysis.
- In the presence of persistent oliguria or azotaemia despite the above manoeuvres, ARF would have set in. The fluids and drugs should be re-evaluated.

Table 73–2. Distinguishing tests between prerenal and intrarenal acute renal failure (ARF)

	Prerenal ARF	Intrarenal ARF
Urine specific gravity	> 1.020	< 1.010
Urine sodium (mmol/L)	< 20	> 20
Urine osmolality (msom/kg)	> 500	< 500
Urine/serum osmolar ratio	> 2 : 1	< 1.1 : 1
Urine/plasma creatinine ratio	> 40 : 1	< 20 : 1
Blood urea nitrogen/serum creatinine ratio	> 20 : 1	< 10 : 1
Urinary sediment	Hyaline casts	Tubular cell, granular casts

- Discontinue all nephrotoxic drugs.
- Reduce dosage of drugs which depend on the kidneys for excretion.
- Commence or continue renal replacement therapy.
- Treat clinical and laboratory manifestations of ARF: fluid overload, altered mental status, nausea, anorexia, pericarditis; acidaemia, hyperkalaemia, hypocalcaemia, hyperphosphataemia, hypermagnesaemia, anaemia.

"RENAL DOSE" DOPAMINE

— The so-called "renal dose" dopamine, at an infusion rate of 0.5–3 μg/kg/min, is widely used in the perioperative period in an attempt to provide renal protection.

— Studies in healthy animals and human volunteers reveal that dopamine causes diuresis and natriuresis as well as some degree of renal vasodilatation.

— However, studies of the perioperative use of dopamine fail to demonstrate any clinically significant benefit as prophylaxis against ARF, or as treatment in established ARF. No benefit other than diuresis is seen in patients with congestive heart failure, critical illness and sepsis.

— Furthermore, dopamine administration is not completely without risk because of its catecholamine and neuroendocrine functions. Side-effects include tachyarrhythmias, myocardial, gut and peripheral vascular ischaemia, over-diuresis in volume depletion, and altered immune responses.

— There is no convincing evidence to support the routine use of prophylactic "renal dose" dopamine, and there are insufficient data to confirm or refute the hypothesis that dopamine is of use as a treatment of ARF.

FURTHER READING

1. Weldon BC, Monk TG. The patient at risk for acute renal failure: Recognition, prevention, and preoperative optimization. Anesthesiol Clin North America 2000; 8:705–17.
2. Jarnberg P. Renal protection strategies in the perioperative period. Best Prac Res Clin Anaesthesiol 2004;18:645–60.
3. Sadovnikoff N. Renal protection. Best Prac Res Clin Anaesthesiol 2000;14:161–71.
4. Burton CJ, Tomson CRV. Can the use of low-dose dopamine for treatment of acute renal failure be justified? Postgrad Med J 1999;75:269–74.
5. Perdue PW, Balser JR, Lipsett PA, Breslow MJ. "Renal dose" dopamine in surgical patients: Dogma or science. Ann Surg 1998;227:470–3.
6. Kellum JA, Decker JM. Use of dopamine in acute renal failure: A meta-analysis. Crit Care Med 2001;29:1526–31.
7. Schetz M. Should we use diuretics in acute renal failure? Best Prac Res Clin Anaesthesiol 2004;18:75–89.

Chapter 74

Postoperative Alteration in Mental Status

INTRODUCTION

Postoperative alteration in mental status following general anaesthesia can be manifested in various ways, such as:

— Confusion, agitation, restlessness, incoherence of speech, hallucinations.

— Disorientation to time, place, person or events.

— Inability to follow simple commands or instructions.

— Failure to recover consciousness or responsiveness within the expected time frame following general anaesthesia.

A patient who is confused or disoriented may be encountered in PACU or in the operating room immediately after extubation, while a patient who fails to awaken is likely to be in the operating room and with the endotracheal tube still *in situ.*

CAUSES

The possible causes are summarized here.

— **Susceptible patients**
- Elderly or demented patient.
- Intoxication with alcohol or drugs.
- Decreased level of consciousness due to raised intracranial pressure or metabolic derangements such as head injury, intracranial space-occupying lesion, cerebral oedema, uraemic or hepatic encephalopathy.
- Significant liver or renal impairment, giving rise to prolonged duration of action of anaesthetic drugs.

— **Drug causes**
- Increased sensitivity to centrally depressant drugs, or prolonged duration of action of such drugs due to various reasons.
- Examples of drugs include premedicant drugs, anaesthetic agents, patient's own medication (e.g., tricyclic antidepressants, sedatives), recreational drugs, alcohol.
- Absolute or relative drug overdose.
- Idiosyncratic response to ketamine, droperidol, scopolamine in the elderly.

— **Metabolic and endocrine causes**
- Hypoxia, hypercarbia, acidosis.
- Electrolyte imbalance involving sodium, potassium, magnesium or calcium.
- Hypo- or hyperosmolality.
- Hypo- or hyperglycaemia.
- Hypothyroidism.
- Hepatic or uraemic encephalopathy.
- Malignant hyperthermia.
- Hypothermia.

— **Neurologic causes**
- Raised intracranial pressure due to cerebral oedema or haemorrhage.
- Cerebrovascular accident: thrombotic, embolic, haemorrhagic.
- Hypoxic encephalopathy.

— **Intraoperative complications resulting in cerebral ischaemia or cerebral oedema**
- Prolonged hypotension secondary to hypovolaemia, cardiac failure.
- Pulmonary embolism (air, carbon dioxide, fat, amniotic fluid, thrombus).
- Water intoxication, hyponatraemia in TURP syndrome.

- Hypoxia, hypercarbia, hypoxic encephalopathy.
- Cerebrovascular accident: thromboembolic or haemorrhagic stroke.

— **Postoperative problems**
- Hypoxia, hypercarbia due to various causes, e.g., hypoventilation, airway obstruction.
- Respiratory insufficiency.
- Inadequate pain relief.
- Bladder distension.
- Metabolic or endocrine abnormalities such as hypoglycaemia, electrolyte imbalance, acidosis, dehydration, hypothyroidism.
- Hypovolaemia secondary to incomplete surgical haemostasis or inadequate volume resuscitation.
- Hypothermia.
- Incomplete reversal of neuromuscular blockade.
- Coronary events: acute myocardial infarction or angina.

Inadequate reversal of neuromuscular blockade may be mistakenly diagnosed as failure to regain consciousness because the patient may be conscious but appears drowsy as a result of ocular and bulbar muscle weakness. These are possible causes for incomplete reversal of neuromuscular blockade.

— Absolute or relative overdosage of neuromuscular blocking drugs.

— Patients with neuromuscular disease, severe hepatic or renal impairment.

— Potentiation of neuromuscular blockade by acidosis, hypothermia, electrolyte imbalance (hypokalaemia, hypermagnesaemia, hypocalcaemia).

— Congenital or acquired pseudocholinesterase deficiency (for suxamethonium apnoea).

PREVENTION

— Identify patients at risk, and opt for local or regional anaesthesia instead of general anaesthesia if feasible.

— Treat and optimize metabolic, endocrine or neurologic abnormalities before surgery.

— Avoid excessive preoperative sedation especially in the elderly and ill patients.

— Careful titration of anaesthetic drugs to avoid overdose.

— Prompt and aggressive resuscitation in the event of any intraoperative complications.

MANAGEMENT

- Attempt to communicate with the patient.
  - Attempt to rouse the patient if he/she is unresponsive, or talk to the patient if he/she is able to vocalize.
  - Use verbal and tactile stimulation, not forceful or painful prodding!
  - If the patient is responsive, he/she may be able to indicate what the problem is: possibly pain at the surgical site, chest pain, distended bladder, cold or respiratory difficulty. Treatment can then be tailored to the specific complaint.
- If the patient is unresponsive, totally confused or disoriented:
  - Quickly check the ABCs: ensure that oxygenation and ventilation are not compromised.
  - Maintain airway support and perform suction to clear secretions as required, checking for the presence of gag reflex in the process.
  - Check respiratory pattern, oxygen saturation, blood pressure and heart rate.
  - Administer supplemental oxygen by face mask: this may be difficult in a confused, combative patient; oxygen delivered via nasal prongs may be better tolerated.
  - Support ventilation or re-intubate if respiration is inadequate.
  - Resuscitate with intravenous fluids, blood or inotropic agents if indicated.
- If the patient is still intubated and connected to the anaesthetic machine, check that all anaesthetic drugs are discontinued.
  - Increase oxygen flow to hasten elimination of inhalational anaesthetics.
  - Check expired anaesthetic concentrations on anaesthetic agent concentration monitor.
- Assess adequacy of recovery from neuromuscular blockade.
  - Inadequate recovery is characterized by jerky, uncoordinated movement with feeble attempts at respiration.
  - Assess clinically and by means of peripheral nerve stimulator, using train of four (TOF) count, TOF ratio or DBS (see Chapter 8).
  - Administer an additional dose of reversal agent if indicated.
  - Support ventilation while the patient regains muscle power; consider additional sedation if this period of recovery is expected to be prolonged: it is terrifying for the patient to be fully awake but unable to breathe.
- Review the anaesthetic history.
  - Review the dose and timing of drugs administered during the course of the anaesthetic.

  - Check syringes and ampoules to rule out the possibility of wrong drug administration.
  - Note any adverse intraoperative events such as hypotension, cardiac dysrhythmias, hypovolaemia and cardiac arrest.
  - Check ECG if myocardial ischaemia is suspected.
- Conduct a careful neurological examination.
  - Check pupil size and reaction to light, gag and cough reflexes, response to tactile or pain stimulus, muscle power, muscle tone, tendon reflexes.
  - Look for any focal neurological signs.
  - Consider referral to a neurologist.
- Bedside and laboratory investigations.
  - Obtain blood samples for glucose, electrolyte concentrations (sodium, potassium, calcium), haematocrit, ABG. These assays can be carried out at the bedside.
  - Send blood samples to clinical laboratory for glucose, urea, electrolytes, serum osmolarity.
  - Do a 12-lead ECG if myocardial ischaemia is suspected.
  - Request for a portable chest X-ray if lung pathology is suspected.
- Treatment for specific disorder.
  - Hypoglycaemia: 50% dextrose bolus, followed by infusion of dextrose solution.
  - Hyperglycaemia: intravenous hydration with normal saline and insulin treatment.
  - Hypo-osmolarity: normal saline, IV frusemide.
  - Hyponatraemia: normal saline, consider hypertonic saline.
- Consider the use of antidotes for reversal of specific drugs.
  - For narcotic analgesic: IV naloxone 0.1 mg increments titrating to effect, maximum 0.4 mg. Beware of risks of pulmonary oedema even with small doses.
  - For benzodiazepines: IV flumazenil 0.2 mg over 15 seconds, repeat until effective (maximum 1 mg in 5 minutes, 3 mg in 1 hour).
  - For anticholinergic agents: IV physostigmine 1 mg, maximum 4 mg.
- If the patient is confused or combative, the tendency is to administer sedative drugs to quieten the patient. Sedation should not be given unless the underlying cause has been identified. It not only masks neurological signs and confuses further neurological assessment, it may also be dangerous in patients with respiratory insufficiency or shock due to any cause.
- Further management in ICU or HDU may be indicated if no improvement occurs.

FURTHER READING

1. O'Keeffe ST, Chonchubhair AN. Postoperative delirium in the elderly. Br J Anaesth 1994;73:673–87
2. Dodds C, Allison J. Postoperative cognitive deficit in the elderly surgical patient. Br J Anaesth 1998;81:449–62.
3. Parr SM, Robinson BJ, Glover PW, Galletly DC. Level of consciousness on arrival in the recovery room and the development of respiratory morbidity. Anaesth Intens Care 1991;19:369–72.
4. Sanders LD, Piggot SE, Isaac PA, et al. Reversal of benzodiazepine sedation with the antagonist flumazenil. Br J Anaesth 1991;66:445–53.

Chapter 75

Seizures

INTRODUCTION

Seizures are paroxysmal neuronal discharges from abnormally excited neuronal foci. There are various clinical presentations, such as tonic-clonic, generalized (grand mal) seizures, partial focal motor seizures, temporal lobe seizures and absence (petit mal) seizures.

Status epilepticus is best defined as a continuous, generalized, convulsive seizure lasting more than 5 minutes, or two or more seizures during which the patient does not return to baseline consciousness. This is a major medical emergency associated with significant morbidity and mortality. Complications include cardiac arrhythmias, neurogenic pulmonary oedema, derangements of metabolic and autonomic function, pulmonary aspiration, hyperthermia, rhabdomyolysis and permanent neurologic damage.

In the perioperative setting, the likelihood of seizures occurring increases in these situations.

— Patients with preexisting seizure disorder.

— Parturients with preeclampsia and with features of impending eclampsia.

— Increased intracranial pressure (ICP) secondary to acute head trauma or other intracranial pathology.
— Hypoxaemia.
— Hypoglycaemia.
— Hyponatraemia/hypo-osmolarity especially during TURP.
— Local anaesthetic toxicity in major regional blockade.
— Drug reaction or overdose, including recreational drugs.
— Children with febrile fits.

PREVENTION

— Identify patients with known history of epilepsy.
- Ensure optimization of treatment. Monitor blood concentration of anticonvulsants in patients with poor seizure control to check whether the therapeutic level is reached.
- Maintain anticonvulsant medication up to the day of surgery; recommence medication as early as feasible in the postoperative period.
- Use benzodiazepine for premedication to raise the seizure threshold.
- Avoid anaesthetic agents which promote abnormal cerebral electrical activity or produce reactions which mimic an epileptic fit (Table 75–1).

— Care in performing regional block.
- Frequent aspiration to exclude intravascular or intrathecal placement of needle or catheter.
- Use of test dose in epidural blocks.
- Inject local anaesthetic slowly and in small aliquots of 3–5 ml each time.
- Close communication and observation of patient during and after regional block.
- Appropriate early management of local anaesthetic toxicity may prevent frank seizure activity.

— Management of preeclampsia (see Chapter 30).
- Close monitoring and control of blood pressure.
- Use magnesium sulphate or phenobarbitone for eclampsia prophylaxis.
- Early recognition and management of prodromal symptoms: headache, nausea, epigastric pain, visual disturbances.

— Prevention, early identification and treatment of TURP syndrome (see Chapter 41).
- Use sodium-containing intravenous fluids for preloading and intraoperative fluid replacement.

Table 75–1. Drugs to be used with caution in epileptics

Drug	Remarks
Enflurane	Associated with abnormal electroencephalographic (EEG) activity especially in the presence of hyperventilation with hypocarbia
Methohexitone	Increased EEG spike activity; thought to be epileptogenic
Ketamine	Best avoided because of cerebral excitatory effects with increased intracranial pressure; but has been used in epileptics without incidence
Etomidate	Non-epileptogenic but high incidence of myoclonus which may be confused with occurrence of seizures
Antiemetics: phenothiazines, dopamine antagonists, butyrophenones	Non-epileptogenic; may be associated with dystonic reactions which may be confused with occurrence of seizures

- Reduce the hydrostatic pressure of irrigation fluid to less than 70 cmH_2O.
- Meticulous haemostasis and prompt surgery to limit the amount of fluid absorbed into the systemic circulation.
- Early recognition of CNS and cardiorespiratory manifestations of TURP syndrome.
- Correct hypervolaemia and hyponatraemia, and other supportive measures as indicated.

MANAGEMENT

Overview of management.

— Rapid termination of seizure activity.

— Airway protection and respiratory support if indicated.

— Measures to prevent pulmonary aspiration.

— Identification and management of precipitating causes.

— Treatment of complications arising from seizure activity.

- Prevention of recurrent seizures.
- Treatment of any underlying conditions.

1. Prevent the patient from falling or inflicting injury to self.

2. Assess and maintain ABCs.
   - Ensure that the airway is patent:
     - Insert an oropharyngeal airway to prevent the tongue from falling back and causing airway obstruction, and to prevent injury to oral structures.
     - Intubate if unable to maintain mask ventilation or to protect airway from aspiration.
   - Ensure adequate oxygenation and ventilation.
   - Support circulation if indicated.

3. Terminate fits with anticonvulsants.
   - Thiopentone, in 25–50 mg increments, is the drug of first choice in seizures during regional anaesthesia since it is readily available on the anaesthetic tray.
   - Benzodiazepine, either midazolam or diazepam 5–10 mg bolus doses, may be used.

4. Use neuromuscular blocking drugs only for specific reasons.
   - To facilitate endotracheal intubation.
   - To abolish unsafe and otherwise uncontrollable muscular activity (e.g., unstable neck fracture).
   - To allow adequate ventilation and oxygenation.

   Avoid prolonged neuromuscular blockade if possible. Remember that when the patient is paralyzed, uncontrolled seizure activities are masked yet can still damage the brain. Some form of cerebral function monitor is indicated if neuromuscular blockade is unavoidable.

5. Identify the possible underlying cause for the seizure.
   - Check blood glucose concentration; correct hypo- or hyperglycaemia if present.
   - Send blood samples for electrolyte concentration and serum osmolarity if TURP syndrome is suspected.
   - Consider possibility of occult head injury, drug reaction or intracranial pathology unrelated to the anaesthetic.

6. Admission to ICU.
   - Mechanical ventilation may be indicated in selected patients, for example:
     - Acute head trauma with raised ICP.
     - Status epilepticus uncontrolled with high doses of anticonvulsants.
     - Significant lung injury due to pulmonary aspiration during seizure.
   - Continue haemodynamic and temperature monitoring; institute active cooling measures if the patient develops significant hyperthermia.
   - Consider brain imaging with CT scan or MRI in patients with previously undiagnosed seizure disorder once seizure activity has been controlled.
   - Institute measures of reducing ICP by hyperventilation, mannitol, dexamethasone, sedation, CSF drainage where appropriate.
   - Continuous motor seizures may lead to muscle breakdown with release of myoglobin.
     - Maintain adequate hydration to prevent myoglobin-induced renal failure.
     - Consider forced saline diuresis and urinary alkalinization in the presence of myoglobinuria or elevated serum creatine kinase levels.

FURTHER READING

1. Chapman MG, Smith M, Hirsch NP. Status epilepticus. Anaesthesia 2001;56:648–59.
2. Marik PE, Varon J. The management of status epilepticus. Chest 2004;126:582–91.

Chapter 76
Venous Air or Gas Embolism

- Introduction
- Monitors for Detection of VAE
- Prevention
- Clinical Manifestations
- Management
- Subsequent Management
- Further Reading

INTRODUCTION

Gas embolism is a clinical condition caused by ingress of air or other gas such as carbon dioxide into the vascular system. The majority of clinical problems are caused by gas entering the venous system and resulting in *venous* air or gas embolism. *Arterial* air embolism can also occur, either in the form of paradoxical air embolism via heart defects, or direct arterial cannulation during cardiac surgery or angiography.

Although classically associated with sitting craniotomy, venous air embolism (VAE) is also a potential complication of laparoscopic, pelvic and orthopaedic procedures. These can occur as a result of:

- Entrainment of air into the venous system when the venous pressure is sub-atmospheric.
  - Surgical field above level of the heart.
  - Central venous cannulation during spontaneous respiration.
- Infusion of air or other gas under pressure into the venous system.
  - Insufflation of CO_2 in laparoscopic surgery.
  - Venturi jet ventilation.
  - Pressurized intravenous infusion sets.

The major cause of fatality in massive VAE is attributed to circulatory obstruction and ultimately arrest resulting from air trapped in the right ventricular outflow tract. On the other end of the spectrum, venous air entrainment may be insidious and with non-specific clinical signs. The time course and severity of VAE are determined by the rate and volume of air entrained, and the position of the patient at the time VAE occurred. Entry of air into the arterial system may present as acute cerebrovascular or coronary event with catastrophic consequences.

MONITORS FOR DETECTION OF VAE

Intraoperative monitoring for VAE is indicated in surgical procedures with increased risks of gas embolism. The monitors listed here are in the order of sensitivity; not all are available for routine use.

1. Transoesophageal echocardiography (TEE)
   - This is the most sensitive monitor as it is able to detect as little as 0.02 ml/kg of air.
   - It is semi-quantitative but requires continuous observation.
   - The monitor is expensive, technically more difficult to place and interpret, and not freely available in locations other than the cardiothoracic OT.

2. Precordial ultrasound Doppler
   - This is the most sensitive non-invasive monitor as it is able to detect 0.2 ml/kg of air.
   - It is non-quantitative and works by detecting flow turbulence and changes in characteristics of heart sounds.
   - Problems exist with significant false negatives, proper positioning of the probe and interference of the signals by diathermy.

3. Pulmonary arterial pressure
   — Increase in PA pressure correlates with the amount and rate of air entrainment.
   — It is slightly more sensitive than capnography but its invasiveness does not justify its routine use.

4. End-expired nitrogen
   — The end-expired nitrogen value is increased in VAE.
   — It is slightly more sensitive than end-tidal CO_2 and highly specific for air, but its accuracy is affected by hypotension.

5. Capnography
   — This is the most convenient, practical, sensitive and reliable monitor in routine use.
   — End-tidal CO_2 decreases as a result of reduction in pulmonary circulation.
   — In CO_2 embolism, a transient increase in end-tidal CO_2 is observed, followed by an exponential decline.

Clinical observation is no less important. One should be vigilant during the surgical procedure, with frequent observation of the surgical field. There should be a high index of suspicion for detection of VAE especially in patients and procedures at risk.

PREVENTION

Various methods are advocated to prevent the occurrence of VAE.

— Steps to minimize pressure gradient between the surgical site and right atrium.
  - Ensure adequate intravascular hydration by volume loading.
  - Intermittent positive pressure ventilation (IPPV) instead of spontaneous ventilation.

— Meticulous surgical haemostasis to minimize the number of venous sinuses open to atmospheric pressure.

— Proper laparoscopic surgical techniques to reduce risk of vessel injury during insertion of Veress needle and trocar.

Even though the incidence of VAE is not increased by the use of nitrous oxide, one should consider using an alternative anaesthetic technique such as total intravenous anaesthesia (TIVA) in high-risk cases. Due to its greater solubility in blood compared to nitrogen, nitrous oxide rapidly diffuses into entrained air bubbles, increases the size of embolus and worsens the effects of VAE.

CLINICAL MANIFESTATIONS

These are the clinical features.

1. Decrease in $ETCO_2$ as described. Fall in SaO_2 due to reduced pulmonary blood flow and V/Q mismatch, with hypercarbia due to carbon dioxide retention.

2. Cardiovascular changes.
   - "Millwheel" murmur via oesophageal or precordial stethoscope.
     - Described as a loud coarse continuous murmur that may obliterate S_1 and S_2.
     - Insensitive monitor but indicates massive air embolism with imminent cardiovascular collapse.
   - Hypotension.
   - Non-specific ECG changes.
     - Tachy- or bradyarrhythmia, atrioventricular block.
     - Right heart strain pattern with peaked P-waves.
     - ST segment elevation or depression, non-specific T-wave changes.
   - Sudden increase in CVP with reduced cardiac output and increased pulmonary vascular resistance.
   - Circulatory collapse with electromechanical dissociation (EMD).

3. Neurological signs may occur secondary to paradoxical air embolism across patent foramen ovale (probe-patent in 25–30% of the population). This include delayed emergence from general anaesthesia, cerebral irritation, convulsions and localizing neurological signs.

MANAGEMENT

Early diagnosis and prompt institution of resuscitative measures are essential to arrest progression to catastrophe and cardiovascular collapse.

- A quick check to rule out breathing system problem such as disconnection, which may account for loss of capnograph trace and falling SpO_2.
- *Inform the surgeon immediately* when venous air embolism is suspected. Attempts should be made to prevent further air entrainment, locate and eliminate possible site of air entry with these manoeuvres.
    - Flood the surgical field with saline.
    - Apply compression to major drainage vessels.
    - Cauterize open veins.
    - Stop reaming and apply bone wax to exposed bone.
    - Prevent further entrainment or infusion of gas.
    - Stop insufflation of carbon dioxide and decompress any gas-pressurized system or cavity.
- Discontinue nitrous oxide and administer 100% oxygen. Rapid infusion of intravenous fluids to increase venous pressure. Vasopressors and inotropes may be needed to support the circulation.
- Perform external cardiac massage according to Advanced Cardiac Life Support (ACLS) protocol if the patient is in EMD (see Chapter 69). This manoeuvre may break up bubbles that cause air lock in the right ventricle and improve pulmonary perfusion.
- Reposition the patient.
    - Lower the surgical site below the level of the heart whenever possible, either in the Trendelenburg position (for head and neck surgery) or reverse Trendelenburg position (for lumbar spine or lower limb surgery).
    - Position the patient in partial left lateral decubitus position in an attempt to relieve the air lock and improve right ventricular outflow.
- Evacuate air from the heart via central venous catheter if this is already *in situ*. This confirms diagnosis even though it is seldom able to aspirate sufficient volume of air to be therapeutic. Effective evacuation of air depends on the optimal positioning of the catheter tip in the right atrium 2 cm below the junction with the superior vena cava (SVC). A multi-orifice catheter is generally more effective than a single-orifice catheter.
- In head and neck surgery, jugular venous compression or moderate Valsalva manoeuvre may prevent more air from entering the chest. The latter may reveal vascular entry site to the surgeon.
- The use of positive end-expiratory pressure (PEEP) or continuous positive airway pressure (CPAP) is controversial. Moderate PEEP or CPAP may limit the extent

and progress of air embolism by increasing intrathoracic pressure and CVP. But this sustained increase in right atrial pressure may predispose to paradoxical air embolism in susceptible individuals.

— Thoracotomy for internal cardiac massage may be indicated in dire emergencies.

SUBSEQUENT MANAGEMENT

— If the situation is rapidly brought under control and the patient is haemodynamically stable, the surgeon may be allowed to proceed with the surgery but nitrous oxide should be avoided for the remainder of the anaesthetic.

— If the patient remains haemodynamically unstable, continue resuscitation, terminate the surgery and transfer the patient to ICU as soon as feasible.

— Correct any preexisting hypovolaemia, establish invasive haemodynamic monitors (if not instituted earlier) and continue cardiovascular support. Perform a 12-lead ECG to look for myocardial ischaemia.

FURTHER READING

1. Muth CM, Shank ES. Primary care: Gas embolism. N Engl J Med 2000;342:476–82.
2. Palmon SC, Moore LE, Lundberg J, Toung T. Venous air embolism: A review. J Clin Anesth 1997;9:251–7.
3. Porter JM, Pidgeon C, Cunningham AJ. The sitting position in neurosurgery: A critical appraisal. Br J Anaesth 1999;82:117–28.

Index

- O -

- P -

- U -

- V -